IMMUNOSUPPRESSION – ROLE IN HEALTH AND DISEASES

Edited by **Suman Kapur**
and **Maristela Barbosa Portela**

Immunosuppression – Role in Health and Diseases
Edited by Suman Kapur and Maristela Barbosa Portela

Published by InTech

Janeza Trdine 9, 51000 Rijeka, Croatia

Publishing Process Manager Ivana Zec

Technical Editor Teodora Smiljanic

Cover Designer InTech Design Team

Additional hard copies can be obtained from orders@intechopen.com

Immunosuppression – Role in Health and Diseases, Edited by Suman Kapur and Maristela Barbosa Portela
p. cm.
ISBN 978-953-51-0152-9

For EU product safety concerns:
IN TECH d.o.o., Prolaz Marije Krucifikse Kozulić 3, 51000 Rijeka, Croatia,
info@intechopen.com or visit our website at intechopen.com.

Meet the editor

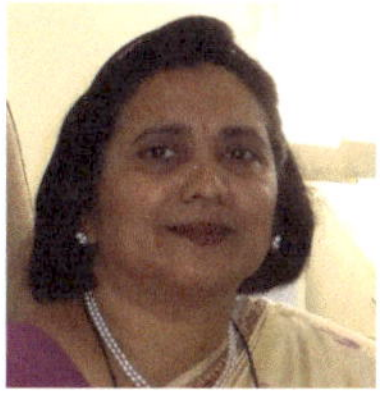

Professor Suman Kapur, currently Dean, Research and Consultancy, at BITS-Pilani Hyderabad Campus obtained her MSc. and Ph.D. degrees from AIIMS, New Delhi. Dr Kapur has authored over 80 peer-reviewed research articles and chapters in several books. She has chaired sessions and delivered over 200 invited lectures in national/international conferences. Dr Kapur has also served as a Jury member for the award of King Faisal International Prize for Excellence in research in Biology, and Ranbaxy Research Scholar award for young scientists. She serves on the editorial boards of several journals and is a life member of numerous professional bodies. Her research interests are studying the role of opiate signaling in immune responses and understanding the link between immune responses and chronic non-infectious diseases. She has mentored more than 10 MD and 15 Ph.D theses.

Contents

Preface XI

Part 1 Suppression and Regulation 1

Chapter 1 **Role of Opioidergic System in Humoral Immune Response 3**
Suman Kapur, Anuradha Pal and Shashwat Sharad

Chapter 2 **Endotoxin Tolerance as a Key Mechanism for Immunosuppression 21**
Subhra K. Biswas and Irina N. Shalova

Chapter 3 **Spleen Tyrosine Kinase: A Novel Target in Autoimmunity 41**
Stephen P. McAdoo and Frederick W. K. Tam

Chapter 4 **Genetic Variation in AhR Gene Related to Dioxin Sensitivity in the Japanese Field Mouse, *Apodemus speciosus* 57**
Hiroko Ishiniwa, Kazuhiro Sogawa, Ken-ichi Yasumoto, Nobuhiko Hoshi, Toshifumi Yokoyama, Ken Tasaka and Tsuneo Sekijima

Chapter 5 **Anti-RhD-Mediated Immunosuppression: Can Monoclonal Antibodies Imitate the Action of Polyclonal Antibodies? 77**
Natalia Olovnikova

Chapter 6 **Immunotropic Properties of GABA-ergic Agents in Suppression 107**
N. Tyurenkov and M. A. Samotrueva

Chapter 7 **Immunodepression and Immunosuppression During Aging 125**
Véronique Thomas-Vaslin, Adrien Six, Hang-Phuong Pham, Cira Dansokho, Wahiba Chaara, Bruno Gouritin, Bertrand Bellier and David Klatzmann

Chapter 8 **Chronic Immune Response Hypothesis for Chronic Fatigue Syndrome: Experimental Results and Literature Overview 147**
E. V. Svirshchevskaya

Chapter 9 **T Cell Suppression in Burn and Septic Injuries 161**
Nadeem Fazal

Chapter 10 **Immunosuppression in Helminth Infection 191**
Maria Doligalska and Katarzyna Donskow-Łysoniewska

Chapter 11 **Microbial Immunosuppression 215**
Mohamed G. Elfaki, Abdullah A. Al-Hokail and Abdelmageed M. Kambal

Chapter 12 **Measles Virus Infection: Mechanisms of Immune Suppression 225**
Xuelian Yu and Reena Ghildyal

Chapter 13 **Immunoregulation: A Proposal for an Experimental Model 255**
Marcela Šperanda and Ivica Valpotić

Part 2 Transplantation and Novel Therapies 291

Chapter 14 **Cellular Therapies for Immunosuppression 293**
Nathalie Cools, Viggo F. I. Van Tendeloo and Zwi N. Berneman

Chapter 15 **Low Immunogenic Potential of Human Neural Stem Cells 317**
L. De Filippis, L. Rota Nodari and Maurizio Gelati

Chapter 16 **Current Immunosuppression in Abdominal Organ Transplantation 335**
Raffaele Girlanda, Cal S. Matsumoto, Keith J. Melancon and Thomas M. Fishbein

Chapter 17 **Induction Therapy in Renal Transplant Recipients 357**
Cheguevara Afaneh, Meredith J. Aull, Sandip Kapur and David B. Leeser

Chapter 18 **Radiotherapy and Immunity – A Mini Review 385**
Rosangela Correa Villar

Chapter 19 **The Role of Cyclosporine A in the Treatment of Prosthetic Vascular Graft Infections with the Use of Arterial Homografts 407**
Artur Pupka and Tomasz Płonek

Chapter 20 **Clinical Immunosuppression in Solid Organ and Composite Tissue Allotransplantation 423**
Barbara Kern and Robert Sucher

Chapter 21 **HIV/AIDS Associated Malignant Disorders: Role of Highly Active Antiretroviral Therapy 433**
Angel Mayor, Yelitza Ruiz, Diana Fernández and Robert Hunter-Mellado

Chapter 22 **E-Health 2.0 Developments in Treatment and Research in Multiple Sclerosis 457**
Peter Joseph Jongen

"Dedicated to my parents, students
and most of all my mentor and guide Prof. G. P Talwar"

Preface

A need for a book on immunology which primarily focuses on the needs of medical and clinical research students was recognized. This book is relatively short and contains topics considered relevant to the understanding of human immune system and its role in health and diseases. Immunology is the study of our protection from foreign macromolecules or invading organisms and our responses to them. These invaders include viruses, bacteria, protozoa or even larger parasites. Certain individuals develop immune responses against their proteins (and other self-molecules) in autoimmunity and against our own aberrant cells as in tumor immunity.

Adaptive immune responses (it takes them days to respond to a primary invasion) such as infection by any pathogen, lead to production of antibodies and cell-mediated responses which recognize foreign pathogens and destroy them as a function of specific immune cell types. The response to a second round of infection is often more rapid than to the primary infection because of the activation of memory B and T cells. These responses are mediated by signals such as lymphokines, cytokines and chemokines produced by various cells and these in turn stimulate cells of the immune system.

When an infection occurs, immune cells flock to the area and secrete large amounts of highly reactive chemicals to combat the invader. But, these inflammatory chemicals also attack normal tissue surrounding the infection and damage critical components of cells, including DNA. During chronic inflammation, DNA damage may lead to mutations or cell death and even to cancer and other diseases. Thus this chronic, and "systemic inflammation," is presently being linked to almost everything from heart disease and diabetes to Alzheimer's and arthritis, and may even be the cause of many other chronic diseases. Nobody knows whether this inflammation is a cause or consequence of chronic disease/s —or perhaps something that just goes along with these conditions. With the growing incidence of chronic human diseases, the role of chronic inflammation and consequently "Therapeutic Immune-suppression" has been getting a lot of attention lately.

Immunosuppression involves an act that reduces the activation or efficacy of the immune system. Some portions of the immune system itself have immuno-suppressive effects on other parts of the immune system, and immunosuppression may occur as an adverse reaction to treatment of other conditions. Deliberately induced immunosuppression is generally done to prevent the body from rejecting an organ transplant, treating graft-versus-host disease after a bone marrow transplant, or for the treatment of auto-immune diseases such as rheumatoid arthritis or Crohn's disease. A person who is undergoing immunosuppression, or whose immune system is weak for other reasons (for example, chemotherapy and HIV patients) is said to be immune-compromised. The downside of immunosuppression is that with such a deactivated immune system, the body is very vulnerable to opportunistic infections, even those usually considered harmless. Also, prolonged use of immune-suppressants increases the risk of cancer.

Therapeutic immunosuppression has very broad applications in clinical medicine, ranging from prevention and treatment of organ and bone marrow transplant rejection, management of various autoimmune disorders (e.g., rheumatoid arthritis), skin diseases, allergies and asthma. Whereas traditionally only a small repertoire of immunosuppressive agents was available for clinical use, recent discoveries have significantly increased the number of approved agents, resulting in numerous trials to further evaluate their potential. In addition, products of the biotechnology industry - monoclonal antibodies, cytokines, cytokine antagonists and other products of genetic engineering that target key molecular pathways in disease pathogenesis - have either already made, or are on the verge of making an important impact on treatment. The present book was planned bearing in mind the recent developments in this growing field. The book brings important developments both in the field of molecular mechanisms involved in Immunosuppression and active therapeutic approaches employed for immune suppression in various human disease conditions.

Researchers have theorized that anti-inflammatory medications may help prevent diseases, such as coronary artery diseases (CAD), cardio vascular diseases (CVD), stroke, colon cancer and Alzheimer's. Several recent findings from different laboratories in the world employing case-control human studies and/or specific animal models for chronic human diseases support these ideas. With the growing developments in stem cell culture and characterization technologies, there is considerable interest in the potential of cell-based therapies (particularly hematopoietic stem and dendritic cell therapy) of allo- and autoimmunity. Important recent advances in the immunotherapy of allergic diseases are also covered in this book. Gene therapy offers considerable promise for suppressing pathogenic processes in either transplantation or autoimmune disorders. The possibility of combining these important new advances to maximize benefit to the patient, and to minimize possible untoward effects (which are also given extensive coverage in this book), is one of the most exciting challenges of contemporary medicine.

This volume is intended both for practicing physicians and surgeons and for biomedical scientists at the graduate/postdoctoral levels. It is designed to provide an insight into various theories behind these various approaches to immunosuppression and provide state-of-the-art reviews of current developments in each area. The contents of the book are organized into two sections: one delineating the current opinions in "Immunosuppression and Regulation of Immune Response" and the other dedicated to strategies adopted in "Transplantation and other Novel Therapies". Each chapter is contributed by one or more experts in the field. There was a need to bring this information together in a single volume, as much of the key recent developments have been dispersed throughout the biomedical literature, largely in specialized journals. Since, as in the past, important developments in immunosuppressive therapy in one branch of medicine (i.e. transplantation) are likely to benefit another (e.g., dermatology, rheumatology, gastroenterology), cross-disciplinary coverage of the mechanistic basis of the various therapeutic strategies in a single volume is likely to convey the potential of advances in therapy in the most coherent manner possible. Hopefully, we will succeed in inducing interest and appreciation among the target readers about the potential for use of therapeutic immunosuppression in improving human life. We hope that the readers will enjoy participating in these advances in immunosuppression and its applications as I and my fellow authors have encountered in our careers.

I would like to acknowledge the help and cooperation extended by all the experts contacted for their indispensable contribution to this book. At the same time I would like to acknowledge the support and editorial help provided by the staff of Intech, especially Ms Ivana Zec and Ms Ana Nikolic, who have done a marvelous job in preparing the layout of each chapter. Without their devoted and persistent help, this book would not have been a reality. I am indebted to one and all.

Suman Kapur
Birla Institute of Technology and Science,
Pilani, Rajasthan,
India

Part 1

Suppression and Regulation

1

Role of Opioidergic System in Humoral Immune Response

Suman Kapur[1], Anuradha Pal[1] and Shashwat Sharad[2]
[1]*Birla Institute of Technology and Science, Pilani, Rajasthan*
[2]*Center for Prostate Disease Research, Department of Surgery, Uniformed Services University of the Health Sciences, Bethesda, MD,*
[1]*India*
[2]*USA*

1. Introduction

The initial idea that exogenous opiates can affect immune function was first floated in 1898 when Cantacuze described the effect of opium on leukocyte phagocytosis in guinea pig model. Recently findings from several investigators (Quaglio et al., 2002; Nath et al., 2002; Georges et al., 1999; Vallejo et al., 2004; Roy et al., 2006; Somaini et al., 2008) support the role of opiates in suppressing a variety of immunological end points in opiate abusers. Endogenous opioids seem to have a physiological role in modulating the Th1/Th2 balance, by reducing Th1 and enhancing Th2 representative cytokines. Exogenous opioids, on the other hand, seem to display various different modulatory profiles on the immune function, according to the drug under consideration. In this regard, available evidence shows that while morphine and heroin are liable to attenuate the immune response, long-acting opioids that are used in withdrawal treatment, such as methadone and buprenorphine, are largely devoid of immunosuppressive activity. Opioids can also influence the immune function through the activation of the descending pathways of the hypothalamus-pituitary axis (HPA) and the sympathetic nervous system (Vallejo et al., 2004). This review on role of opioidergic system in humoral immune response summarizes the effect of opiate receptor polymorphism on innate and adaptive immunity, identifies the role of the mu opioid receptor in these functions, and finally discusses how changes in these parameters may increase the risk for opportune infections in drug dependent subjects or attenuate the symptoms of rheumatoid arthritis.

2. Immune system and immune response

The immune system is composed of many interdependent cell types that collectively protect the body from bacterial, parasitic, fungal, viral infections and from the growth of tumor cells. Many of these cell types have specialized functions. The cells of the immune system can engulf bacteria, kill parasites or tumor cells, or viral-infected cells. The immune system protects us from potentially harmful substances by recognizing and responding to their presence, invoking a specific and targeted response. An immune response is thus the mechanism by which the body recognizes and defends itself against foreign or non-self substances and organisms such as bacteria, viruses, and other substances that appear harmful to the body. Taken together these substances are known as antigens and the immune system recognizes and destroys substances that contain any antigens.

Immune system works as a layered defence system of increasing specificity. It can be divided into two major components:

- The Innate immune system forming the first line of defence providing an immediate, non-specific response (Litman et al., 2005)
- The Adaptive immune system, which becomes activated in case of failure/inadequacy of the innate immunity to contain the infection, recognizes the pathogen mounting a specific response, leading to formation of an immunological memory, enabling a stronger and faster response each time this pathogen is re-encountered (Mayer, 2006) in the life course of the individual.

The role of innate and adaptive immunity is tabulated below:

Function/Immunity	Innate	Adaptive Immunity
Kinetics	Immediate	Delayed
Nature of Response	Non -Specific	Specific
Cells Types Involved	Leucocytes : NK cells, Basophils, Mast cells	Lymphocytes: T-cells and B-cells
Immune memory	No immunological memory on exposure	Immunological memory is generated on exposure
Receptor Reorganization	Limited number of target conserved domains	Larger number of both conserved and novel domains

Table 1. Differences between Innate and Adaptive immunity

An immune response to foreign antigen requires the presence of an antigen-presenting cell (APC), (usually either a macrophage or dendritic cell) in combination with a B cell or T cell. When an APC presents an antigen on its cell surface to a B cell, the B cell is signalled to proliferate and produce antibodies that specifically bind to that antigen and become an agent for removal of the antigen from the host organism.

3. Humoral response and its role

Humoral immunity is so named because it involves substances found in the humours, or body fluids. It is mediated by antibodies produced by cells of the B lymphocyte lineage. B cells, activated by the adaptive immune responses, transform into plasma cells which secrete antibodies. This process is aided by CD4+ T-helper 2 cells, which provide active co-stimulation. The secreted antibodies bind to antigens present on the surfaces of invading microbes, which marks them for subsequent destruction (Pier et al., 2004). Another important function of antibodies is to initiate the "complement destruction cascade."

Antibodies are glycoproteins belonging to the molecular superfamily of immunoglobulins which are often used interchangeably. In structure, they are large Y-shaped globular proteins and are classified into five types: IgA, IgD, IgE, IgG, and IgM. Each immunoglobulin class differs in its biological properties in targeting different types of antigens (Pier et al., 2004). Each antibody recognizes a specific antigen unique to its target. By binding their specific antigens, antibodies can cause agglutination and precipitation of antigen-antibody products, prime for phagocytosis by macrophages and other cells, block viral receptors, and stimulate other immune responses, such as the complement pathway.

Name	Type	Complex	Primary Function	Special properties
IgA	2	Dimer	Prevents gut and airways colonization by pathogens	
IgD	1	Monomer	Functions as an antigen receptor on B-cells unexposed to antigens	
IgE	1	Monomer	Binds to allergens and triggers histamine release	
IgG	4	Monomer	Provides the majority of antibody-based immunity	Can crossover from placenta to provide passive immunity
IgM	1	Pentamer	Eliminates pathogens in the early stages of B cell mediated IR	

Table 2. Antibody types and their functions

4. Expression of Mu opioid receptor on immune cells

4.1 Opioid system and its components

Opioids are chemicals that work by binding to opioid receptors, found in the central and peripheral nervous system and the gastrointestinal tract. Opioids play diverse biological functions, including reward, analgesia, and stress responsivity (Kreek and Koob, 1998; Vaccarino et al., 2000) and have been extensively studied for their therapeutic properties.
For opioids to be biologically active they must engage with any of the three principal classes of opioid receptors, namely, μ, κ, δ (mu, kappa, and delta). In all about seventeen different receptor types are reported, which include the ε, ι, λ, and ζ (Epsilon, Iota, Lambda and Zeta) receptors. These receptors share the common feature of binding to opioids/opiates with high affinity and classical stereo-selectivity. Cloning of the opioid receptors allowed their classification into the super-family of seven trans-membrane domain guanine-protein (G-protein) coupled receptors and are known to be involved in GABAnergic neurotransmission and their activation is reversed by the opioid inverse-agonist naloxone. The opioid receptors show a very high degree of sequence similarity at both nucleotide and protein levels. The homology is particularly striking in the seven trans-membrane domains and three intracellular loops. The extra-cellular N-terminal domain, three extra-cellular loops and the intra-cellular carboxy-terminal domains are less conserved among the three receptor types. Chromosomal locations for the human opioid receptors and opioid peptide genes have been established and are summarised in Table 3.

Protein	Gene	Location
Mu opioid recptor	*OPRM1*	6q24-25[d]
Kappa opioid recptor	*OPRK1*	8q11.2 [e, g]
Delta opioid recptor	*OPRD1*	1p34.3-36.1[f]
Preproopiomelanocortin	*POMC*	2p23.3 [a, b, h]
Preproenkephalin	*PENK*	8q23-q24[c]
Preprodynorphin	*PDYN*	20p12-pter[c]

Table 3. Chromosomal locations of human genes coding for opiate receptors & endogenous opioid peptides

Endogenous opioid peptides and their receptors form a neuromodulatory system that impacts several physiological processes, such as cognition, pain control, emotions, response to stress, and pathophysiology of both addiction to and immunosuppressive effects of opiates (Olson et al., 1996). Despite a number of side effects, such as respiratory depression, constipation, tolerance and dependence, morphine remains one of the most valuable therapeutic drugs (Schug SA et al., 1992).
Clinicians have long known that apart from being addictive opiates also cause immunosuppression. Present knowledge of interaction between opiates and the immune system is based on pharmacological studies and several mechanisms have been proposed. *In vitro* experiments suggest that opiates act directly upon immune cells (Sibinga and Goldstein, 1988; Chuang et al., 1995). Some reports indicate detectable expression of μ opioid receptor (MOR) mRNA in immune cells suggesting that these cells are targets for direct opioid action (Smolka and Schmidt, 1999). Others have proposed the existence of non-classical receptors, which specifically bind β-endorphin or recognize alkaloids but not peptidic opioid ligands (Pasternak., 1993). Pharmacology of opiates on immune responses seems complex, due to presence of a wide diversity of opiate receptors and therefore the molecular basis of opiate action on the immune system needs to be further studied.
Allelic variants in the opioid receptor and/or opioid peptide genes may lead to an altered endogenous opioid system. More than 100 polymorphisms have been identified in the human *OPRM1* gene and at least 10 single nucleotide polymorphisms (SNPs) have been reported in *OPRM1*-translated regions (Bond et al., 1998; Hoehe et al., 2000). Of these 10 SNPs, the A118G variant (rs 1799971) is the most prevalent and widely studied. The 118G allele is reported to increase the affinity of MOR for β-endorphin, an endogenous opiate, and activate inwardly rectifying potassium channels with three times greater potency than the most prevalent A118 allele (Bond et al., 1998). Although pharmacological studies suggest that the inhibitory action of opiates on immunity is mediated by opioid receptors, however molecular evidence for individual differences remains elusive.

4.2 Opioid receptors and immune functions

Opiates are immunosuppressive drugs and cause a decrease in several immune components (Brown et al., 1974). Jankovic and Maric (1987) showed that the neuropeptides, methionine-enkephalin, leucine-enkephalin, especially the former, exhibit a protective action against anaphylactic shock in rats sensitized to ovalbumin. On the other hand small doses of enkephalins stimulated humoral immune responses in rats. Thus, it appears that enkephalins both suppress and potentiate immune responsiveness. Naloxone, a blocker of opioid receptors, enhanced humoral immune reactions in rats.

Sibinga and Goldstein (1988) first showed that opioid receptors are expressed on cells from the immune system as determined by receptor binding and functional assays. Opioid alkaloids and peptides, such as morphine and endogenous opioid peptides, namely β-endorphin, have been shown to modulate the function of lymphocytes and other cells involved in host defence and immunity. Results from several laboratories have indicated that opioids can operate as cytokines, the principal communicating signals among the immunocytes. Indeed, all of the major properties of cytokines are shared by opioids, i.e., production by immune cells with paracrine, autocrine, and endocrine sites of action, functional redundancy, pleiotropy, and effects that are both dose and time dependent (Peterson et al., 1998). The μ-selective opioid, DAMGO, has been shown to increase the release of the monocyte chemoattractant protein-1 (MCP-1), RANTES, and interferon-γ from human peripheral mononuclear cells. Buprenorphine, another compound, known to have both agonist and antagonist properties at the MOR, has been shown to suppress splenic NK-cell activity, lymphocyte proliferation, and IFN-γ production in rats in a naltrexone-reversible manner suggesting a role of MOR in immune-modulations (Bidlack, 2006). Opiates like morphine, heroin, fentanyl and methadone are known to induce immune-suppression and affect both innate and adaptive immunity defining a role of MOR in these functions (Roy et al., 2006). Immune cells at different stages of differentiation express MOR differentially. Morphine affects the development, differentiation and function of various immune cells (Roy et al., 2006). Opiates directly bind to both classical and non-classical opioid receptors on immune cells and thus modulate their function. They also bind to classical opioid receptors in the CNS, causing the release of catecholamines and/or steroids, which in turn further affect the immune cell functions. They play a role in suppressing a variety of immunological end points such as proliferation, functions and responses of both T and B cells and attenuating the cytokine system (Vallejo et al., 2004;). They also suppress movement and number of circulating white blood cells (Miyagi et al., 2000; Perez-Castrillon et al., 1992).

5. Clinical observations

5.1 In opiate dependent subjects

Heroin addicts have been repeatedly documented to have an increased susceptibility to a variety of infectious diseases, and also depict alterations in a wide variety of immune cell parameters. These subjects manifest a variety of changes in the immune system indicative of both decreased and increased immune responses. While the absolute number and percentage of total and active T lymphocytes in the peripheral blood of opiate addicts and T-cell rosette formation were found to be significantly depressed in one study, an increase in the absolute number of T-cells in the blood of heroin addicts was reported in another. Similar conflicting results have been reported concerning the functional activity of T lymphocytes from heroin addicts. Brown et al. (1974) found impaired responsiveness, in vitro, of lymphocytes to each of the three mitogens (PHA, concavanalin A, pokeweed mitogen) in heroin addicts relative to control values but another group reported normal T-proliferative responses to both concavanalin A and tetanus toxoid antigen in another group of healthy addicts. Immunophenotypic markers on lymphoid cells in human addicts have been studied using flow-cytometric analysis and a profound decrease in the T-helper/cytotoxic T- cell (CD4/CD8) ratio in heroin addicts as well as a normal pattern of T-cell subsets and a normal CD4/CD8 ratio in another group of healthy intravenous drug abusers and methadone patients has been reported by separate groups. More, recent studies have further established the immunosuppressive effects of opioids. Morphine has been shown to antagonize IL-1α and TNF-α induced chemotaxis in human leucocytes as well decrease levels of IL-2 and IFN-γ and increase levels of IL-4 and IL-5. They have also been shown to suppress expression of antigenic markers on T- helper cells.

Opiate use is known to depress E-rossette formation, indicating clinical immunosuppression. Long-term use of opiates produces atrophy of lymphoid organs, decreases lymphoid content, alters antigen-specific antibody production, causes loss of T helper (Th) cells (McDonough et al., 1980; Donahoe et al., 1987) and decreases T cell reactivity, T helper/T cytotoxic cell ratios and T helper cell function specifically (Thomas et al., 1995; Rouveix, 1992). Opiates are known to impair both immunoglobulin synthesis, function and induce immunonutritional deficiencies (Varela et al., 1997). Humoral immunity can be assessed by determining the levels of immunoglobulins, which are antigenic receptors, secreted by B-cells. Alterations of normal immunoglobulin concentration in opiate users are an indication of immunologic impairment (Rho 1972). Alterations in immunoglobulin (Ig) synthesis, concentration and function (Thomas et al., 1995; Islam et al., 2004) are indication of immunologic impairment in opiate users (Rho, 1972; Islam et al., 2001; 2002).

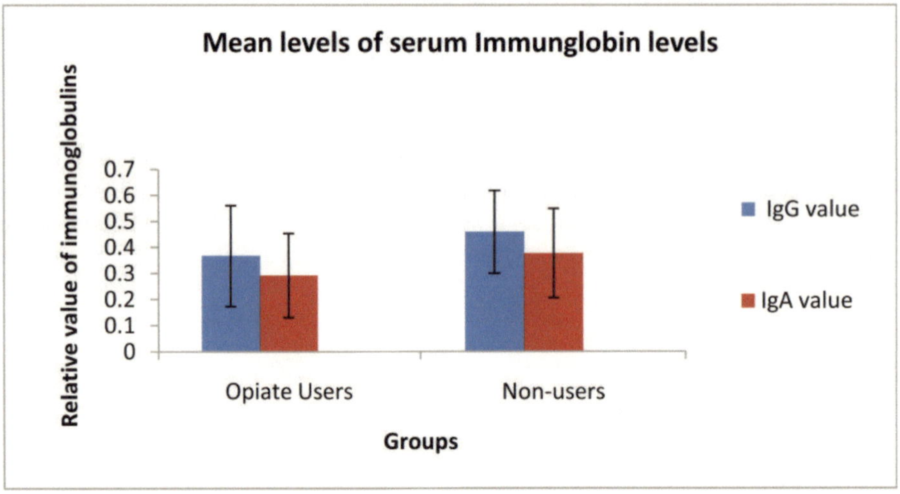

Fig. 1. Serum IgG, IgA levels in Opiate users & Nonusers

A decrease of IgA levels and increase of IgG and IgM levels has also been reported in Indian opiate users as compared to non-users (Naik et al., 2001; Islam et al., 2004). We used a genetic approach to correlate a functional *OPRM1* gene polymorphism with known action of opiates on immunity and a prospective study was undertaken to address the relationship of the A118G variation with the amount of exogenous opiates consumed and correlate the immunosuppressive effects of exogenous opiates with the MOR alleletype among opiate-dependent and control subjects from northern India. We investigated the immune status of opiate users by measuring serum Ig (IgG and IgA) levels, in association with specific MOR genotype of the study subjects (Sharad et al., 2007). Our findings confirmed that the mean circulating levels of Ig were significantly lower in opiate users when compared with levels in cohort controls (Figure 1). Among opiate dependent subjects, individuals with AA genotypetype were found to have the lowest levels of circulating Igs, both IgG and IgA (p=0.0001) while the AG genotype carrying individuals had a higher level of both Igs. The homozygous GG genotype was in between the AA and AG genotypes (Figure 2).

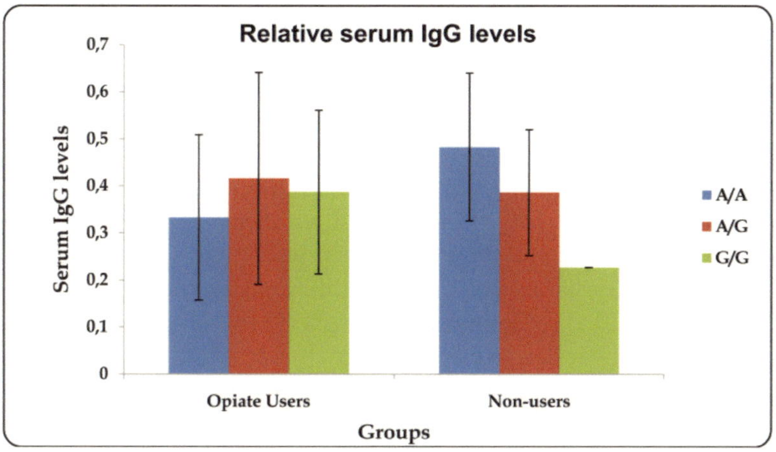

Fig. 2. Serum IgG Values in Opiate users and Non-users with different MOR genotypes

5.2 Auto-antibodies in individuals with different MOR alleles

Autoantibodies (aAbs) is a greek derived word meaning against the self as "auto" means "self", "anti" means "against" and "body". They are produced by the immune system but recognise the proteins produced in the individual's own body. The antibodies that usually attack the proteins present in the nucleus of the cell are called antinuclear antibodies (ANA). It is a known that about 15% of the completely normal population tests positive for ANA.

The interactions between these receptors and immune system, including autoimmune responses, are poorly understood. Granstrem and his co-workers (2006) showed that administration of morphine significantly elevate the levels of aAbs to mu delta-opiate receptor (MDOR). At the same time psycho-stimulant drug, d-amphetamine, or a commonly abused substance, nicotine, had no effect on these aAbs levels. Such observations support the hypothesis that, opiates could be common mediators between the nervous and the immune system. The high levels of aAbs to MDOR were also observed in heroin self-administering rats as well as in human addicts and shown as a function of severity of opiate addiction (Dambinova and Izykenova, 2002), suggesting that opiate addiction may be somehow associated with autoimmune response/processes.

Koziol and collègues (1997) compared the range of ANA in "healthy" individuals in comparison with patients with autoimmune disorders such as systemic lupus erythematosus, systemic sclerosis, sjogren's syndrome and rheumatoid arthritis, or soft tissue rheumatism. Their findings revealed that in healthy individuals, the frequency of ANA did not differ significantly across the 4 age subgroups spanning 20-60 years of age. This putatively normal population was ANA positive in 31.7% of individuals at 1:40 serum dilution, 13.3% at 1:80, 5.0% at 1:160, and 3.3% at 1:320 (Koziol, 1997). Experiments by Bendtzen and co-workers (1993) confirmed the presence of nano-to-picomolar concentrations of high affinity IgG antibody to interleukin 6 (IL-6ab) in sera of 15% normal Danish blood donors. The same group had earlier shown presence of detectable autoantibodies against IL-1α in sera from 10% of normal human subjects (Bendtzen, et al., 1989).

To study the functional consequences of OPRM1 genotype as early modifiers of auto-immune response we estimated ANA in opiate dependent subjects with A118 or G118 MOR allele (unpublished data; Kapur S and co-workers). A sandwich ELISA assay was performed using Nuclear S100 extract prepared from lymphocytes of normal individuals. The whole complement of the nuclear fraction was used to increase the antigen repertoire. In order to test the impact of OPRM1 genotype, plasma from diagnosed cases of Rheumatoid Arthritis, clinically known to have a higher level of circulating ANA, were also tested for comparison. True to our projections our findings confirmed significantly higher titres of ANA in the rheumatoid arthritis subjects in comparison to those seen in plasma of opiate dependent and control subjects. The mean titres of ANA in the different groups are shown in Figure 3. The mean anti ANA titres in AA genotype bearing subjects were higher than those observed in GG genotype bearing subjects in all three groups studied.

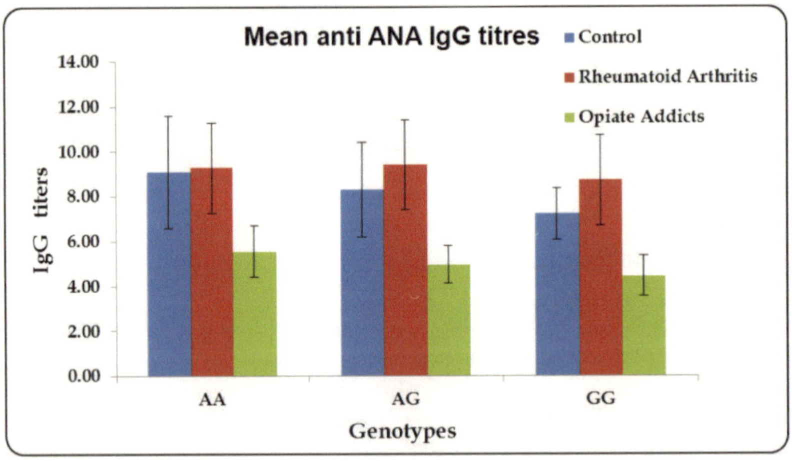

Fig. 3. Bar graph showing relative levels of ANA titres in the groups under study

5.3 Chemokines in relation to MOR genotype

Chemokines consist of a family of 8-16 kDa cytokines that are generated very early in a wide variety of inflammatory responses and attract leukocytes to local sites. At nanomolar concentration chemokines initiate signal transduction and activate leukocytes through seven transmembrane (STM) receptors, but higher micromolar doses result in homologous desensitizing effects. Chemokines along with adhesion molecules orchestrate the migration of opioid peptide-containing leukocytes to inflamed tissue. Leukocytes secrete opioid peptides under stressful conditions or in response to releasing agents such as corticotropin-releasing factor and other chemokines. Due to the crucial role of chemokines in recruitment of leukocytes to sites of inflammation they play a vital role in a variety of infective/anti-inflammatory diseases. Chemokines are subdivided according to their structure into two subgroups, of which the largest are the CXC, or alpha, and CC, or beta groups defined by the presence or absence of an additional amino acid ("X") respectively between the first two cysteine residues in a conserved four cysteine motif. The alpha chemokines are further subdivided according to the presence or absence of a glutamine-leucine-arginine (ELR) amino-acid sequence near the active site. Those possessing this sequence are potent chemoattractants for neutrophils while those that do not possess the motif are chemotactic for lymphocytes.

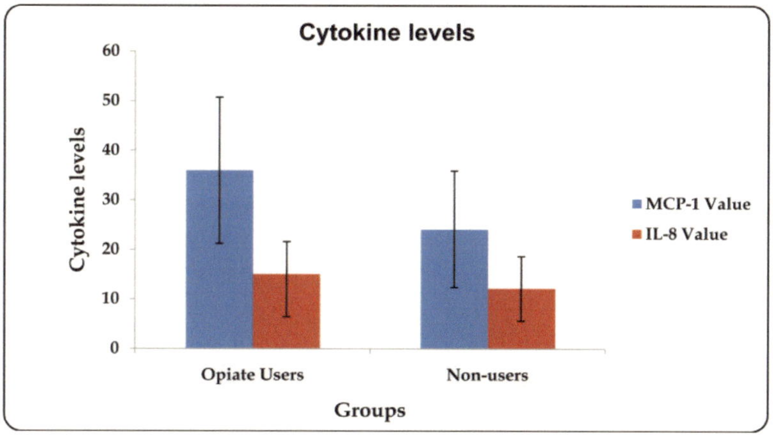

Fig. 4. Mean levels of cytokines (MCP-1and IL-8 values (pg/ml)) in Opiate users and Non-users

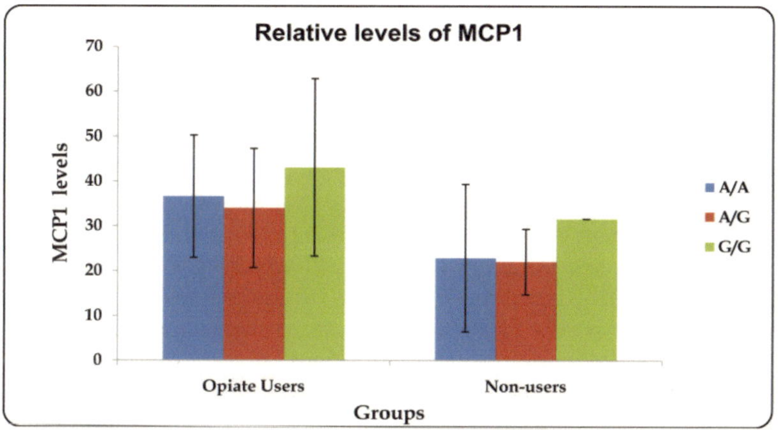

Fig. 5. MCP-1 Values (pg/ml) in Opiate users and Non-users with different MOR genotypes

Interleukin 8 (IL-8) possesses an ELR amino acid-sequence and is the prototype alpha chemokine, being exclusively chemotactic for neutrophils. IL-8 is produced by macrophages and other cell types such as epithelial cells and is also synthesized by endothelial cells, which store IL-8 as storage vesicles. IL-8 has potent chemotactic activity at nanomolar and picomolar concentrations for neutrophils and lymphocytes, respectively (Larsen et al., 1989) and induces leukocyte trans-endothelial transmigration (Zoja et al., 2002). Thus, IL-8 is better known for its role in inflammatory diseases, where it attracts white blood cells into an area of tissue injury and sites of inflammation. On the basis of reports that opiates have anti-inflammatory effects and also use STM, it has been postulated that they may cross-desensitize the response of leukocytes to chemokines. Met-enkephalin (MET) is chemotactic for human peripheral blood monocytes. Indeed it has been observed that preincubation of monocytes or neutrophils with MET or morphine prevented their subsequent chemotactic response to chemokines (MIP1 or IL-8). However, MET does not inhibit the chemotactic response of PMN to NAP-2, a homologous chemokine that is less potent than IL-8 but cannot be desensitized. The inhibitory effect of opiates on chemokine-induced chemotaxis was also antagonized by naloxone. Since MIP-1 and IL-8, unlike NAP-2, have the capacity to desensitize leukocytes, it is reasonable to expect that opiates, by desensitizing some chemokine responses, can suppress inflammatory reactions.

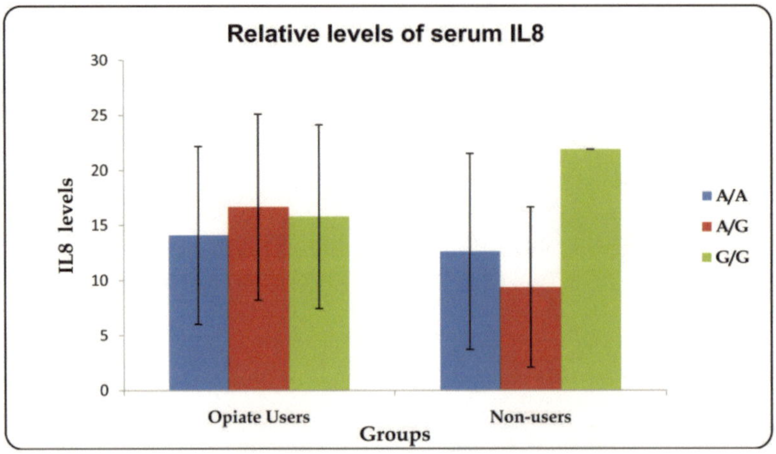

Fig. 6. IL-8 Values (pg/ml) in Opiate users and Non-users with different MOR genotypes

Mu opioids have been shown to alter the release of chemokines important for both host defence and inflammatory response. Exposure to morphine has been shown to suppress production of IFN-α, IL-2 and IL-4 by lymphocytes (Lysle et al., 1993; Geber et al., 1975; Bhargava et al., 1994). Wetzel et al., (2000) showed that mu selective agonists increased the expression of the CC chemokine, MCP-1. MCP-1 plays a major role in two distinctly different host responses: cellular immune reactions and responses to active tissue injury (Leonard et al., 1990). MCP-1 can be produced by leukocytes of both lymphocyte and monocyte lineages and is specific for monocytes, macrophages and activated T cells. MCP-1 can both initiate and amplify monocyte recruitment to the microvascular walls, and let monocyte enter into the tissues and be transformed into macrophages (Sozzani et al., 1995). Recruitment of macrophages into tissues is an important process in inflammation and host defence and thus both MCP-1 and IL-8 both play a significant role in inflammation and host defence. Mean MCP-1 levels in dependent subjects were 35.87 pg/ml (ranging between 8.95-80.81 pg/ml) while in non-users it was 24.12 pg/ml (5.87-109.1) and were significantly higher in opiate users as compared to control subjects ($p = 0.0001$, $t = 6.398$). The mean IL-8 in opiate dependent subjects was 15.08 pg/ml (ranging between 1.580-44.38) and 12.13 pg/ml (ranged from 3.390-37.60) in control subjects (non users). The levels in addicts were significantly higher in comparison to control subjects ($p = 0.0061$, $t = 2.773$) as shown in Figures 4-6. The presence of 118G allele was found to be associated with increased levels of both MCP1 and IL-8 and can be envisaged to play a critical role in chemotactic migration of both lymphocytes and neutrophils to site of inflammation and tissue injury.

6. Observations in cases of therapeutic use of opiates as analgesics

One of the most frequent conditions for which morphine is used is the treatment of pain. Hashiguchi and colleagues (Hashiguchi et al., 2005) published a study with a limited

number of patients who were receiving morphine therapy for advanced cancer pain. Although not conclusive, this work suggests that both humoral and cellular immunity are modulated by morphine and its metabolites during the early phases of therapy, and that such immune-modulation can have long-term detrimental effects.
The immunosuppressive properties of another potent opioid fentanyl have been shown to affect cellular immune responses in humans in a dose related manner (Jacobs et al., 1999 & Beilin et al., 1996). In another study, patients with a long history of heroin intake when switched to high doses of buprenorphine showed significant immuno-suppression. Endogenous opiates lead to elevated plasma levels of corticotrophin releasing hormone, adrenocorticoid hormone and glucocorticoids, which further lead to immune suppression and increased incidence of opportunistic infections. Inhibitory action of morphine on immune responses, demonstrated both in animal models and humans (Quaglio et al., 2002; Nath et al., 2002) accounts for increased susceptibility to opportunistic infections in opiate dependent subjects (Vallejo et al., 2004).
MOR is expressed in ileal and colonic enteric neurons as well as in immunocytes such as myeloid cells and CD4+ and CD8+ T cells. Specific host defense in the intestine is mediated by the gut-associated lymphoid tissue (GALT), which comprises the largest mass of immune cells in the body. GALT, which consists of both organized and diffuse lymphoid tissue mediates immune protection at both local and distant anatomical sites through local dimeric IgA secretion and the ability of lymphocytes activated at one mucosal site to recirculate and home to other mucosal surfaces (Mowat & Viney, 1997). Thus, humoral immunity in GALT is conveyed by plasma cells committed to IgA synthesis and IgA-producing plasma cells circulate throughout the lymphatic system and protect other mucosal surfaces (Croitoru & Bienenstock., 1994). Polymeric IgA is transported into epithelial cells via secretary component and released into the lumen as secretary IgA (sIgA) where it can neutralize viruses and prevent bacterial adherence to the activated mucosa.

7. Epigenetics and *OPRM1* gene

Genetic studies have revealed the existence of several common susceptibility genes for autoimmune/inflammatory disorders. However, genetic variation represents only half of the story. Recent studies have unequivocally established that epigenetic mechanisms regulate gene expression and are sensitive to external stimuli, bridging the gap between environmental and genetic factors. Thus, gene function depends not only on DNA sequence, but also on epigenetic modifications, including both DNA methylation and histone post-translational modifications. These modifications are influenced by environmental factors and are known to contribute to the pathogenesis of several autoimmune diseases. Several studies have highlighted the importance of the tissue-specificity of DNA methylation changes. Over and above the expression of basic genetic variability, the contribution of genetic factors to disease risk can be modulated by the environment. A number of internal and external environmental factors have been associated with the etiopathology of inflammatory disorders, including viral infection, nutrition, and exposure to chemicals and radiation. Such factors influence or modify the profile of epigenetic modifications, which, in turn, have a direct relationship with the regulation of gene expression, and ultimately the function of the immune system. Active demethylation has been described, particularly in cell (de)differentiation and reprogramming processes, and in the context of the activation of immune cells (Bhutani et al., 2010; Bruniquel & Schwartz., 2003). The first suggestions of a potential role for DNA methylation in autoimmune disease came from studies in which

small compounds that result in decreased DNA methylation, such as 5-azacytidine, hydralazine or procainamide, induced symptoms that are associated with autoimmune disease. For example, these drugs induce autoreactivity in CD4+ T cells, or antinuclear factors in both human and mouse models (Cannat & Seligmann, 1968; Richardson, 1986; Cornacchia et al. , 1988). Most of the genes for which DNA hypomethylation has been reported are from the cluster of differentiation (CD) group, including *ITGAL* (also known as *CD11A*), (Lu et al., 2002) which is important for cell–cell adhesion, *CD70* (encoding CD70, also known as tumor necrosis factor ligand superfamily member 7), (Oelke et al., 2004) which is required for T cell proliferation, clonal expansion and the promotion of effector T cell formation, and *CD40LG* (encoding CD40 ligand), (Lu et al., 2007) which stimulates B cell IgG overproduction.
On the other hand in case of hypermethylation of promoter sequences, transcription factor-binding sites have reduced binding affinity for their cognate transcription factors. Nielson et al (2009) examined whether there are differences in cytosine: guanine (CpG) dinucleotide methylation in the OPRM1 promoter between former heroin dependent subjects and controls. Analysis of methylation at 16 CpG dinucleotides in DNA obtained from lymphocytes of 194 Caucasian former severe heroin addicts stabilized in methadone maintenance treatment and 135 Caucasian control subjects revealed significant methylation differences at the -18 CpG and +84 CpG dinucleotide sites in the propmoter region of the OPRM1 gene. Both the -18 and the + 84 CpG sites are located in potential Sp1 transcription factor-binding sites. Methylation of these CpG sites may lead to reduced OPRM1 expression in the lymphocytes of these former heroin addicts and in turn impact the immune response mounted to both auto and external antigens.

8. Failing to protect: Immune dysfunction spells trouble

Immune suppression has been seen in patients suffering from heroin dependence (Naik et al., 2001). Opiate drug and its psychonutritional consequences have been reported to suppress movement and number of white blood cells (Perez-Castrillon et al., 1992; Herbert and Cohen, 1993; Scrimshaw and SanGiovanni 1997; Miyagi et al 2000). Opioid abuse is directly associated with some severe intestinal complications, including toxic megacolon, necrotizing enterides and necrotizing angiitis (Roszler et al., 1991). In addition, Gram-negative enteric bacteria have been implicated as causative agents in enterococcal endocarditis and other severe infections associated with opiate abuse. Recent studies with MOR deficient mice support a physiological anti-inflammatory effect of MOR at the colon interface (Philippe et al., 2006). Exogenous morphine reduces IgA production in the intestinal tract of mice in response to oral administration of cholera toxin (Dinari et al., 1989). Our own findings show that subjects with the prototypical A118A (AA) genotype are at a greater risk for active immuno-suppression by exogenous opiates. The marked reduction in circulating IgA observed in the AA genotype bearing dependent subjects suggests that such individuals could be at a higher risk for developing opiate-induced intestinal complications and/or defects in mucosal defence. This study also provides an insight into the probable molecular basis for differential adverse reactions, specifically gastrointestinal complications in different individuals. However, more studies are required to further elucidate whether MOR genotype differences contribute to an individual's vulnerability to develop gastrointestinal disorders linked with opiate addictions and /or the course and outcome of inflammatory/infectious diseases due to active immuno-suppression by exogenous opiates. This review also provides an insight into the probable molecular basis for differential adverse immune reactions and gastrointestinal complications in different individuals.

9. Conclusion

Opioid receptors are expressed in cells of the immune system, and potent immunomodulatory effects of their natural and synthetic ligands have been reported. Opiate drugs are known to possess direct suppressive effects on cellular and humoral immunity by influencing both the function of immunocompetent cells and inflammation mediator gene/s expression and secretion (Shin and Masato, 2008). In turn, the major source of local endogenous opioid ligands (beta-endorphin, enkephalins, endomorphins and dynorphin) are leukocytes themselves. Both in vivo and in vitro opioids affect activity of leukocytes and expression of inflammatory molecules, such as chemokines and chemokine receptors, in leukocytes. Chemokines induce cellular migration and are crucial players in initiating both innate and adaptive immune response (Figure 7).

A series of very early inflammatory events induce activation of tissue and endothelial cells and culminates in production of chemokines such as interleukin-8 (IL-8) that induce migration of neutrophils to the affected site where they inactivate pathogens by phagocytosis or release of microbicides (Shen et al., 2006). U87 (astrocytoma), normal human astrocyte (NHAs) (Neudeck and Loeb, 2002) and Caco2 (Neudeck et al., 2003) cells treated with morphine showed significant down-regulation of proinflammatory chemokines such as IL-8, MCP-1, and MIP-1 beta and this was inhibited by treatment with MOR antagonist, beta-funaltrexamine (Mahajan et al., 2005).

Opioid receptors activate several intracellular pathways, such as closing of voltage-sensitive calcium channels, opening of potassium channels leading to cellular hyper-polarization and decrease in cyclic AMP production through inhibition of adenylate cyclase. Predominant channels found in lymphocytes are voltage-gated K+ channels and several lines of evidence suggest that these channels are involved in lymphocyte function/s. Vassou et al (2008) have suggested that the effects of opioids on B-lymphocytes may be attributed to interplay between distinct cell populations. Findings from our lab show that the presence 118G allele not only impacts the amount of drug consumed, but also influences the immunomodulation caused by exogenous opiates. The individuals homozygous for AA genotype seem to be more vulnerable to suppression of humoral immunity (antibody production by B cells) while those with GG genotype could be protected against such depression of B-cell function. Indeed, Vassou et al. (2008) have shown that opiates like morphine, alpha$_{S1}$-casomorphin and ethylketocyclazocine modulate antibody and cytokine secretion by multiple myeloma cells in a cell line-dependent manner and decrease antibody secretion by normal B-lymphocytes. Data from both transfected cells and human autopsy brain tissue from carriers of 118G allele indicate that this allele may produce deleterious effect on mRNA and corresponding MOR protein yield (Janicki et al., 2006). Based on the literature reviewed here it can be conclusively said that the complete repertoire of molecular consequence of the 118G SNP on receptor function in various immune cells and nevous tissue still remain unelucidated. A larger study to delineate the effect of AG and GG alleles on suppression of B cell function in the carriers, increasing susceptibility to consequent metabolic compromises leading to diseases and to establish the utility of of this SNP as a marker for estimating adverse immune-modulation in opiate dependent subjects and patients under treatment with opiate drugs needs to be undertaken in different ethnic populations world wide.

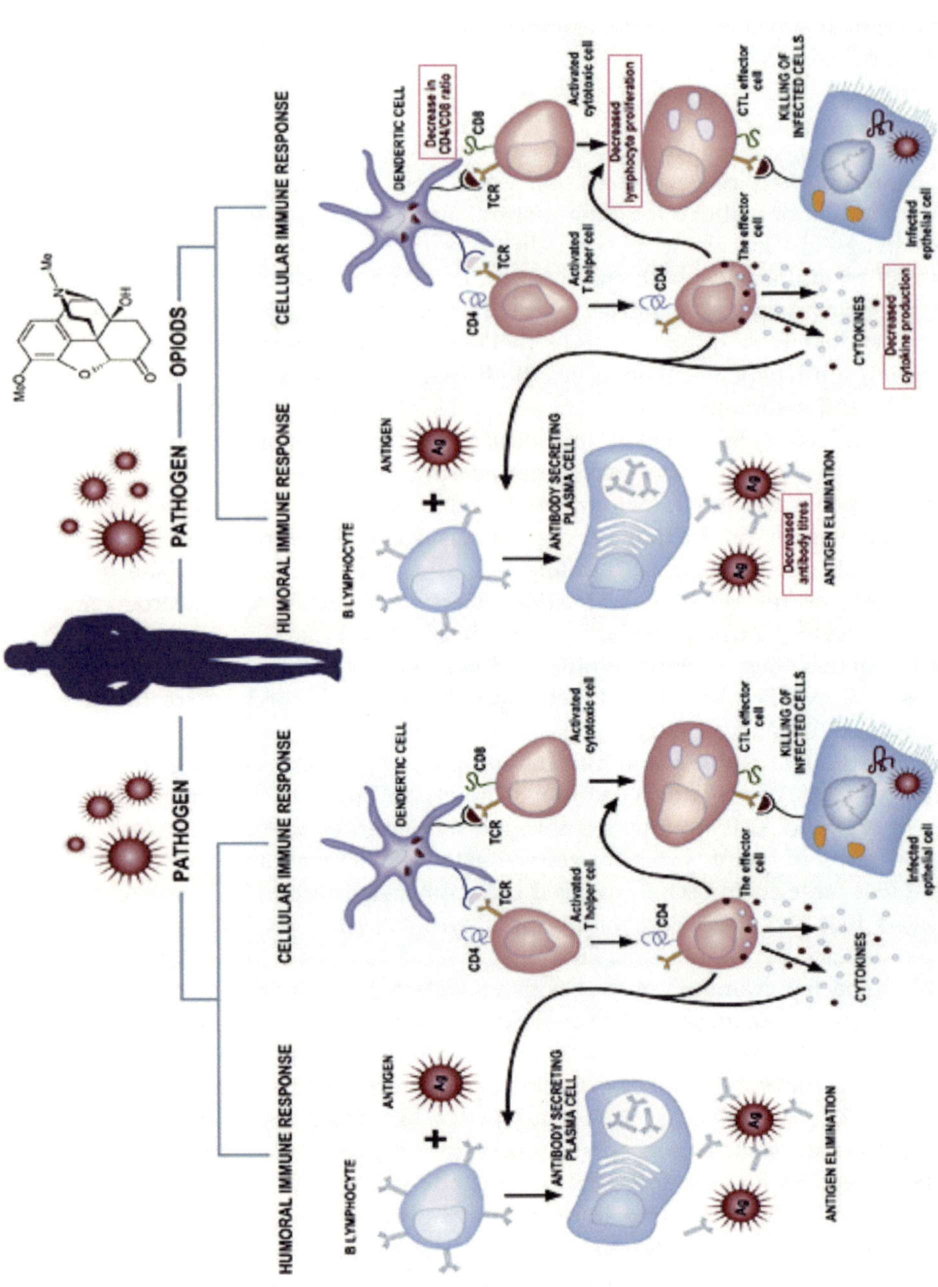

Fig. 7. Effect of opioid intake on immune system

10. Acknowledgment

This work was supported by an extramural grant to Dr Suman Kapur and fellowship to Dr. Shashwat Sharad from Indian Council Medical Research, New Delhi, and to Council of Scientific and Industrial Research, New Delhi for fellowship awarded to Ms. Anuradha Pal.

11. References

Befort, K., et al. (1994). Chromosomal localization of the delta opioid receptor gene to human 1p:14.3-p36.1 and mouse 4D bands by in sim hybridization. *Genomics* 20:143-145.

Beilin, B., et al. (1996). Effects of anesthesia based on large versus small doses of fentanyl on natural killer cell cytotoxicity in the perioperative period. *Anesth Analg*. 82:492–497.

Bendtzen K., et al. (1989). IgG Autoantibodies against Interleukin 1α in Sera of Normal Individuals. *Scandinavian Journal of Immunology*. 29(4):489–492.

Bendtzen K., et al. (1993). High-affinity IgG autoantibodies to IL-6 in sera of normal individuals are competitive inhibitors of IL-6 in vitro. *Cytokine*. 5(1):72-80.

Bhargava, H.N., et al. (1994). Effects of morphine tolerance and abstinence on cellular immune function. *Brain Res*. 642:1- 10.

Bhutani, N., et al.(2010). Reprogramming towards pluripotency requires AID-dependent DNA demethylation. *Nature*. 463:1042–1047.

Bidlack, J.M., et al. (2006). Opioid Receptors and Signaling on Cells from the Immune System. *Journal of Neuroimmune Pharmacology*. 1(3):260-269.

Bond, C., et al. (1998). Single-nucleotide polymorphism in the human mu opioid receptor gene alters beta-endorphin binding and activity: possible implications for opiate addiction. *Proc Natl Acad Sci USA*. 95:9608–9613.

Brown, S.M., et al. (1974). Immunologic dysfunction in heroin addicts. *Arch Intern Med*. 134(6):1-6.

Bruniquel, D., & Schwartz, R.H. (2003). Selective, stable demethylation of the interleukin-2 gene enhances transcription by an active process. *Nat. Immunol*. 4:235–240.

Cannat, A., & Seligmann, M. (1968). Induction by isoniazid and hydralazine of antinuclear factors in mice. *Clin. Exp. Immunol*. 3:99–105.

Cantacuzene, J. (1898). Nouvelles recherches sur le monde de destruction des vibrions dans l'organisme. *Ann Inst Pasteur*. 12:273–300.

Chuang, T.K., et al. (1995). Mu Opioid Receptor Gene Expression in Immune Cells. *Biochem Biophys Res Commun*. 216:922-930.

Cornacchia, E., et al. (1988). Hydralazine and procainamide inhibit T cell DNA methylation and induce autoreactivity. *J. Immunol*. 140:2197–2200.

Croitoru, K. & Bienenstock, J. (1994). Characteristics and functions of mucosa-associated lymphoid tissue. In Add edition. *Handbook of Mucosal Immunology* (ed. Ogra, P. L. et al). 141-149, San Diego: Academic Press.

Dambinova, S.A. & Izykenova, G.A. (2002). Recombinant mu-delta receptor as a marker of opiate abuse. *Ann. N. Y. Acad. Sci*. 965:497–514.

Dinari, G., et al. (1989). The effect of opiates on the intestinal immune response to cholera toxin in mice. *Digestion*. 44:14-19.

Donahoe, R. M., et al. (1987). Mechanistic Implications of the Findings That Opiates and Other Drugs of Abuse Moderate T-Cell Surface Receptors and Antigenic Markers. *Am NY Acad Sci*. 496:711-721.

Geber, W.F., Lefkowitz, S.S. &. Hung, C.Y. (1975). Effect of morphine, hydromorphone, methadone, mescaline, trypanblue, vitaminA, sodiumsalicylate, and caffeine on the serum interferon level in response to viral infection. *Arch. Int. Pharmacodyn*. 214:322- 327.

Georges, H., Leroy, O., Vandenbussche, C., Guery, B., Alfandari, S., Tronchon, L., Beaucaire, G. (1999). Epidemiological features and prognosis of severe community-acquired pneumococcal pneumonia. *Intensive Care Med*. 25 (2): 198- 206.

Hashiguchi, S., et al. (2005). Effects of morphine and its metabolites on immune function in advanced cancer patients. *J Clin Anesth.* 17:575–580.

Herbert, T.B. & Cohen, S. (1993). Stress and immunity in humans: a meta-analytic review. *Psychosom Med.* 55(4):364-79.

Hoehe, M.R., et al. (2000). Sequence variability and candidate gene analysis in complex disease: association of mu opioid receptor gene variation with substance dependence. *Hum Mol Genet.* 9:2895–2908.

Islam, S. N. et al. (2002). Nutritional Status of the Drug Addicts undergoing detoxification: prevalence of malnutrition and influence of illicit drugs and life style. *Br J Nutr.* 88:507-513.

Islam, S. N., Hossain, K. J. & Ahsan, M. (2001). Original Communication: Serum vitamin E, C and A status of the drug addicts undergoing detoxification: influence of drug habit, sexual practice and lifestyle factors. *Eur J Clin Nutr.* 55:1022-1027.

Islam, S.K., et al. (2004). Serum immunoglobulins and white blood cells status of drug addicts: influence of illicit drugs and sex habit. *Addict Biol.* 9(1):27-33.

Jacobs, R., et al. (1999). Effects of fentanyl on cellular immune in man. *Int J Immunopharmacol.* 21: 45–454.

Janicki, P.K., et al. (2006). A genetic association study of the functional A118G polymorphism of the human mu-opioid receptor gene in patients with acute and chronic pain. *Anesth Analg.* 103(4):1011-7.

Janković, B.D. & Marić, D. (1987). Enkephalins and immunity. I: In vivo suppression and potentiation of humoral immune response. *Ann N Y Acad Sci.* 496:115-25.

Koziol, J.A., et al. (1997). Range of antinuclear antibodies in "healthy" individuals. *Arthritis Rheum.* 40(9):1601-11.

Kreek, M.J. & Koob, G.F. (1998). Drug dependence: stress and dys-regulation of brain reward pathways. *Drug Alcohol Depend.* 51: 23-47.

Larsen, C.G., et al. (1989). The neutrophil-activating protein (NAP-1) is also chemotactic for T lymphocytes. *Science.* 243:1464–1466.

Leonard, W.J., Gnarra, J.R. & Sharon, M. (1990). The multisubunit interleukin-2 receptor. *Ann N Y Acad Sci* . 594:200-206.

Litman G.W., Cannon J.P. & Dishaw L.J. (2005). Reconstructing immune phylogeny: new perspectives. *Nature Reviews. Immunology.* 5(11):866–79.

Litt, M., et al. (1988). Chromosomal localization of the human proenkephalin and prodynorphin genes. *Am J Hum Genet.* 42(2): 327-334.

Lu, Q., et al. (2002). Demethylation of ITGAL (CD11a) regulatory sequences in systemic lupus erythematosus. *Arthritis Rheum.* 46:1282–1291.

Lu, Q., et al. (2007). Demethylation of CD40LG on the inactive X in T cells from women with lupus. *J. Immunol.* 179:6352–6358.

Lysle, D.T., et al. (1993). Morphine induced alterations of immune status: dose dependency, compartment specificity and antagonism by naltrexone. *J.Pharmacol.Exp.Ther* 265 (3):1071- 1078.

Mahajan, S.D., et al. (2005). Morphine modulates chemokine gene regulation in normal human astrocytes. *Clin Immunol* . 115(3):323-32.

Mayer, G. (2006). *Innate (non-specific) Immunity.* In : Immunology. Microbiology and Immunology On-Line Textbook. USC School of Medicine.

McDonough, R.J., et al. (1980). Alteration of T and null lymphocyte frequencies in the peripheral blood of human opiate addicts: in vivo evidence for opiate receptor sites on T lymphocytes. *J Immunol.* 125 (6):2539-2543.

Miyagi, A.U., et al. (2000). Opioids suppress chemokine-mediated migration of monkey neutrophils and monocytes - an instant response. *Immunopharmacology.* 47:53-62.

Mowat, A.M. & Viney, J.L. (1997). The anatomical basis of intestinal immunity. *Immunol Rev.* 156: 145-166.

Naik, S., Vaswani, M., & Desai, N.G. (2001). Humoral immune function in non-parenteral heroin dependence: Indian data. *Alcoholism.* 37(1):25-34.

Nath, A., et al. (2002). Molecular basis for interactions of HIV and drugs of abuse. *J Acquir Immune Defic Syndr.* 31(Suppl 2): S62-69.

Neudeck, B.L. & Loeb. J.M. (2002). Endomorphin-1 alters interleukin-8 secretion in Caco-2 cells via a receptor mediated process. *Immunol Lett.* 84(3): 217-21.

Neudeck, B.L., Loeb, J., Buck, J. (2003). Activation of the κ-opioid receptor in Caco-2 cells decreases interleukin-8 secretion. *Eur J Pharmacol.* 467(1-3): 81-84.

Oelke, K., et al. (2004). Overexpression of CD70 and overstimulation of IgG synthesis by lupus T cells and T cells treated with DNA methylation inhibitors. *Arthritis Rheum.* 50:1850–1860.

Olson, G.A., Olson, R.D. & Kastin, A.J. (1996). Endogenous opiates. *Peptide.* 17:1421-1466.

Owerbach, D., et al. (1981). The proopiocortin (adrenocorticotropin/beta-lipoprotein) gene is located on chromosome 2 in humans. *Somatic Cell Genet.* 7(3):359-69.

Pasternak, G.W. (1993). Pharmacological mechanisms of opioid analgesics. *Clin Neuropharmacol.* 1:1–18.

Perez-Castrillon, J. L., et al. (1992). Opioids depress in vitro human monocyte chemotaxis. *Immunopharmacology.* 23(1):57-61.

Peterson, P.K., Molitor, T.W. & Chao, C.C. (1998). The opioid-cytokine connection. *J. Neuroimmunol.* 83:63–69.

Philippe, D., et al. (2006). Mu opioid receptor expression is increased in inflammatory bowel diseases: implications for homeostatic intestinal inflammation. *Gut.* 55(6): 815-823.

Pier, G.B., Lyczak, J.B., & Wetzler, L.M. (2004). *Immunology, Infection, and Immunity.* ASM Press. ISBN 1-55581-246-5.

Quaglio, G., et al. (2002). Prevalence of tuberculosis infection and comparison of multiple-puncture liquid tuberculin test and Mantoux test among drug users. *Scand J Infect Dis.* 34(8):574–576.

Rho, Y.M. (1972). Infections as fatal complications of narcotism. *NY St J Med.* 72(7):823-830.

Roszler, M. H., McCarroll, K. A. & Jacobs, I. J. (1991) *Radiologic study of intravenous drug abuse complications, in Infections in Intravenous Drug Abusers,* Oxford Univ. Press. New York. pp 96-151

Rouveix, B. (1992). Opiates and immune function. Consequences on infectious diseases with special reference to AIDS.*Therapie.* 47(6):503-512.

Roy, S., et al. (2006). Modulation of Immune Function by Morphine: Implications for Susceptibility to Infection. *J Neuroimmune Pharmacol.* 1:77–89.

Satoh, I.I. & Mori, S. (1997). Subregional assignment of the proopiomelanocortin gene (POMC) to human chromosome band 2p23.3 by fluorescence in situ hybridization. *Cytogenet Cell Genet.* 76:221-222.

Schug, S.A., Zech, D. & Grond, S. (1992) Adverse effects of systemic opioid analgesics. *Drug Safety.* 7:200-13.

Scrimshaw, N.S. & SanGiovanni, J.P. (1997). Synergism of nutrition, infection, and immunity: an overview. *Am J Clin Nutr.* 66(2):464S-477S.

Sharad, S., et al.. (2007). Correlation of circulatory immunoglobulin levels with Mu opiate receptor allele. *Indian J Biochem Biophys.* 44(5):394-400.

Shen, L., et al. (2006). Differential regulation of neutrophil chemotaxis to IL-8 and fMLP by GM-CSF: lack of direct effect of oestradiol. *Immunology.* 117(2):205–212.

Shin, K. & Masato, K. (2008). Anesthetics, immune cells, and immune responses. *J Anesth.* 22:263-277.

Sibinga, N.S. & Goldstein, A. (1988). Opioid Peptides and Opioid Receptors in Cells of the Immune System. *Annual Review of Immunology.* 6:219-249.

Simonin, F., et al. (1995). K-opioid receptor in humans: cDNA and genomic cloning, chromosomal assignment, functional expression, pharmacology, and expression pattern in the central nervous system. *Proc Natl Acad Sci USA.* 92:1006-1010.

Smolka, M., & Schmidt, L.G. (1999). The influence of heroin dose and route of administration on the severity of the opiate withdrawal syndrome. *Addiction.* 94: 1191-1198.

Somaini., L, Giaroni, C. & Gerra, G. (2008). Opioid Therapy and Restoration of the Immune Function in Heroin-Addicted Patients. *Heroin Addict Relat Clin Probl.* 10(4):39-44.

Sozzani, S., et al. (1995). Receptors, signal transduction, and spectrum of action of monocyte chemotactic protein-1 and related chemokines. *J Leukoc Biol.* 57(5):788-794.

Thomas, P.T., Bhargava, H.N. & House, R.V. (1995). Immunomodulatory effects of in vitro exposure to morphine and its metabolites. *Pharmacology.* 50(1):51-62.

Vaccarino, A.L., et al. (2000). Analgesic effects of endomorphin-1 and endomorphin-2 in the formalin test in mice. *Pharmacology letters.* 67(8):907-912.

Vallejo, R., de Leon-Casasola, O. & Benyamin, R. (2004) Opioid therapy and immunosuppression: a review. *Am J Ther.* 11(5):354–365.

Varela, P., et al. (1997). Human immunodeficiency virus infection and nutritional status in female drug addicts undergoing detoxification: anthropometric and immunologic assessments. *Am J Clin Nutr.* 66(2):504S-508S.

Vassou, D., et al. (2008). Opioids modulate constitutive B lymphocyte secretion. *Int Immunopharmacol.* 8:634-644.

Wang, J.B., et al. (1994). Human mu opiate receptor: cDNA and genomic clones, pharmacologic characterization and chromosomal assignment. *FEBS Lett.* 338: 217–222.

Wetzel, M.A., et al. (2000). µ-Opioid Induction of Monocyte Chemoattractant Protein-1, RANTES, and IFN-{gamma}-Inducible Protein-10 Expression in Human Peripheral Blood Mononuclear Cells. *J. Immuno.* 165: 6519-6524.

Yasuda, K., et al. (1994). Localization of the kappa opioid receptor gene to human chromosome band 8q11.2. *Genomics.* 19: 596¬597.

Zabel, B.U., et al. (1983). High-resolution chromosomal localization of human genes for amylase, proopiomelanoconin, soma¬tostatin, and a DNA fragment (D3SI) by in situ hybridization. *Proc Nad Acad Sci USA.* 80:6932-6936.

Zoja, C., et al. (2002). Shiga toxin-2 triggers endothelial leukocyte adhesion and transmigration via NF-kappaB dependent up-regulation of IL-8 and MCP-1. *Kidney Int.* 62:846–856.

2

Endotoxin Tolerance as a Key Mechanism for Immunosuppression

Subhra K. Biswas and Irina N. Shalova
*Singapore Immunology Network, BMSI, A*STAR*
Singapore

1. Introduction

Inflammation is a complex pathophysiological phenomenon orchestrated by immune cells in response to infection and/or tissue damage (Nathan, 2002; Foster & Medzhitov, 2009). It serves protective mechanism against pathological insults and aims to re-instate homeostasis. Monocytes/macrophages are the first line of immune cells to detect and response to "danger signals" in an organism (e.g. pathogens, tissue damage). The detection of pathogens and/or endotoxins by these cells is mediated through pattern recognition receptors (PRRs) such as Toll-like receptors (TLRs) which triggers a robust and inflammatory reaction (Figure 1). However, uncontrolled inflammation can lead to extensive tissue damage and manifestation of pathological states like sepsis, autoimmune diseases, metabolic diseases and cancer (Foster & Medzhitov, 2009). Thus, the innate immune cells 'adapt' themselves in the later phase of inflammation to tune down this response and promote resolution of inflammation leading to healing and tissue repair (Figure 1).

Organisms as well as their immune cells have developed mechanisms to protect themselves from excessive inflammation in response to endotoxins. Endotoxin tolerance (ET) is such an adaptation wherein organisms or their innate immune cells (like monocytes/macrophages) show diminished response to endotoxins as a result of prior exposure to low doses of endotoxins (Foster & Medzhitov, 2009; Biswas et al., 2007; Dobrovolskaia & Vogel, 2002; Fan & Cook, 2004; Cavaillon & Adib-Conquy, 2006). In other words, the organism or their immune cells have developed a "tolerance" to endotoxin. Clinically, this phenomenon can be observed in monocytes/macrophages in patients with sepsis, trauma, surgery or pancreatitis (Cavaillon et al., 2003; Monneret et al., 2008). In most of these cases ET contributes to immunosuppression, while in sepsis it has been linked to mortality as well (Figure 1) (Monneret et al., 2008). These and other facts have suggested ET as a key mechanism for immunosuppression associated with diverse pathological conditions. In this chapter, we will review the *in vitro* and *in vivo* evidences for ET, as well as an insight into the cellular and molecular basis of this phenomenon. In addition, the pathophysiological implications of ET will be also discussed.

2. *In vitro* and *in vivo* evidences for ET

ET has been observed both *in vitro* and *in vivo* in animal models as well as in humans (Biswas et al., 2007; Dobrovolskaia & Vogel, 2002; Cavaillon & Adib-Conquy, 2006; Biswas &

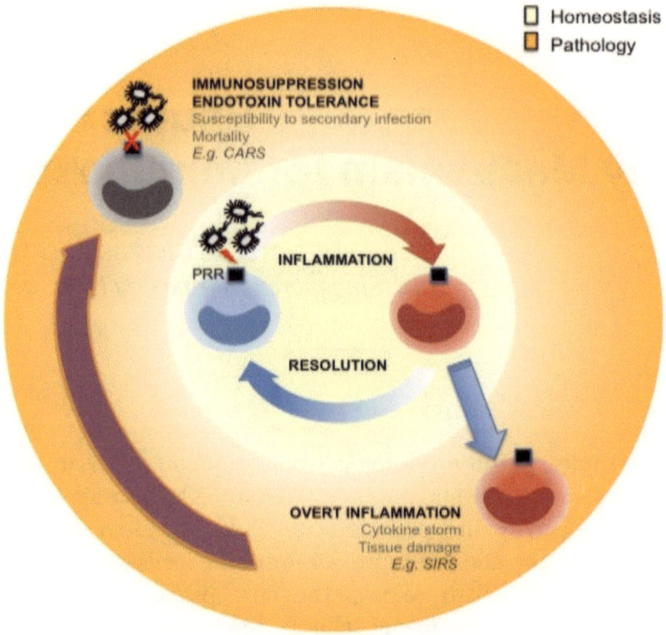

Fig. 1. Inflammation and resolution are pathophysiological responses in host defense and homeostasis. Inflammation is necessary to trigger a defense response against pathogens, while resolution promotes healing and re-instates homeostatic conditions. Monocytes/macrophages detect and respond to pathogens via PRRs to mediate both inflammation and resolution. However, exaggerated inflammation can lead to deleterious effects like cytokine storm and tissue damage (e.g. in SIRS). As a protective response to this overt inflammation, an immunosuppressive or endotoxin tolerant phase (e.g. CARS) ensues, which in the case of sepsis leads to susceptibility to secondary infection and even mortality. SIRS: Systemic inflammatory response syndrome; CARS: Compensatory anti- inflammatory response syndrome

Tergaonkar, 2007; del Fresno et al., 2009; Foster et al., 2007; Dobrovolskaia et al., 2003; Medvedev et al., 2000). The first report of ET was by Paul Beeson in 1946. He observed that repeated injection of typhoid vaccine in rabbits caused a progressive reduction of fever induced by the vaccine (Foster & Medzhitov, 2009). Similarly, in humans who were recovering from typhoid fever or malaria, wherein re-challenge with endotoxin showed reduced fever (Cavaillon & Adib-Conquy, 2006). In mice, prior injection with a sublethal dose of Lipopolysaccharide (LPS) protected them from a subsequent and otherwise lethal dose of LPS (Cavaillon & Adib-Conquy, 2006). This study also showed monocytes/macrophages as the principal cells responsible for the induction of ET *in vivo*. Subsequently, several *in vitro* studies have confirmed ET in murine macrophages as well as human monocytes when re-challenged *in vitro* with LPS, following a prior exposure to suboptimal levels of endotoxin (e.g. LPS). The key readout for ET in these cells was the drastic reduction of TNFα production as compared to the cells exposed to endotoxin only once (Biswas et al., 2007; Dobrovolskaia & Vogel, 2002; Cavaillon & Adib-Conquy, 2006; del Fresno et al., 2009; Foster et al., 2007). Transcriptome studies have expanded our understanding of the gene expression response related to ET in murine macrophages (Dobrovolskaia & Vogel, 2002; Dobrovolskaia et al., 2003; Medvedev et al., 2000) and human monocytes (Cavaillon & Adib-Conquy, 2006; Chan et al., 2005; Chen et al., 2009; El Gazzar et al., 2009; Melo et al., 2010; Pena et al., 2011). These studies have not only shown the downregulation of a large panel of pro-inflammatory genes (the "tolerized" genes), but also defined a subset of "non-tolerant" whose transcription remained unaffected or even upregulated in the tolerized cells. For example, inflammatory cytokines/chemokines like TNFα, IL-6, IL-12, IL-1β, CCL3 and CCL4 were downregulated upon LPS re-stimulation of the endotoxin tolerized cells. In contrast, the upregulated genes were more varied, consisting of anti-inflammatory cytokines such as IL-10, TGFβ and IL-1RA; scavenging C-type lectin receptors such as MARCO, CLEC4α, CD136, CD23, and CD64; negative regulators such as IRAK-M and a variety of anti-microbial genes (e.g. FPR1, AOAH and RNASET2) (del Fresno et al., 2009; Foster et al., 2007; Mages et al., 2007; Draisma et al., 2009; Pena et al., 2011). Several genes related to tissue remodeling and repair (e.g. VEGF, MMP, FGF2) were also upregulated. Transcriptomic analysis of murine macrophages from an *in vivo* LPS tolerance model confirmed some of the above findings as well as the downregulation of genes related to the cell death pathway (e.g. PARP-1, caspase 3, FASL and TRAIL) in LPS tolerant macrophages (Melo et al., 2010). These results have prompted the idea of ET as a case of gene re-programming rather than "tolerance" which suggests an overall downregulation of responses.

Functionally, endotoxin-tolerant monocytes are characterized by increased phagocytic ability but an impaired antigen presentation capacity (del Fresno et al., 2009; Monneret et al., 2004). Increased phagocytosis was suggested in this study to be due to the upregulated expression of the cell surface receptor CD64, whereas impaired antigen presentation was possibly due to downregulated expression of several MHC Class II molecules (e.g. HLA-DRs) and the master regulator of MHC Class II expression, CIITA (del Fresno et al., 2009; Monneret et al., 2004). IL-10 and TGFβ have been implicated in downregulate MHC Class II and the CD86 co-stimulatory molecule in endotoxin-tolerant human monocytes (Wolk et al., 2000; Wolk et al., 2003; Schroder et al., 2003). Increased production of tissue remodeling factors like VEGF, MMPs and FGF2 was related to the enhanced capacity of endotoxin tolerized monocytes in wound healing assays (Pena et al., 2011). Collectively, these studies observations may imply some functional relevance. For example, downregulation of inflammatory cytokines coupled with upregulation of anti-inflammatory cytokines as well as tissue remodeling factors may help to check against an overt inflammation and promote tissue repair, while increased phagocytic capability may be crucial to killing and clearance of bacteria. Additionally, downregulation of death-related genes would protect macrophages from death with possible implications on survival (Melo et al., 2010). However, further studies would be needed to demonstrate the occurrence of mechanism *in vivo* in animal models of sepsis progression.

In the line with the observations in monocytes/macrophages, ET affects dendritic cells (DC), neutrophils as well as some non-immune cells, like endothelial cells of the intestine (Ogawa et al., 2003). Endotoxin-tolerant DC show a downregulation of IL-12, TNFα and IL-6 expression, but enhanced IL-10 expression and endocytosis (Sharabi et al., 2008; Albrecht et al., 2008). Endotoxin-tolerant neutrophils demonstrate loss of TLR4 expression and impaired respiratory burst, but retain their proinflammatory cytokine phenotype (Parker et al., 2005). However, a full scale dissection of ET in different blood cell lineages and tissues would be particularly important to better understand the impact of this phenomenon at the organism level.

3. Polarization of myelomonocytic cells in ET

A characteristic feature of monocytes and macrophages is their functional diversity and plasticity whereby these cells can display a variety of functional phenotypes depending on the microenvironment stimuli they encounter (Gordon & Taylor, 2005; Biswas and Mantovani, 2010). Analogous to the Th1 and Th2 polarization scheme, two distinct activation states of macrophages have been defined, namely, classical or M1 activation and alternative or M2 activation state (Mantovani et al., 2004; Biswas & Mantovani, 2010) (Figure 2).

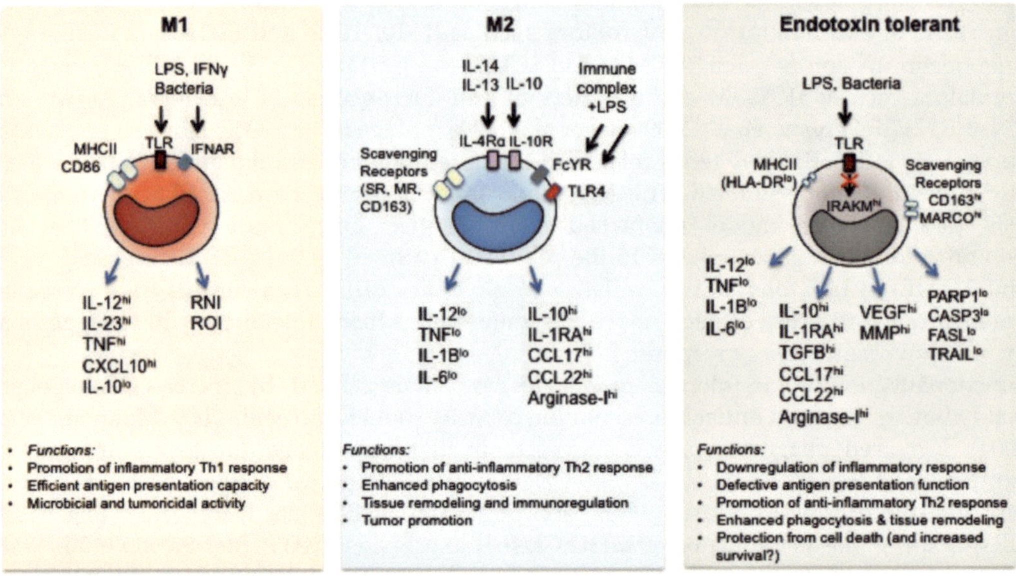

Fig. 2. Polarization states of monocytes and macrophages. Figure summaries the salient characteristics and functional properties defining the M1 and M2 polarization states. The figure also shows the salient properties of endotoxin tolerized monocytes and macrophages (as revealed by current studies) indicating them to be an M2 polarized population. SR: Scavenging receptor; MR: Mannose receptor

Th1 cytokines like IFNγ as well as microbial stimuli (e.g. LPS) polarize macrophages to an M1 state whereas Th2 cytokines like IL-4, IL-13 or IL-10, glucocorticoids and immune complexes plus LPS, polarize macrophages to an M2 state. M1 macrophages show inflammatory characteristics with increased expression of proinflammatory cytokines like IL-12, TNFα, IL-23, CXCL10, reactive nitrogen and oxygen intermediates (RNI/ROI) but downregulate IL-10 expression. These cells display microbicidal and tumoricidal activity. In contrast, M2 macrophages produce very less inflammatory cytokines but upregulate the expression of anti-inflammatory cytokines (e.g. IL-10), arginase I, as well as factors which promote tissue remodeling, angiogenesis, wound healing and tumor promotion. It may be emphasized that M1 and M2 phenotypes represent extremes of a spectrum of macrophage functional states (Mantovani et al., 2004; Mosser & Edwards, 2008). The occurrence of mixed phenotype with overlapping M1 and M2 characteristics as well as plasticity between these two phenotypes have been observed *in vivo* (Biswas & Mantovani, 2010). In fact, the plasticity of macrophages from an M1 to an M2-like state is integral to their role in inflammation and resolution.

Several lines of evidences suggest endotoxin-tolerant monocytes/macrophages to resemble an M2 polarized population (Figure 2). These characteristics include downregulation of inflammatory cytokines (e.g. IL-12, TNFα) and upregulation of anti-inflammatory cytokines (e.g. IL-10), scavenging receptor and efficient phagocytosis (del Fresno et al., 2009; Mantovani et al., 2005). Further, endotoxin tolerized mouse macrophages to express typical markers of M2 polarization like Arg1, CCL17 and CCL22 (Porta et al., 2009). Similarly, M2-like Gr1+CD11b+ myeloid suppressor cells with increase IL-10 production and T-cell suppressive phenotype has also been reported in a murine polymicrobial sepsis model (Delano et al., 2007). More recent study on human monocytes confirmed its M2 polarization characterized by upregulation of scavenging receptors (MARCO, CD163, CD23), tissue remodeling genes (VEGF, FGF, MMPs) and M2-specific cytokine/chemokine genes (IL-10, CCL22 and CCL24) (Pena et al., 2011). The fact that endotoxin tolerized monocytes/macrophages are M2 polarized population is also in line with the observation of a Th2-polarized adaptive immune response in LPS-injected healthy donors and in murine polymicrobial sepsis (Delano et al., 2007; Lauw et al., 2000). However, the actual polarization state of monocytes and macrophages during endotoxin tolerance *in vivo* may be more complex, as with most pathological situations.

4. Sepsis is a paradigm for ET

Sepsis is a complex syndrome characterized by dysregulated inflammation and systemic bacterial infection. It consists from two phases. The first early phase is called Systemic inflammatory response syndrome or SIRS (Figure 1). It is characterized by leukocytes activation, rapid release of cytokines (also called 'Cytokine Storm') and tissue injury (Adib-Conquy & Cavaillon, 2009). The second late phase of sepsis is called Compensatory anti-inflammatory response syndrome or CARS (Figure 1). The CARS is characterized by leukocyte deactivation, immunosuppression and endothelial/epithelial dysfunction. This phase resembles an endotoxin-tolerant state (Monneret et al., 2008; Buras et al., 2005). In fact, some studies have linked this immunosuppressive or ET phase to mortality in sepsis patients (Monneret et al., 2008; Adib-Conquy & Cavaillon, 2009; Hotchkiss et al., 2009; Pachot et al., 2006). In line with the above observation, sepsis blood monocytes show a phenotype similar to ET. This is characterized by i) a downregulation of proinflammatory cytokines like TNFα, IL-6, IL-1α, IL-1β and IL-12 upon *ex vivo* LPS challenge as compared to that of monocytes from healthy donors (Monneret et al., 2008; Draisma et al., 2009; Munoz et al., 1991a,b); ii) downregulation of expression of MHC Class II molecules, CD86 and CIITA (Pachot et al., 2006; Manjuck et al., 2000); and iii) upregulation of anti-inflammatory cytokines like IL-10, TGFβ and IL-1RA (Draisma et al., 2009; Monneret et al., 2004; Cavaillon et al., 2005). Further, the decreased monocyte IL-12 production in trauma patients correlates to impaired T-cell proliferation and a polarization towards a Th2 response (Monneret et al., 2008; Hotchkiss & Karl, 2003).

Paralleling the biphasic nature of sepsis progression from SIRS to CARS, monocytes are also believed to mirror a plasticity of their phenotype from an inflammatory to an anti-inflammatory endotoxin tolerant. However, whether this is a cause or effect of the biphasic nature of sepsis and what are the triggers for this switch in the monocyte/macrophage phenotype remains to be investigated. It is believed that exposure to chronicle level of inflammatory substances as well as products of tissue damage at the early phase of sepsis may trigger mechanisms which stimulate endotoxin tolerance of monocytes in the later phase of sepsis. One of the examples of such dual regulation could be hyaluronic acid (HA), a component of the extracellular matrix. At the early phase of inflammation macrophages and neutrophils release hyaluronase that degrade HA. At the same time, HA inhibit TNFα expression and activate IL10 production in macrophages that help to block inflammation (Kuang et al., 2007). Moreover HA activates Matrix metalloprotease (MMP) which, in turn, activates the anti-inflammatory cytokine TGFβ (Nathan, 2002; Adair-Kirk & Senior, 2008). Another interesting molecule is COX2, which is responsible for prostaglandin E2 (PGE2) production. Sepsis macrophages show high expression of COX2; however accumulation of PGE2 can inhibit COX2 expression in a negative feedback manner and stimulate the production of anti-inflammatory compounds like lipoxins (Serhan et al., 2007). Even the phagocytosis of apoptotic neutrophils, that take place at late phase of inflammation, can stimulate macrophages in anti-inflammatory mode that includes the production of TGFβ (Fadok et al., 1998). In contrast to the biphasic nature of sepsis discussed above, some authors have suggested host response to sepsis as concurrent process of overt inflammatory and immunosuppression. This seems plausible since sepsis monocytes show an inflammatory phenotype (as compared to normal monocytes), yet displaying an endotoxin phenotype upon further activation.

5. Molecular mechanisms driving ET

5.1 Role of MyD88 and TRIF pathways

Innate immune cells detect pathogen through pattern recognition receptors (PRR). While there exist a diverse array of secreted, transmembrane and cytosolic PRRs which respond to various danger signals (Iwasaki & Medzhitov, 2010), we focus on Toll-like receptor 4 (TLR4), the major PRR involved in the detection of Gram-negative bacteria and their associated endotoxins (e.g. Lipopolysaccharide, LPS; Lipid A) (Beutler, 2004; O'Neill & Bowie, 2007). TLR4 signaling is mediated by two distinct adaptors, namely, MyD88 and TRIF [1] (Figure 3) (Kawai & Akira, 2011).

The MyD88-dependent pathway leads to the activation of the transcription factor NF-κB and inflammatory genes like TNFA, IL1B, IL6 and IL12A (Figure 3). The TRIF-dependent pathway upregulates the transcription factor IRF3 which induces expression of IFNβ and this, in turn, activates transcription factor STAT1 and expression of interferon-inducible genes like CCL5 and CXCL10 (Figure 3) (Kawai & Akira, 2011; Yamamoto et al., 2003; Biswas & Lopez-Collazo, 2009). However, crosstalk exists between both these pathways.

Several studies have indicated defects in the TLR4 pathways as a mechanistic basis of ET in monocytes and macrophages. These defects can be at multiple levels starting from the receptor, adaptors, signaling molecules, and transcription factors (Biswas & Lopez-Collazo, 2009). For example, downregulation of TLR4, decrease in TLR4-MyD88 complex formation,

---

[1] ***Abbreviation for** signaling molecules:* **AP1**: activator protein 1; **ATF3**: Activating transcription factor 3; **BCL3**: B-cell CLL/lymphoma 3; **FLN29**: TRAF-type zinc finger domain containing 1(TRAFD1); **GAS6**: Growth arrest-specific 6; **HA**: Hyaluronic acid; **IRAK-M**: interleukin-1 receptor-associated kinase 3; **IRF3**: Interferon regulatory factor 3; **JNK**: Jun N-terminal kinase; **LPS**: Lipopolysaccharide; **MKP1**: MAP kinase phosphatase 1; **MyD88**: Myeloid differentiation 88; **NF-kB**: Nuclear factor-kappa B; **SIGIRR**: Single immunoglobulin IL-IR-related; **SOCS**: Suppressor of cytokine signaling; **ST2**: Suppression of tumorigenicity 2; **STAT**: Signal transducer and activator of transcription; **TBK1**: TANK-binding kinase 1; **TRAF3**: TNF receptor-associated factor 3; **TRIF**: TIR domain-containing adapter protein inducing IFN-beta.

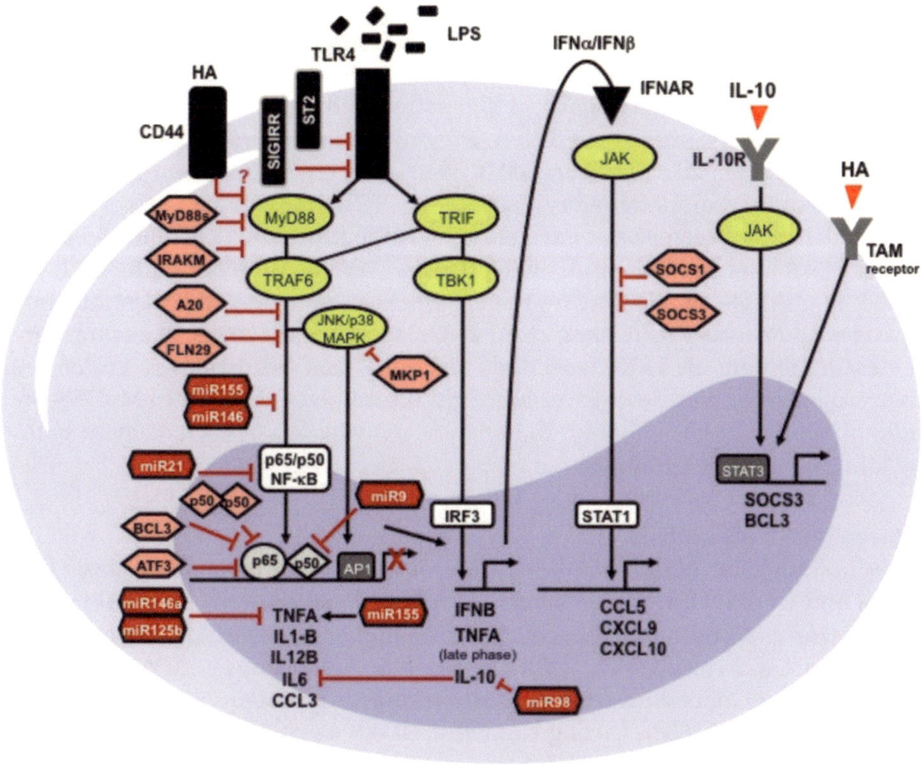

Fig. 3. Toll-like receptor 4 (TLR4) pathway and its negative regulators implicated in endotoxin tolerance. TLR4 signaling is mediated by two distinct adaptor proteins, namely, MyD88 and TRIF. Signaling via MyD88 leads to phosphorylation-mediated degradation of IκBα, nuclear translocation of p65/p50 NF-kB and transcription of proinflammatory genes like TNFA, IL1B, IL12B, IL6, and CCL3. The MyD88 pathway activates MAPKs (e.g JNK, p38) and their downstream transcription factor, AP-1 which also regulates proinflammatory cytokine gene transcription. Signaling though TRIF pathway induces a phosphorylation cascade involving activation of TBK1 and the downstream transcription factor IRF3 leading to the expression of IFNB. Late-phase TNFA is transcribed through this pathway (Covert et al., 2005). IL-10 is induced through the TRIF pathway via TRAF3 or Type I Interferon (Chang et al., 2007; Hacker et al., 2006). Signaling though IL-10R and TAM receptors activates STAT3 which transcribes SOCS3 and BCL3. Both these molecules negatively regulate STAT1 and NF-κB. Several negative regulators of the TLR4/IL-1R/NF-kB pathway (shown by pink boxes) as well as MicroRNAs (shown by red boxes) with relevance in ET are indicated on the figure. Hyaluronic acid (HA) signals though CD44 and is reported to downregulate TLR4 signaling and expression of proinflammatory genes (del Fresno et al., 2005; Kuang et al., 2007; Kuang et al., 2007). It may be noted that not all negative regulators shown on the figure have been validated in human. "⊥" denotes inhibition; "→" denotes stimulation; "?" -denotes pathways not fully characterized

inhibition of IRAK-1 activity, as well as mitogen-activated protein kinases (MAPKs) and NF-kB have been noted in endotoxin tolerized monocytes/macrophages (Fan & Cook, 2004; Biswas & Tergaonkar, 2007). While a majority of the above events are linked to defects in the

MyD88-dependent pathway, several evidences point towards a non-redundant role for TRIF pathway in ET. The majority of the LPS-induced transcriptome in macrophages is TRIF-dependent with several proinflammatory genes being controlled through this pathway (Bjorkbacka et al., 2004). In particular, TRIF pathway has been suggested to mediate the sustained, late-phase expression of TNFα, a cytokine known to induce ET upon chronic exposure (Covert et al., 2005; Beutler, 2004). Thus, it is possible that through the sustained expression of such proinflammatory factors the TRIF pathway may contribute to the induction of ET. In agreement, we have shown TRIF pathway to contribute to ET in mouse embryonal fibroblasts (Biswas et al., 2007). Further, the TRIF/IFNβ pathway is also been implicated to mediate expression of IL-10, which is upregulated in endotoxin tolerant macrophages and monocytes (Chang et al., 2007; Hacker et al., 2006). In contrast, in human monocytes, inhibition of TRIF-dependent signaling has been shown under endotoxin tolerance. Collectively, these evidences highlight the involvement of both MyD88- and TRIF-dependent pathway in ET, although the relative contribution of each of these pathways in driving ET remains to be addressed.

5.2 Differential NF-κB activity

The transcription factor NF-κB is a key regulator of many inflammatory genes like TNFα, IL-1β, IL-6 and COX2. However, a switch in NF-κB function from an inflammatory to an anti-inflammatory has been noted in course of inflammation, which could be relevant to the mechanism of ET (Lawrence et al., 2001; Cavaillon & Adib-Conquy, 2006). NF-kB functions as hetero- or homodimers with the Rel family transacting proteins p65, p50, c-rel, relB and p52 (Hayden & Ghosh, 2008). During canonical NF-kB signaling, phosphorylation-induced proteosomal degradation of the inhibitor protein, IκBα, releases the p65/p50 NF-κB heterodimer to translocate to the nucleus. There, it binds to the target gene promoter and induces gene transcription (Figure3). In contrast, the p50/p50 NF-κB homodimers have an inhibitory effect wherein they compete with p65/p50 NF-κB heterodimers and prevent their binding to inflammatory gene promoter, thereby inhibiting the transcription of these genes (Hayden & Ghosh, 2008). In agreement, endotoxin-tolerant murine macrophages and human monocytes as well as monocytes from sepsis and trauma patients characterize by decreased NF-κB activity due to over-expression of p50 NF-κB homodimers and decreased level of the active p65-p50 NF-κB heterodimers (Cavaillon & Adib-Conquy, 2006; Ziegler-Heitbrock, 2001; Adib-Conquy et al., 2000). The impact of p50/p50 homodimers in the induction of ET is further justified by results from p50 -/- murine macrophages which cannot be rendered endotoxin tolerant upon prolonged treatment with LPS (Bohuslav et al., 1998; Wysocka et al., 2001). p50/p50 NF-κB homodimers besides inhibiting the expression of inflammatory genes like IL12p40, TNFA, NOS2 can also induce the expression of anti-inflammatory genes like TGFβ and IL-10 which are also known to be upregulated in ET (Lawrence et al., 2001). Thus, the switching of NF-κB from p65/p50 to a p50/p50 dimer may be a possible mechanism for converting inflammatory monocytes/macrophages to an endotoxin tolerant state. In addition, other members of the NF-κB family such as IkBα, IkBε and RelB have also been proposed in ET. Indeed, high level of inhibitory proteins IkBα and IkBε was reported in ET mouse macrophages, at the same time ET human monocytes were characterized by overexpression of RelB (Dobrovolskaia et al., 2003; Chen et al., 2009). However, the interplay of different NF-κB-IκB family members in sepsis-induced immunosuppression and ET warrants further investigation.

5.3 Negative regulators of TLR4 pathway

Many of the defects in the TLR4 pathway during ET have been attributed to the overexpression of negative regulators of this pathway. Endotoxin tolerant cells show high expression of negative regulators of TLR4 pathway, such as IRAK-M, MKP1, FLN29, ST2, SOCS1, short version of MyD88 (MyD88sh) (Liew et al., 2005; Lopez-Collazo et al., 2006; Escoll et al., 2003; Kobayashi et al., 2002) and SHIP (Rauh et al., 2005) (Figure 3). IRAK-M is the only molecule that is consistently overexpressed in human monocytes and mouse macrophages during ET as well as in low-grade endotoxemia in humans (del Fresno et al., 2009; van 't Veer et al., 2007; Kobayashi et al., 2002). For all others negative regulators the mechanism differs in human and mice. For example, ST2, SOCS1, and SHIP were not upregulated in human endotoxemia while their knockout mice failed to develop ET (del Fresno et al., 2009; van 't Veer et al., 2007; Liew et al., 2005; Rauh et al., 2005). Other negative regulators like A20 and MKP1 have not been considered as candidates in human ET, due to their very early induction during endotoxemia (van 't Veer et al., 2007).
The list of putative negative regulators with relevance to ET is expanding. TREM-1 has been shown to play an important role in the developing of ET in leukocytes from Cystic Fibrosis patients (del Fresno et al., 2008). In particular, the soluble form of TREM-1 which plays an anti-inflammatory role may be the likely candidate (Gibot et al., 2004). TAM receptors (viz. Axl, Tyro3, Mer) are induced by Type I interferons downstream of TLR pathways and act as a negative feedback loop for TLR signaling through the induction of SOCS1 and SOCS3 (Rothlin et al., 2007). Thus, TAM receptors qualify as possible candidates that may contribute to ET. In accordance, TAM receptors have been implicated in the induction of immunosuppression in sepsis patients (Rothlin et al., 2007). Another new molecule called Twist-2 may also be implicated in ET via its regulatory role on IL-10 expression, which is upregulated in most endotoxin tolerant cells (Sharabi et al., 2008). Similarly, ATF3 is reported to downregulate IL-6 production and protect from LPS shock in mice, but its role in ET is still unknown (Figure 3) (Gilchrist et al., 2006).

6. Chromatin modification and gene reprogramming in ET

Transcriptomic analysis of human monocytes as well as mouse macrophages under ET state has shown profound gene reprogramming. Foster et al. demonstrated that epigenetic regulation was responsible for this gene reprogramming during ET (Foster et al., 2007). Histone modifications can lead to changes in the degree of coiling of the DNA which affects their accessibility to transcription. This constitutes an important epigenetic regulatory mechanism. Accordingly, deacetylation or methylation of histones promotes gene silencing, while acetylation or demethylation of histones stimulates transcription of target genes (Wilson, 2008). In the study by Foster et al., two sets of genes were identified: i) genes which were inhibited (i.e. Tolerant genes; e.g. inflammatory genes) and ii) genes which remained inducible or upregulated (i.e. Non-tolerant; e.g. antimicrobial genes) upon the second LPS challenge. LPS provoke histone methylation of Tolerant as well as Non-tolerant gene promoters (Foster et al., 2007). However, upon a second challenge with LPS, re-acetylation of histones was only observed for the promoter of Non-tolerant genes which led to RNA polymerase recruitment and their transcription. In contrast, no such event was observed for Tolerant gene promoters which remained inactive (Beutler, 2004). The upregulation of Non-tolerant genes during the second LPS challenge was explained by histone modifications of their promoters during the initial LPS activation which primed them for subsequent transcription. Other evidences for histone modification causing the suppression of inflammatory genes during ET are also available. For example, binding of high-mobility group box 1 proteins (HMGB1) and histone H1 linker at the promoters of TNFα and IL-1β genes induces chromatin remodeling and gene silencing during ET (El Gazzar et al., 2009). Similarly, RelB directed histone H3K9 demethylation caused impaired p65 NF-κB transactivation at the IL1B promoter and silencing of the gene in endotoxin-tolerant human monocytic cell lines (Chan et al., 2005). It may be envisaged that chromatin remodeling in ET may depend on *de novo* synthesis of one or more factors during the initial LPS exposure (Foster et al., 2007). Supporting this idea, many LPS-induced primary gene products such as Brg1 and IkBζ can modulate chromatin remodeling at the promoters of secondary response genes, thereby allowing their subsequent re-programming (Kayama et al., 2008; Ramirez-Carrozzi et al., 2006). In this context, the LPS-induced histone demethylase, JMJD3 has been shown to cause chromatin remodeling and transcription of M2 macrophage specific genes, suggesting a potential mechanism of how inflammatory macrophages may switch to an M2 phenotype during endotoxin tolerance (De Santa et al., 2007; Satoh et al., 2010). Collectively, the facts discussed here point towards an important role for epigenetic regulation in shaping the gene expression response in ET. However, the epigenetic landscape and the upstream signaling molecules that regulate this process remain to be characterized.

7. MicroRNA-mediated regulation of ET

MicroRNA is another important post-transcriptional regulatory mechanism for gene expression in many cellular processes including immune response (Bartel, 2009; Baltimore, 2008). Proinflammatory stimuli such as LPS, TNFα, and IL-1β as well as ligands for TLR2 and TLR5 induce the expression of specific microRNAs that modulate TLR4 and IL-1 receptor (IL-1R) signaling pathways in monocytes/macrophages (Baltimore, 2008; O'Connell et al., 2007; Taganov et al., 2006). As reviewed recently, several microRNAs play a crucial role in the ET mechanism (Biswas & Lopez-Collazo, 2009; Nahid et al., 2011). miR146 and miR155 were the first identified microRNAs, that could be stimulated by LPS in human monocytic cells (O'Connell et al., 2007; Taganov et al., 2006). miR146 was shown to inhibit TLR4/IL-1R signaling through post-transcriptional regulation of the signaling proteins, IRAK-1 and TRAF6 (Figure 3) (Baltimore et al., 2008; Taganov et al., 2006). Indeed, decrease of IRAK-1 protein but not its mRNA was observed during ET (Baltimore et al., 2008). Further, miR146a also was shown to inhibit TNFα at transcription as well as translation level during TLR4-induced gene reprogramming (Figure 3) (El Gazzar et al., 2011).

miR155 is another microRNA induced by LPS and double-stranded RNA through an autocrine and/or paracrine induction of TNFα (O'Connell et al., 2007). miR155 inhibits TLR4 signaling by targeting IKKε and promotes TNFα at the translational level (Figure 3) (Tili et al., 2007). In fact, mir155 knock-in mice are highly susceptible to LPS shock as a result of high levels of TNFα (Costinean et al., 2006). Contrary to this, miR125b is another LPS-inducible microRNA that promotes TNFα degradation during LPS stimulation (Figure 3) (Tili et al., 2007). miR9 is also induced by LPS in monocytes and targets NF-kB1 (p105/p50NF-κB) transcript thereby serving as a possible negative feedback mechanism on the inflammation (Bazzoni et al., 2009). A more recent study found miR98 to be involved in post-transcriptional control of IL-10 production during ET in macrophages (Liu et al., 2011). miR21 has been suggested to enhance IL-10 and inhibit NF-κB via regulation of the proinflammatory protein PDCD4 in LPS-treated human peripheral blood monocytes and hence be a possible candidate in mediating ET (Figure 3) (Sheedy et al., 2010). The growing list of microRNAs clearly shows them to act at multiple levels of the inflammatory pathway. However, the actual role of microRNAs in the control of ET could be at the late phase of inflammation wherein microRNAs act as a negative feedback loop inhibiting the TLR4 pathway and inflammatory cytokines at a post-transcriptional and translation level and thus promoting ET (El Gazzar & McCall, 2010; Biswas & Collazo, 2009).

8. Contribution of immune cell apoptosis to ET

Apoptosis of immune cells has been suggested to contribute to immunosuppression and ET in sepsis. Apoptosis of several types of cells like CD4+ T-cells, B-cells and follicular DCs was reported in the spleen for sepsis patients (Hotchkiss & Karl, 2003). Interestingly, CD8+ T cells, NK cells, monocytes or macrophages showed no apoptosis during ET. Recent studies have shown that differential modulation of the gene expression of cell death pathway during *in vivo* LPS tolerance helps to protect macrophages from apoptosis and results in enhanced survival of mice (Melo et al., 2010). In line with this, LPS-tolerant macrophages were found to have reduced apoptosis compared to naive macrophages, during polymicrobial sepsis. Depletion of DCs has been noted in human and mice sepsis (Hotchkiss et al., 2002; Efron et al., 2004), whereas, increased DC survival in mice stimulates resistance to endotoxin shock and attenuate LPS-induced immunosuppression (Gautier et al., 2008). Although, the role of apoptosis in ET still warrants investigation, the evidence at hand emphasize the importance of immune cell apoptosis in mediating sepsis-induced immunosuppression.

9. ET as an 'adaptive' response of innate immunity

One of the defining paradigms of the adaptive immunity is the ability to mount an enhanced and tailored immune response upon secondary exposure to the same antigen. Similarly, sensing of microbial components by macrophages not only results in their functional activation, but also in reshaping subsequent responses to microbes. Thus, innate immunity also has a built-in 'adaptive' component (Bowdish et al., 2007; Mantovani, 2008). Supporting this concept, studies with in germ-free mice indicated their inability to trigger an inflammatory response following endotoxin challenge (Souza et al., 2004). Further studies revealed that innate immune sensing by commensal bacteria was essential for mounting an acute inflammatory response to subsequent endotoxin stimulation (Amaral et al., 2008). Similarly, bacterial components can induce an upregulation of the scavenging receptor MARCO in macrophages which in turn influences their phagocytic and cytokine secreting ability, poising them for an enhanced immune response to subsequent pathogenic challenge (Bowdish et al., 2007; Willment et al., 2003). ET presents an analogous situation where exposure to endotoxins influences subsequent responses to endotoxins by dampening inflammatory response. While we have restricted our discussion to ET mediated through TLR4 receptor by LPS or Gram-negative sepsis, stimulation by other TLR ligands and Gram-positive sepsis can also lead to ET. This phenomenon is referred to heterotolerance or crosstolerance (Dobrovolskaia et al., 2003). Pretreatment of macrophages with TLR2 ligands like lipoteichoic acid (LTA), Pam3Cysk4 or MALP2 stimulates ET to LPS in these cells (Dobrovolskaia et al., 2003; Sato et al., 2000). Damage-associated molecular patterns (DAMPs), such as HA, HMGB1, fibronectin, NOD2, also stimulate ET under certain conditions (Kuang et al., 2007; Liu et al., 2008; Adair-Kirk & Senior, 2008; Kwon et al., 2004; Kim et al., 2008). Interestingly, the fact that macrophages can 'remember' a prior exposure to endotoxin (as seen in ET) is reminiscent of an 'immunological memory', another feature of the adaptive immune system. Based on the above observations, it may be suggested that ET represents an 'adaptive' response of innate immunity and a part of the so-called 'trained immunity' (Biswas & Mantovani, 2010; Netea et al., 2011).

10. ET as a common paradigm for immunosuppression in many diseases

One of the key characteristics defining ET is a downregulation of the inflammatory response of innate immune cells like monocytes/macrophages subsequently challenged with endotoxin. Such endotoxin refractory state has been observed in the innate immune cells associated with various pathologies like hepatic and renal ischemia, coronary occlusion, acute coronary syndromes, cystic fibrosis and even cancer (del Fresno et al., 2009; Nimah et al., 2005; Ziegler-Heitbrock, 2001; Wilson, 2008).

Similar to ET associated with sepsis, the incidence of such refractory states in acute pulmonary syndromes and cystic fibrosis induces susceptibility to nosocomial infections and complications. Further, mechanistic paradigms common to ET (and sepsis) have also been observed in other diseases. For example, IRAK-M, a major mediator of ET in monocytes/macrophages (Biswas & Lopez-Collazo, 2009), is upregulated in circulating monocytes of patients with gram-negative sepsis, acute coronary syndrome and cystic fibrosis, together with poor TNFα induction to LPS challenge (Palsson-McDermott et al., 2009; Ziegler-Heitbrock, 2001; del Fresno et al., 2009). In addition to their refractoriness to endotoxins, cystic fibrosis monocytes also show impaired antigen presentation but potent phagocytic activity similar to the endotoxin tolerant human monocytes (del Fresno et al., 2009). In cancer the induction of tumor-induced immunosuppression is widely known phenomenon. In line with this, tumor associated macrophages (TAMs) show an immunosuppressive phenotype similar to ET. TAMs are refractory to *ex vivo* LPS challenge and show decreased production of inflammatory cytokines like IL-12p40 and TNFα, but upregulation of anti-inflammatory cytokines, IL-10 and TGFβ, similar to ET macrophages (Wilson, 2008). At the mechanistic levels defective NF-κB activation, p50/p50 NF-κB homodimers overexpression and a functional TRIF pathway have been observed in these cells, similar to ET (Biswas et al., 2007; Wilson, 2008; Kayama et al., 2008). Co-culturing human monocytes with cancer cells causes refractoriness to endotoxin which is suggested to be linked to the upregulation of IRAKM, as known for ET (del Fresno et al., 2005). These observations show tumor-induced immunosuppression and ET to share many common characteristics. It may be possible that analogous to the chronic inflammation induced by exposure to low doses of endotoxin, smouldered inflammation associated with cancer may also induce a "tolerance" in the associated immune cells, thus giving rise to the immunosuppressive phenotype (Mantovani & Sica, 2010). Taken together, the above observations strongly suggest the endotoxin tolerant state as a general paradigm for immunosuppression across different diseases. Importantly, this finding potentially enables to apply the lessons learnt from ET to provide clues in explaining immunosuppression associated with other pathologies.

11. Conclusion

Based on the evidences discussed in this review, it is clear that ET represents an 'adaptive' response of the innate immune system that protects against exaggerated inflammation.

Accordingly, ET involves extensive gene reprogramming that supports the functional polarization of monocytes and macrophages, tuning down inflammatory response, but promoting phagocytosis, tissue repair and immunoregulatory functions. Besides being a protective response, ET is also associated with a variety of pathological conditions where it serves as a mechanism for immunosuppression. Such conditions often contribute to immune evasion, increased susceptibility to secondary infection and even mortality. Thus, a cellular and molecular understanding of ET will serve as a key step towards understanding of immunosuppression and its targeting in many diseases.

12. Acknowledgment

SKB and INS are supported by funding from Biomedical Research Council (BMRC), A*STAR, Singapore. The authors sincerely apologize to all those authors whose original works could not be quoted in this review due to space constraints.

13. Reference

Adair-Kirk, T.L. & Senior, R.M. (2008) Fragments of extracellular matrix as mediators of inflammation. *Int. J. Biochem. Cell Biol.*, 40, 6-7, 1101–1110.

Adib-Conquy, M. & Cavaillon, J.M. (2009) Compensatory anti-inflammatory response syndrome. *Thromb. Haemost.*, 101, 1, (January 2009), 36–47.

Adib-Conquy, M., Adrie, C., Moine, P., Asehnoune, K., Fitting, C., Pinsky, M.R., Dhainaut, J.F., & Cavaillon, J.M. (2000) NF-kappaB expression in mononuclear cells of patients with sepsis resembles that observed in lipopolysaccharide tolerance. *Am. J. Resp. Crit. Care Med.*, 162, 5, (November 2000), 1877–1883.

Albrecht, V., Hofer, T.P., Foxwell, B., Frankenberger, M., & Ziegler-Heitbrock, L. (2008) Tolerance induced via TLR2 and TLR4 in human dendritic cells: role of IRAK-1. *BMC Immunol.*, 9, (November 2008), 69.

Amaral, F.A., Sachs, D., Costa, V.V., Fagundes, C.T., Cisalpino, D., Cunha, T.M., Ferreira, S.H., Cunha, F.Q., Silva, T.A., Nicoli, J.R., Vieira, L.Q., Souza, D.G., & Teixeira, M.M. (2008) Commensal microbiota is fundamental for the development of inflammatory pain. *Proc Natl Acad Sci U S A.*, 105, 6, (February 2008), 2193 - 2197.

Baltimore, D., Boldin, M.P., O'Connell, R.M., Rao, D.S., & Taganov, K.D. (2008) MicroRNAs: new regulators of immune cell development and function. *Nat Immunol.*, 9, 8, (August 2008), 839–845.

Bartel, D.P. (2009) MicroRNAs: target recognition and regulatory functions. *Cell*, 136, 2, (January 2009), 215-233.

Bazzoni, F., Rossato, M., Fabbri, M., Gaudiosi, D., Mirolo, M., Mori, L., Tamassia, N., Mantovani, A., Cassatella, M.A., & Locati, M. (2009) Induction and regulatory function of miR-9 in human monocytes and neutrophils exposed to proinflammatory signals. *Proc Natl Acad Sci U S A*, 106, 13, (March 2009), 5282–5287.

Beutler, B. (2004) SHIP, TGF-beta, and endotoxin tolerance. *Immunity*, 21, 2, (August 2004), 134–135.

Biswas, S.K. & Mantovani, A. (2010) Macrophage plasticity and interaction with lymphocyte subsets: cancer as a paradigm. *Nat Immunol.* 11, 10, 889–896.

Biswas, S.K. & Tergaonkar, V. (2007) Myeloid differentiation factor 88-independent toll-like receptor pathway: sustaining inflammation or promoting tolerance. *International Journal of Biochemistry and Cell Biology*, 39, 9, 1582-1592.

Biswas, S.K. & Lopez-Collazo, E. (2009) Endotoxin tolerance: new mechanisms, molecules and clinical significance. *Trends Immunol.*, 30, 10, (October 2009), 475-487.

Biswas, S.K., Bist, P., Dhillon, M.K., Kajiji, T., Del Fresno, C., Yamamoto, M., Lopez-Collazo, E., Akira, S., & Tergaonkar, V. (2007) Role for MyD88-independent, TRIF pathway in lipid A/TLR4-induced endotoxin tolerance. *J Immunol.*, 179, 6, (September 2007), 4083-4092.

Björkbacka, H., Fitzgerald, K.A., Huet, F., Li, X., Gregory, J.A., Lee, M.A., Ordija, C.M., Dowley, N.E., Golenbock, D.T., & Freeman, M.W. (2004) The induction of macrophage gene expression by LPS predominantly utilizes Myd88-independent signaling cascades. *Physiol Genomics*, 19, 3, (November 2004), 319-330.

Bohuslav, J., Kravchenko, V.V., Parry, G.C., Erlich, J.H., Gerondakis, S., Mackman, N., & Ulevitch, R.J. (1998) Regulation of an essential innate immune response by the p50 subunit of NF-kappaB. *J. Clin. Invest.*, 102, 9, (November 1998), 1645–1652.

Bowdish, D.M., Loffredo, M.S., Mukhopadhyay, S., Mantovani, A. & Gordon, S. (2007) Macrophage receptors implicated in the 'adaptive' form of innate immunity. *Microbes Infect.*, 9, 14-15, (November-December 2007), 1680–1687.

Buras, J.A., Holzmann, B., & Sitkovsky, M. (2005) Animal models of sepsis: setting the stage. *Nat Rev Drug Discov.*, 4, 10, (October 2005), 854–865.

Cavaillon, J.M. & Adib-Conquy, M. (2006) Bench-to-bedside review: endotoxin tolerance as a model of leukocyte reprogramming in sepsis. *Critical care (London, England)*, 10, 5, 233.

Cavaillon, J.M., Adrie, C., Fitting, C., & Adib-Conquy, M. (2003) Endotoxin tolerance: is there a clinical relevance? *J. Endotoxin Res.*, 9, 2, 101–107.

Cavaillon, J.M., Adrie, C., Fitting, C., & Adib-Conquy, M. (2005) Reprogramming of circulatory cells in sepsis and SIRS. *J Endotoxin Res.*, 11, 5, 311-320.

Chan, C., Li, L., McCall, C.E., & Yoza, B.K. (2005) Endotoxin tolerance disrupts chromatin remodeling and NF-kappaB transactivation at the IL-1beta promoter. *J. Immunol.*, 175, 1, (July 2005), 461–468.

Chang, E.Y., Guo, B., Doyle, S.E., & Cheng, G. (2007) Cutting edge: involvement of the type I IFN production and signaling pathway in lipopolysaccharide-induced IL-10 production. *J. Immunol.*, 178, 11, (June 2007), 6705–6709.

Chen, X., Yoza, B.K., El Gazzar, M., Hu, J.Y., Cousart, S.L., & McCall, C.E. (2009) RelB sustains IkappaBalpha expression during endotoxin tolerance. *Clin. Vaccine Immunol.*, 16, 1, (January 2009), 104–110.

Costinean, S., Zanesi, N., Pekarsky, Y., Tili, E., Volinia, S., Heerema, N., & Croce, C.M. (2006) Pre-B cell proliferation and lymphoblastic leukemia/high-grade lymphoma in E(mu)-miR155 transgenic mice. *Proc Natl Acad Sci U S A*, 103, 18, (May 2006), 7024–7029.

Covert, M.W., Leung, T.H., Gaston, J.E., & Baltimore, D. (2005) Achieving stability of lipopolysaccharideinduced NF-kappaB activation. *Science*, 309, 5742, (September 2005), 1854–1857.

De Santa, F., Totaro, M.G., Prosperini, E., Notarbartolo, S., Testa, G., & Natoli G. (2007) The histone H3 lysine-27 demethylase Jmjd3 links inflammation to inhibition of polycomb-mediated gene silencing. *Cell*, 130, 6, (September 2007), 1083-1094.

del Fresno, C., García-Rio, F., Gómez-Piña, V., Soares-Schanoski, A., Fernández-Ruíz, I., Jurado, T., Kajiji, T., Shu, C., Marín, E., Gutierrez del Arroyo, A., Prados, C., Arnalich, F., Fuentes-Prior, P., Biswas, S.K., & López-Collazo, E. (2009) Potent phagocytic activity with impaired antigen presentation identifying lipopolysaccharide-tolerant human monocytes: demonstration in isolated monocytes from cystic fibrosis patients. *J Immunol.*, 182, 10, (May 2009), 6494-6507.

del Fresno, C., Gómez-Piña, V., Lores, V., Soares-Schanoski, A., Fernández-Ruiz, I., Rojo, B., Alvarez-Sala, R., Caballero-Garrido, E., García, F., Veliz, T., Arnalich, F., Fuentes-Prior, P., García-Río, F., & López-Collazo, E. (2008) Monocytes from cystic fibrosis patients are locked in an LPS tolerance state: down-regulation of TREM-1 as putative underlying mechanism. *PLoS ONE*, 3, 7, (July 2008), e2667.

del Fresno, C., Otero, K., Gómez-García, L., González-León, M.C., Soler-Ranger, L., Fuentes-Prior, P., Escoll, P., Baos, R., Caveda, L., García, F., Arnalich, F., & López-Collazo, E. (2005) Tumor cells deactivate human monocytes by up-regulating IL-1 receptor associated kinase-M expression via CD44 and TLR4. *J. Immunol.*, 174, 5, (March 2005), 3032–3040.

Delano, M.J., Scumpia, P.O., Weinstein, J.S., Coco, D., Nagaraj, S., Kelly-Scumpia, K.M., O'Malley, K.A., Wynn, J.L., Antonenko, S., Al-Quran, S.Z., Swan, R., Chung, C.S., Atkinson, M.A., Ramphal, R., Gabrilovich, D.I., Reeves, W.H., Ayala, A., Phillips, J., Laface, D., Heyworth, P.G., Clare-Salzler, M., & Moldawer LL. (2007) MyD88-dependent expansion of an immature GR-1(+)CD11b(+) population induces T cell suppression and Th2 polarization in sepsis. *J. Exp. Med.*, 204, 6, (June 2007), 1463–1474.

Dobrovolskaia, M.A. & Vogel, S.N. (2002) Toll receptors, CD14, and macrophage activation and deactivation by LPS. *Microbes Infect.*, 4, 9, (July 2002), 903-914.

Dobrovolskaia, M.A., Medvedev, A.E., Thomas, K.E., Cuesta, N., Toshchakov, V., Ren, T., Cody, M.J., Michalek, S.M., Rice, N.R., & Vogel, S.N. (2003) Induction of in vitro reprogramming by Toll-like receptor (TLR)2 and TLR4 agonists in murine macrophages: effects of TLR "homotolerance" versus "heterotolerance" on NF-kappa B signaling pathway components. *J Immunol.*, 170, 1, (January 2003), 508-519.

Draisma, A., Pickkers, P., Bouw, M.P., & van der Hoeven, J.G. (2009) Development of endotoxin tolerance in humans in vivo. *Crit Care Med.*, 37, 4, (April 2009), 1261-1267.

Efron, P.A., Martins, A., Minnich, D., Tinsley, K., Ungaro, R., Bahjat, F.R., Hotchkiss, R., Clare-Salzler, M., & Moldawer, L.L. (2004) Characterization of the systemic loss of dendritic cells in murine lymph nodes during polymicrobial sepsis. *J. Immunol.*, 173, 5, (September 2004), 3035–3043.

El Gazzar, M., Yoza, B.K., Chen, X., Garcia, B.A., Young, N.L., & McCall, C.E. (2009) Chromatin-specific remodeling by HMGB1 and linker histone H1 silences proinflammatory genes during endotoxin tolerance. Mol. *Cell Biol.*, 29, 7, (April 2009), 1959–1971.

El Gazzar, M. & McCall, C.E. (2010) MicroRNAs distinguish translational from transcriptional silencing during endotoxin tolerance. *J Biol Chem.*, 285, 27, (July 2010), 20940-20951.

El Gazzar, M., Church, A., Liu, T., & McCall, C.E. (2011) MicroRNA-146a regulates both transcription silencing and translation disruption of TNF-{alpha} during TLR4-induced gene reprogramming. *J Leukoc Biol.*, 90, 3, September 2011), 509-519.

Escoll, P., del Fresno, C., García, L., Vallés, G., Lendínez, M.J., Arnalich, F., & López-Collazo, E. (2003) Rapid up-regulation of IRAK-M expression following a second endotoxin challenge in human monocytes and in monocytes isolated from septic patients. *Biochem Biophys Res Commun.*, 311, 2, (November 2003), 465–472.

Fadok, V.A., Bratton, D.L., Konowal, A., Freed, P.W., Westcott, J.Y., & Henson, P.M. (1998) Macrophages that have ingested apoptotic cells in vitro inhibit proinflammatory cytokine production through autocrine/paracrine mechanisms involving TGF-beta, PGE2, and PAF. *J. Clin. Invest.*, 101, 4, (February 1998), 890–898.

Fan, H. & Cook, J.A. (2004) Molecular mechanisms of endotoxin tolerance. *J Endotoxin Res.*, 10, 2, 71-84.

Foster, S.L. & Medzhitov, R. (2009) Gene-specific control of the TLR-induced inflammatory response. *Clin Immunol.*, 130, 1, (January 2009), 7-15.

Foster, S.L., Hargreaves, D.C., & Medzhitov, R. (2007) Gene-specific control of inflammation by TLR-induced chromatin modifications. *Nature*, 447, 7147, (June 2007), 972-978.

Gautier, E.L., Huby, T., Saint-Charles, F., Ouzilleau, B., Chapman, M.J., & Lesnik, P. (2008) Enhanced dendritic cell survival attenuates lipopolysaccharide-induced immunosuppression and increases resistance to lethal endotoxic shock. *J. Immunol.*, 180, 10, (May 2008), 6941–6946.

Gibot, S., Kolopp-Sarda, M.N., Béné, M.C., Bollaert, P.E., Lozniewski, A., Mory, F., Levy, B., & Faure, G.C. (2004) A soluble form of the triggering receptor expressed on myeloid cells-1 modulates the inflammatory response in murine sepsis. *J Exp Med.*, 200, 11, (December 2004), 1419–1426.

Gilchrist, M., Thorsson ,V., Li ,B., Rust, A.G., Korb, M., Roach, J.C., Kennedy, K., Hai, T., Bolouri, H., & Aderem, A. (2006) Systems biology approaches identify ATF3 as a negative regulator of Toll-like receptor 4. *Nature*, 441, 7090, (May 2006), 173–178.

Gordon, S. & Taylor, P.R. (2005) Monocyte and macrophage heterogeneity. *Nat Rev Immunol.*, 5, 12, (December 2005), 953–964.

Hacker, H., Redecke, V., Blagoev, B., Kratchmarova, I., Hsu, L.C., Wang, G.G., Kamps, M.P., Raz, E., Wagner, H., Häcker, G., Mann, M., & Karin, M. (2006) Specificity in Toll-like receptor signaling through distinct effector functions of TRAF3 and TRAF6. *Nature*, 439, 7073, (January 2006), 204–207.

Hayden, M.S. & Ghosh, S. (2008) Shared principles in NF-kappaB signaling. *Cell*, 132, 3, (February 2008), 344–362.

Hotchkiss, R.S. & Karl, I.E. (2003) The pathophysiology and treatment of sepsis. *N. Engl. J. Med.*, 348, 2, (January 2003), 138–150.

Hotchkiss, R.S., Tinsley, K.W., Swanson, P.E., Grayson, M.H., Osborne, D.F., Wagner, T.H., Cobb, J.P., Coopersmith, C., & Karl, I.E. (2002) Depletion of dendritic cells, but not macrophages, in patients with sepsis. *J. Immunol.*, 168, 5, (March 2002), 2493–2500.

Hotchkiss, R.S., Coopersmith, C.M., McDunn, J.E., & Ferguson T.A. (2009) The sepsis seesaw: tilting toward immunosuppression. *Nat Med.*, 15, 5, (May 2009), 496-497.

Iwasaki, A. & Medzhitov, R. (2010) Regulation of adaptive immunity by the innate immune system. *Science*, 327, 5963, (January 2010), 291–295.

Kawai, T. & Akira, S. (2011) Toll-like receptors and their crosstalk with other innate receptors in infection and immunity. *Immunity, 34, 5, (May 2011)*, 637-650.

Kayama, H., Ramirez-Carrozzi, V.R., Yamamoto, M., Mizutani, T., Kuwata, H., Iba, H., Matsumoto, M., Honda, K., Smale, S.T., & Takeda, K. (2008) Class-specific regulation of pro-inflammatory genes by MyD88 pathways and IkappaBzeta. *J. Biol. Chem.*, 283, 18, (May 2008), 12468–12477.

Kim, Y.G., Park, J.H., Daignault, S., Fukase, K., & Núñez, G. (2008) Cross-tolerization between Nod1 and Nod2 signaling results in reduced refractoriness to bacterial infection in Nod2-deficient macrophages. *J Immunol.*, 181, 6, (September 2008), 4340–4346.

Kobayashi, K., Hernandez, L.D., Galán, J.E., Janeway, C.A. Jr., Medzhitov, R., & Flavell, R.A. (2002) IRAK-M is a negative regulator of Toll-like receptor signaling. *Cell*, 110, 2, (July 2002), 191–202.

Kuang, D.M., Wu, Y., Chen, N., Cheng, J., Zhuang, S.M., & Zheng, L. (2007) Tumor-derived hyaluronan induces formation of immunosuppressive macrophages through transient early activation of monocytes. *Blood*, 110, 2, (July 2007), 587–595.

Kwon, A.H., Qiu, Z., Nagahama, H., Kaibori, M., & Kamiyama, Y. (2004) Fibronectin suppresses apoptosis and protects mice from endotoxic shock. *Transplantation proceedings*, 36, 8, (October 2004), 2432–2435.

Lauw, F.N., ten Hove, T., Dekkers, P.E., de Jonge, E., van Deventer, S.J., & van Der Poll, T. (2000) Reduced Th1, but not Th2, cytokine production by lymphocytes after in vivo exposure of healthy subjects to endotoxin. *Infect. Immun.*, 68, 3, (March 2000), 1014–1018.

Lawrence, T. Gilroy, D.W., Colville-Nash, P.R., & Willoughby, D.A. (2001) Possible new role for NF-kappaB in the resolution of inflammation. *Nat. Med.*, 7, 12, (December 2001), 1291–1297.

Liew, F.Y., Xu, D., Brint, E.K., & O'Neill, L.A. (2005) Negative regulation of toll-like receptormediated immune responses. *Nat. Rev. Immunol.*, 5, 6, (June 2005), 446–458.

Liu, Y.Y., Lee, C.H., Dedaj, R., Zhao, H., Mrabat, H., Sheidlin, A., Syrkina, O., Huang, P.M., Garg, H.G., Hales, C.A., & Quinn, D.A. (2008) High-molecular-weight hyaluronan–a possible new treatment for sepsis-induced lung injury: a preclinical study in mechanically ventilated rats. *Crit. Care (London, England)*, 12, 4, R102.

Liu, Y., Chen, Q., Song, Y., Lai, L., Wang, J., Yu, H., Cao, X., & Wang, Q. (2011) MicroRNA-98 negatively regulates IL-10 production and endotoxin tolerance in macrophages after LPS stimulation. *FEBS Lett.*, 585, 12, (June 2011), 1963-1968.

Lopez-Collazo, E., Fuentes-Prior, P., Arnalich, F., & del Fresno, C. (2006) Pathophysiology of interleukin-1 receptor-associated kinase-M: implications in refractory state. *Curr. Opin. Infect. Dis.*, 19, 3, (June 2006), 237–244.

Mages, J., Dietrich, H., & Lang, R. (2007) A genome-wide analysis of LPS tolerance in macrophages. *Immunobiology*, 212, 9-10, 723-737.

Manjuck, J., Saha, D.C., Astiz, M., Eales, L.J., & Rackow, E.C. (2000) Decreased response to recall antigens is associated with depressed costimulatory receptor expression in septic critically ill patients. *J. Lab. Clin. Med.*, 135, 2, (February 2000), 153–160.

Mantovani, A. (2008) From phagocyte diversity and activation to probiotics: back to Metchnikoff. *Eur. J. Immunol.*, 38, 12, (December 2008), 3269–3273.

Mantovani, A., Sica, A., & Locati, M. (2005) Macrophage polarization comes of age. *Immunity*, 23, 4, (October 2005), 344–346.

Mantovani, A., Sica, A., Sozzani, S., Allavena, P., Vecchi, A., & Locati, M. (2004) The chemokine system in diverse forms of macrophage activation and polarization. *Trends Immunol.*, 25, 12, (December 2004), 677 - 686.

Mantovani, A. & Sica, A. (2010) Macrophages, innate immunity and cancer: balance, tolerance, and diversity. *Curr Opin Immunol.*, 22, 2, (April 2010), 231-237.

Medvedev, A.E., Kopydlowski, K.M., & Vogel, S.N. (2000) Inhibition of lipopolysaccharide-induced signal transduction in endotoxin-tolerized mouse macrophages: dysregulation of cytokine, chemokine, and toll-like receptor 2 and 4 gene expression. *J Immunol.*, 164, 11, (June 2000), 5564-5574.

Melo, E.S., Barbeiro, D.F., Gorjão, R., Rios, E.C., Vasconcelos, D., Velasco, I.T., Szabo, C., Curi, R., de Lima-Salgado, T.M., & Soriano, F.G. (2010) Gene expression reprogramming protects macrophage from septic-induced cell death. *Mol Immunol.*, 47, 16, (October 2010), 2587-2593.

Monneret, G., Finck, M.E., Venet, F., Debard, A.L., Bohé, J., Bienvenu, J., & Lepape, A. (2004) The anti-inflammatory response dominates after septic shock: association of low monocyte HLA-DR expression and high interleukin-10 concentration. *Immunol Lett.*, 95, 2, (September 2004), 193-198.

Monneret, G., Venet, F., Pachot, A., & Lepape A. (2008) Monitoring immune dysfunctions in the septic patient: a new skin for the old ceremony. *Molecular medicine (Cambridge, Mass)*, 14, 1-2, (January-February 2008), 64-78.

Mosser, D.M. & Edwards, J.P. (2008) Exploring the full spectrum of macrophage activation. *Nat Rev Immunol.*, 8, 12, (December 2008), 958-969.

Munoz, C., Carlet, J., Fitting, C., Misset, B., Blériot, J.P., & Cavaillon, J.M. (1991a) Dysregulation of in vitro cytokine production by monocytes during sepsis. *J. Clin. Invest.*, 88, 5, (November 1991), 1747–1754.

Munoz, C., Misset, B., Fitting, C., Blériot, J.P., Carlet, J., & Cavaillon, J.M. (1991b) Dissociation between plasma and monocyte-associated cytokines during sepsis. *Eur. J. Immunol.*, 21, 9, (September 1991), 2177–2184.

Nahid, M.A, Satoh, M., & Chan E.K.L. (2011) MicroRNA in TLR signalling and endotoxin tolerance. *Cellular & Molecular Immunology*, In press (doi: 10.1038/cmi.2011.26).

Nathan, C. (2002) Points of control in inflammation. *Nature*, 420, 6917, (December 2002), 846-852.

Netea, M.G., Quintin, J., & van der Meer, J.W. (2011) Trained immunity: a memory for innate host defense. *Cell Host Microbe.*, 9, 5, (May 2011), 355-361.

Nimah, M., Zhao, B., Denenberg, A.G., Bueno, O., Molkentin, J., Wong, H.R., & Shanley, T.P. (2005) Contribution of MKP-1 regulation of p38 to endotoxin tolerance. *Shock*, 23, 1, (January 2005), 80–87.

O'Connell, R.M. Taganov, K.D., Boldin, M.P., Cheng, G., & Baltimore, D. (2007) MicroRNA-155 is induced during the macrophage inflammatory response. *Proc Natl Acad Sci U S A*, 104, 5, (January 2007), 1604–1609.

Ogawa, H., Rafiee, P., Heidemann, J., Fisher, P.J., Johnson, N.A., Otterson, M.F., Kalyanaraman, B., Pritchard, K.A.Jr., & Binion, D.G. (2003) Mechanisms of endotoxin tolerance in human intestinal microvascular endothelial cells. *J. Immunol.*, 170, 12, (June 2003), 5956–5964.

O'Neill, L.A. & Bowie, A.G. (2007) The family of five: TIR-domain-containing adaptors in Toll-like receptor signalling. *Nat Rev Immunol.*, 7, 5, (May 2007), 353-364.

Pachot, A., Lepape, A., Vey, S., Bienvenu, J., Mougin, B., & Monneret, G. (2006) Systemic transcriptional analysis in survivor and non-survivor septic shock patients: a preliminary study. *Immunol. Lett.*, 106, 1, (July 2006), 63–71.

Palsson-McDermott, E.M., Doyle, S.L., McGettrick, A.F., Hardy, M., Husebye, H., Banahan, K., Gong, M., Golenbock, D., Espevik, T., & O'Neill, L.A. (2009) TAG, a splice variant of the adaptor TRAM, negatively regulates the adaptor MyD88-independent TLR4 pathway. *Nat. Immunol.*, 10, 6, (June 2009), 579–586.

Parker, L.C., Jones, E.C., Prince, L.R., Dower, S.K., Whyte, M.K., & Sabroe, I. (2005) Endotoxin tolerance induces selective alterations in neutrophil function. *J. Leukoc. Biol.*, 78, 6, (December 2005), 1301–1305.

Pena, O.M., Pistolic, J., Raj, D., Fjell, C.D., & Hancock, R.E. (2011) Endotoxin tolerance represents a distinctive state of alternative polarization (M2) in human mononuclear cells. *J Immunol.*, 186, 12, (June 2011), 7243-7254.

Porta, C., Rimoldi, M., Raes, G., Brys, L., Ghezzi, P., Di Liberto, D., Dieli, F., Ghisletti, S., Natoli, G., De Baetselier, P., Mantovani, A., & Sica, A. (2009) Tolerance and M2 (alternative) macrophage polarization are related processes orchestrated by p50 nuclear factor kappaB. *Proc Natl Acad Sci U S A*, 106, 35, (September 2009), 14978-14983.

Ramirez-Carrozzi, V.R., Nazarian, A.A., Li, C.C., Gore, S.L., Sridharan, R. Imbalzano, A.N., & Smale, S.T. (2006) Selective and antagonistic functions of SWI/SNF and Mi-2beta nucleosome remodeling complexes during an inflammatory response. *Genes Dev.*, 20, 3, (February 2006), 282–296.

Rauh, M.J., Ho, V., Pereira, C., Sham, A., Sly, L.M., Lam, V., Huxham, L., Minchinton, A.I., Mui, A., & Krystal, G. (2005) SHIP represses the generation of alternatively activated macrophages. *Immunity*, 23, 4, (October 2005), 361–374.

Rothlin, C.V., Ghosh, S., Zuniga, E.I., Oldstone, M.B., & Lemke, G. (2007) TAM receptors are pleiotropic inhibitors of the innate immune response. *Cell*, 131, 6, (December 2007), 1124–1136.

Sato, S., Nomura, F., Kawai, T., Takeuchi, O., Mühlradt, P.F., Takeda, K., & Akira, S. (2000) Synergy and cross-tolerance between toll-like receptor (TLR) 2- and TLR4-mediated signaling pathways. *J Immunol.*, 165, 12, (December 2000), 7096–7101.

Satoh, T., Takeuchi, O., Vandenbon, A., Yasuda, K., Tanaka, Y., Kumagai, Y., Miyake, T., Matsushita, K., Okazaki, T., Saitoh, T., Honma, K., Matsuyama, T., Yui, K., Tsujimura, T., Standley, D.M., Nakanishi, K., Nakai, K., & Akira, S. (2010) The Jmjd3-Irf4 axis regulates M2 macrophage polarization and host responses against helminth infection. *Nat Immunol.*, 11, 10, (October 2010), 936-944.

Schroder, M., Meisel, C., Buhl, K., Profanter, N., Sievert, N., Volk, H.D., & Grütz, G. (2003) Different modes of IL-10 and TGF-beta to inhibit cytokine-dependent IFN-gamma production: consequences for reversal of lipopolysaccharide desensitization. *J Immunol.*, 170, 10, (May 2003), 5260-5267.

Serhan, C.N., Brain, S.D., Buckley, C.D., Gilroy, D.W., Haslett, C., O'Neill, L.A., Perretti, M., Rossi, A.G., & Wallace, J.L. (2007) Resolution of inflammation: state of the art, definitions and terms. *FASEB J.*, 21, 2, (February 2007), 325–332.

Sharabi, A.B., Aldrich, M., Sosic, D., Olson, E.N., Friedman, A.D., Lee, S.H., & Chen, S.Y. (2008) Twist-2 controls myeloid lineage development and function. *PLoS Biol.*, 6, 12, (December 2008), e316.

Sheedy, F.J., Palsson-McDermott, E., Hennessy, E.J., Martin, C., O'Leary, J.J., Ruan, Q., Johnson, D.S., Chen, Y., & O'Neill, L.A. (2010) Negative regulation of TLR4 via targeting of the proinflammatory tumor suppressor PDCD4 by the microRNA miR-21. *Nat Immunol.*, 11, 2, (February 2010), 141-147.

Souza, D.G., Vieira, A.T., Soares, A.C., Pinho, V., Nicoli, J.R., Vieira, L.Q., & Teixeira, M.M. (2004) The essential role of the intestinal microbiota in facilitating acute inflammatory responses. *J Immunol.*, 173, 6, (September 2004), 4137-4146.

Taganov, K.D. Boldin, M.P., Chang, K.J., & Baltimore, D. (2006) NF-kappaB-dependent induction of microRNA miR-146, an inhibitor targeted to signaling proteins of innate immune responses. *Proc Natl Acad Sci U S A*, 103, 33, (August 2006), 12481–12486.

Tili, E., Michaille, J.J., Cimino, A., Costinean, S., Dumitru, C.D., Adair, B., Fabbri, M., Alder, H., Liu, C.G., Calin, G.A., & Croce, C.M. (2007) Modulation of miR-155 and miR-125b levels following lipopolysaccharide/TNF-alpha stimulation and their possible roles in regulating the response to endotoxin shock. *J. Immunol.*, 179, 8, (October 2007), 5082–5089.

van 't Veer, C., van den Pangaart, P.S., van Zoelen, M.A., de Kruif, M., Birjmohun, R.S., Stroes, E.S., de Vos, A.F., & van der Poll, T. (2007) Induction of IRAK-M is associated with lipopolysaccharide tolerance in a human endotoxemia model. *J Immunol.*, 179, 10, (November 2007), 7110–7120.

Willment, J.A., Lin, H.H., Reid, D.M., Taylor, P.R., Williams, D.L., Wong, S.Y., Gordon, S., & Brown, G.D. (2003) Dectin-1 expression and function are enhanced on alternatively activated and GM-CSF-treated macrophages and are negatively regulated by IL-10, dexamethasone, and lipopolysaccharide. *J. Immunol.*, 171, 9, (November 2003), 4569–4573.

Wilson, A.G. (2008) Epigenetic regulation of gene expression in the inflammatory response and relevance to common diseases. *J. Periodontol.*, 79, 8 Suppl, (August 2008), 1514–1519.

Wolk, K., Döcke, W.D., von Baehr, V., Volk, H.D., & Sabat, R. (2000) Impaired antigen presentation by human monocytes during endotoxin tolerance. *Blood*, 96, 1, (July 2000), 218-223.

Wolk, K., Kunz, S., Crompton, N.E., Volk, H.D., & Sabat, R. (2003) Multiple mechanisms of reduced major histocompatibility complex class II expression in endotoxin tolerance. *J Biol Chem.*, 278, 20, May 2003, 18030-18036.

Wysocka, M., Robertson, S., Riemann, H., Caamano, J., Hunter, C., Mackiewicz, A., Montaner, L.J., Trinchieri, G., & Karp, C.L. (2001) IL-12 suppression during experimental endotoxin tolerance: dendritic cell loss and macrophage hyporesponsiveness. *J. Immunol.*, 166, 12, (June 2001), 7504–7513.

Yamamoto, M., Sato, S., Hemmi, H., Hoshino, K., Kaisho, T., Sanjo, H., Takeuchi, O., Sugiyama, M., Okabe, M., Takeda, K., Akira, S. (2003) Role of adaptor TRIF in the MyD88-independent toll-like receptor signaling pathway. *Science*, 301, 5633, (August 2003), 640–643.

Ziegler-Heitbrock, L. (2001) The p50-homodimer mechanism in tolerance to LPS. *J. Endotoxin Res.*, 7, 3, 219–222.

3

Spleen Tyrosine Kinase: A Novel Target in Autoimmunity

Stephen P. McAdoo and Frederick W. K. Tam
Imperial College Kidney and Transplant Institute, London
United Kingdom

1. Introduction

Spleen tyrosine kinase (Syk) is a non-receptor tyrosine kinase that is highly expressed in cells of haematopoietic lineage, where it has an important role in the intra-cellular signalling cascades for various immunoreceptors, such as the B cell receptor and the Fc receptor. As such, it is a potential target in allergic and autoimmune diseases. Emerging evidence also suggests that Syk may have additional roles beyond its well defined functions in classical immunoreceptor signalling, which may have implications, potentially useful or harmful, for therapies directed at this protein. Given these diverse functions in numerous cell types, it is unsurprising that Syk has been the subject of hundreds of original research articles, as well as several excellent reviews in recent years (Sada, Takano et al. 2001; Ruzza, Biondi et al. 2009; Mocsai, Ruland et al. 2010; Riccaboni, Bianchi et al. 2010). In this chapter we aim to summarise current understanding of the basic structure and function for Syk, before developing a rationale for targeting Syk in autoimmune disease. We will then review progress towards Syk-directed therapies in clinical practice, and finally we shall consider the emerging functions of Syk beyond the adaptive immune response, and what implications these may have for therapy.

2. Discovery

Syk was identified in the early 1990s in the cytostolic fractions of lysates from porcine spleen and bovine thymus as a 40kDa protein with intrinsic kinase activity. This 40kDa protein was subsequently shown to be a fragment, containing only the catalytic domain, of a larger 72kDa protein that was identified from a porcine spleen cDNA library (from whence it gained its name) using oligonucleotides designed according to the partial sequence of the purified 40kDa fragment (Taniguchi, Kobayashi et al. 1991). The *Syk* gene was subsequently mapped to chromosome 9q22 in humans (Ku, Malissen et al. 1994).

3. Basic structure and function

The Syk molecule has a multi-domain structure (Figure 1a) containing two N-terminal tandem Src Homology 2 (SH2) domains and a C-terminal kinase domain (Sada, Takano et al. 2001). Interdomains A and B connect the SH2-SH2 and SH2-kinase domains, respectively. At least 10 major phosphorylation sites have been identified within the molecule (Furlong,

Mahrenholz et al. 1997) - one located in interdomain A, five within interdomain B, two within the kinase domain, and two near the extreme C-terminus. An alternatively spliced form of Syk - SykB - lacks a 23 amino acid sequence in interdomain B, and in this respect is similar to ZAP-70, the only other member of the Syk family of kinases. ZAP-70 has approximately 60% overall homology to Syk and its expression appears to be more restricted, in particular to T lymphocytes and natural killer (NK) cells (Au-Yeung, Deindl et al. 2009).

In the resting state, it is thought that Syk assumes a closed, auto-inhibited structure (Figure 1b), wherein interdomain A and interdomain B bind to the C-terminal kinase domain, preventing its interaction with potential substrates, in what is termed a 'linker-kinase sandwich' (Deindl, Kadlecek et al. 2007; Kulathu, Grothe et al. 2009). Upon activation, structural changes within the molecule result in an open conformation that allows the exposed catalytic kinase domain to interact with downstream targets.

The canonical mechanism of Syk activation is via its interaction with immunoreceptor tyrosine-based activation motifs (ITAMs) (Turner, Schweighoffer et al. 2000). ITAMs are short peptide sequences characterised by a consensus sequence that contains two tyrosine residues 6-12 amino acids apart. As their name suggests, they are found in association with the cytoplasmic components of classical immunoreceptors, including the T-cell receptor (TCR), B-cell receptor (BCR) and Fc-receptor (FcR) for immunoglobulins, either as an associated adapter protein, or within the cytoplasmic region of the receptor itself.

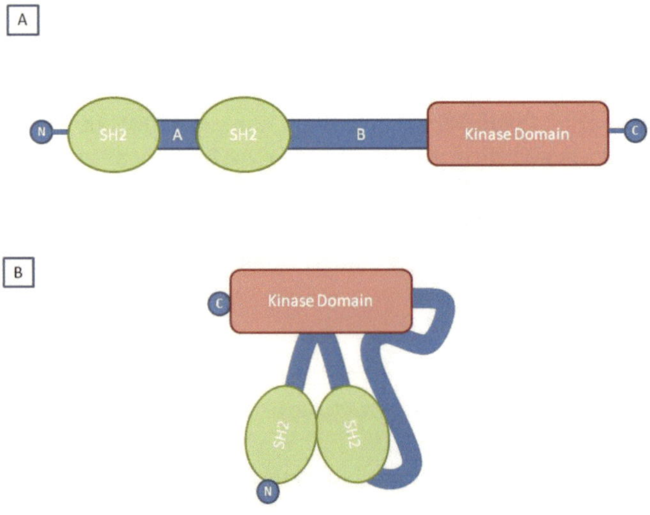

Fig. 1. a. Schematic diagram showing the multi-domain structure of Syk, including two N-terminal SH2-domains, C-terminal kinase domain, and interdomains A and B. Figure 1b: Schematic diagram of the 'linker-kinase sandwich' conformation that has been suggested for resting Syk (see text for details)

Upon receptor engagement, the tyrosine residues on ITAMs are rapidly phosphorylated, primarily by Lyn and other members of the Src family of kinases (Figure 2). The phosphorylated ITAM can now act as a docking site for the SH2 domains of Syk, resulting in conformational changes, exposure of the kinase domain, autophosphorylation and propagation of downstream signalling. In addition, disruption of the 'linker-kinase sandwich' may occur upon phosphorylation of tyrosine residues alone, particularly those within interdomain B. This may occur by autophosphorylation following ITAM-mediated activation, or by transphosphorylation by other kinases, such as Lyn or other Src family kinases that are often co-localised with ITAMs at the cell membrane. As a consequence, positive feedback and sustained Syk activity is possible in the absence of phosphorylated ITAMs. This 'dual' mechanism of activation has recently lead to the proposal of Syk as an 'OR' gate in signalling pathways (Tsang, Giannetti et al. 2008; Bradshaw 2010).

In addition to releasing the enzymatic domain of the protein from the 'linker-kinase sandwich', these changes in structure and phosphorylation, particularly within the tyrosine-rich interdomain B, create docking sites for downstream targets of Syk, for which it can perform both enzymatic and adapter functions (Kulathu, Grothe et al. 2009). These downstream targets include a host of adapter proteins and other enzyme targets (including LAT, SLP76, Vav1, PLC-γ, PI3K and MAP kinases) that are then able to effect complex cellular responses including proliferation, differentiation, phagocytosis and cytokine production (Mocsai, Ruland et al. 2010).

Two groups simultaneously reported the effects of targeted disruption of the *Syk* gene in mice in the mid-90s (Cheng, Rowley et al. 1995; Turner, Mee et al. 1995). *Syk* knockout resulted in perinatal death with a severe haemorrhagic phenotype. This was subsequently shown to be due to a failure of communication between developing vasculature and lymphatics during embryogenesis (Abtahian, Guerriero et al. 2003). Analysis of Syk-deficient lymphoid cells derived from these knock-out animals was critical in developing our early understanding of the functional role of Syk in immunoreceptor signalling in various cell types.

Bone marrow chimera animals, reconstituted with haematopoietic stem cells from Syk-deficient mice, showed no reduction in the numbers of circulating erythrocytes, platelets and total leucocytes. These animals had relatively normal reconstitution of T cells, however detailed analysis revealed impaired differentiation of the B cell lineage, with development arrested at the pro-B to pre-B cell stage, consistent with a role for Syk in pre-BCR signalling (Cheng, Rowley et al. 1995; Turner, Mee et al. 1995). Subsequent *in vitro* work, using a variety of cell lines and cell-based reconstitution systems, has defined a clear role for Syk in initiating downstream signalling following engagement of the BCR (Geahlen 2009), and indeed it was study in this area that was responsible for much of our understanding of the basic structure and function of Syk. The functional role of Syk in mature B cells (such as on antibody production by plasma cells) *in vivo*, however, is less well defined and future studies using small molecule inhibitors, or potentially conditional knockout in this cellular compartment, will be informative.

Analysis of myeloid cells, such as macrophages and neutrophils, from *Syk* knockout bone marrow chimeras showed ablation of FcR-mediated responses including phagocytosis and the generation of reactive oxygen intermediates (Crowley, Costello et al. 1997; Kiefer, Brumell et al. 1998). The role of Syk in signal transduction for activatory FcR in these and a variety of other cell types is now well established, including mast cells bearing FcεR (de Castro 2011). A critical role for Syk in FcγR-mediated antigen internalisation and maturation by dendritic cells has also been described (Sedlik, Orbach et al. 2003), and is notable given the important role of dendritic cells in initiating adaptive immune responses.

In addition to FcR-mediated responses, Syk has been implicated in integrin signalling in myeloid cells (Mocsai, Zhou et al. 2002; Mocsai, Abram et al. 2006). Integrins are transmembrane receptors that have a critical role in cell adhesion and migration, via their interaction with adhesion molecules expressed on other cells, particularly the vascular endothelium. Syk deficient myeloid cells show impaired integrin-mediated responses, thought to be dependent on the association of integrins with ITAM-containing adapter proteins such as FcRγ-chain and DAP12, as myeloid cells deficient in these adapter proteins show similar defects.

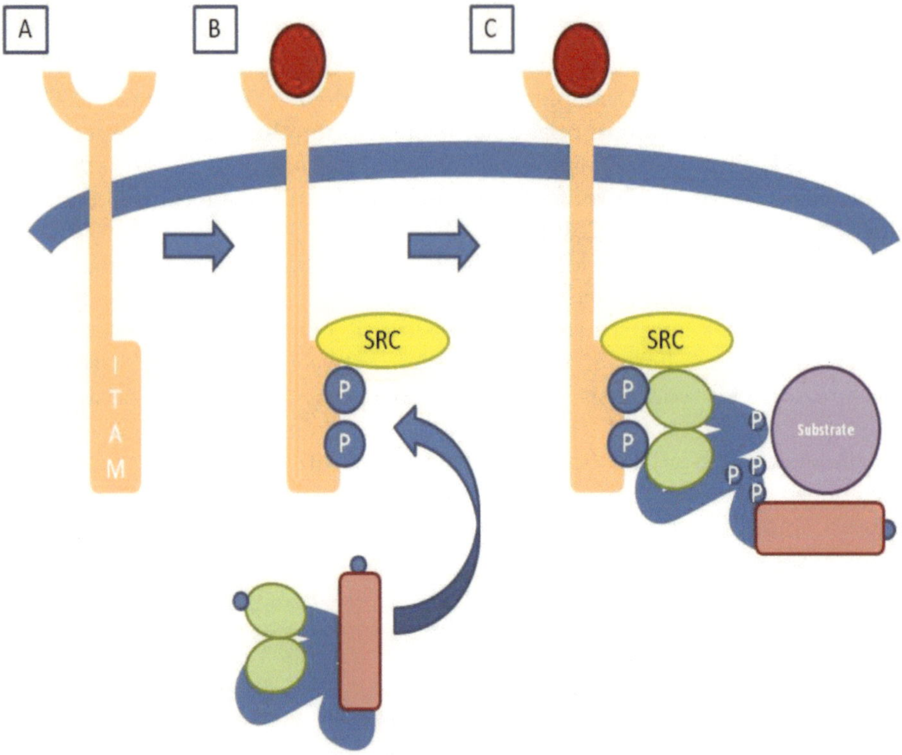

Fig. 2. Simplified schematic showing activation of Syk by interaction with ITAM.
2a: Unengaged receptor bearing non-phosphorylated ITAM motif within its cytoplasmic tail. 2b: Upon receptor engagement Src family kinases (SRC) phosphorylate (P) tyrosine residues within the ITAM motif. 2c: Phosphorylated ITAM motif acts as a docking site for the SH2 domains of Syk, resulting in conformational changes, auto- and transphosphorylation of tyrosines within Syk, thus resulting in activation and phosphorylation of downstream targets

4. Syk in autoimmunity

Given our understanding of its role in BCR- and FcR-mediated signalling, the rationale for targeting Syk in autoimmunity is clear. The presence of autoantibodies is the hallmark of many autoimmune diseases. Whilst not universally pathogenic, these antibodies often contribute to disease via their interaction with FcR expressed on many immune effector cells (and other mechanisms including complement activation). Notably, FcR-deficient mice are resistant to a variety of animal models of autoimmunity, and FcR polymorphisms have been shown to be important determinants of human autoimmune disease (Takai 2002; Nimmerjahn 2006). Syk inhibition may, therefore, have the desirable double effect of preventing the production of pathogenic autoantibodies, via inhibiting B cell activation via the BCR, and simultaneously inhibiting their downstream effects via disrupting signalling from their receptors.

It is encouraging that other therapeutic approaches that target B-cells have recently shown efficacy in clinical practice (Townsend, Monroe et al. 2010). Interestingly, however, clinical benefit cannot always be attributed to eradication of circulating autoantibody, and it is probable that effects on other B cell functions, such as antigen presentation, cytokine production, and provision of co-stimulation to other immune cells, contribute to the benefit seen. Disruption of Syk-dependent BCR signalling may provide similar benefits.

In addition, Syk inhibition may have the additional effect of inhibiting migration and recruitment of immune effector cells to sites of tissue inflammation, via inhibited integrin signalling.

Therapeutic strategies to target Syk, therefore, are desirable and can be broadly classified into two main approaches: pharmacological inhibition of Syk activity, and gene-based therapies aiming to silence Syk expression (Ruzza, Biondi et al. 2009). Whilst the application of the latter has yet to advance to clinical studies, we shall briefly review their future potential, before focusing on the progress of Syk inhibition therapies.

5. Gene-based therapies targeting Syk

5.1 Antisense oligonucleotides (ASO)

ASO are short, single stranded nucleic acid sequences that bind sense mRNA via complementary base-pairing, and thus inhibit the translation of the relevant protein. ASO directed against Syk have shown activity in a variety of cell types *in vitro*, including inhibitory effects of FcγR-mediated signalling in monocytes (Matsuda, Park et al. 1996). Published *in vivo* studies using Syk ASO are limited to animal models of allergic inflammation (Stenton, Kim et al. 2000; Stenton, Ulanova et al. 2002). These have shown that aerosolized Syk ASO, delivered in a liposomal complex, suppress Syk expression in, and inflammatory mediator release from, alveolar macrophages. In addition, markers of pulmonary inflammation were reduced in two distinct animal models. Whilst there have been no *in vivo* studies in autoimmune models, the proposed mechanism of action in these allergic models is via inhibition of activatory FcR-mediated responses, suggesting similar approaches my be effective in autoimmune disease. However, progress in the clinical use of ASO based therapy has been frustratingly slow since the introduction of Fomivirsen, the first antisense therapy to be licensed by the Food and Drug Administration (FDA), being approved for use in AIDS-related cytomegalovirus (CMV) retinitis over 10 years ago. This is due, in part, to the difficulty of producing reliable delivery systems to target the cells, tissues or organs of choice (White, Anastasopoulos et al. 2009) - a not insignificant problem given the multi-system nature of many autoimmune diseases.

5.2 RNA interference (RNAi)

RNAi is an innate cellular process that is thought to regulate endogenous gene expression and protect against viral infection. A variety of small RNA molecules, such as endogenous, genetically encoded microRNA (miRNA) or exogenous small interfering RNA (siRNA), may bind target mRNA via Watson-Crick complementary base pairing, and then direct this target mRNA into an RNA-induced silencing complex (RISC), a natural degradation pathway, thus effecting gene silencing prior to translation. Since this first description of RNAi in 1998, advance in the field has been rapid, and there have been promising early phase clinical studies in a number of conditions, including retinal diseases, malignancies and viral infections. The most commonly used technique to harness RNAi for therapy has been to transfect siRNA into target cells. siRNA specific to Syk, for example, have been shown to inhibit antibody-mediated phagocytosis by human macrophages (Lu, Wang et al. 2011). Again, *in vivo* studies in this field are limited to models of allergic inflammation, and to date are only reported in international patent applications. Aerosolised delivery of Syk siRNA, using similar methods as used for ASO delivery, resulted in decreased pulmonary inflammation, as determined by recruitment of cells to bronchoalveolar lavage fluid, in a rat model of ovalbumin-induced asthma. Again, these findings augur well for the translation and use of RNAi in autoimmune disease. As with antisense therapy, outstanding challenges for harnessing RNAi include the development of effective delivery systems, escape of the innate 'interferon' response directed against foreign nucleic acids, and avoidance of 'off-target' gene silencing (Davidson and McCray 2011).

6. Pharmacological inhibition

A number of biotechnology and pharmaceutical companies are working to develop compounds to inhibit Syk (Ruzza, Biondi et al. 2009; Riccaboni, Bianchi et al. 2010). To date, two such inhibitors, both identified by Rigel Pharmaceuticals, and now in development by AstraZeneca, have progressed to clinical trials - initially R112, and more recently the related compound, R406 (and its respective prodrug, R788).

6.1 Preclinical studies with small molecule inhibitors

Cell based high-throughput screening of small molecules identified R112 as a potent inhibitor of Syk activity, as assayed by production and release of inflammatory mediators following FcRε crosslinking by anti-IgE (Rossi, Herlaar et al. 2006). Subsequent characterization showed that R112 is an ATP-competitive inhibitor of Syk activity, as demonstrated by *in vitro* kinase assays (IC_{50} = 226 nmol/l). These assays also showed activity against other kinases such as Lyn (IC_{50} = 300nmol/l) and Lck (IC_{50} =645 nmol/l). However, when tested in cell-based assays, R112 was shown to be relatively selective for Syk as determined by phosphorylation of target proteins, despite the similar IC_{50} values in the *in vitro* assays.

Rigel subsequently developed the related compound R406, another potent competitive ATP inhibitor for Syk (*in vitro* IC_{50} = 41 nmol/l) (Braselmann, Taylor et al. 2006). Again, selectivity assessments using over 90 *in vitro* kinase assays showed an inhibitory effect on other kinases, although cell based assays confirmed selectivity for Syk - FLT3 was the next most potently inhibited kinase, though at 5-fold less activity. R406 has been shown to inhibit FcR-mediated responses in a variety of cell types *in vitro*, including mast cells, macrophages, neutrophils and dendritic cells (Braselmann, Taylor et al. 2006; Matsubara, Koya et al. 2006). In addition, activity against BCR-mediated responses has been shown in primary human B cells *in vitro*. Notably, R406 did not show significant activity in Syk-independent pathways (such as following lipopolysaccharide stimulation) at the concentrations necessary to inhibit

FcR- and BCR-mediated pathways, in keeping with the selectivity for Syk seen in the cell based phosphorylation assays. R788, or fostamatinib disodium (see McAdoo and Tam 2011 for review) was then developed as the methylene phosphate prodrug of R406, to improve its solubility and potential for oral dosing.

The efficacy of R406/R788 has been studied in numerous animal models of autoimmunity. In a murine model of immune cytopenias, for example, treatment with R788 prevented haemolysis and the development of thrombocytopenia following the administration of anti-red blood cell and anti-platelet antibodies respectively (Podolanczuk, Lazarus et al. 2009). Treatment with R406/R788 reduced clinical, histological and radiographic evidence of joint inflammation following the induction of collagen-induced arthritis, a rodent model of rheumatoid arthritis (Pine, Chang et al. 2007). R788 has shown efficacy in three animal models of SLE (Bahjat, Pine et al. 2008; Deng, Liu et al. 2010). Treatment of the lupus-prone NZB/NZW mouse strain reduced kidney disease, as determined by proteinuria and renal histology, and improved platelet counts and survival. In the BAK/BAX knockout mouse, treatment with R788 reduced lupus-like skin disease and lymphadenopathy. Similarly, in the MRL/lpr strain, treatment improved renal and skin disease, in addition to reducing lymphadenopathy. In a rodent model of antibody-mediated glomerulonephritis, treatment with R788 prevented the induction of disease (Smith, McDaid et al. 2010). In addition, treatment had a profound effect on established disease, reversing the histological features of crescentic glomerulonephritis even when initiated after the induction of disease. Finally, in an autoimmune diabetes model, R788 delayed the onset of insulinitis and spontaneous diabetes in NOD mice (Colonna, Catalano et al. 2010). Again, significant effects were seen even when treatment was initiated after the onset of glucose intolerance. Though not strictly a model of autoimmunity, treatment with R788 reduced local and remote inflammation in mesenteric ischaemia-reperfusion in mice (Pamuk, Lapchak et al. 2010), suggesting effects independent of the FcR and BCR, such as inhibition of leucocyte migration.

The safety of R788/R406 has also been assessed in detailed rodent toxicity and immunotoxicology studies (Zhu, Herlaar et al. 2007). At high doses, R406 was associated with a reduction in circulating lymphocyte count, bone marrow cellularity, and thymic and spleen weight. These changes generally resolved during a drug-withdrawal recovery period. In murine host resistance models, treatment with R788 did not significantly impair clearance of influenza, Listeria or streptococcal infection.

Other pharmaceutical companies have developed a number of other small molecule inhibitors. The majority of these, like R112 and R406, are competitive inhibitors for the ATP binding site of the catalytic domain. Bayer, for example, has developed the imidazopyrimidine analogue BAY 61-3606, which inhibits Syk-mediated responses *in vitro* and has demonstrated efficacy in animal models of allergy *in vivo (Yamamoto, Takeshita et al. 2003)*. However, the published selectivity profile is limited to only 6 other kinases, and comparison with genetic knockdown suggests that BAY 61-3606 may have significant off-target effects (Lin, Huang et al. 2010).

Other groups have chosen to target the non-kinase domains of the Syk molecule. By inhibiting the interaction of the SH2-domains with their docking proteins, it has been proposed that Syk inhibition may be achieved whilst avoiding off-target effects on other kinases, and one such approach has been shown to inhibit IgE-mediated responses *in vitro* and *in vivo (Mazuc, Villoutreix et al. 2008)*. Whilst the precise molecular mechanism of the inhibitory effects of this molecule are yet to be definitively described, it should be noted that the SH2-domain is a highly conserved motif found in a large number of proteins involved in signal transduction, and targeting this domain may in turn have diverse off target effects.

6.2 Clinical studies

R112 was the first Syk inhibitor treatment to be assessed in clinical studies, where it showed benefit in relieving symptoms of allergic rhinitis when delivered as an intranasal preparation (Meltzer, Berkowitz et al. 2005). Subsequent work focused on R406/R788, with early phase clinical studies confirming that R406/788 is highly bioavailable following oral administration, rapidly absorbed systemically, and well tolerated at doses needed to achieve biological effects such as inhibition of basophil activation in response to anti-IgE *ex vivo* (IC_{50} 1.06 microM) (Braselmann, Taylor et al. 2006; Sweeny, Li et al. 2010).

To date, the results of five phase II studies with R788 (fostamatinib) have been published. Three of these investigated the effects of fostamatinib in rheumatoid arthritis (RA) (Table 1). The first recruited almost 200 patients with active disease despite standard therapy with methotrexate (Weinblatt, Kavanaugh et al. 2008). Clinical responses were seen as early as one week following the initiation of treatment, and sustained at three months, with significant improvements in disease activity scores in the treatment groups versus placebo. The second study enrolled over 450 patients with active disease despite long-term methotrexate therapy, and this confirmed benefit at six months, with improved American College of Rheumatology 20% improvement criteria (ACR20), ACR50, ACR70 and DAS28 scores (Weinblatt, Kavanaugh et al. 2010). Notably, both these studies included a significant proportion of patients who had failed biological therapy with anti-TNF or anti-CD20 agents, and benefit with fostamatinib was seen in these subgroups (although overall response rates were lower than for the whole study population). A subsequent trial designed specifically to examine the efficacy of fostamatinib in this group of patients failing biologic therapy, however, did not achieve its primary endpoint of improved ACR20 in the treatment group (Genovese, Kavanaugh et al. 2011). There were, however, significant improvements in radiographic and biochemical markers of inflammation.

A small open label study in immune thrombocytopenic purpura (ITP) has also shown promising results (Podolanczuk, Lazarus et al. 2009). Although the numbers are small (n=16), the majority of patients had refractory disease with multiple previous ITP treatments (commonly steroids, intravenous immunoglobulin, rituximab and splenectomy). As such, the sustained (50%) and transient (25%) response rates seen during the average follow up time of 36 weeks represent encouraging results and further studies are planned.

In addition to these studies in autoimmune disease, a fifth phase II study examined the effects of fostamatinib in haematological malignancy (Friedberg, Sharman et al. 2010), the rationale for which is discussed below. Again, in a study population that included a significant proportion of patients with heavily pre-treated, relapsed or refractory disease, fostamatinib showed modest but significant clinical activity and a manageable side-effect profile.

The most frequent adverse event seen in these clinical studies was gastrointestinal toxicity, a common side effect of many kinase inhibitors. Symptoms were dose-related, and seen at rates of up to 45% in groups receiving the highest doses of fostamatinib, and this was the most common reason for patient withdrawal from the RA trials.

REF	N	ENTRY CRITERIA	FOLLOW UP	ENDPOINT	OUTCOMES	COMMENTS
Weinblatt, Kavanaugh et al. 2008)	189	Active RA (≥ 12 months from diagnosis) despite ≥ 6 months methotrexate therapy	12 weeks	ACR20 response rate (ACR50, ACR70, DAS28 response rates)	Significant benefits in all disease activity scores in patients treated with fostamatinib 100-150mg bd. Clinical responses notes as early as one week after initiation of treatment.	Approximately 1/3 of patients continued to receive other DMARDs during the study; Approximately 20% had received prior biologic therapy (with appropriate washout period before entering study).
Weinblatt, Kavanaugh et al. 2010)	457	Active RA (≥ 6 months from diagnosis) despite ≥ 3 months methotrexate therapy	6 months	ACR20 response rate (ACR50, ACR70, DAS28 response rates)	Significant benefits in all disease activity scores in patients treated with fostamatinib 100-150mg bd. Again, responses noted as early as one week.	15% of patients in this study had received prior biologic therapy. Although overall response rates were lower in this subgroup, still significantly more patients demonstrated responses than the equivalent placebo group.
Genovese, Kavanaugh et al. 2011)	229	Active RA (≥ 12 months from diagnosis) with disease unresponsive to current or previous biologic therapy	3 months	ACR20 response rate (ACR50, ACR70, DAS28 response rates; synovitis scores on MRI)	No difference in disease activity scores across treatment and placebo groups. Significant improvements in circulating inflammatory markers and synovitis scores on MRI noted in treatment groups.	Despite randomisation, baseline differences in steroid dose, previous biologic exposure and synovitis scores were noted between groups, which authors suggest may account for lack of efficacy.

Table 1. Summary of Phase II trials with fostamatinib in patients with rheumatoid arthritis (RA). ACR20/50/70, American College of Rheumatology 20/50/70% improvement criteria; DAS28, disease activity score using 28 joint counts; MRI, magnetic resonance imaging; DMARD, disease modifying anti-rheumatic drug

Neutropenia occurred in up to 30% of patients receiving fostamatinib in the RA trials. Again, this finding appeared to be dose-related and responded to dose reduction or temporary withdrawal of the drug. Although no direct pharmacokinetic interaction has been detected between fostamatinib and methotrexate (Baluom, Samara et al. 2011), synergistic effects on haematopoiesis beyond individual pharmacokinetic parameters (along with underlying bone marrow disease or other concomitant immunosuppressant therapy) may have contributed to this phenomenon, as neutropenia was not reported in the ITP trial. An increased rate of uncomplicated upper respiratory tract infections was seen in the treatment group of the largest RA trial. However, this was not associated with neutropenia. In addition, no opportunistic or atypical infections were reported in any of the clinical trials.

7. Beyond adaptive immunity: problems and potential for Syk-directed therapy

Recently, Syk has been implicated in a number of signalling pathways beyond the adaptive immune response that may have implications for Syk-directed therapy in clinical practice. These include the aforementioned role in cell adhesion, as well as possible roles in innate immunity, platelet function, bone metabolism and tumorigenesis (Mocsai, Ruland et al. 2010). Disruption of these functions may lead to significant toxicity, or alternatively open novel therapeutic avenues, in targeting Syk. The basic mechanism of these functions has been reviewed in detail elsewhere (Mocsai, Ruland et al. 2010); we shall here consider the potential clinical implications.

7.1 Innate Immunity and Infection

Given its diverse effects on adaptive immune responses, coupled to a role in inflammatory cell adhesion and migration, the preeminent concern with Syk directed therapies must be of over-immunosuppression and the associated risk of infection. It is also notable that Syk has recently been associated with a variety of pathogen recognition receptors (PRRs), important components of the innate immune response that recognise pathogen-associated molecular patterns (PAMPs). C-type Lectins, one such class of PRR, play an important role in antifungal immunity in particular, and Syk has been implicated in the intracellular signalling cascades for these receptors (Drummond, Saijo et al. 2011). Some, such as Dectin-1, contain an ITAM motif on their cytoplasmic domain, and others may associate with ITAM containing adaptor proteins such as FcRγ chain or DAP12. As such, Syk inhibition may potentially lead to excessive downregulation of multiple inflammatory, innate and adaptive immune responses, resulting in risk of overwhelming infection. The results of the preclinical toxicity assessments and host resistance models are reassuring in this respect (although a host resistance model of fungal infection has not been studied), as is the absence of severe, atypical or opportunistic infection in the clinical studies thus far. Larger and longer clinical studies are, however, needed to establish the long term and cumulative effects of Syk inhibition on innate immune responses and infection risk, particularly in patient groups who have had extensive treatment histories with other immunosuppressant agents.

7.2 Platelet function

Syk has been shown to be involved in a number of platelet activation pathways, including via the glycoprotein GPVI receptor (an FcRγ chain-associated receptor that bears an ITAM motif), integrin αIIbβ3, and C-type Lectin 2 (CLEC-2; a type II membrane protein containing a single tyrosine-based motif in its cytoplasmic tail that has been termed a hemITAM) (Watson, Auger et al. 2005; Watson, Herbert et al. 2010). In addition, R406 has demonstrated inhibitory activity in these pathways (Spalton, Mori et al. 2009). Notably, however, very high dose exposure to R406 did not prolong bleeding time in mice, and in phase I human studies, R406 did not inhibit collagen or ADP-induced platelet aggregation *ex vivo (Braselmann, Taylor et al. 2006)*, perhaps suggesting redundancy of Syk dependent pathways *in vivo*. Based on these observations, it would appear that targeting Syk in isolation would not be an effective anti-thrombotic therapy. However, synergistic effects, potentially both therapeutic and harmful, with other anti-platelet agents have not been explored in clinical studies.

7.3 Bone metabolism

Syk has been shown to regulate osteoclastic bone resorption, via its association with integrin $\alpha v\beta 3$ and ITAM bearing proteins, such as DAP12 and FcRγ chain, expressed at the osteoclast cell surface (Zou, Kitaura et al. 2007). In addition, Syk has recently been implicated in the suppression of osteoblast differentiation (Yoshida, Higuchi et al. 2011). Thus, Syk may represent a therapeutic target in disorders of bone metabolism such as osteoporosis, although potential effects of Syk inhibition on normal bone, such as osteosclerosis and increased fragility and fracture risk, have yet to be investigated *in vivo* or in clinical studies.

7.4 Tumorigenesis

It has been suggested that Syk is a negative regulator of progression in various types of malignancy (including breast, gastric and melanoma) based on the observation of decreased Syk expression in these tumour types and experimental studies where Syk transfection and re-expression in tumour cell lines suggested a tumour- and metastasis- suppressive effect (Coopman and Mueller 2006). The molecular mechanism of this suppressive role has yet to be established. Conversely, fostamatinib has shown activity in NCI-60 (a panel of 60 diverse human cancer cell lines), although this may be due to off-target effects, rather than Syk inhibition specifically. On this basis, however, a broad multi-histology Phase II study is currently recruiting (NCT00923481).

Syk signalling through the BCR has also been implicated as an important survival signal in various lymphoid malignancies, and R406 has shown antiproliferative and proapoptotic activity in B cell lymphoma and CLL lines *in vitro* (Chen, Monti et al. 2008; Buchner, Fuchs et al. 2009; Quiroga, Balakrishnan et al. 2009). Furthermore, R788 is highly active in animal models of non-Hodgkin's lymphoma (NHL) and chronic lymphocytic leukaemia (CLL) (Young, Hardy et al. 2009; Suljagic, Longo et al. 2010), and in a Phase II clinical trial, fostamatinib showed significant clinical activity in a heterogeneous group of NHL and CLL (Friedberg, Sharman et al. 2010). Based on these findings, larger Phase II trials in haematological malignancy are ongoing (NCT00446095, NCT00798096). Interestingly, some oncogenic viruses have been shown to encode ITAM-containing proteins - for example, Epstein Barr virus (EBV) latent membrane protein 2A (LMP2A) contains an ITAM motif, and has been shown to promote B cell development and survival (Caldwell, Wilson et al. 1998).

7.5 Cardiovascular risk

Hypertension was a commonly reported adverse event in clinical studies with fostamatinib. It is unclear whether this was due to Syk inhibition *per se*, or potentially due to off-target effects on other kinases – the vascular endothelial growth factor receptor 2 being a putative candidate. Whilst usually mild, and responsive to dose reduction of fostamatinib or augmented antihypertensive therapy, the long-term effects of even small increases in blood pressure in patients with autoimmune rheumatic diseases such as RA and lupus, who already have dramatically increased cardiovascular risk, need to be considered. Interestingly, administration of fostamatinib was recently shown to attenuate plaque development in a rodent model of atherosclerosis, an effect thought to be mediated by impaired recruitment of inflammatory cells, suggesting that Syk inhibition is a potential target in atherosclerotic cardiovascular disease (Hilgendorf, Eisele et al. 2011). Syk has also been implicated in the mechanism of high-glucose induced NF-κB activation in glomerular endothelial cells, suggesting a potential role of Syk inhibition in preventing end-organ complications of diabetes mellitus (Yang, Seo et al. 2008).

8. Conclusions

The rationale, the experimental data, and the clinical experience to date augur well for the efficacy of Syk inhibition in autoimmune disease. Several large phase II-III trials in RA are currently in progress (NCT01242514, NCT01264770, NCT01197521, NCT01197534, NCT01197755) and it is hoped that if successful, efficacy could translate to a wide range of organ-specific and systemic autoimmune diseases. Indeed, it is tempting to propose that Syk-directed therapy, with its proven clinical efficacy in early trials, along with potential benefits in cardiovascular disease, hyperglycaemia, bone metabolism and malignancy (particularly those related to oncogenic viruses) is the proverbial 'Holy Grail' of immunosuppressant therapy following 40 years of steroid- and cytotoxic-based regimes complicated by hypertension, diabetes, osteoporosis and lymphoproliferative disease. However, the widespread role of Syk in numerous immune functions raises serious concerns regarding the risk of opportunistic infection, and some questions about the oncogenic potential of Syk disruption in certain cell types remain unanswered. In addition, it is disappointing that Syk inhibition with fostamatinib, the drug furthest through clinical development, showed only improvement by objective assessment using MRI or biochemical markers, rather than clinical benefit in patients who had not responded to biologic therapy. Future clinical studies will need to establish both the long-term safety and superiority of Syk inhibition in practice.

9. Acknowledgements

S.P.M. is in receipt on an MRC Research Training Fellowship
F.W.K.T. has been supported by the Diamond Fund from Imperial College Healthcare Charity, MRC and the Wellcome Trust. F.W.K.T. has received research project grants from Roche Palo Alto, AstraZeneca Limited and Baxter Biosciences.

10. References

Abtahian, F., A. Guerriero, et al. (2003). Regulation of blood and lymphatic vascular separation by signaling proteins SLP-76 and Syk. *Science* 299(5604): 247-251.

Au-Yeung, B. B., S. Deindl, et al. (2009). The structure, regulation, and function of ZAP-70. *Immunol Rev* 228(1): 41-57.

Bahjat, F. R., P. R. Pine, et al. (2008). An orally bioavailable spleen tyrosine kinase inhibitor delays disease progression and prolongs survival in murine lupus. *Arthritis Rheum* 58(5): 1433-1444.

Baluom, M., E. Samara, et al. (2011). Fostamatinib, a syk-kinase inhibitor, does not affect methotrexate pharmacokinetics in patients with rheumatoid arthritis. *J Clin Pharmacol* 51(9): 1310-1318.

Bradshaw, J. M. (2010). The Src, Syk, and Tec family kinases: distinct types of molecular switches. *Cell Signal* 22(8): 1175-1184.

Braselmann, S., V. Taylor, et al. (2006). R406, an orally available spleen tyrosine kinase inhibitor blocks fc receptor signaling and reduces immune complex-mediated inflammation. *J Pharmacol Exp Ther* 319(3): 998-1008.

Buchner, M., S. Fuchs, et al. (2009). Spleen tyrosine kinase is overexpressed and represents a potential therapeutic target in chronic lymphocytic leukemia. *Cancer Res* 69(13): 5424-5432.

Caldwell, R. G., J. B. Wilson, et al. (1998). Epstein-Barr virus LMP2A drives B cell development and survival in the absence of normal B cell receptor signals. *Immunity* 9(3): 405-411.

Chen, L., S. Monti, et al. (2008). SYK-dependent tonic B-cell receptor signaling is a rational treatment target in diffuse large B-cell lymphoma. *Blood* 111(4): 2230-2237.

Cheng, A. M., B. Rowley, et al. (1995). Syk tyrosine kinase required for mouse viability and B-cell development. *Nature* 378(6554): 303-306.

Colonna, L., G. Catalano, et al. (2010). Therapeutic targeting of Syk in autoimmune diabetes. *J Immunol* 185(3): 1532-1543.

Coopman, P. J. and S. C. Mueller (2006). The Syk tyrosine kinase: a new negative regulator in tumor growth and progression. *Cancer Lett* 241(2): 159-173.

Crowley, M. T., P. S. Costello, et al. (1997). A critical role for Syk in signal transduction and phagocytosis mediated by Fcgamma receptors on macrophages. *J Exp Med* 186(7): 1027-1039.

Davidson, B. L. and P. B. McCray, Jr. (2011). Current prospects for RNA interference-based therapies. *Nat Rev Genet* 12(5): 329-340.

de Castro, R. O. (2011). Regulation and function of syk tyrosine kinase in mast cell signaling and beyond. *J Signal Transduct* 2011: 507291.

Deindl, S., T. A. Kadlecek, et al. (2007). Structural basis for the inhibition of tyrosine kinase activity of ZAP-70. *Cell* 129(4): 735-746.

Deng, G. M., L. Liu, et al. (2010). Suppression of skin and kidney disease by inhibition of spleen tyrosine kinase in lupus-prone mice. *Arthritis Rheum* 62(7): 2086-2092.

Drummond, R. A., S. Saijo, et al. (2011). The role of Syk/CARD9 coupled C-type lectins in antifungal immunity. *Eur J Immunol* 41(2): 276-281.

Friedberg, J. W., J. Sharman, et al. (2010). Inhibition of Syk with fostamatinib disodium has significant clinical activity in non-Hodgkin lymphoma and chronic lymphocytic leukemia. *Blood* 115(13): 2578-2585.

Furlong, M. T., A. M. Mahrenholz, et al. (1997). Identification of the major sites of autophosphorylation of the murine protein-tyrosine kinase *Syk. Biochim Biophys Acta* 1355(2): 177-190.

Geahlen, R. L. (2009). Syk and pTyr'd: Signaling through the B cell antigen receptor. *Biochim Biophys Acta* 1793(7): 1115-1127.

Genovese, M. C., A. Kavanaugh, et al. (2011). An oral Syk kinase inhibitor in the treatment of rheumatoid arthritis: a three-month randomized, placebo-controlled, phase II study in patients with active rheumatoid arthritis that did not respond to biologic agents. *Arthritis Rheum* 63(2): 337-345.

Hilgendorf, I., S. Eisele, et al. (2011). The Oral Spleen Tyrosine Kinase Inhibitor Fostamatinib Attenuates Inflammation and Atherogenesis in Low-Density Lipoprotein Receptor-Deficient Mice. *Arterioscler Thromb Vasc Biol.*

Kiefer, F., J. Brumell, et al. (1998). The Syk protein tyrosine kinase is essential for Fcgamma receptor signaling in macrophages and neutrophils. *Mol Cell Biol* 18(7): 4209-4220.

Ku, G., B. Malissen, et al. (1994). Chromosomal location of the Syk and ZAP-70 tyrosine kinase genes in mice and humans. *Immunogenetics* 40(4): 300-302.

Kulathu, Y., G. Grothe, et al. (2009). Autoinhibition and adapter function of Syk. *Immunol Rev* 232(1): 286-299.

Lin, Y. C., D. Y. Huang, et al. (2010). Anti-inflammatory actions of Syk inhibitors in macrophages involve non-specific inhibition of toll-like receptors-mediated JNK signaling pathway. *Mol Immunol* 47(7-8): 1569-1578.

Lu, Y., W. Wang, et al. (2011). Antibody-mediated platelet phagocytosis by human macrophages is inhibited by siRNA specific for sequences in the SH2 tyrosine kinase, *Syk. Cell Immunol* 268(1): 1-3.

Matsubara, S., T. Koya, et al. (2006). Syk activation in dendritic cells is essential for airway hyperresponsiveness and inflammation. *Am J Respir Cell Mol Biol* 34(4): 426-433.

Matsuda, M., J. G. Park, et al. (1996). Abrogation of the Fc gamma receptor IIA-mediated phagocytic signal by stem-loop Syk antisense oligonucleotides. *Mol Biol Cell* 7(7): 1095-1106.

Mazuc, E., B. O. Villoutreix, et al. (2008). A novel druglike spleen tyrosine kinase binder prevents anaphylactic shock when administered orally. *J Allergy Clin Immunol* 122(1): 188-194, 194 e181-183.

McAdoo, S. P. and F. W. K. Tam (2011). FOSTAMATINIB DISODIUM Tyrosine-Protein Kinase SYK/FLT3 Inhibitor Treatment of Rheumatoid Arthritis Oncolytic. *Drugs of the Future* 36(4): 273-280.

Meltzer, E. O., R. B. Berkowitz, et al. (2005). An intranasal Syk-kinase inhibitor (R112) improves the symptoms of seasonal allergic rhinitis in a park environment. *J Allergy Clin Immunol* 115(4): 791-796.

Mocsai, A., C. L. Abram, et al. (2006). Integrin signaling in neutrophils and macrophages uses adaptors containing immunoreceptor tyrosine-based activation motifs. *Nat Immunol* 7(12): 1326-1333.

Mocsai, A., J. Ruland, et al. (2010). The SYK tyrosine kinase: a crucial player in diverse biological functions. *Nat Rev Immunol* 10(6): 387-402.

Mocsai, A., M. Zhou, et al. (2002). Syk is required for integrin signaling in neutrophils. *Immunity* 16(4): 547-558.

Nimmerjahn, F. (2006). Activating and inhibitory FcgammaRs in autoimmune disorders. *Springer Semin Immunopathol* 28(4): 305-319.

Pamuk, O. N., P. H. Lapchak, et al. (2010). Spleen tyrosine kinase inhibition prevents tissue damage after ischemia-reperfusion. *Am J Physiol Gastrointest Liver Physiol* 299(2): G391-399.

Pine, P. R., B. Chang, et al. (2007). Inflammation and bone erosion are suppressed in models of rheumatoid arthritis following treatment with a novel Syk inhibitor. *Clin Immunol* 124(3): 244-257.

Podolanczuk, A., A. H. Lazarus, et al. (2009). Of mice and men: an open-label pilot study for treatment of immune thrombocytopenic purpura by an inhibitor of Syk. *Blood* 113(14): 3154-3160.

Quiroga, M. P., K. Balakrishnan, et al. (2009). B-cell antigen receptor signaling enhances chronic lymphocytic leukemia cell migration and survival: specific targeting with a novel spleen tyrosine kinase inhibitor, R406. *Blood* 114(5): 1029-1037.

Riccaboni, M., I. Bianchi, et al. (2010). Spleen tyrosine kinases: biology, therapeutic targets and drugs. *Drug Discov Today* 15(13-14): 517-530.

Rossi, A. B., E. Herlaar, et al. (2006). Identification of the Syk kinase inhibitor R112 by a human mast cell screen. *J Allergy Clin Immunol* 118(3): 749-755.

Ruzza, P., B. Biondi, et al. (2009). Therapeutic prospect of Syk inhibitors. *Expert Opin Ther Pat* 19(10): 1361-1376.

Sada, K., T. Takano, et al. (2001). Structure and function of Syk protein-tyrosine kinase. *J Biochem* 130(2): 177-186.

Sedlik, C., D. Orbach, et al. (2003). A critical role for Syk protein tyrosine kinase in Fc receptor-mediated antigen presentation and induction of dendritic cell maturation. *J Immunol* 170(2): 846-852.

Smith, J., J. P. McDaid, et al. (2010). A spleen tyrosine kinase inhibitor reduces the severity of established glomerulonephritis. *J Am Soc Nephrol* 21(2): 231-236.

Spalton, J. C., J. Mori, et al. (2009). The novel Syk inhibitor R406 reveals mechanistic differences in the initiation of GPVI and CLEC-2 signaling in platelets. *J Thromb Haemost* 7(7): 1192-1199.

Stenton, G. R., M. K. Kim, et al. (2000). Aerosolized Syk antisense suppresses Syk expression, mediator release from macrophages, and pulmonary inflammation. *J Immunol* 164(7): 3790-3797.

Stenton, G. R., M. Ulanova, et al. (2002). Inhibition of allergic inflammation in the airways using aerosolized antisense to Syk kinase. *J Immunol* 169(2): 1028-1036.

Suljagic, M., P. G. Longo, et al. (2010). The Syk inhibitor fostamatinib disodium (R788) inhibits tumor growth in the Emu- TCL1 transgenic mouse model of CLL by blocking antigen-dependent B-cell receptor signaling. *Blood* 116(23): 4894-4905.

Sweeny, D. J., W. Li, et al. (2010). Metabolism of fostamatinib, the oral methylene phosphate prodrug of the spleen tyrosine kinase inhibitor R406 in humans: contribution of hepatic and gut bacterial processes to the overall biotransformation. *Drug Metab Dispos* 38(7): 1166-1176.

Takai, T. (2002). Roles of Fc receptors in autoimmunity. *Nat Rev Immunol* 2(8): 580-592.

Taniguchi, T., T. Kobayashi, et al. (1991). Molecular cloning of a porcine gene syk that encodes a 72-kDa protein-tyrosine kinase showing high susceptibility to proteolysis. *J Biol Chem* 266(24): 15790-15796.

Townsend, M. J., J. G. Monroe, et al. (2010). B-cell targeted therapies in human autoimmune diseases: an updated perspective. *Immunol Rev* 237(1): 264-283.

Tsang, E., A. M. Giannetti, et al. (2008). Molecular mechanism of the Syk activation switch. *J Biol Chem* 283(47): 32650-32659.

Turner, M., P. J. Mee, et al. (1995). Perinatal lethality and blocked B-cell development in mice lacking the tyrosine kinase Syk. *Nature* 378(6554): 298-302.

Turner, M., E. Schweighoffer, et al. (2000). Tyrosine kinase SYK: essential functions for immunoreceptor signalling. *Immunol Today* 21(3): 148-154.

Watson, S. P., J. M. Auger, et al. (2005). GPVI and integrin alphaIIb beta3 signaling in platelets. *J Thromb Haemost* 3(8): 1752-1762.

Watson, S. P., J. M. Herbert, et al. (2010). GPVI and CLEC-2 in hemostasis and vascular integrity. *J Thromb Haemost* 8(7): 1456-1467.

Weinblatt, M. E., A. Kavanaugh, et al. (2008). Treatment of rheumatoid arthritis with a Syk kinase inhibitor: a twelve-week, randomized, placebo-controlled trial. *Arthritis Rheum* 58(11): 3309-3318.

Weinblatt, M. E., A. Kavanaugh, et al. (2010). An oral spleen tyrosine kinase (Syk) inhibitor for rheumatoid arthritis. *N Engl J Med* 363(14): 1303-1312.

White, P. J., F. Anastasopoulos, et al. (2009). Overcoming biological barriers to in vivo efficacy of antisense oligonucleotides. *Expert Rev Mol Med* 11: e10.

Yamamoto, N., K. Takeshita, et al. (2003). The orally available spleen tyrosine kinase inhibitor 2-[7-(3,4-dimethoxyphenyl)-imidazo[1,2-c]pyrimidin-5-ylamino]nicotinamide dihydrochloride (BAY 61-3606) blocks antigen-induced airway inflammation in rodents. *J Pharmacol Exp The*r 306(3): 1174-1181.

Yang, W. S., J. W. Seo, et al. (2008). High glucose-induced NF-kappaB activation occurs via tyrosine phosphorylation of IkappaBalpha in human glomerular endothelial cells: involvement of Syk tyrosine kinase. *Am J Physiol Renal Physiol* 294(5): F1065-1075.

Yoshida, K., C. Higuchi, et al. (2011). Spleen tyrosine kinase suppresses osteoblastic differentiation through MAPK and PKCalpha. *Biochem Biophys Res Commun.*

Young, R. M., I. R. Hardy, et al. (2009). Mouse models of non-Hodgkin lymphoma reveal Syk as an important therapeutic target. *Blood* 113(11): 2508-2516.

Zhu, Y., E. Herlaar, et al. (2007). Immunotoxicity assessment for the novel Spleen tyrosine kinase inhibitor R406. *Toxicol Appl Pharmacol* 221(3): 268-277.

Zou, W., H. Kitaura, et al. (2007). Syk, c-Src, the alphavbeta3 integrin, and ITAM immunoreceptors, in concert, regulate osteoclastic bone resorption. *J Cell Biol* 176(6): 877-888.

4

Genetic Variation in AhR Gene Related to Dioxin Sensitivity in the Japanese Field Mouse, *Apodemus speciosus*

Hiroko Ishiniwa[1], Kazuhiro Sogawa[2], Ken-ichi Yasumoto[2], Nobuhiko Hoshi[3], Toshifumi Yokoyama[3], Ken Tasaka[3] and Tsuneo Sekijima[1]

[1]*Niigata University,*
[2]*Tohoku University,*
[3]*Kobe University*
Japan

1. Introduction

Human beings have developed many tools, technologies, and chemicals for their convenience and comfort. For example, herbicides and/or insecticides that are sprayed on crop lands prevent damage from pests and have resulted in remarkable increases in crop yield. Polychlorinated biphenyls (PCBs), which have insulating properties and are incombustible, were widely used in the past in electronic instruments and by the electric industry. However, some of these chemicals have harmful effects on organisms. In Seveso, Italy, a large amount of dioxins was emitted by explosion of an agrochemical factory. This accidental release of dioxins killed a lot of farm animals and many people living near the factory developed skin inflammation due to exposure to the high concentrations of dioxins. As seen above, many similar chemical spill disasters have occurred and new chemicals are still being produced. Dioxins are one of the most toxic groups of manmade chemicals known. Dioxins are not only highly toxic, but they also insidiously disrupt reproductive function by mimicking the actions of hormones in the body. Their effects on reproduction, such as reducing the number of sperm and affecting the sex ratio in offspring, may impair the fitness of individuals. Decreased reproductive success of individuals in a population may result in the extinction of local populations and eventually species extinction.
In this chapter, we describe the effects of the most toxic chemical pollutant, dioxins, on the Japanese field mouse, *Apodemus speciosus*. We also discuss the diversity of dioxin sensitivity and attempted to identify dioxin sensitivity in mice using a molecular indicator. Our findings suggest that it is important to take into consideration the differences in dioxin response in each mouse for an accurate estimation of the impact of the pollution.

1.1 Dioxins, benzofurans, and PCBs

1.1.1 Physical and chemical properties

Dioxin is a generic term for polychlorinated dibenzo-*p*-dioxins (PCDDs), dibenzofurans (PCDFs), and coplanar polychlorinated biphenyls (co-PCBs), all of which are halogenated aromatic compounds. Among them, PCDDs are comprised of two benzene rings interconnected by two oxygen bridges. PCDFs also consist of two benzene rings interconnected by a carbon bond and an oxygen bridge. The generic structures of PCDDs and PCDFs are shown in Figure 1a and b. PCDDs and PCDFs have 75 and 135 congeners, respectively. Each compound differs in the number and position of the chlorine atoms. PCBs comprise two benzene rings joined by a carbon bond and have 209 congeners (Fig. 1c). Among these, the congeners with a coplanar conformation that shows chlorine substitution in the non-*ortho* (2, 2′, 6, and 6′) or mono-*ortho* position are called dioxins. Dioxins exhibit extremely low water solubility but are highly soluble in organic solvents. Their lipophilic and hydrophobic properties explain their high concentrations in lipids and organic compounds, and consequently their high degree of biomagnification through food webs.

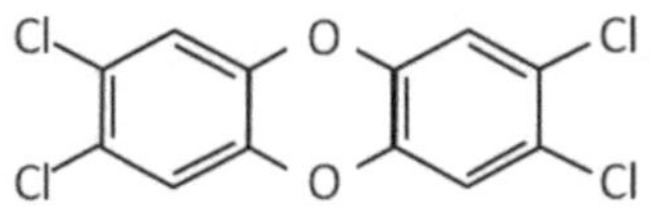

(a) 2,3,7,8-tetrachlorodibenzo-p-dioxin (2,3,7,8-TCDD)

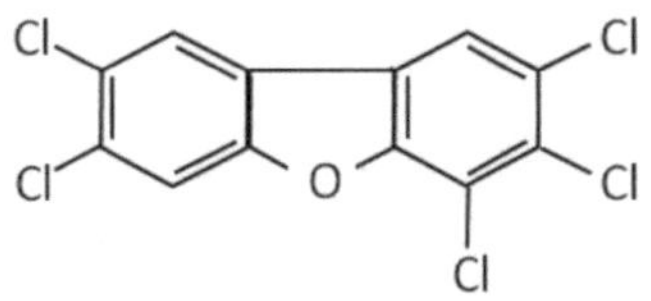

(b) 2,3,4,7,8-pentachlorodibenzofuran (2,3,7,8-PCDF)

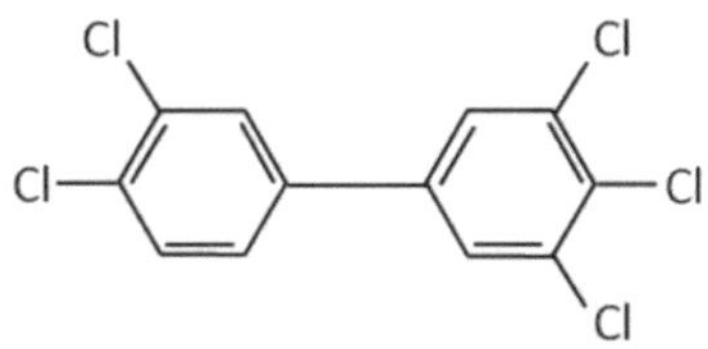

(c) 3,3′,4,4′,5-pentachlorobiphenyl (PCB 126)

Fig. 1. Chemical structures of a dioxin, dibenzofuran, and co-PCB

1.1.2 Overview of pollution

Dioxins are unintentionally generated chemical compounds. They were present in minute amounts as a byproduct in previous herbicides. The first time dioxins were recognized worldwide was the Vietnam War. Between 1961 and 1971, nearly 19.5 million gallons (approximately 78 million liters) of herbicides were aerially-sprayed in Vietnam by the United States Armed Forces for tactical defoliation and crop destruction (Stellman et al., 2003). The most commonly used herbicide was Agent Orange, which was constructed of esters of 2,4-dichlorophenoxyacetic acid and 2,4,5-trichlorophenoxyacetic acid (2,4,5-T). The 2,4,5-T contained in herbicides included 2,3,7,8-tetrachlorodibenzo-*p*-dioxin and resulted in serious harm to human health, such as birth defects. Thereafter, many accidental seepages and spillages during the production of chlorine and organochlorine compounds, such as bleach, herbicides, and pesticides, were reported (Roland et al., 2008). Furthermore, solid residues emitted by chemical companies have been discharged into landfills and dumps. Some landfills and dumps that were not adequately prepared to prevent pollution leaked PCDD/Fs into the environment. Hazardous waste incinerators and other thermal processes produce high proportions of of PCDD/Fs from these precursors, resulting in a considerable impact on the local environment by high emission of PCDD/Fs. Although new cases of pollution due to dioxin emissions rarely occur these days, previous contaminations have not yet been adequately remediated because it is not easy to completely eliminate a pollutant once it has been emitted.

1.2 Effect of dioxin on organisms is mediated by AhR

Dioxin absorption into the body results in various toxic effects, such as induction of various drug metabolizing enzymes, wasting syndrome, immune suppression, tumor promotion, inflammation, teratogenesis, homeostasis disruption, alterations in cell proliferation, apoptosis, adipose differentiation, and endocrine disruption (Masunaga, 2009; Pohjanvirta & Tuomisto, 1994; Poland & Knutson, 1982; Puga et al., 2000; Stevens et al., 2009; Vos et al., 2000). Although the toxic effects of dioxins are widespread, most are controlled by one protein, aryl hydrocarbon receptor (AhR).

AhR is a ligand-activated transcription factor which mediates most of the dioxin-derived toxic effects (Sogawa & Fujii-Kuriyama, 1997). AhR initially forms a complex with heat shock protein 90 (HSP90), X-associated protein 2 (XAP2), and telomerase binding protein (p23) in cytoplasm (Fig. 2). When an AhR ligand such as TCDD enters the cytoplasm and binds to AhR, the activated AhR translocates into the nucleus, where it dissociates from chaperone proteins and interacts with a number of different proteins.

1.2.1 Induction of various drug metabolizing enzymes

The ligand-activated AhR taken up into the nucleus forms a heterodimer with AhR nuclear translocator (Arnt) (Fig. 2). AhR-Arnt heterodimers bind to the xenobiotic responsive element (XRE), and activate transcription of various drug metabolizing genes such as the cytochrome P450-1A1 (CYP1A1), -1A2, and -1B1, uridine diphosphate glycosyltransferase 1 family polypeptide A1 (UGT1A1), glutathione S-transferase (GST)-Ya subunit and NADPH-quinon-oxidoreductase (Denison et al., 1988; Elferink et al., 1990; Fujisawa-Sehara et al., 1987, 1988) (Fig. 2). The CYP1-family (-1A1, -1A2, and -1B1) consists of phase I drug metabolizing enzymes and they oxidize extraneous substances like dioxins to metabolites and finally excrete them from the body. However, in the process of metabolism, oxidation by CYP enzymes activates xenobiotics and produces reactive oxygen species (ROS), which cause cellular oxidative stress and ultimately result in DNA damage by DNA-single strand break and sometimes cancer promotion (Dalton et al., 2002; Nebert et al., 2000). Furthermore, Latchoumycandane et al. (2002) reported a TCDD dose-dependent reduction of sperm number in rats by oxidative stress. The sperm plasma membrane is rich in polyunsaturated fatty acids so lipid peroxidation of the polyunsaturated fatty acids adversely affects sperm.

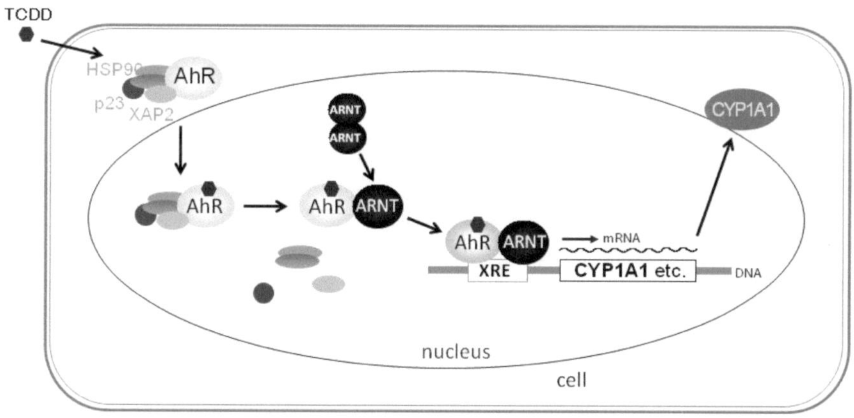

Fig. 2. Simplified scheme of gene regulation by AhR in terms of drug metabolizing enzymes

1.2.2 Disruption of reproductive function

Originally it was believed that AhR regulated the expression of ovarian cytochrome P450 aromatase (CYP19), which is a key enzyme in estrogen synthesis (Baba et al., 2005). AhR regulates the ovarian biological clock and ultimately governs the estrus cycle with AhR repressor (AhRR), which is a negative feedback modulator of the AhR. The AhR also regulates the expression of testicular cytochrome P450 side chain cleavage (P450scc), which is a key enzyme in testosterone synthesis (Fukuzawa et al., 2004). If TCDD invades the cell and binds to AhR, it would disrupt the functions of AhR, such as hormonal synthesis. Furthermore, AhR acts on steroid receptors, such as the oestrogen receptor (ER) and androgen receptor (AR), by two opposite pathways (Ohtake et al., 2003, 2007). In one pathway, ligand-activated AhR activates the expression of ER and AR mediated target genes without hormonal stimulation, while in the other pathway, ligand-activated AhR degrades ER and AR through an ubiquitin-proteasomal system. These actions of AhR induced by TCDD disrupt usual hormonal action and ultimately reproductive function as well.

1.2.3 Cell cycle regulation, tumor promotion, and apoptosis

AhR dimerizes with the RelA subunit of nuclear factor-kappa B (NF-κB). NF-κB/Rel transcription factors regulate many genes involved in control of cellular proliferation, neoplastic transformation, and apoptosis (Kim et al., 2000). Also, AhR and RelA cooperate to activate c-myc oncogene, which is associated with cellular proliferation and tumor promotion. Furthermore, it is known that AhR promotes progression of the cell through the cell cycle (Puga et al., 2002). The gap1 (G1) phase of the cell cycle is inhibited by TCDD-induced AhR. In the DNA synthesis (S) phase, AhR forms protein-protein complexes with the retinoblastoma protein (RB), which is critical for transfer into S-phase. Thus, AhR directly affect cell cycle regulation. Therefore, exposure to TCDD is likely to disrupt the cell cycle and stimulate tumorigenesis.

1.2.4 Cellular inflammatory response

AhR is involved in cellular inflammatory signaling through a non-genomic pathway (Matsumura, 2009). This non-genomic pathway does not require dimer formation with Arnt. The ligand activated AhR regulates rapid increases in intracellular Ca2+ concentration, as well as increases in enzymatic activation of cytosolic phospholipase A2 (cPLA2) and cyclooxygenase-2 (Cox-2). These factors are associated with inflammatory action and cause wasting syndrome and hydronephrosis.

1.2.5 Immunotoxicity

The immune system is one of the most sensitive targets of dioxin (Birnbaum and Tuomisto, 2000). However, conflicting findings have been reported regarding the immunological effects of dioxin. One adverse effect is suppression of the immune system. TCDD inhibits immunoglobulin secretion and decreases resistance to bacterial, viral, and parasitic infections in TCDD-exposed animals (Birnbaum and Tuomist, 2000; Holsapple et al., 1991; Nohara et al., 2002). Also, AhR has been recognized as a key factor in the immunotoxicity of dioxin because AhR plays an important role in the development of liver and the immune system (Fernandez-Salguero et al., 1995). Meanwhile, another advantageous effect is its promotion of immunity. AhR regulates regulatory T (T_{reg}) cells and interleukin (IL)-17-producing T (T_H17) cell differentiation in a ligand-specific manner (Quintana et al., 2008).

The former cells suppress autoimmune conditions such as encephalomyelitis, while the latter cells increase the conditions. Since AhR activation by TCDD has been shown to induce functional T_{reg} cells and improve immunity, AhR is being focused on as a unique property for therapeutic immune-modulation.

1.3 AhR diversity

As above mentioned, AhR is a vital factor because its functions are wide-ranging, from cell cycle regulation to hormonal synthesis. In fact, AhR have been present for a long time in various organisms such as invertebrates, fish, birds, and mammals. Meanwhile, in any single species, the genetic diversity of AhR, which may alter protein function, is always maintained.

1.3.1 History of AhR

Many mammal, bird, fish, insect, and nematode species possess AhR (Hahn, 2002). In invertebrates like nematodes and flies that have ancestral AhR protein, AhR homologs lack specific binding ability to dioxin-like compounds (Butler et al., 2001). Originally in evolutionary history, AhR only had a physiological function without ligand-induced activity. This is why invertebrates are not affected by dioxin related chemicals. AhR subsequently developed into a ligand-inducible biotransformation system in some lineages. Vertebrates like birds and fish have at least two AhR genes, designated AhR1 and AhR2 (Hahn, 2002). In fish AhR genes, AhR1 shows a lower mRNA expression level than AhR2. Also, AhR1 has inactive or reduced TCDD sensitivity as compared with AhR2 (Hansson & Hahn, 2008). Therefore, AhR 2 has been considered as the predominant form in fish. In birds, meanwhile, AhR2 is a recessive form and AhR1 is the major form (Yasui et al., 2007). Although both forms exhibited specific binding to TCDD and induced genes, AhR2 showed a lower binding efficiency than AhR1. In mammals, just a single AhR gene has been confirmed. The mammalian AhR exhibited high binding affinity to TCDD in laboratory rodents to marine wild mammals such as beluga whales and harbor seals (Hahn, 2002).
These studies on AhR indicated that ancestral AhR was duplicated in at least the fish lineage with dioxin-binding ability and disappearance of one AhR gene in the mammalian lineage. The AhR gene was widely conserved among animals, but has evolved by acquiring a new function or functions in each lineage.

1.3.2 AhR structure and function

AhR is a member of the structurally similar gene family with structural motifs designated as bHLH (basic helix–loop–helix) and PAS (Per, Arnt/AhR, Sim homology) (Gu et al., 2000; Taylor & Zhulin, 1999). In the NH2-terminal region, AhR proteins contain a bHLH motif, which is involved in DNA binding and hetero- or homodimerization (Fig. 3). bHLH includes both a nuclear localization signal (NLS) and a nuclear export signal (NES) (Davarinos & Pollenz, 1999; Lees & Whitelaw, 1999). The sequence of nearly 250 amino acids adjacent to the COOH-terminus of the bHLH region is called the PAS domain, which was initially identified as a sequence conserved among *Drosophila* PER, human ARNT and *Drosophila* SIM (Gu et al., 2000; Taylor & Zhulin, 1999). The PAS domain consists of the two imperfect repeats of 50 amino acids, PAS-A and PAS-B, and has been considered to function as an interactive surface for hetero or homodimer formation. The ligand binding domain of AhR is located in the sequence overlapping in part with the PAS-B region, and also with the binding site for Hsp90 which keeps AhR structurally competent to bind a ligand

(Coumailleau et al., 1995). The Hsp90 interacts with the bHLH region to mask the NLS of AhR, resulting in the cytoplasmic maintenance of AhR. Ligand binding to AhR protein changes the conformation of the Hsp90/AhR complex to expose the NLS of AhR, leading to nuclear translocation of the complex (Lees & Whitelaw, 1999). The COOH-terminal half of AhR possesses transactivation activity that is mediated through CBP/p300 and RIP140 coactivators (Sogawa et al., 1995).

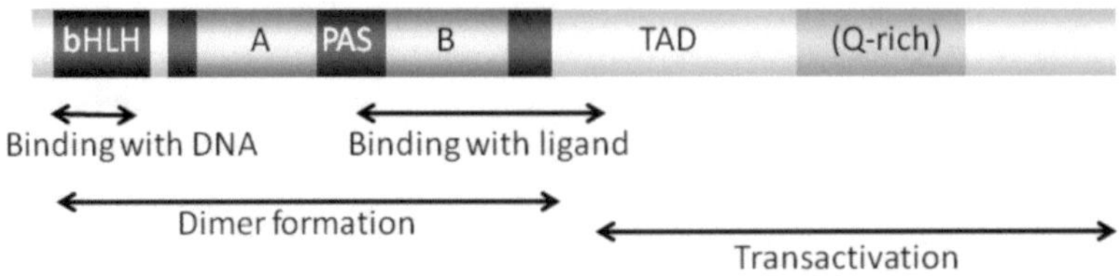

Fig. 3. Schematic representation of functional domain of AhR
bHLH (basic helix-loop- helix); PAS (Per- Arnt- Sim) domain; A and B (PAS A and B repeats); TAD (Transactivation domain); Q-rich (glutamine rich) region. The locations of functional domains are indicated by bars.

1.3.3 Dioxin sensitivity and AhR polymorphism

Remarkable differences in sensitivity to TCDD have been reported among species and strains (Bello et al., 2001; Enan et al., 1996; Kleeman et al., 1988; Pohjanvirta et al., 1993; Pohjanvirta and Tuomisto, 1994; Poland and Knutson, 1982). For example, the lethal dose 50 % (LD50) values vary from 1 μg/kg for guinea pig, the most sensitive animal, to >5000 μg/kg for hamster, the most resistant (Poland and Knutson, 1982). Also, aquatic birds including the common tern (*Sterna hirundo*) are up to 250-fold less sensitive to dioxins than the typical avian model, the domestic chicken (*Gallus gallus*) (Hoffman et al., 1998; Lorenzen et al., 1997). In the case of same species, LD50 value varies from 182 μg/kg for dioxin-sensitive C57/BL6 strain mice to 2570 μg/kg for mouse DBA strain that is resistant (Poland and Knutson, 1982).

Some of these differences have been explained by genetic variations in AhR which are related to significant protein function. In congeneric mouse strains, C57/BL6 and DBA, the difference in sensitivity is due to a difference in ligand-binding affinity from the difference in the primary structures by only one amino acid substitution (Ema et al., 1994). Similar findings have been reported in 2 bird species, chicken and common tern (Karchner et al., 2006). Furthermore, deletion of 38 or 43 amino acids in the transactivation domain due to one base substitution in an intronic region resulted in different susceptibility to TCDD in congeneric rat strains (Pohjanvirta et al., 1998).

1.3.4 Significance of genetic diversity

As mentioned above, AhR has high diversity among and within species. These genetic variations are linked to differences in protein function that had an important effect on ecological processes such as population recovery from a disturbance (Pearman & Garner, 2005; Reusch et al., 2005), interspecific competition (Booth & Grime, 2003; Yoshida et al., 2003), and local adaptation (Kron & Husband, 2006; de Roode et al., 2005). If an environment is changed by an accident like chemical pollution and warming temperatures, native

organisms would find it difficult to survive in such as altered environment. However, if organisms can maintain genetic diversity that is reflected in differences in response to environmental change, local adaptation would occur and the species would be maintained.
Dioxin pollution is one example of environmental change. Although many toxic effects of dioxin have been clarified, the disruption of reproductive function may have a serious impact on the offspring of adult animals and ultimately may cause local extinction. AhR is a useful gene with which to conduct field studies of dioxin pollution because the functional cascade of AhR is well-known and actual variations including functional differences have been reported. Furthermore, because AhR plays a very important role in a variety of biological processes, AhR variation that alters the action of a protein would have a strong effect on an organism. If we can find a mutation related to AhR ability, the mutation may be a useful molecular indicator for differentiating between dioxin sensitivity and insensitivity.

1.4 Present situation and past examples of dioxin pollution in Japan

1.4.1 Dioxin Pollution in Japan

Large amounts of dioxins have been released into the Japanese environment since the 1950s (Masunaga et al., 2001, 2003; Yoshida & Nakanishi, 2003). The major sources of pollution from the 1960s to 1970s were derived from two herbicides used in rice paddy fields, pentachlorophenol (PCP) and chlornitrofen (CNP). Since the 1980s, however, municipal and industrial waste incinerators have become the major sources of dioxin emissions. Illegal incinerators and dumpsites built in lowland areas in particular have released large amounts of dioxins into the environment and thereby may have seriously affected wildlife living in the vicinity of these polluted sites.

1.4.2 Japanese field mouse

The Japanese field mouse, *Apodemus speciosus*, is broadly distributed in secondary forest in Japanese lowlands, including polluted areas where a lot of dioxins have been illegally released by herbicide spraying and illegally constructed waste incinerators. Furthermore, this species possesses the species-specific characteristic of accumulating higher levels of dioxins in the liver than higher order predators in the same food web (Ministry of Environment, Government of Japan, 2008; Yasuda et al., 2003). According to a previous study, the dioxin concentration in the Japanese field mouse was 4,900 pg-TEQ/g-lipid, which was higher than the Japanese weasel (2,900 pg-TEQ/g-lipid) and the red fox (2,300 pg-TEQ/g-lipid) (Yasuda et al., 2003). Additionally, it is easier to develop a genetic study because the Japanese field mouse is phylogenetically closer to other mice that have been used as a model animal in the field of life science. Therefore, this species is useful when studying the physiological and ecological effects of dioxin on wildlife.
The aim of this study is to clarify the effects of dioxin pollution on Japanese wildlife in terms of genetic background. Therefore, our focus was mutation of the Aryl hydrocarbon receptor gene as a molecular marker that reflects the degree of response to dioxin. We also selected the Japanese field mouse as a bioindicator because of their high accumulation of dioxin, broad distribution in the Japanese environment, and ease of genetic analysis.
First, we identified polymorphisms of *Apodemus speciosus* AhR (*As*-AhR) and a critical mutation related to functional differences. Then we estimated the toxic effect of dioxin on Japanese field mice in terms of the degree of dioxin sensitivity using AhR mutation as a molecular indicator.

2. Searching for critical mutation in *As*-AhR

2.1 Analysis of *As*-AhR sequence and polymorphisms

We examined the full-length of the *As*-AhR sequence and found a lot of variation in the nucleotide sequences. *As*-AhR consists of 857 to 875 amino acids with calculated molecular masses of 96.0 to 97.9 kDa, and exhibited the highest degree of similarity to the mouse AhR by a database search (DDBJ). The variations in sequence length were due to the insertion of 8 to 23 repeats of glutamines (Glns) at codon 596 in the transactivation domain (TAD). In comparison to mouse C57BL/6J strain AhR (Ema et al., 1992), *As*-AhR showed a high similarity (approximately 88.2%) of the amino acid sequence. Also, it shared 100% sequence identity in the basic helix-loop-helix (bHLH) motif (aa 36 - 82 for *As*-AhR and mouse AhR), and high sequence identity of 98 % in the Per-AhR/Arnt-Sim homology (PAS)-A and 95.2 % in the PAS-B domains (PAS-A, aa 130 - 186 for *As*-AhR, aa 130 - 182 for mouse AhR; PAS-B, aa 292 - 343 for *As*-AhR, aa 288 - 339 for mouse AhR). As for TAD (aa 384 – stop codon for *As*-AhR, aa 381 – stop codon for mouse AhR), the sequence homology between *As*-AhR and mouse AhR was 82.9 %.

As-AhR exhibited a variety of polymorphisms in the coding region. Seventy-one SNPs were found within 63 individuals that underwent sequencing. Forty-four of 71 SNPs were synonymous, while 27 non-synonymous changes produced 25 amino acid substitutions. The N-terminal half of *As*-AhR, aa 1 - 383 including bHLH and PAS domains, contained 27 SNPs and 8 amino acid substitutions. On the other hand, the C-terminal half of *As*-AhR, aa 384 - stop codon including TAD, had 44 SNPs and 17 amino acid substitutions. Variations of Gln repeats were found in TAD. Like the Japanese field mouse, such a large number of variations in a species living in the wild have never been reported. For example, the human AhR variation which was studied in various ethnic groups around the world had only four amino acid substitutions (Harper et al., 2002).

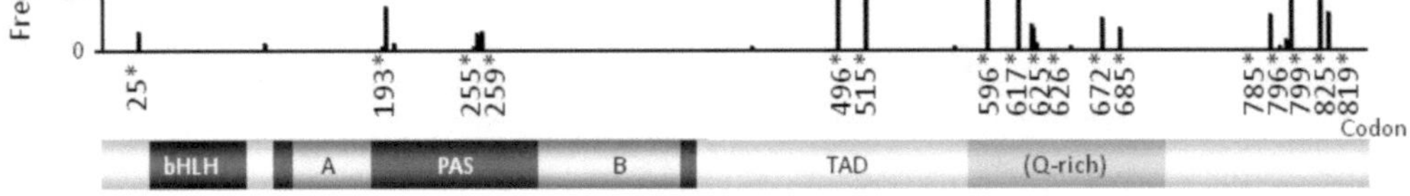

Fig. 4. Frequency of mutation
These bars indicate the number of mutations on the basis of major sequences among 63 individuals analyzed (126 *As*-AhR genes). Horizontal axis shows codon number of *As*-AhR. * indicates significant mutation site calculated by binominal test with probability 1/850 and Bonferroni correction

Next, to identify the key region for mutation in *As*-AhR, the frequencies of mutations at each codon were counted (Fig. 4). In the N-terminal half of AhR, genes which had a mutation at each codon were very few, although four sites showed a significant difference by binomial test. In TAD, many codons had a significantly higher mutation rate. In codon 596 having Gln repeats especially, the frequency of variation was the highest (88.1 %). The bHLH, PAS-A, and PAS-B regions that shared high sequence identity with mouse AhR revealed no amino acid variations (Fig. 4). These regions were highly conserved within and among species. In contrast, almost all amino acid substitutions were found in TAD and the region between PAS-A and -B. These results agree with previous studies on AhR variations among laboratory strains of rodent species (Hahn et al., 2004; Harper et al., 2002; Thomas et al., 2002). bHLH and PAS domains in the AhR may be under a physicochemical constraint that does not permit amino acid substitutions. Therefore, a mutation in these regions may potentially cause a critical change in protein function. On the other hand, a mutation in bHLH and PAS domains always implies extreme risk since these regions of AhR are essential for survival. In TAD, many mutations were observed and provided diversity of AhR. In *As*-AhR, nearly 70 % amino acid substitution was observed in TAD. The highest frequency of variation was Gln repeats at codon 596 in which 8 to 23 repeats of poly-Gln were found. Poly-Gln repeats encoded on DNA have been recognized as a medically important trigger because some neurological disorders were found to be associated with unstable expanded trinucleotide repeats, which are called trinucleotide repeat diseases, examples of which are fragile X syndrome and spinobulbar muscular atrophy. These diseases develop when the number of uninterrupted repeats exceeds a constant number and thereby lead to a worsening phenotype into subsequent generation by repeat expansion (Cummings & Zoghbi, 2000). On the other hand, the extended CAG repeats in androgen receptors (AR) have been known to prevent a decrease in sperm number and loss of DNA integrity that were caused by persistent organohalogen pollutant (POP) exposure as a beneficial effect of poly-Gln repeats in human male reproductive function (Giwercman et al., 2007). The expanding Gln repeats found in *As*-AhR might cause a functional change in activity of *As*-AhR protein, as suggested by trinucleotide repeat diseases and CAG repeats in AR gene.

2.2 Functional analysis of *As*-AhR polymorphism *in vitro*

To identify mutations that play a critical role in functional differences in *As*-AhR protein, we initially clarified functional domains altering protein activity by mutation. Comparison of the protein activity of *As*-AhR between the N-terminal and C-terminal regions by reporter assays revealed that mutations detected in the N-terminal region had no functional differences while mutations in the C-terminal region caused functional differences in protein activity (Ishiniwa et al., 2010). Therefore, we focused on polymorphisms in the C-terminal region including TAD which had a higher variation rate than the PAS region. We constructed expression plasmids fused to the C-terminal region (aa 423 to C-terminus) of 9 *As*-AhR alleles into the 3′ end of GAL4 DNA binding sequence (pGAL4DBD-*As*-AhR-TAD), which covered all 17 amino acid mutations detected in TAD. The transcriptional activity of the transactivation domain of AhR (*As*-AhR-TAD) was then measured (Fig. 5).

A significant difference in transactivation was observed among the *As*-AhR-TAD alleles (one-way ANOVA, $F=3.806$, $p=0.002$). Insertion of different numbers of Gln repeats into codon 596 had no apparent effect on the transactivation activity (Fig. 5). Also, comparison of alleles that showed higher and lower activity in reporter assay revealed a residue was common in three alleles which exhibited lower activity, allele 7, 8, and 9 (Fig. 5). The shared residue was arginine (Arg) at codon 799. On the other hand, other alleles, allele 1 to 6, which showed higher activity, shared glutamine (Gln) at codon 799. Therefore, we focused on the substitution at codon 799.

allele	Codon																	
	439	496	515	574	596Q	617	625	626	629	652	672	685	785	792	796	**799**	819	825
1	A	T	T	T	21	H	A	P	Q	N	E	T	P	G	P	**Q**	V	A
2	.	A	M	.	18	Q	.	.	.	D	.	.	H	D	.	.	L	.
3	.	E	.	.	9	Q	.	.	.	D	.	.	.	.	.	.	L	.
4	.	A	M	.	14	.	.	.	.	D	.	.	.	.	.	.	.	S
5	.	A	.	M	10	.	.	.	.	D	D	.	H	.	.	.	.	.
6	.	A	.	.	9	.	G	.	.	D	.	.	.	.	S	.	L	.
7	.	.	.	.	8	.	.	.	K	D	.	.	.	.	.	**R**	L	.
8	.	A	M	.	17	R	.	Q	.	D	.	.	.	.	.	**R**	.	.
9	T	A	M	.	12	.	.	.	.	D	.	A	.	.	.	**R**	.	.

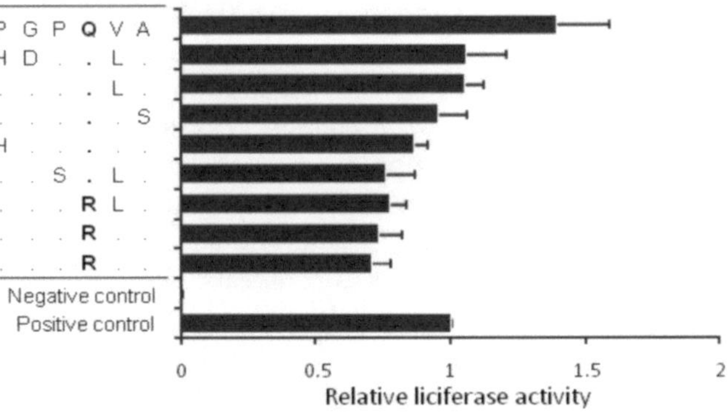

Fig. 5. Functional analysis of *As*-AhR-TAD *in vitro*
The left diagram shows the *As*-AhR-TAD alleles used in the functional analysis. A dot indicates the same residue as the top sequence. The numbers in the 596Q line show the Gln repeat number at codon 596. The right bars indicated the degree of transactivation mediated by *As*-AhR-TAD alleles. HeLa cells were transfected with pG5E-luc, pBOS-LacZ along with expression constructs for mouse AhR-TAD (Positive control), *As*-AhR-TAD, or no TAD (Negative control.; empty GAL4DBD vector). Luciferase activity was measured after 44 h. Relative luciferase activity was calculated by normalizing firefly luciferase activity to the control of mouse AhR-TAD. The values are expressed as the mean and standard error calculated from seven replicates (one-way ANOVA, p=0.002).

To compare the functional difference between Gln-799 and Arg-799 mutants in the same background, pBOS-HA-*As*-AhR-Gln-799 and Arg-799 were constructed and ligand-inducible luciferase expression was quantified. The reporter activity of Gln-799 showed significantly higher activity than Arg-799 (Fig. 6; t-test, p=0.015).
According to Ko et al. (1997), the mouse AhR-TAD can be divided into three subdomains: acidic-rich (aa 515 - 583), proline-rich (aa 643 - 740), and serine-rich (aa 726 - 805) regions. Similarly, the human AhR-TAD also contains three subdomains: an acidic subdomain (aa 500 - 600), a Q-rich subdomain (aa 600 - 713), and a P/S/T subdomain (aa 713 - 848) (Rowlands et al., 1996). In *As*-AhR-TAD, codon 799 is localized in a region orthologous to the serine-rich subdomain of mouse AhR-TAD and P/S/T subdomain of human AhR-TAD. Both of these subdomains act as a repression domain of AhR transactivation (Ko et al., 1997; Kumar et al., 2001). Although the protein structure of the AhR-TAD region is not yet fully understood, differences in the chemical properties between Gln and Arg might change the protein structure and interaction with coactivators, and result in repressive function in transcription. In summary, we succeeded in finding a critical point mutation in *As*-AhR that causes a functional difference in protein activity *in vitro*, which may be related to dioxin sensitivity.

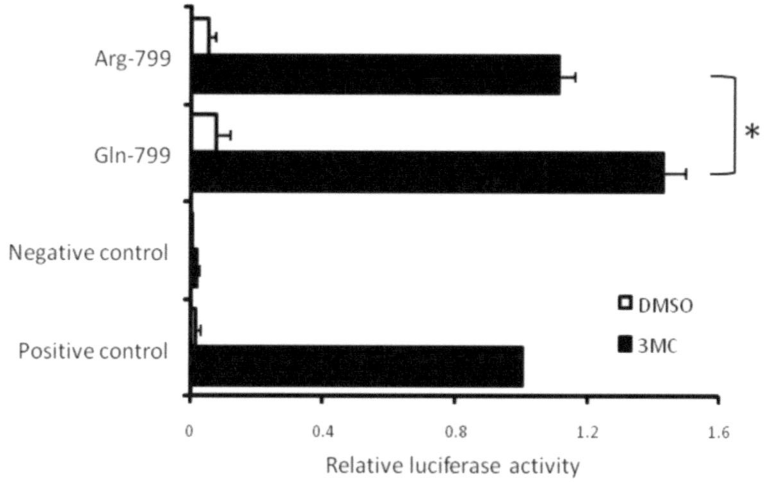

Fig. 6. Functional analysis of mutant AhR, Arg-799 and Gln-799
HeLa cells were transfected with pXREtk-Luc, mouse Arnt, and pBOS-LacZ along with expression constructs for mouse AhR; positive control, As-AhR (Arg-799 and Gln-799), or no AhR (negative control). Transfected cells were treated with DMSO or 3MC (3 mM final concentration), and luciferase activity was measured after 44 h. Relative luciferase activity was calculated by normalizing firefly luciferase activity to the control of mouse AhR. The values are expressed as the mean and standard error calculated from three replicates. A significant difference between mutant As-AhRs was detected by the t-test (*$p < 0.05$).

2.3 Functional analysis of *As*-AhR polymorphism *in vivo*

Does the mutation found *in vitro*, Gln and Arg at codon 799, cause differences in dioxin sensitivity *in vivo*? We examined this question by TCDD administration to Japanese field mice, whose genotype has been identified. Male mice (n=14) were divided into the two genotypes, Q/Q and R/R, by restriction fragment length polymorphism (RFLP) -PCR. TCDD was then administered orally by gastric sonde with an initial loading dose of 200 ng TCDD/kg body weight or an equivalent volume of sesame oil (vehicle) as control, followed by a weekly maintenance dose of 40 ng TCDD/kg body weight or an equivalent volume of sesame oil for three weeks. One week after the last exposure, male mice were deeply anesthetized with diethyl ether, and then the major organs including the testis, epididymis, and liver were removed.

The CYP1A1 mRNA expression level was measured in liver. Here, CYP1A1 was used as a marker enzyme to evaluate the toxic effects of dioxins because it has been reported that CYP1A1 was a sensitive dioxin induced gene (Hirakawa et al., 2007; Watanabe et al., 2005). In both genotypes, an increase in hepatic CYP1A1 mRNA expression was observed at a dose of 200/40 (Fig. 7). However, a comparison between genotypes showed that Q/Q was higher in CYP1A1 expression than R/R at doses of 200/40 ng/kg body weight and a significant difference in the expression between Q/Q and R/R was observed (Mann-Whitney U-test, $p<0.05$). Furthermore, we evaluated the reproductive effects caused by oxidative stress through the AhR-CYP1A1 pathway. In histological analysis, morphological abnormality and the number of single strand DNA breaks in the testis were not observed, while the number of spermatozoa in the epididymis showed a clear difference between genotypes.

Specifically, genotype Q/Q showed a 20 % reduction in the number of spermatozoa after TCDD exposure, while R/R showed no response (data not shown). In genotype Q/Q, the reduction of the number of spermatozoa was most likely due to the high activity of AhR protein observed in CYP1A1 expression. Meanwhile, reproduction in genotype R/R was not affected by TCDD exposure because the activity of AhR protein would be low, as shown in terms of CYP1A1 expression.

As a result, a single mutation at the gene level caused a difference in reproductive function between the two genotypes through an AhR mediated physiological response. Thus, genotype R/R was dioxin-resistant and Q/Q had high sensitivity, which indicates that the Japanese field mouse has a diverse TCDD sensitivity that is mediated by AhR. The mutation in *As*-AhR would be a useful indicator for making a decision about whether a mouse is susceptible or resistant to dioxin.

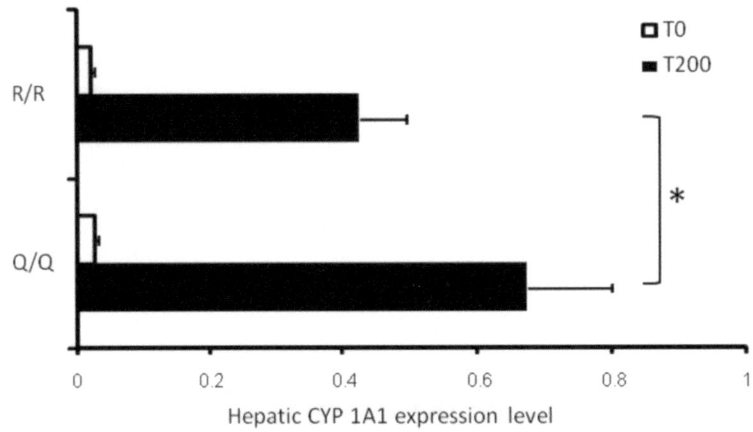

Fig. 7. Induction of CYP1A1 mRNA expression level in genotype Q/Q and R/R mouse
The animals were treated with 0 and 200 ng TCDD/kg as an initial dose followed by weekly maintenance doses of 0 and 40 ng TCDD/kg. The mRNA levels were corrected by β-actin expression. The values are expressed as the mean ± SE for 7 mice per treatment group. A significant difference between Q/Q and R/R at each exposure dose was detected by the U-test (*$P<0.05$)

3. Application of the critical mutation in *As*-AhR to field study

3.1 Overview of study sites

The sampling was conducted from 2003 to 2004 at six different sites in Japan. Four of six sites were chosen as dioxin-polluted sites. Sanwa (San) in Niigata Prefecture and Kunugi-yama (Kun) in Saitama Prefecture were near garbage incineration plants. Nagaoka (Nag) in Niigata Prefecture was located downstream of industrial waste disposal plants. Sakata (Sak) in Niigata Prefecture was a lagoon contaminated by an influx of agrichemicals. The remaining two sites, Kakuda (Kak) which is secondary forest located in Niigata Prefecture and Nukumidaira (Nuk) which is a primary beech forest in Yamagata Prefecture, were chosen as non-polluted background sites. At each site, the mice were captured using Sherman-type live traps baited with sunflower seeds and soil samples were obtained. A total of 92 mice were caught; 55 at polluted sites and 37 at non-polluted sites.

The dioxin concentrations in soil were 78.5 ± 2.3 pg-TEQ/g dw-ignition-loss (average ± standard error) in non-polluted sites (n=2) and 1140.6 ± 749.5 pg-TEQ/g dw-ignition-loss in polluted sites (n=4). The concentrations in liver were 411.6 ± 6.4 pg-TEQ/g-lipid in non-polluted sites (n=2) and 1847.3 ± 547.6 pg-TEQ/g-lipid in polluted sites (n=4). The CYP1A1 expression as physical reaction to dioxin pollution showed 0.05 ± 0.01 in non-polluted sites (n=37) and 0.11 ± 0.01 in polluted sites (n=55). These values are presented as levels of CYP1A1 mRNA relative to control. A significant difference in the CYP1A1 level was observed between polluted and non-polluted sites (Mann-Whitney U-test, p=0.007).

Polluted sites had higher dioxin levels in both soil and mice. Furthermore, higher CYP1A1 expression as a toxic reaction was observed in polluted sites. However, these chemical and physiological analytical results were not considered to represent the diversity of mouse sensitivity to dioxin. We decided to determine what would happen if these results were re-analyzed using AhR polymorphism as a molecular indicator.

3.2 Effects of dioxin pollution on the Japanese field mouse –Reanalysis using molecular indicator related to dioxin sensitivity-

To clarify differences in the response to dioxin exposure between dioxin-sensitive mice and dioxin-resistant mice, we divided the mice into three genotypes, Q/Q, Q/R, and R/R at codon 799 of *As*-AhR by RFLP-PCR. The CYP1A1 level in each genotype between non-polluted and dioxin-polluted sites was analyzed again. For genotype Q/Q, the Japanese field mice collected from polluted sites showed significantly higher CYP1A1 mRNA expression levels than those from non-polluted sites (Fig. 8, U-test, p=0.009). For genotype Q/R, mice from polluted sites showed higher CYP1A1 expression levels than those from non-polluted sites, although a significant difference was not observed. For genotype R/R, there was no difference between the two sites. Also, the difference in CYP1A1 mRNA expression level between polluted and non-polluted sites became smaller from genotype Q/Q to R/R (Fig. 8). The result which pooled data from all genotypes in section 3.1 was similar to the result for genotype Q/Q mice because both showed remarkable differences in CYP1A1 expression between non-polluted and polluted sites. Then, after calculating the frequency of each genotype at non-polluted and polluted sites, it was revealed that both sites were occupied by the genotypes Q/Q and Q/R (Fig. 9). At dioxin-polluted sites, genotype Q/Q constituted more than half of all individuals, while the frequency of genotype R/R was very low at both sites.

These results suggest that the difference in CYP1A1 expression level between non-polluted and polluted sites in pooled data of all genotypes was due to the proportion of genotype Q/Q and Q/R to the total population. In this study, the mice from dioxin-polluted sites were predominantly genotype Q/Q, which had a high sensitivity to dioxin, thereby revealing a critical difference between non-polluted and polluted sites. If genotype R/R is a major constituent member in mice from polluted sites, CYP1A1 expression levels will not appear to be so high, leading us to conclude that the mice were not exposed to dioxin exposure. Therefore, when comparing the toxic effect of dioxin exposure among various populations, information concerning population structure with respect to dioxin sensitivity is important for discussing the result because the implication of the response to dioxin exposure is different between mice that are susceptible and resistant to dioxin.

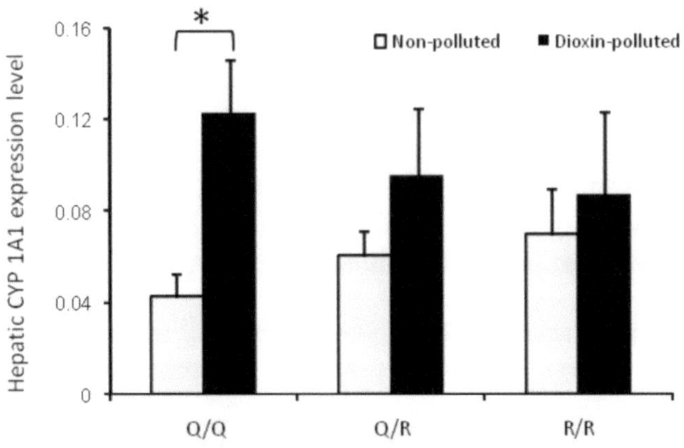

Fig. 8. Hepatic CYP1A1 mRNA expression level of Japanese field mice captured in non-polluted and polluted forests
Hepatic CYP1A1 mRNA expression levels were estimated by quantitative real-time RT-PCR analysis. The histogram represents relative levels of CYP1A1 to β-actin mRNA. The values are expressed as the mean ± standard error. Q/Q, Q/R, and R/R indicate the genotypes at codon 799 of As-AhR. A significant difference between non-polluted and polluted forests was detected by the U-test (* $p < 0.05$)

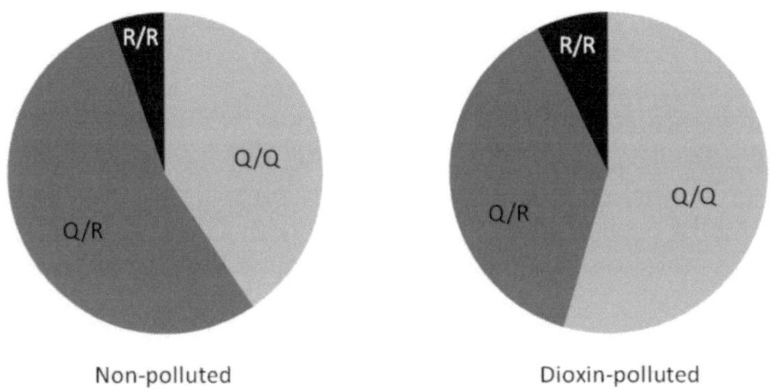

Fig. 9. Frequency of genotype Q/Q, Q/R, and R/R in dioxin polluted and non-polluted sites

4. Conclusion

In this chapter, we have described the toxic reaction to dioxin pollution in Japanese field mice based on their genetic background related to dioxin sensitivity. As a molecular indicator, we focused on the AhR gene, which plays an important role in dioxin-induced toxicity and consequently detected mutations, Q and R, at codon 799 in *As*-AhR that resulted in functional differences between alleles *in vitro* and *in vivo*. Mice with the Q allele showed high dioxin sensitivity, while those with the R allele showed resistance. Furthermore, we applied the mutation to wild mice and found that mice collected from dioxin-polluted sites exhibited a significantly higher toxic reaction than mice from non-polluted sites because mice from polluted sites were predominantly genotype Q/Q. AhR polymorphism was useful as an indicator for evaluating the effects of dioxin pollution on wildlife.

5. Acknowledgement

The authors gratefully acknowledge the editor and publishing process managers for giving us this opportunity and their generous support. We would also like to thank Professor Yukio Takahashi and Dr. Mizuki Sakai for their technical assistance with the HRGC-HRMS analysis for the determination of PCDD/Fs and PCBs concentrations. This study was supported by Grants-in-Aid for Scientific Research (B) (No. 18380089) and (C) (No. 16580119) from the Japan Society for the Promotion of Science. Reprinted from Ishiniwa, H.; Sogawa, K.; Yasumoto, K.; Sekijima, T., Polymorphisms and functional differences in aryl hydrocarbon receptors (AhR) in Japanese field mice, *Apodemus speciosus, in Environmental Toxicology and Pharmacology* vol. 29, pp. 280-289, Copyright (2010), with permission from Elsevier.

6. References

Baba, T.; Mimura, J.; Nakamura, N.; Harada, N.; Yamamoto, M.; Morohashi, K. & Fujii-Kuriyama, Y. (2005). Intrinsic function of the aryl hydrocarbon (dioxin) receptor as a key factor in female reproduction, *Molecular and cellular biology*, Vol.25, pp. 10040-10051, ISSN 0270-7306

Bello, S.M.; Franks, D.G.; Stegeman, J.J. & Hahn, M.E. (2001). Acquired resistance to Ah receptor agonists in a population of Atlantic Killifish (Fundulus heteroclitus) inhabiting a marine superfund site: in vivo and in vitro studies on the inducibility of xenobiotic metabolizing enzymes. *Toxicological Sciences*, Vol.60, pp.77-91, ISSN 1096-6080

Birnbaum L. S. & Tuomisto, J. (2000). Non-cancer effects of dioxins. *Food additives and contaminants*, Vol.17, pp.275–288, ISSN 0265-203X

Booth, R.E. & Grime, J.P. (2003). Effects of genetic impoverishment on plant community diversity. *The Journal of Ecology*, Vol.91, pp.721-730, ISSN 0022-0477

Butler, R.B.; Kelley, M.L.; Powell, W.H.; Hahn, M.E. & Van Beneden, R.J. (2001). An aryl hydrocarbon receptor homologue from the soft-shell clam, *Mya arenaria*: evidence that invertebrate AHR homologues lack TCDD and BNF binding. *Gene*, Vol.278, pp.223-234, ISSN 0378-1119

Coumailleau, P.; Poellinger, L.; Gustafsson, J.A. & Whitelaw, M.L. (1995). Difinition of a minimal domain of the dioxin receptor that is associated with Hsp90 and maintains wild type ligand binding affinity and specificity. *The Journal of Biological chemistry*, Vol.270, pp.25291-25300, ISSN 0021-9258

Cummings, C.J. & Zoghbi, H.Y. (2000). Trinucleotide repeats: mechanisms and pathophysiology. *Annual Review of Genomics and Human Genetics*, Vol.1, pp.281-328, ISSN 1527-8204

Dalton T.P.; Puga, A. & Shertzer H.G. (2002). Induction of cellular oxidative stress by aryl hydrocarbon receptor activation. *Chemico-Biological Interactions*, Vol.141, pp.77-95, ISSN 0009-2797

Davarinos, N.A. & Pollenz, R.S. (1999). Aryl hydrocarbon receptor imported into the nucleus following ligand binding is rapidly degraded via the cytosplasmic proteasome following nuclear export. *The Journal of Biological Chemistry*, Vol.274, pp.28708-28715, ISSN 0021-9258

de Roode, J.C.; Pansini, R.; Cheesman, S.J.; Helinski, M.E.H.; Huijben, S.; Wargo, A.R.; Bell, A.S.; Chan, B.H.K., Walliker, D. & Read, A.F. (2005), Virulence and competitive ability in genetically diverse malaria infections. *Proceedings of the National Academy of Science of the United States of America*, Vol.102, pp.7264-7628, ISSN 0027-8424

Denison, M.S.; Fisher, J.M. & Whitlock Jr., J.P. (1988). The DNA recognition site for the dioxin-Ah receptor complex. Nucleotide sequence and functional analysis. *The Journal of Biological Chemistry*, Vol.263, pp.17221-17224, ISSN 0021-9258

Elferink, C.J.; Gasiewicz, T.A. & Whitlock, Jr. J.P. (1990) Protein-DNA interactions at a dioxin-responsive enhancer. Evidence that the transformed Ah receptor is heteromeric. *The Journal of Biological Chemistry*, Vol.265, pp.27078-27012, ISSN 0021-9258

Ema, M.; Ohe, N.; Suzuki, M.; Mimura, J.; Sogawa, K.; Ikawa, S. & Fujii-Kuriyama, Y. (1994). Dioxin binding activities of polymorphic forms of mouse and human arylhydrocarbon receptors. *The Journal of Biological Chemistry*, Vol.269, pp.27337-27343, ISSN 0021-9258

Ema, M.; Sogawa, K.; Watanabe, N.; Chujoh, Y.; Matsushita, N.; Gotoh, O.; Funae, Y. & Fujii-Kuriyama, Y. (1992). cDNA cloning and structure of mouse putative Ah receptor. *Biochemical and Biophysical Research Communications*, Vol.184, pp.246-253, ISSN 0006-291X

Enan, E.; Overstreet, J.W.; Matsumura, F.; VandeVoort C.A. & Lasley B.L. (1996). Gender differences in the mechanism of dioxin toxicity in rodents and in nonhuman primates. *Reproductive Toxicology*, Vol.10, pp.401-411, ISSN 0890-6238

Fernandez-Salguero, P.; Pineau, T.; Hilbert, D.M.; McPhail, T.; Lee, S.S.; Kimura, S.; Nebert, D.W.; Rudikoff, S.; Ward, J.M. & Gonzalez, F.J. (1995). Immune system impairment and hepatic fibrosis in mice lacking the dioxin-binding Ah receptor. *Science*, Vol.268, pp.722-726, ISSN 0036-8075

Fujisawa-Sahara, A.; Yamane, M. & Fujii-Kuriyama, Y. (1988). A DNA-binding factor specific for xenobiotic responsive elements of P-450c gene exists as a cryptic form in cytoplasm: Its possible translocation to nucleus. *Proceedings of the National Academy of Science of the United States of America*, Vol.85, pp.5859-5863, ISSN 0027-8424

Fujisawa-Sehara, A.; Sogawa, K.; Yamane M. & Fujii-Kuriyama, Y. (1987). Characterization of xenobiotic responsive elements upstream from the drug-metabolizing cytochrome P-450c gene: a similarity to glucocorticoid regulatory elements. *Nucleic Acids Research*, Vol.15, pp.4179-4191, ISSN 0305-1048

Fukuzawa, N.H.; Ohsako, S.; Wu, Q.; Sakaue, M.; Fujii-Kuriyama, Y.; Baba, T. & Tohyama, C. (2004). Testicular cytochrome P450scc and LHR as possible targets of 2,3,7,8-tetrachlorodibenzo-p-dioxin (TCDD) in the mouse. *Molecular and Cellular Endochrinology*, Vol.221, pp.87-96, ISSN 0303-7207

Giwercman, A.; Rylander, L.; Rignell-Hydbom, A.; Jönsson, B.A.G.; Pedersen, H.S.; Ludwicki, J.K.; Lesovoy, V.; Zvyezday, V.; Spano, M.; Manicardi, G.C.; Bizzaro, D.; Bonefeld-Jørgensen, E.C.; Toft, G.; Bonde, J.P.; Giwercman, C.; Tiido, T.; Giwercman, Y.L. & INUENDO. (2007). Androgen receptor gene CAG repeat length as a modifier of the association between persistent organohalogen pollutant exposure markers and semen characteristics. *Pharmacogenetics and Genomics*, Vol.17, pp.391-401, ISSN 1744-6872

Gu, Y.Z.; Hogenesch, J.B. & Bradfield, C.A. (2000). The PAS superfamily: Sensors of environmental and developmental signals. *Annual Review of Pharmacology and Toxicology*, Vol.40, pp.519-561, ISSN 0362-1642

Hahn, M.E. (2002). Aryl hydrocarbon receptors: diversity and evolution. *Chemico-Biological Interactions*, Vol.141, pp.131-160, ISSN 0009-2797

Hahn, M.E.; Karchner, S.I.; Franks, D.G. & Merson, R.R. (2004). Aryl hydrocarbon receptor polymorphisms and dioxin resistance in Atlantic killifish (Fundulus heteroclitus). *Pharmacogenetics and Genomics*, Vol.14, pp.131-143, ISSN 1744-6872

Hansson, M.C. & Hahn, M.E. (2008). Functional properties of the four Atlantic Salmon (*Salmo Salar*) aryl hydrocarbon receptor type 2 (AHR2) isoforms. *Aquatic Toxicology*, Vol.86, pp.121-130, ISSN 0166-445X

Harper, P.A.; Wong, J.M.Y.; Lam, M.S.M. & Okey, A.B. (2002). Polymorphisms in the human AH receptor. *Chemico-Biological Interactions*, Vol.141, pp.161-187, ISSN 0009-2797

Hirakawa, S.; Iwata, H.; Takeshita Y.; Kim, E.Y.; Sakamoto, T.; Okajima, Y.; Amano, M.; Miyazaki, N.; Petrov, E.A. & Tanabe, S. (2007). Molecular characterization of cytochrome P450 1A1, 1A2, and 1B1, and effects of polychlorinated dibenzo-p-dioxin, dibenzofuran, and biphenyl congeners on their hepatic expression in Baikal Seal (Pusa sibirica). *Toxicological Sciences*, Vol.97, pp.318-335, ISSN 1096-6080

Hoffman, D.J.; Melancon, M.J.; Klein, P.N.; Eisemann, J.D.; Spann, J.W. (1998). Comparative developmental toxicity of planar polychlorinated biphenyl congeners in chickens, American kestrels, and common terns. *Environmental toxicology and chemistry*, Vol.17, pp.747-757, ISSN 0730-7268

Holsapple, M.P.; Snyder N.K.; Wood S.C. & Morris D.L. (1991). A review of 2,3,7,8-tetrachlorodibenzo-p-dioxin-induced changes in immunocompetence: 1991 update. *Toxicology*, Vol.69, pp.219-255, ISSN 0300-483X

Ishiniwa, H.; Sogawa, K.; Yasumoto, K. & Sekijima, T. (2010). Polymorphisms and functional differences in aryl hydrocarbon receptor(AhR) in Japanese field mice, *Apodemus speciosus*. *Environmental Toxicology and Pharmacolgy*, Vol.29, pp.280-289, ISSN 1382-6689

Karchner S.I.; Franks D.G.; Kennedy S.W.; Hahn M.E. (2006). The molecular basis for differential dioxin sensitivity in birds: Role of the aryl hydrocarbon receptor. *Proceedings of the National Academy of Sciences of the United States of America*, Vol.103, pp.6252-6257, ISSN 1091-6490

Kim, D.W.; Gazourian, L.; Quadri, S.A.; Romieu-Mourez, R.; Sherr D.H. & Sonenshein, G.E. (2000). The RelA NF-κB subunit and the aryl hydrocarbon receptor (AhR) cooperate to transactivate the c-myc promoter in mammary cells. *Oncogene*, Vol.19, pp.5498-5506, ISSN 0950-9232

Kleeman J.M.; Olson J.R. & Peterson R.E. (1988). Species differences in 2,3,7,8-tetrachlorodibenzo-p-dioxin toxicity and biotransformation in fish. *Fundamental and Applied Toxicology*, Vol.10, pp.206-213, ISSN 0272-0590

Ko, H.P.; Okino, S.T.; Ma, Q. & Whitlock, J.P. Jr. (1997). Transactivation domains facilitate promoter occupancy for the dioxin-inducible CYP1A1 gene in vivo. *Molecular and Cellular Biology*, Vol.17, pp.3497-3507, ISSN 0270-7306

Kron, P. & Husband, B.C. (2006). The effects of pollen diversity on plant reproduction: Insights from apple. *Sexual plant reproduction*, Vol.19, pp.125-131, ISSN 0934-0882

Kumar, M.B.; Ramadoss, P.; Reen, R.K.; Vanden-Heuvel, J.P. & Perdew, G.H. (2001). The Q-rich subdomain of the human Ah receptor transactivation domain is required for dioxin-mediated transcriptional activity. *The Journal of Biological Chemistry*, Vol.276, pp.42302-42310, ISSN 0021-9258

Latchoumycandane, C.; Chitra, K.C. & Mathur, P.P. (2002). Induction of oxidative stress in rat epididymal sperm after exposure to 2,3,7,8-tetrachlorodibenzo-p-dioxin. *Archives of Toxicology*, Vol.76, pp.113-118, ISSN 0340-5761

Lees, M.J. & Whitelaw, M.L. (1999). Multiple roles of ligand in transforming the dioxin receptor to an active basic Helix-Loop-Helix/PAS transcription factor complex with the nuclear protein Arnt. *Molecular and Cellular Biology*, Vol.19, pp5811-5822, ISSN 0270-7306

Lorenzen, A.; Shutt, J.L.; Kennedy, S.W. (1997). Sensitivity of common tern (Sterna hirundo) embryo hepatocyte cultures to CYP1A induction and porphyrin accumulation by halogenated aromatic hydrocarbons and common tern egg extracts. *Archives of Environmental Contamination and Toxicology*, Vol.32, pp.126-134, ISSN 0090-4341

Masunaga, S.; Takasuga, T. & Nakanishi, J. (2001). Dioxin and dioxin-like PCB impurities in some Japanese agrochemical formulations. *Chemosphere*, Vol.44, pp.873-885, ISSN 0045-6535

Masunaga, S.; Yao, Y.; Ogura, I.; Sakurai, T.;& Nakanishi, J. (2003). Source and behavior analyses of dioxins based on congener-specific information and their application to Tokyo Bay basin. *Chemosphere*, Vol.53, pp.315-324, ISSN 0045-6535

Matsumura, F. (2009). The significance of the nongenomic pathway in mediating inflammatory signaling of the dioxin-activated Ah receptor to cause toxic effects. *Biochemical Pharmacology*, Vol.77, pp.608-626, ISSN 0006-2952

Ministry of the Environment Government of Japan, (2008). Bioaccumulation and exposure of dioxins and research result of bromo-dioxins in 2006. Report of dioxin accumulation on wildlife. (in Japanese)

Nebert, D.W.; Roe, A.L.; Dieter, M.Z.; Solis, W.A.; Yang, Y. & Dalton, T.P. (2000). Role of the aromatic hydrocarbon receptor and [Ah] gene battery in the oxidative stress response, cell cycle control, and apoptosis. *Biochemical Pharmacology*, Vol.59, pp.65-85, ISSN 0006-2952

Nohara, K.; Fujimaki, H.; Tsukumo, S.; Inouye, K.; Sone, H. & Tohyama, C. (2002). Effects of 2,3,7,8-tetrachlorodibenzo-p-dioxin (TCDD) on T cell-derived cytokine production in ovalbumin (OVA)-immunized C57BL/6 mice. *Toxicology*, Vol.172, pp.49-58, ISSN 0300-483X

Ohtake, F.; Baba, A.; Takada, I.; Okada, M.; Iwasaki, K.; Miki, H.; Takahashi, S.; Kouzmenko, A.; Nohara, K.; Chiba, T.; Fujii-Kuriyama, Y. & Kato, S. (2007). Dioxin receptor is a ligand-dependent E3 ubiquitin ligase. *Nature*, Vol.446, pp.562-566, ISSN 0028-0836

Ohtake, F.; Takeyama, K.; Matsumoto, T.; Kitagawa, H.; Yamamoto, Y.; Nohara, K.; Tohyama, C.; Krust, A.; Mimura, J.; Chambon, P.; Yanagisawa, J.; Fujii-Kuriyama, Y. & Kato, S. (2003). Modulation of oestrogen receptor signalling by association with the activated dioxin receptor. *Nature*, Vol.423, pp.545-550, ISSN 0028-0836

Pearman, P.B. & Garner, T.W.J. (2005). Susceptibility of Italian agile frog population to an emerging strain of *Ranavirus* parallels population genetic diversity. *Ecology Letters*, Vol.8, pp. 401-408, ISSN 1461-0248

Pohjanvirta, R. & Tuomisto, J. (1994). Short-term toxicity of 2,3,7,8-tetrachlorodibenzo-p-dioxin in laboratory animals: effects, mechanisms, and animal models. *Pharmacological Reviews*, Vol.46, pp.483-549, ISSN 0031-6997

Pohjanvirta, R.; Unkila, M. & Tuomisto, J. (1993). Comparative acute lethality of 2,3,7,8-tetrachlorodibenzo-p-dioxin (TCDD), 1,2,3,7,8-pentachlorodibenzo-p-dioxin and 1,2,3,4,7,8-hexachlorodibenzo-p-dioxin in the most TCDD-susceptible and the most TCDD-resistant rat strain. *Pharmacology & Toxicology*, Vol.73, pp.52-56, ISSN 0901-9928

Pohjanvirta, R.; Wong, J.M.Y.; Li, W.; Harper, P.A.; Tuomisto, J. & Okey, A.B. (1998). Point mutation in intron sequence causes altered carboxyl-terminal structure in the aryl hydrocarbon receptor of the most 2,3,7,8-tetrachlorodibenzo-p-dioxin-resistant rat strain. *Molecular Pharmacology*, Vol.54, pp.86-93, ISSN 0026-895X

Poland, A. & Knutson, J.C. (1982). 2,3,7,8-tetrachlorodibenzo-p-dioxin and related halogenated aromatic hydrocarbons: examination of the mechanism of toxicity. *Annual Review of Pharmacology and Toxicology*, Vol.22, pp.517-554, ISSN 0362-1642

Puga, A.; Xia, Y. & Elferink, C. (2002). Role of the aryl hydrocarbon receptor in cell cycle regulation. *Chemico- Biological Interactions*, Vol.141, pp.117-130, ISSN 0009-2797

Quintana, F.J.; Basso, A.S.; Iglesias, A.H.; Korn, T.; Farez, M.F.; Bettelli, E.; Caccamo, M.; Oukka, M. & Weiner, H.L. (2008). Control of Treg and T_H17 cell differentiation by the aryl hydrocarbon receptor. *Nature*, Vol.453, pp65-71, ISSN 0028-0836

Reusch, T.B.H.; Ehlers, A.; Haemmerli, A. & Worm, B. (2005). Ecosystem recovery after climatic extremes enhanced by genotypic diversity. *Proceedings of the National Academy of Science of the United States of America*, Vol.102, pp.2826-2831, ISSN 0027-8424

Rowlands, J.C.; McEwan, I.J. & Gustafsson, J.A. (1996). Trans-activation by the human aryl hydrocarbon receptor and aryl hydrocarbon receptor nuclear translocator proteins: direct interactions with basal transcription factors. *Molecular Pharmacology*, Vol.50, pp.538-548, ISSN 0026-895X

Sogawa, K. & Fujii-Kuriyama, Y. (1997). Ah receptor, a novel ligand-activated transcription factor. *The Journal of Biochemistry*, Vol.122, pp.1075-1079, ISSN 0021-924X

Sogawa, K.; Iwabuchi, K.; Abe, H. & Fujii-Kuriyama, Y. (1995). Transcriptional activation domains of the Ah receptor and Ah receptor nuclear translocator. *Journal of Cancer Research and Clinical Oncology*, Vol.121, pp.612-620, ISSN 0171-5216

Stellman, J.M.; Stellman, S.D.; Christian, R.; Weber, T. & Tomasallo, C. (2003). The extent and patterns of usage of Agent Orange and other herbicides in Vietnam. *Nature*, Vol.422, pp681-687, ISSN 0028-0836

Stevens, E.A.; Mezrich J.D. & Bradfield, C.A. (2009). The aryl hydrocarbon receptor: a perspective on potential roles in the immune system. *Immunology*, Vol.127, pp.299-311, ISSN 0019-2805

Taylor, B.L. & Zhulin, I.B. (1999). PAS domains: Internal sensors of oxygen, redox potential, and light. *Microbiology and Molecular Biology Reviews*, Vol.63, pp.479-506, ISSN 1092-2172

Thomas, R.S.; Penn, S.G.; Holden, K.; Bradfield, C.A. & Rank, D.R. (2002). Sequence variation and phylogenetic history of the mouse Ahr gene. *Pharmacogenetics and Genomics*, Vol.12, pp.151-163, ISSN 1744-6872

Vos, J.G.; Dybing, E.; Greim, H.A.; Ladefoged, O.; Lambre, G.; Tarazona, J.V.; Brandt, I. & Vethaak, A.D. (2000). Health effects of endocrine-disrupting chemicals on wildlife, with special reference to the European situation. *Critical Reviews in Toxicology*, Vol.30, pp.71-133, ISSN 1040-8444

Watanabe, M.X.; Iwata, H.; Okamoto, M.; Kim, E.Y.; Yoneda, K.; Hashimoto, T. & Tanabe, S. (2005). Induction of cytochrome P450 1A5 mRNA, protein and enzymatic activities by dioxin-like compounds, and congener-specific metabolism and sequestration in the liver of wild jungle crow (*Corvus macrorhynchos*) from Tokyo, Japan. *Toxicological Sciences*, Vol.88, pp.384-399, ISSN 1096-6080

Weber R.; Gaus, C.; Tysklind, M.; Johnston, P.; Forter, M.; Hollert, H.; Heinisch, E.; Holoubek, I.; Lloyd-Smith, M.; Masunaga, S.; Moccarelli, P.; Santillo, D.; Seike, N.; Symons, R.; Torres, J.P.M.; Verta, M.; Varbelow, G.; Vijgen, J.; Watson, A.; Costner, P.; Woelz, J.; Wycisk, P. & Zennegg, M. (2008). Dioxin- and POP-contaminated sites - contemporary and future relevance and challenges. *Environmental Science and Pollution Research*, Vol. 15, pp.363-393, ISSN 0944-1344

Yasuda, M.; Yamada, F.; Kawaji, N.; Okochi, I.; Yamazaki, K.; Nakajima, M.; Ishizuka, T.; Takasuga, T. & Kumar, K.S. (2003). Concentration of POPs in wildlife from central Japan. Abstracts of 12th Symposium on Environmental Chemistry, pp.448-449. (in Japanese)

Yasui, T.; Kim, E.Y.; Iwata, H.; Franks, D.G.; Karchner, S.I.; Hahn, M.E. & Tanabe, S. (2007). Functional characterization and evolutionary history of two aryl hydrocarbon receptor isoforms (AhR1 and AhR2) from avian species. *Toxicological Science*, Vol.99, pp.101-117, ISSN 1096-6080

Yoshida, K. & Nakanishi, J. (2003). Estimation of dioxin risk of Japanese from the past to the future. *Chemosphere*, Vol.53, pp.427-436. ISSN 0045-6535

5

Anti-RhD-Mediated Immunosuppression: Can Monoclonal Antibodies Imitate the Action of Polyclonal Antibodies?

Natalia Olovnikova
Hematology Research Center, Laboratory for Physiology of Hematopoiesis, Moscow Russia

1. Introduction

Passively administered IgG antibodies can temporary prevent the antibody response to the corresponding antigen. This phenomenon of antibody-mediated immune suppression has been successfully applied in clinical practice: administration of polyclonal anti-RhD immunoglobulin to Rh-negative women during and after pregnancy is a very effective measure for the preventing D immunization by D-positive fetal red blood cells and, as a result, the hemolytic disease of the next D-positive fetus or newborn. Anti-D immunoglobulin is derived from sera of immune donors. Plenty of human monoclonal and recombinant anti-D antibodies have been obtained around the world and some of them have passed initial stages of clinical trials; however, none of the monoclonal preparations can be used as a surrogate for polyclonal ones. Evaluation has revealed the two major obstacles that limit the development of an effective monoclonal preparation. They are a low clinical activity of monoclonal anti-D and the lack of a suitable cell line-producer that will be able to provide a "correct" glycosylation of monoclonal antibodies.

Despite a long period of anti-Rh immunoglobulin application we still fail to determine a precise list of the cellular and molecular participants involved in the mechanism for immunosuppression. To date, the overwhelming evidence points to the key role of immune complexes and the peculiarities of their interaction with Fcgamma-receptors (FcγR) on immune cells. The most convincing is the mechanism for a temporal switch-off of the immune response to the antigen due to co-ligation by immune complexes of the B cell receptor and inhibitory low-affinity receptor FcγRIIB on specific B cells (effect of clonal silencing). We investigated *in vitro* into the interaction of human monoclonal anti-D antibodies with different types of FcγR, as well as into the molecular structure of genes of anti-D antibodies and the composition of the sugar which, as known, does exert a significant influence on the efficiency of interaction between the antibody Fc fragment and FcγR. We have received a series of anti-D antibody counterparts and shown that the effector function crucially varies depending on the nature of the host cells. The original research data provide information valuable for developing a strategy of creation of monoclonal drugs with anti-inflammatory properties; moreover, they may help with clarifying some still elusive aspects of regulation of the humoral immune response in general. The data obtained make it possible to speculate that the immunosuppressive activity of polyclonal antibodies and inability of peripheral B cells to produce antibodies with a similar property may be attributed to the fact that B cells of different subpopulations secrete antibodies with different functional properties. According to the hypothesis proposed here, only long-lived plasma cells are able to synthesize anti-inflammatory immunosuppressive antibodies that are an essential element of the feedback regulation of antibody production.

2. Prevention of D sensitization: Clinical application of antibody-mediated antigen-specific immunosuppression

Prevention of RhD-sensitization - a mandatory procedure in obstetrics now - is currently the only example of a conventional clinical application of antibody-mediated antigen-specific immune suppression. This procedure involves administration of anti-D immunoglobulin to Rh-negative women after delivery of an Rh-positive infant and is required for prophylaxis of the Rh hemolytic disease of the next Rh-positive fetus and newborn.

The erythrocyte D antigen determines the Rh phenotype of human blood: individuals with D are Rh-positive, those without D are Rh-negative. The D antigen is highly immunogenic and present in part of population (about 85% of the European ethnicity are D positive), which creates conditions for incompatible transfusions and immunization of Rh-negative women with fetal D positive (D+) red cells during or after pregnancy. Despite a very small volume of the fetal blood that enters a maternal organism during pregnancy or delivery (it is less than 1 ml at uncomplicated delivery), this amount is quite sufficient for about 16% of Rh negative women to be immunized after their first ABO-compatible Rh-positive pregnancy (Bowman, 1988). During next pregnancies immune anti-D IgG antibodies cross the placenta and destroy fetal D positive red cells, provoking a severe pathology of the fetus /newborn - hemolytic disease. About 10% of neonatal deaths were due to hemolytic disease of the newborn before the era of immunoprophylaxis had begun (Bowman, 2003).

The idea to apply anti-D antibodies for the prevention of D-sensitization was experimentally supported in the 1950s-60s by several groups of researchers. By that time, it had been known from clinical observations that the ABO incompatibility of an Rh-positive fetus with its Rh-negative mother could reduce the incidence of D-immunization (Levin, 1943). It was assumed that suppression might be related to the destruction of D+ red cells by natural anti-A or anti-B antibodies, as well as to their fast clearance in liver before they reached immunocompetent sites. This clinical observation was experimentally checked, and the experiment proved that the ABO incompatibility did provide a partial protection against D sensitization (Stern et al., 1956). The same study also demonstrated that the injection into Rh-negative men of Rh-positive red cells coated *in vitro* with anti-D antibodies was completely ineffective in inducing the anti-D immune response. Based on these findings, a group of British researchers from Liverpool carried out a study when D-negative volunteers were given an injection of D+ red cells followed by anti-D immune serum and showed that IgM anti-D was ineffective, whereas anti-D IgG had a high protective effectiveness (Clarke et al., 1963). At the same time, similar studies were undertaken in New York; however, their theoretical rationale was different (Freda et al., 1964; Gorman et al., 1966). The authors decided to apply a phenomenon that was described by the first Nobel Prize Laureate in Physiology or Medicine Emil Adolf von Behring over 100 years ago (von Behring, 1892) and is currently called the antibody-mediated immune suppression (AMIS). This phenomenon is based on the ability of antisera to the antigen to suppress the immune response to this antigen after their simultaneous administration. A specific antibody injected passively, either with its antigen or separately, has been found to prevent the active immunity that follows injections of the antigen alone in many different antigen-antibody systems in various species of animals, including humans. Suppression of the immune response to sheep red cells in rabbits and mice by antiserum or monoclonal antibodies against sheep red cells is a classical example of AMIS (Heyman & Wigzell, 1984). Based on the AMIS phenomenon, it could be expected that anti-D antibodies introduced simultaneously with D+ red cells would also block the anti-D immune response. The remarkable result of the studies on both sides of the Atlantic and following successful clinical trials resulted in that prevention of D sensitization with anti-D immunoglobulin became a mandatory procedure in obstetrics, thus turning the hemolytic disease of the newborn into a rare pathology in developed countries (Bowman, 1988; 2003). At present, every D-negative unimmunized woman must be given one prophylactic dose of anti-D immunoglobulin (the dose ranges from 150 to 300 mcg of anti-D in different countries) after the delivery of a D-positive infant, irrespective of the ABO blood group of the infant.

The most striking characteristic of a polyclonal anti-D preparation is its ability to induce a fast clearance of D+ red cells and their sequestration in the spleen (Mollison et al., 1965). Unlike the liver where red cells are sequestered after exposure to natural anti-A and anti-B antibodies, spleen is an organ of the active immune response; nevertheless, D+ red cells entering this lymphoid organ do not cause sensitization but, instead, lead to the suppression of the immune response. Anti-D immunoglobulin is able to prevent the primary anti-D response, but it is ineffective or low effective in the case of the secondary response (Tovey & Robinson, 1975; de Silva et al, 1985). Despite a long history of anti-D immunoglobulin usage we still fail to fully understand which of the two assumptions - fast clearance or AMIS - is closer to the truth and what particular process (or a set of processes) is crucial and leads to immunosuppression. The answer to this question may be interesting not only from the general scientific standpoint but is also essential in terms of its practical usage. Widespread prophylaxis of D-sensitization requires a large amount of preparation that is administered not only after delivery, but also in the last trimester of pregnancy, after abortion, after therapeutic and diagnostic amniocentesis and other episodes of transplacental hemorrhage. Anti-D immunoglobulin is produced by isolating the IgG fraction from pooled immune donor plasma. Obviously, the development of biotechnologies for obtaining monoclonal anti-D human antibodies has generated great optimism and expectations that the alternative source for the anti-D immunoglobulin production may be found. So, what is the reason for why the effective monoclonal anti-D is not yet developed, while a whole range of therapeutic monoclonal antibodies of other specificities is now used in oncology, rheumatology, etc.?

3. The mechanism for antibody mediated immune suppression

Some mechanisms are proposed to clarify the phenomenon of AMIS; among the most discussed are the following:

- the mechanism of antigen camouflage, that is, masking of antigen determinants due to the excessive dose of antibodies;
- a fast clearance of the antigen-antibody complex before it can activate specific B cells;
- a selective suppression of antigen specific B cells and lack of anti-D antibody production.

While the first mechanism does not require Fc fragments of antibodies for its work, and masking of antigens can be induced by the Fab parts of antibodies, the other two

mechanisms depend on the properties of the Fc fragments of immunoglobulins and the type of their interplay with Fc receptors. The effect of a large number of immune preparations is mainly based on the bipolarity of antibodies, that is, the ability of the antigen-binding site of antibodies to bind to a relevant antigen and the ability of the Fc fragment to mediate both recognition of the antigen-antibody complex by the immunocompetent effector cells bearing Fcγ receptors and elimination of these complexes from the organism.
What arguments are there "pro" and "contra" the involvement of the above mechanisms in AMIS and preventing anti-D sensitization?

3.1 The mechanism of antigen camouflage

Investigations of the primary immune response to the antigen in the presence of antibodies to this antigen used excessive dose of antibodies usually sufficient for binding all antigen determinants. "The determination of which effect of antibody will predominate probably depends on many factors, but if large amounts of antibody with high binding affinity are employed, suppression will usually occur" (Uhr & Möller, 1968). AMIS in transgenic mice lacking the known receptors for IgG (the fact that initially raised much confusion since the involvement of FcγR in regulation of the immune response had been thought unquestionable by that time) can most likely be accounted for by the masking of antigen (Heyman, 1999). The data indicating that F(ab)2 fragments as well as IgE are efficient suppressors of antibody responses in FcγR–deficient mice argue in favor of the antigen masking (Karlsson et al., 1999; Karlsson et al., 2001).
Interestingly, we accidentally found the masking effect of anti-D monoclonal antibodies during clinical trails of their efficacy (Olovnikova et al., 2000). One of the anti-D IgG1 monoclonal antibodies, G17, administered at the same dose as the other anti-D demonstrated the unique capability of binding *in vivo* the maximum D sites and making D+ red cells fully saturated. It was not possible to stain red cells sensitized *in vivo* by either other monoclonal or polyclonal anti-D antibodies. Irrespective of this property, G17 poorly accelerated the clearance of D+ red cells from the circulation in D-negative individuals, so we observed sensitized D+ red cells in the blood of the individuals during several months. None of the 5 subjects who had received G17 produced anti-D within 6 months; however, three in this group showed the secondary immune response after rechallenge with D+ red cells. Studies of AMIS, in FcR-deficient mice including, are often limited to investigations of the primary immune response (Heyman, 2000); meanwhile, it is quite possible that the results similar to ours may be obtained in the case of reimmunization.
These findings strongly suggest that IgG is able to efficiently suppress antibody response independently of the Fc part and argue in favor of an important role of antigen masking under some experimental conditions. However, the mechanism of antigen masking can not be relevant to explanation of the anti-D immune suppression since only about 10% of D antigen sites are found to be occupied after administration of an effective dose of a polyclonal or monoclonal anti-D antibodies. Moreover, approximately 200 anti-D IgG molecules per erythrocyte are sufficient to effectively suppress the anti-D immune response (Kumpel et al., 1995; 2006). It was shown that Fab can not prevent the anti-D immune response (Nicholas, 1969). The ability of antibodies to one blood group antigen to suppress the immune response to the other blood group antigen simultaneously expressing on the red cell also can not be accounted for by the mechanism of antigen blocking. For example, polyclonal IgG anti-K (Kell system antigen) was shown to prevent immunization against both K and D antigens after immunization of Rh-negative K-negative individuals with

D+K+ red cells (Woodrow et al., 1975). It is known that IgG can induce nonepitope-specific suppression; however, the effect requires a high epitope density (Heyman & Wigzell, 1984). D and K antigens have a relatively low density (approximately 20,000 molecules per erythrocyte), their positions in the membrane are not related to each other; this is the reason for why inhibition of the anti-D response by anti-K antibodies can not be explained simply by steric screening of D epitopes.

3.2 Fcγ receptors and assays for evaluation of the functional properties of anti-D antibodies

The immune response of an organism to a foreign agent is the process of activation and development of the system of specific protection, that is, recognition, neutralization, destruction and elimination of the foreign object. When antibodies form a complex with a soluble or membrane antigen, they activate the effector cells and molecules that destroy foreign cells and remove immune complexes from the organism. The interaction between a complement or Fc-receptors on effector cells and the Fc region of IgG forming complexes with the antigen plays the key role in the physiological response to the presence of immune complexes. Although the ability to activate the complement system underlies the action of many therapeutic cytotoxic antibodies, we do not consider this aspect here due to the fact that anti-D antibodies do not activate the complement, and this mechanism is not involved in the clearance of D+ red cells in the presence of anti-D.

Cellular receptors for IgG, FcγR, a group of surface glycoproteins belonging to the Ig superfamily and expressed mostly on immune cells, are divided into three classes: FcγRI (CD64), FcγR II (CD32) and FcγRIII (CD16). Some of the FcγR features that may be involved in the processing of sensitized red blood cells are presented in Table 1.

The important characterstics of FcγRs are their affinity for IgG and the nature of the signal transduced, i.e. whether they initiate activating or inhibitory signalling cascades. FcγRI has a high affinity for IgG and has the capacity to bind not only IgG within the complexes but also monomeric molecules. The other FcγRs are of low to medium affinity and recognize only the IgG in the form of immune complex (Aschermann et al., 2010). The reaction of an effector cell in response to binding the complex is determined by the cytoplasmic part of the receptor that bears the immunoreceptor tyrosine-based activation motif (ITAM) in activating receptors and the immunoreceptor tyrosine-based inhibitory motif (ITIM) in inhibitory receptors (Amigorena et al., 1992; Isakov, 1997). Interaction of the immune complex with the FcγRI, FcγRIIA and FcγRIII containing both a ligand-binding subunit and the associated signaling part ITAM leads to the cellular activation. The nature of the responses primarily depends on the cell type; these can be antibody-dependent cellular cytotoxicity (ADCC), phagocytosis, endocytosis and cytokine or the inflammatory mediator release (Daëron, 1997; Clynes et al., 1999; Siberil et al., 2007). In contrast, the ITIM-containing receptor FcγRIIB, a transducer of inhibitory signals, down regulates the ITAM-mediated cellular activation when it co-ligates with the activating receptors (Ono et al., 1996). As an example, coligation of FcγRIIB and an ITAM-containing B cell receptor leads to aborted activation in B cells (Phillips &Parker, 1984).

The ADCC test using human peripheral blood mononuclear cells as effector cells is a multipurpose *in vitro* assay that makes it possible to determine the ability of antibodies to mediate cytolysis and to estimate the contribution of different types of receptors to this process (Engelfriet et al., 1994). The scheme of the ADCC assay adapted for the research of antibody-mediated hemolysis is shown in Fig. 1; the effector cells are listed in Table 1.

Receptor	Affinity	Affinity for IgG isotype	IgG bound form: monomeric/ complex	Signal	Mediating process	Localization on cells in the organism	Localization on effector cells in ADCC
FcγRI	High	IgG3 > IgG1>> IgG4>>> IgG2	Monomeric and within the complex	Activating	ADCC, endocytosis, phagocytosis	Monocytes, macrophages, CD34+ cells	Monocytes
FcγRIIA	Low	IgG1> IgG2 (depends on FcγRIIA poly-morphism) >>> IgG3	Within the complex	Activating	ADCC, endocytosis, phagocytosis, inflammatory mediator release	Monocytes, macrophages, neutrophils, platelets	Monocytes
FcγRIIB	Low	IgG3 ≥ IgG1> IgG4 >>> IgG2	Within the complex	Inhibiting	Blockade of B cell activation, internalization of immune complexes	B cells, basophils, monocytes, macrophages mast cells, dendritic cells	
FcγRIIC	Low	IgG1, IgG3	Within the complex	Activating	ADCC (some isoform)	NK * lymphocytes	NK lymphocytes
FcγRIIIA	Inter-mediate	IgG1= IgG3 >>>IgG2, IgG4	Within the complex	Activating	Cytotoxicity, endocytosis, phagocytosis, cytokine release	NK lymphocytes, T cells, monocytes, macrophages	NK lymphocytes, monocytes
FcγRIIIB	Inter-mediate	IgG1, IgG3	Within the complex	Activating	Generation of reactive oxygen species	Neutrophils	

Table 1. Human Fcγ receptors. The papers used in preparation of the table (Ravetch & Kinet, 1991; Engelfriet et al., 1994; de Haas et al., 1995; Ernst et al., 2002; Siberil et al., 2007; Kumpel, 2007)

*NK – natural killer lymphocytes

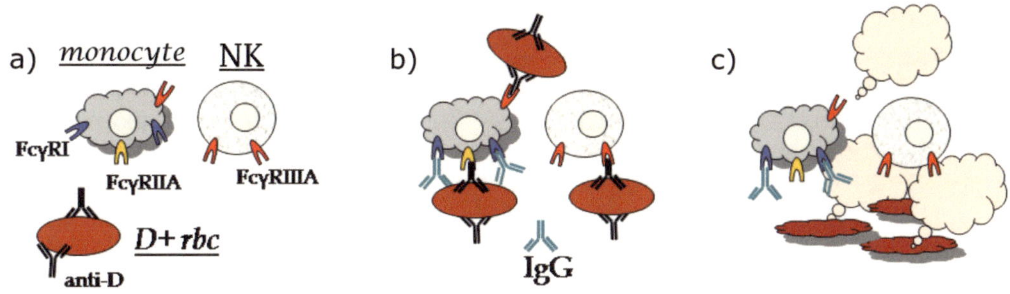

Fig. 1. Antibody-dependent cellular cytotoxicity assay. a) Participants of the ADCC assay are: effector cells bearing FcγRs (NK lymphocytes and monocytes); target cells (D+ red cells); anti-D antibodies. b) Intravenous Immunoglobulin (IG) is added as a source of monomeric IgG to block FcγRI. Only FcγRIIA and FcγRIIIA take part in the interaction with anti-D in this variant of the test that will be denoted as ADCC+IG. c) The concentration of free hemoglobin correlates with the hemolytic efficiency of anti-D in the standard formulation of the reaction

The concentration of free hemoglobin in the medium, being proportional to the number of destroyed target red blood cells, reflects the ability of antibodies to mediate ADCC. The non-immune IgG blocking the high-affinity FcγRI is added to the medium to estimate the ability of antibodies for triggering hemolysis via low-affinity FcγRIIA and FcγRIIIA (Fig. 1b). Antibody interactions with different types of FcγR can be studied using blocking antibodies against corresponding receptors (Kumpel et al., 2002a). Sometimes researchers apply a modification of the test, the so-called K-ADCC, which is designed to evaluate the interaction of antibodies with FcγRIIIA only. The fraction of nonadherent peripheral blood mononuclear cells containing FcγRIIIA-positive NK lymphocytes is used as effector cells in this test (Urbaniak, 1979a). It is worth noting that the test for the ability of anti-D to mediate lysis via FcγRIIIA is quite artificial: it is conducted with red cells treated with proteases only since native red cells do not work in this reaction (Urbaniak, 1979b). Irrespective of this, ADCC was found to be very useful for the evaluation and comparison of the functional activity of polyclonal and monoclonal anti-D antibodies. In the absence of a proper animal model of the Rh-conflict pregnancy, the efficacy of antibodies in ADCC serves a crucial factor before clinical trials.

Functional assay for the estimation of the IgG affinity for inhibitory receptor FcγRIIB is absent; the measurement of the IgG affinity for human FcγRIIB expressed on transfected cells or bound to beads may be used (Siberil et al., 2006; Lazar et al., 2006).

3.3 Clearance of D+ red cells *in vivo* upon the treatment with polyclonal anti-D immunoglobulin

The ability to accelerate the clearance of cells or target molecules is an important indicator for the effectiveness of the majority of immunopreparations. The ability of anti-D immunoglobulin to accelerate the clearance of coated D+ red cells is also considered to be its essential feature. Relation between the rate of clearance and the degree of red cell coating, on the one hand, and correlation between the rate of clearance and suppression, on the other hand, were found many years ago (Mollison et al., 1965; Mollison, 1984).

Anti-D prophylaxis was thought to be successful due to the efficient clearance of RhD-positive RBCs from the circulation and phagocytosis of anti-RhD-coated RBCs by macrophages in the spleen (Pollack, 1984). The role of spleen in the non-inflammatory removal of antibody-coated cells was reviewed in (Kumpel, 2006). The participation of the FcγRI in this process still remains elusive, since high-affinity FcγRI *in vivo* should be fully saturated with the circulating monomer IgG whose concentration in the serum is more than 10 mg/ml. One cannot exclude the possibility that the administered anti-D antibodies may be captured by FcγRI on macrophages along with other IgG. Sensitized ("arming") macrophages will in turn catch D+ red cells, thereby causing the *in vivo* destruction of the unsensitized red cells expressing the corresponding antigen (Griffiths et al., 1994). Nonetheless, it is highly probable that FcγRIII plays the key part in the clearance of sensitized cells. It was shown that intravenous infusion in chimpanzees of monoclonal antibodies which block 51-73 kD FcyRs that is similar to human FcγRIIIA dramatically prolongs the clearance of IgG-sensitized red cells (Clarkson et al., 1986). Strong association between the rate of removal of sensitized red cells and the allelic variant of human FcγRIIIA suggests, though indirectly, the engagement of this receptor in eliminating the antibody coated red cells. It has been demonstrated that the FcγRIIA polymorphism also has an effect on the rate of clearance (Miescher et al., 2004). However, FcγRIIA is considered to make no significant contribution to the red cells clearance *in vivo*, and FcγRIIIA is therefore likely to be the primary receptor utilized by macrophages *in vivo* for sequestration of anti-D-coated red cells (Kumpel, 2007). A set of data supports the role of FcγRIII in the cancer therapy with monoclonal antibodies and the relationship between the Fc - FcγRIII affinity and cytotoxic potency of antibody. For example, antitumor antibodies were unable to arrest tumor growth in FcγRIII-deficient mice (Clynes et al., 2000). A number of studies have documented a correlation between the clinical efficacy of anti-CD20 in humans and the allotype of their FcγRIIIA (Cartron et al., 2002; Weng & Levy, 2003).

The above data demonstrate that FcγR-dependent mechanisms substantially contribute to the action of cytotoxic antibodies and the clearance of target cells, but fail to answer the key question concerning the mechanism of AMIS: whether a fast clearance of the antigen can, by itself, make it possible to escape from the immunological surveillance and cause a temporal non-responsiveness to this antigen. On the one hand, two different processes such as an accelerated removal through the liver of the D+ red cells by natural IgM anti-A or anti-B antibodies and an accelerated removal through the spleen of the D+ red cells by IgG anti-D lead to the same result - the temporal tolerance to the D antigen, and this result indicates the importance of a fast removal of D+ red cells from the circulation. That is why the ability to interact with FcγRIIIA and induce a fast clearance of D+ red cells *in vivo* are the main features that should be taken into account during anti-D monoclonal antibodies selection. On the other hand, it was observed that the immune response could be suppressed if anti-D was given as late as two weeks after D+ red cells entered the circulation (Contreras, 1998), and that the initial rate of the red cells clearance did not appear to influence the effectiveness of protection (Kumpel et al., 1995). Our data providing evidence that a fast clearance is not sufficient for inducing immunosuppression will be discussed below (Olovnikova et al., 2000).

3.4 FcγRIIB is a negative regulator of the B cell differentiation and the antibody level

To date, there is a lot of data suggesting that AMIS can be regulated by a special mechanism mediated by the FcγRIIB inhibitory receptor. This is the only FcγR receptor expressed on B cells, and it plays a major role in the negative feedback regulation of B cell responses (Heyman, 2003; Hjelm et al., 2006).

At the beginning of an immune response, the primary contact with antigen leads to the activation of B cells expressing the specific B-cell receptor (BCR). After the BCR activation, naïve B cells proliferate and differentiate rapidly into IgM-secreting plasma cells or mature after class-switching into IgG-B cells which differentiate into IgG-secreting plasma cells or join the memory B cell compartment (Igarashi et al., 2007; Fournier et al., 2008). The differentiation and expansion of B cells is tightly controlled, thus preventing inadequate levels of circulating antibodies, plasma cells, and memory B cells. The control is ensured through the IgG immune complexes that can bind simultaneously to the BCR and FcγRIIB, leading to the inhibition of the IgG-B cell response (Phillips & Parker, 1984). The cross-linking of FcγRIIB and BCR induces the ITIM-associated recruitment of the phosphatase SHIP (SH2 domain-containing inositol 5'-phosphatase) which dephosphorylates and thus inactivates mediators of the BCR signalling, thereby dampening the B cell activation (Ono et al., 1996). There is evidence that FcγRIIB can control the bone marrow plasma cell persistence also in the absence of BCR triggering (Xiang et al., 2007). The role of inhibitory FcγRIIB in the regulation of the BCR signalling has been convincingly shown by using FcγRIIB-deficient mice (Takai et al., 1996). For example, the mice lacking this receptor display elevated levels of antibodies after immunization with both thymus-dependent and thymus-independent antigens, as well as have increased anaphylactic reactions and more severe symptoms in various models for autoimmunity (Heyman, 2003). This perhaps is related to that FcγRIIB limits the activation of high affinity autoreactive B cells and can influence the activation of dendrite cells through an immune complex-mediated mechanism (Venkatesh et al., 2009). It has also been shown that the only FcγR that is important for the anti-inflammatory activity of IVIG is the inhibitory FcγRIIB. Mice deficient in FcγRIIB no longer respond to the IVIG therapy in models of idiopathic thrombocytopenic purpura, serum transfer arthritis and nephrotoxic nephritis (Aschermann et al., 2010). A lot of evidence has recently appeared in support of the disturbances of the FcγRIIB expression in human autoimmune diseases. FcγRIIB has been shown to be up-regulated on memory B cells in normal humans, but this upregulation is significantly decreased in systemic lupus erythematosus patients (Mackay et al., 2006). Accordingly, there is a decreased FcγRIIB-mediated suppression of the BCR activation in B cells from lupus erythematosus patients (Nashi et al., 2010). Studies of the receptor expression in healthy individuals compared with rheumatoid arthritis patients have demonstrated that rheumatoid arthritis patients have fewer FcγRIIB positive B cells and decreased receptor expressions in contrast to healthy subjects. Their B cells display a significantly increased proliferative response *in vitro*. Interestingly, healthy women have overall lower FcγRIIB expression on B cells than men and it significantly decreases with age. The reduced FcγRIIB expression on B cells in women may account for the increased frequency of autoimmunity in women in comparison to men (Prokopec et al., 2010).

As concerns prevention of the anti-D immune response, the involvement of FcγRIIB in this process still remains unclear. As discussed above, AMIS in FcγRIIB-deficient mice that can be accounted for by the antigen masking does not argue against the engagement of this receptor in the establishment of the antigen-specific immunosuppression. If we assume that the immune antibodies can block B cell maturation and limit their own production through the interaction of immune complexes with FcγRIIB, it follows that the polyclonal anti-D prepared from the plasma of hyperimmune donors should also have this property. Whereas neither the antigen masking nor the accelerated clearance can explain the protective activity of anti-D immunoglobulin, the mechanism of a selective inactivation of antigen-specific B cells can elucidate all the known experimental facts related to AMIS. This mechanism, although being schematic, can give reasons for why antibodies to the Kell antigen prevent the immune response to the other antigens that are present on the erythrocyte, particularly the D antigen (Woodrow et al., 1975): while BCR specifically recognizes the D antigen, FcγRIIB interacts with the Fc region of the antibody bound to any antigen on the same red cell. Thus the cross-linking of "nonspecific"FcγRIIB and anti-D BCR leads to suppression of the anti-D response. D prophylaxis, in its turn, appears to prevent the synthesis of antibodies of other specificities (Pollack, 1984).

The issue concerning whether a preventive effect of the polyclonal anti-D preparation results from the action of the anti-D antibody fraction or is associated with a nonspecific immunomodulating effect has arisen many times (Petri et al., 1984; Branch et al., 2006). The immunosuppressive and anti-inflammatory effect of a nonspecific intravenous immunoglobulin has been reliably evaluated in many autoimmune diseases (Bayry et al., 2002; Simon & Spath, 2003). Nonetheless, it is not quite justified to expect common mechanisms of anti-D and intravenous immunoglobulin action since intravenous immunoglobulin is administered repeatedly at a high dose (generally 1-2 grams per kg body weight), while anti-D is used as a single dose of 1-2 ml 10% IgG solution, that is, 100-200 mg IgG. The following facts argue in favor of anti-D being the main triggering factor. In the classical experiment that first showed the immunosuppressive effect of anti-D, Rh-negative recipients received red cells sensitized *in vitro* when all other components of the preparation had been removed (Stern et al., 1961). The ability of the monoclonal anti-D to prevent D-sensitization is one more piece of evidence that it is anti-D antibodies that play a key part in suppression of the anti-D immune response (Kumpel et al., 1995).

4. Effector activity of poly- and monoclonal antibodies in ADCC

4.1 Monoclonal anti-D antibodies

Lymphocytes from immune Rh-negative donors are the only source for generation of the antibody-producing cell lines and isolation of genes of anti-D antibodies because the animals conventionally intended for immunization do not respond to the human Rh antigens. Thus, the development of therapeutic anti-D antibodies does not encounter the bioengineering problem of humanization. The lymphoblastoid cell lines producing anti-D antibodies are usually established by the Epstein-Barr virus infection of human B cells (Koskimies, 1980). Epstein-Barr virus is a B-lymphotropic human herpesvirus which initiates the infection of B lymphocytes by binding to CD21, a complement receptor. A scheme of development of the cell lines producing anti-D monoclonal antibodies is as follows. An immune Rh-negative donor is given a booster injection of D+ red cells 7-10 days before blood collection to have a higher yield of the anti-D cell line (Deriugina et al., 1991). Mononuclear cells isolated from the peripheral blood are seeded into 96-well plates, followed by the addition to the medium of the virus and the agent, for example, cyclosporine A suppressing the cytotoxic attack against the virus-infected B-cells. After 2-3 weeks, when the colonies of transformed cells have grown in the wells, the supernatants are tested for the presence of anti-D antibodies in the agglutination tests with D+ red cells for the selection of anti-D producers. Lymphocytes immortalized by the Epstein-Barr virus may be cloned and then can grow for some period of time in the culture without ceasing antibody secretion; however, for the purposes of stability and a higher yield of antibodies, they are usually fused with the mouse myeloma to derive stable heterohybridomas. Almost all anti-D monoclonal antibodies currently used in immunoserological testing are produced by heterohybridoma cell lines. An alternative approach to obtain anti-D is transfection and production of recombinant antibodies in rodent (Chinese hamster ovary - CHO, rat myeloma -YB2/0) or human (PER.C6) cell lines.

4.2 Characteristic features of poly- and monoclonal antibodies in ADCC

All polyclonal anti-D, either commercial products or individual sera from immune donors, as well as anti-D sera from pregnant women, have except rare instances the ability to mediate hemolysis in ADCC not only through FcγRI but also through FcγRIIIA (Armstrong-Fisher et al., 1995; Hadley et al.,1995). In contrast, only a few monoclonals have this property, which was demonstrated, for example, by a study of the functional activity of monoclonal anti-D IgGs submitted to the Fourth International Workshop on Monoclonal Antibodies against Human Red Blood Cells (Kumpel et al., 2002a). Only 8 out of 64 anti-D were shown to be able to mediate hemolysis in ADCC in the presence of monomeric IgG (ADCC+IG, Fig. 1b), but all of them could promote hemolysis through interaction with FcγRI.

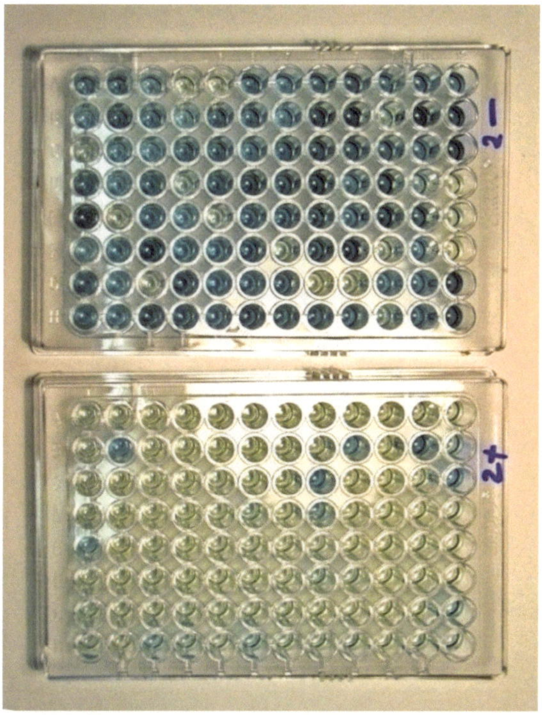

Fig. 2. Parallel testing of supernatants in ADCC (upper plate) and ADCC+IG (lower plate) three weeks after Epstein-Barr virus transformation of lymphocytes from anti-D donor. The effectiveness of hemolysis was estimated according to the concentration of free hemoglobin in the wells. The principle of this colorimetric assay is based on the oxydization of the 2.7-diaminofluorene by the pseudoperoxidase activity of free hemoglobin; the intensity of blue color is proportional to the hemoglobin concentration (Ducrot et al., 1996). Monomeric immunoglobulin is seen to fully or strongly inhibit ADCC (lower plate)

In order to find FcγRIIA / FcγRIIIA-binding antibodies and to evaluate the frequency of their occurrence, we performed ADCC+IG simultaneously with testing of anti-D in supernatants after transformation of lymphocytes by the Epstein-Barr virus (Olovnikova et al., 2006). The required anti-D were very rare: we could not detect them from some donors at all or detected only in 1-2% of wells with the anti-D, although the yield of FcγRI-active anti-D from the cells of the same donors was high (Fig. 2). Similar results were reported by Kumpel: only 5 out of 37 monoclonal anti-D IgG had a hemolytic activity in K-ADCC, and they were all obtained from one donor (Kumpel et al., 1989). A blend of the FcγRIIIA-nonactive monoclonal anti-D antibodies (pseudo-polyclonal anti-D) remained nonactive in ADCC+IG (data not shown). Possible reasons for this inconsistency, i.e., a high activity in ADCC+IG of all polyclonal anti-D antibodies and the absence of the monoclonals with the same hemolytic features, will be discussed in Section 8.
Nevertheless, we have received some lymphoblastoid cell lines that secrete anti-D IgG1 promoting hemolysis in ADCC+IG (Fig. 3) and compared them with anti-D IgG1 binding only FcγRI.

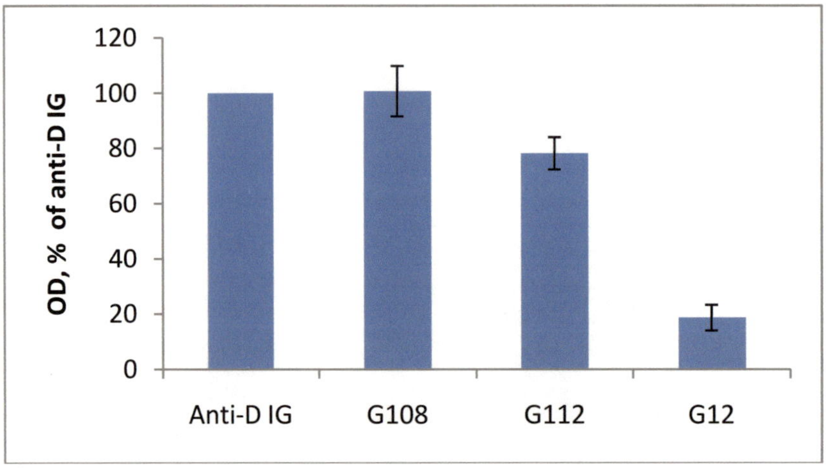

Fig. 3. ADCC+IG mediated by three anti-D IgG1 monoclonal antibodies (G108, G112, G12) produced by lymphoblastoid cell lines or the polyclonal product (anti-D IG). Concentration of anti-D in all the samples was 250 mcg/ml. Y axis: the optical density as percentage of the activity of polyclonal antibodies

Anti-D	Light chain	Isotype	Producing cell line	Activity in ADCC+IG (% of anti-D IG)	Sequencing of Fc
G108	κ	IgG1	Lymphoblastoid	101	IGHG1*03
G112	κ	IgG1	Lymphoblastoid	78	IGHG1*03
G12	κ	IgG1	Lymphoblastoid	19	IGHG1*03

Table 2. Structural and functional properties of anti-D IgG1 monoclonal antibodies
IGHG1*03 is the IgG1 allotype

The analysis of the primary sequence of genes of anti-D monoclonal antibodies with different activity in ADCC+IG did not reveal any differences in their Fc fragments (Olovnikova et al., 2009). Table 2 represents the characteristics of the three IgG1 anti-D having a different effector activity and obtained from lymphocytes of a single donor. We also did not find a correlation between the functional properties and the epitope specificity in the analysis of a set of IgG1 anti-D (data not shown).

5. Glycosylation of IgG. Ways of modifying the effector properties of antibodies

Interaction with the FcγR on an effector cell is the prerogative of the Fc fragment of IgG. IgG is a glycopeptide; it is known that oligosaccharide bound to the Fc fragment of an immunoglobulin molecule through Asn^{297} influences pharmacokinetics and plays an important role in the interaction of antibodies with the Fc receptors on effector cells (Raju, 2008), although the sugar does not, by itself, directly contact the receptor (Radaev & Sun, 2001). Aglycosylated antibodies lose the possibility to interact with Fc receptors (Nose & Wigzell, 1983; Walker et al., 1989). The largest sugar chain of a human IgG is shown in Fig. 4. About 25% of the sugar chains are sialylated; the high heterogeneity of neutral glycans is produced by the presence or absence of the two terminal galactoses, the bisecting N-acetylglucosamin and the fucose residue. Despite this high multiplicity, the molar ratio of each oligosaccharide in IgG of a healthy individual is quite constant (Kobata, 1990) but can vary widely in different diseases: the rheumatoid arthritis, heavy-chain deposition disease, multiple myeloma (Furukawa & Kobata, 1991; Omtvedt et al., 2006).

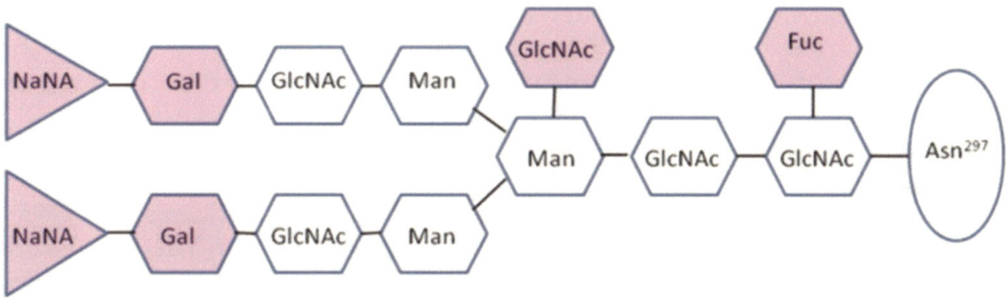

Fig. 4. The structure of the Asn ^{297}-bound oligosaccharide of human IgG
NaNA – N-acetylneuraminic acid; Gal - galactose; GlcNAc – N-acetylglucosamine;
Man - mannose; Fuc - fucose; Asn^{297} - asparagine of the Fc fragment of IgG
Neutral sugars do not contain sialic acids (NaNA); G2, G1 and G0 are neutral sugars with two, one and without terminal galactose. Carbohydrate residues that can be absent are color-marked

The structure of glycans that are synthesized in cells of various species of rodents has well been investigated due to a wide usage of rodent cell lines in the biopharmaceutical industry to produce recombinant proteins (Hossler et al., 2009). The glycosylation machinery of the mouse cells is dominant in heterohybridomas obtained by the fusion of antibody-producing human cells with myelomas; human IgGs from heterohybridomas contain monoantennary complex-type and high mannose-type oligosaccharides which have never been detected in human serum IgGs (Tandai et al., 1991). In hamster cells, as well as in murine cells, antibodies contain N-Glycolylneuraminic acid or some types of glycan that are not normally found, or found at low levels, in human IgG and can be immunogenic for humans (Hossler et al., 2009). For example, mannose can be bound by the circulating mannose receptor and recognized as being foreign by natural killer and macrophage cells (Rademacher, 1993).

At present, it is the carbohydrate moiety of IgG that is the main target for the modulation of the antibody effector properties. Numerous studies have provided evidence that fucose has a significant impact on the ability of monoclonal antibodies to interact with FcγRIIIA; defucosylated antibodies display an enhanced ADCC independent of the polymorphism of FcγRIIIA compared with their fucosylated counterparts (Shields et al., 2002; Shinkawa et al., 2003; Niwa et al., 2004). It has been shown that the antigenic density required to induce an efficient ADCC is lower for the low-fucose IgG1 as compared to a highly fucosylated antibodies (Niwa et al., 2005). This field of engineering is being actively elaborated due to the fact that it is the cytotoxic activity that underlies the action of many anti-cancer monoclonal antibodies. Antibodies with low fucose can be produced by the cell lines with a reduced fucosylation activity such as rat myeloma YB2/0 cells or the CHO variant cell line, Lec13 (Shields et al., 2002; Shinkawa et al., 2003). New host cell lines which produce completely defucosylated antibodies with enhanced effector functions were generated by knockout of the fucosyltransferase gene (Yamane-Ohnuki et al., 2004; Kanda et al., 2006). A number of other approaches to improve the FcγRIIIA affinity are being developed: for example, human IgG1 bearing immature oligomannose-type glycans also display an increased ADCC (Crispin et al., 2009).

An example of one anti-D given below shows a considerable magnitude at which the functional activity of its counterparts can vary both in different host cells and in the presence of the substances affecting the pattern of glycosylation. G12, anti-D IgG1, had a low activity in ADCC+IG when produced by the human lymphoblastoid cells (Fig. 5). Lymphoblastoid cells were fused with the mouse myeloma X63.Ag8.653 or the rat myeloma YB2/0; recombinant G12 were expressed in the retinal human cell line PER.C6® (Jones et al., 2003). Our special goal was to test the applicability of non-lymphoid human cell line PER.C6® (Olovnikova et al., in press) since the majority of industrial host cell lines have rodents cells origin.

Fig. 5 shows that the G12 expression in human-mouse heterohybridoma as well as in PER.C6® did not affect the activity in ADCC+IG, but the fusion with YB2/0 dramatically changed G12 properties: an inactive G12/LBL became highly active under the influence of the rat myeloma cells (Olovnikova et al., 2009). The same effect was attained by adding kifunensine to the G12/PER.C6® cell culture. Kifunensine is a potent inhibitor of α-mannosidase I, which leads to the synthesis of non-fucosylated oligomannose-type glycans (Zhou et al., 2008). This type of glycosylation totally transformed G12/PER.C6®, providing them with improved ability to trigger ADCC via low-affinity receptors. The effect of kifunensine can be explained by the two factors: the absence of fucose and a high content of olygomannoses that also enhances the affinity of the Fc fragment for FcγRIII (Raju, 2008; Zhou et al., 2008). However, a similar effect of the YB2/0 myeloma indirectly suggests the crucial contribution made by fucose.

Obviously, it is reasonable to increase the affinity of anti-tumor antibodies to FcγRIIIA since a high cytotoxicity of antibodies leads to a better anti-tumor effect. However, D antibodies are intended for another purpose. The tendency to improve FcγRIII binding is explained not only by our desire to achieve the fastest possible clearance of red cells, but also by the hope that the binding of other low-affinity receptors, FcγRIIB including, will also be enhanced. There is sufficient evidence in support of this correlation. Thus, low fucosylated anti-D produced by YB2/0 binds strongly to both activating FcγRIII and inhibitory FcγRIIB, as opposed to its highly fucosylated counterpart produced by CHO (Siberil et al., 2006). Fc variants of anti-tumor MoAb trastuzumab with the greatest enhancements in the FcγRIIIA affinity also significantly increased binding to FcγRIIB (Lazar et al., 2006).

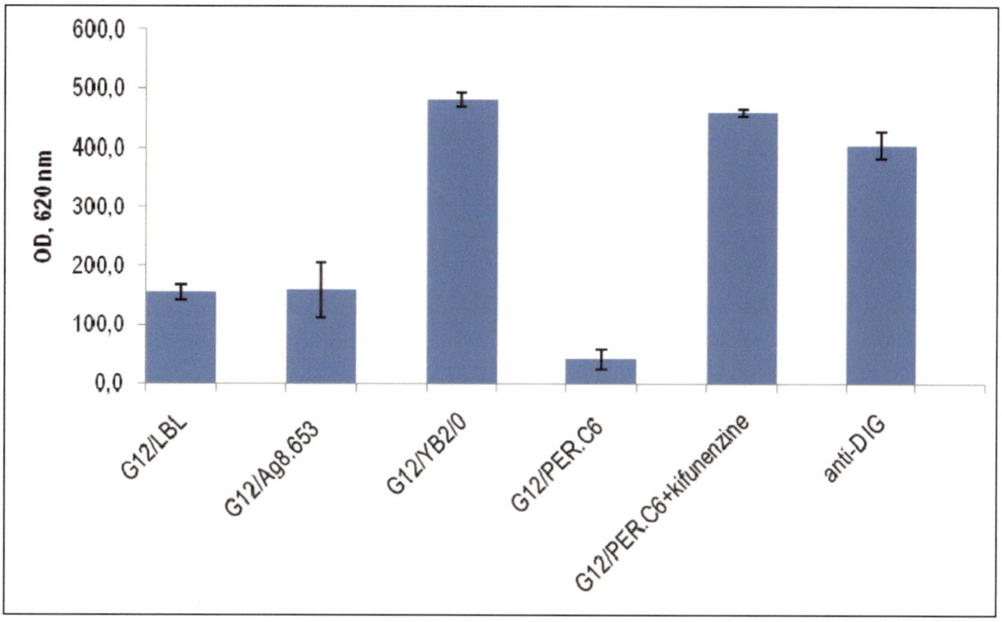

Fig. 5. The effect of host cells and metabolic modulation on the hemolytic activity of anti-D G12 in the ADCC+IG

Y axis: optical density at 620 nm; the concentration of all anti-D is 100 mcg / ml. G12/LBL - G12 from lymphoblastoid B-cell line; G12/Ag8.653 and G12/YB2/0 - G12 from corresponding heterhybridomas; G12/PER.C6® - recombinant G12 from PER.C6®; G12/PER.C6® + kifunensine - recombinant G12 from PER.C6 ®with 1 mcg/ ml of kifunensine in culture medium; anti-D IG - anti-D immunoglobulin

We have shown that a pattern of interaction with FcγRs of low-fucosylated G12/YB2/0 was different from polyclonal anti-D and the G108 produced by lymphoblastoid cells. Polyclonal anti-D and the G108/LBL utilized both FcγRIIA and FcγRIIIA in ADCC+IG. The hemolytic activity of G12/YB2/0 in ADCC+IG was predominantly mediated through FcγRIIIA; the low fucose content had a negative effect on the affinity to FcγRIIA (Fig. 6).

Despite a high affinity for FcγRIIIA, anti-D/YB2/0 and anti-D/PER.C6 ®synthesized in the presence of kifunensine have an uncommon for human IgG oligosaccharide structure: anti-D /YB2/0 may contain rodent IgG sugar moieties whereas the cultivation with kifunensine leads to the synthesis of oligomannoses-type glycans. Such structures can be recognized in the organism not only by FcγRs, but also by the receptors of the innate immunity, which can lead to immunization, rather than immunosuppression.

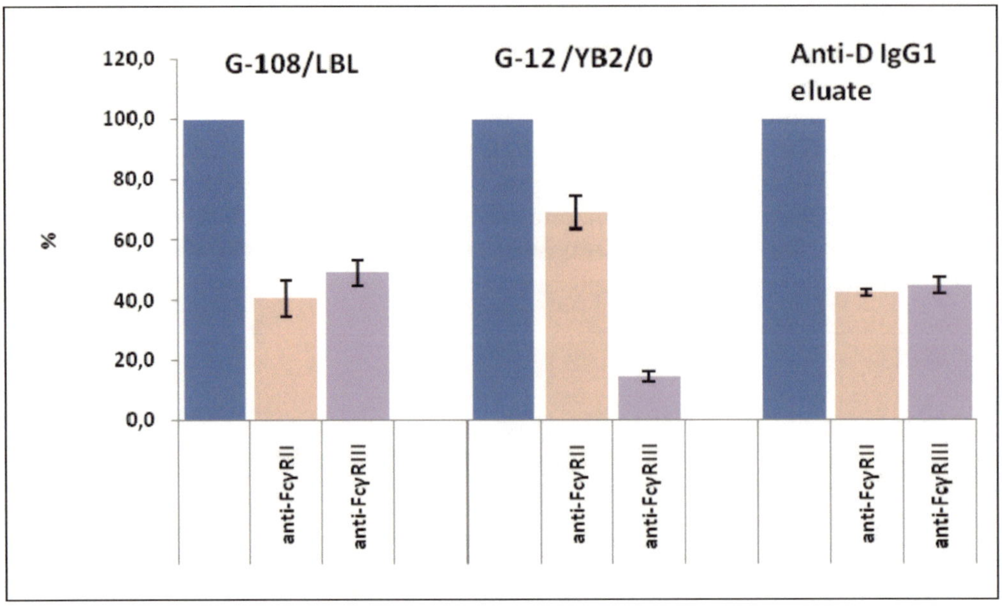

Fig. 6. ADCC+IG with the blocking antibodies to CD16 (FcγRII) and CD32 (FcγRIII) (Dako, Denmark). The activity of each anti-D in ADCC+IG (the first column) is taken as 100%. The second and third columns show the contribution of FcγRIII and FcγRII to ADCC+IG. Purified polyclonal anti-D IgG antibodies were prepared by adsorption of anti-D immunoglobulin on D+ red cells, followed by elution and isolation on Protein A. This control polyclonal preparation containing predominantly anti-D IgG1 is more adequate than total anti-D immunoglobulin in which the fraction of anti-D antibodies is about 0,1% (1 dose of anti-D is usually 1-2 ml of 10% IgG solution containing 200-300 mcg of anti-D antibodies). The concentration of each anti-D was 250 mcg/ml

6. The analysis of the glycan structure of anti-D antibodies

Comparison of the four anti-D IgG1, produced by human lymphoblastoid cell lines and having a different activity in ADCC+IG (G12 and G17 with a low activity, G112 and G108 with an intermediate and high activity, correspondingly), was performed to estimate whether the hemolytic activity correlates with the peculiarities of the composition of sugars (Table 3).

Earlier studies reported about the correlation between the ADCC activity and sialylation of monoclonal anti-D (Kumpel et al., 1994). Sialic acids were shown to have negative effect on the affinity of Fc fragments for FcγRIII (Scallon et al., 2007). However, we found no such connection. Apparently, both inactive and active monoclonal and purified polyclonal anti-D antibodies are almost equally sialylated (Table 3). Study of sugar moieties of the four anti-D/LBLs did not reveal any significant differences between the structures of FcγRIIIA-active and FcγRIIIA-nonactive anti-D. Table 3 allows comparison of glycosylation of the two anti-D polyclonal antibody products. One can see that the content of sialylated sugars and the neutral G2F form in anti-D IgG eluate is higher than in the total anti-D IG, while the G0F fraction is on the contrary sufficiently higher in the total anti-D IG. It is notable that the content of non-fucosylated neutral sugars in the eluate is higher than in other preparations:

9.2% vs. 2.6% in anti-D IG. As concerns glycosylation of IgG1 in human PER.C6® cells, there is a significant deviation in its profile in relation to a normal range of IgG glycans. An example of G12/PER.C6® shows that PER.C6® produces antibodies without sialic acids and completely fucosylated. This structure of glycan transformed FcγRIIIA-active anti-D G108/LBL into FcγRIIIA-inactive G108/PER.C6® (data not shown), despite the absence of sialic acids, which again points out the key role of fucose.

		G12/ PER.C6®	G12/ LBL	G17/ LBL	G112/ LBL	G108/ LBL	Anti-D IG	Anti-D IgG eluate
ADCC+IG		low	low	low	Inter-mediate	high	high	high
Fucosylated	G2F	5,7*	41,1	28,7	41,3	33,1	24,0	31
	G1F	29,1	13,0	26,2	21,8	27,1	35,0	20
	G0F	60,9	2,0	4,9	2,2	4,5	20,0	5,6
	total	95,7	56,1	59,8	65,3	64,7	79	56,6
Not fucosylated	G2	0,0	1,4	2,5	1,7	2,4	1,5	7,3
	G1	0,5	0,6	0,8	0,6	1,3	0,8	1,2
	G0	0,2	0,2	0,0	0,0	0,8	0,3	0,7
	total	0,7	2,2	3,3	2,3	4,5	2,6	9,2
Sialylated**		0,5	28,8	34,4	25,7	24,6	15	28
Unassigned		3,1	12,9	2,5	6,7	6,2	3,4	6,2

Table 3. Oligosaccharides of mono- and polyclonal D antibodies

The samples were analyzed following the SOP "AA Fluorescent N-linked Oligosaccharide Profiling of Neutral Monosaccharides using an Aqueous Chromatographic Separation;

* In % of all glycans;

** The structure of sialylated glycans was not analyzed.

Interestingly, none of the cloned lines secretes a really monoclonal antibody in terms of glycosylation: each monoclonal anti-D demonstrates a wide range of glycoforms (Table 3).

7. What *in vivo* investigations of monoclonal and recombinant anti-D antibodies have shown

Study of immunosuppressive properties of monoclonal and recombinant anti-D antibodies was carried out following evaluations of their safety, pharmacokinetics, as well as the ability to accelerate the clearance of sensitized red cells (Thomson et al., 1990; Blancher et al., 1993; Goodrick et al., 1994; Bichler et al., 2004). To date, over ten anti-D IgG1 and two IgG3 of different origin (lymphoblastoid cell lines, human-mouse heterohybridomas, CHO, YB2/0) have been tested on volunteers. Kumpel in the detailed reviews reported on the results of the research into anti-D monoclonal antibodies on volunteers (Kumpel, 2007; 2008). Although the design of testing varied in details in different laboratories, its general outline was as follows. After the administration of 1-10 ml D+ red cells to a Rh-negative recipient, a blood sample is taken to measure the initial content of D+ red cells. Following intravenous or intramuscular injection of the anti-D antibody, blood samples are collected every few hours during the first three days. The level of residual radioactivity, taking the initial sample as 100%, is evaluated when using red blood cells labeled with a radioactive isotope; in the case of injection of native unlabeled red cells, a number of D+ red cells is directly calculated using flow cytometry after labeling red cells with antibodies conjugated with fluorescein isothiocyanate. These data allow researchers to estimate the effect of anti-D on the clearance of D+ red cells, as well as the number of anti-D molecules bound to the D+ red cells if flow cytometry is used. Subsequent blood samples are regularly taken approximately every 2 weeks for the period of time up to 6 months in order to find the immune anti-D antibodies and to detect the time of their appearance, their class and titer. The boost, that is, unprotected red cells challenge, is eventually given no earlier than after 6 months to determine the state of sensitization in those subjects in whom antibodies were not detected: the secondary-type immune response indicates a state of sensitization and non-effectiveness of anti-D prophylaxis. Although the studies on volunteers have left many questions unanswered, they permitted detection of some features of monoclonal anti-D antibodies that were impossible to predict neither theoretically nor based on their properties in tests *in vitro*.

1. Although acceleration of the clearance is the most distinctive characteristic of the polyclonal anti-D, and designers of anti-D preparations initially tried to get just this property, a fast clearance is not the only requirement for the prevention of anti-D sensitization. Our study of the preventive activity of the four monoclonal IgG1 anti-D antibodies of the human-mouse heterohybridoma origin and the blends of these anti-Ds has found that the clearance of D+ red cells in the group of recipients given a blend of G7 and G12 anti-Ds was as fast as that in the group given polyclonal anti-D IG. Nonetheless, all the subjects treated with the G7 + G12 blend rapidly became D immunized (Olovnikova et al., 2000).
2. Acceleration of the red cell clearance usually directly correlates with the ability of antibodies to mediate ADCC through FcγRIIIA. This rule may have exceptions: our anti-Ds G7 and G12 that caused an effective clearance of D+ red cells had a low activity in ADCC + IG.
3. In the groups of volunteers given anti-Ds produced by human-mouse heterohybridomas, a percentage of sensitized subjects was higher than in the control unprotected group, irrespective of the rate of clearance of the red cells injected. Moreover, unusually for the anti-D response, most of the responders formed IgM anti-D and developed them more rapidly than would be expected after red cells alone. In other words, monoclonal anti-Ds had an adjuvant effect enhancing the immune response instead of suppressing it (Olovnikova et al., 2000; Beliard, 2006). It seems quite reasonable to agree with the opinion that monoclonals of the heterohybridoma origin containing foreign glycans may be recognized by Toll-like receptors of the innate immunity and direct the immune response in the pro-inflammatory way that stimulates the antibody production (Kumpel, 2007). These receptors do not participate in the destruction of the red cells sensitized by polyclonal anti-D or anti-D from human lymphoblastoid cells. In light of this assumption, a high *in vitro* and *in vivo* hemolytic activity of low-fucosylated anti-Ds secreted by rodent cells does not ensure their immunosuppressive effectiveness. Clinical trials of anti-D expressed in the YB2/0 myeloma that were announced in France are to give an answer to this question (Urbain et al., 2009).
4. Only anti-Ds produced by human lymphoblastoid lines that are able to mediate hemolysis via FcγRIIIA in ADCC showed a high protective activity among any of the

monoclonal preparations tested *in vivo*. Their immunosuppressive effectiveness was the same as that of polyclonal antibodies, and the absence of anti-D response in a large percentage of subjects after the next unprotected immunization indicated a long-term character of the anti-D suppression (Kumpel, 2002b).

5. There is no reliable answer to the question of which class of anti-D, IgG1 or IgG3, is more effective and whether it is essential to mix monoclonal antibodies of different classes. The experimental data did not allow conclusions about the benefits of the IgG1 + IgG3 mixture containing antibodies in a physiological proportion compared with a single IgG1 (Kumpel et al., 1995, 2002b).
6. The question of whether the oligoclonal mixture of antibodies of the same class can be more effective than a single antibody still remains unanswered. The first pseudo-polyclonal preparation Rozrolimupab that comprises 25 recombinant unique IgG1 antibodies expressed in CHO cells (Symphogen) is being investigated for the prevention of hemolytic disease of the fetus and newborn and for the treatment of idiopathic thrombocytopenic purpura (Stasi, 2010).
7. We lack a sustainable cell line that can stably grow in the culture and give a high-yield output of rightly glycosylated antibodies. Although some lymphoblastoid lines secrete the "right" antibodies, their unstable growth make them inadequate to allow a large-scale production.
8. As concerns a polyclonal anti-D preparation, it is still unclear whether it is a fraction of anti-D antibodies that is responsible for its immunosuppressive impact, or it is due to a cumulative effect of anti-Ds with different FcγR affinity.

8. Differential glycosylation of antibodies produced by different subpopulations of B cells as a mechanism for regulating the humoral immune response: A hypothesis

The amount of antibodies formed to a particular antigen can not rise for a limitlessly long period of time; in general, it appears to be restricted over a wide range of antigen dosage and a variety of immunization regimens and as a rule reaches a predictable maximal level, despite continued immunization (Uhr & Möller, 1968). The regulation of the antibody synthesis is assumed to be consistent with the feedback principle, and the ability of antibodies to enhance or suppress the immune response reflects this physiological mechanism. An insightful hypothesis of the mechanism for anti-D AMIS was proposed by Gorman and Pollack (Pollack, 1984). The authors speculated that, in particular, in the presence of early IgM antibodies the formation of IgM - antigen complexes stimulates the committed B cells, whereas after the switching to IgG production, the formation of IgG - antigen complexes limits further expansion of the plasma cell clones.

A primary contact with an antigen leads to the formation of Ab-secreting plasmablasts with a lifespan of less than one week and results in short-term Ab responses, but most Ab-secreting cells are generated during the secondary immune response (Smith et al., 1996, Odendahl et al., 2005). As a result of the secondary contact with the antigen, memory B cells undergo a massive expansion and differentiation toward short-lived plasma cells. Some plasma cells become long-lived if rescued in available niches such as bone marrow. These cells can survive, continue to secrete antibodies and sustain serum antibody levels for extended periods of time (> 1 year) even in the absence of any detectable memory B cells (Slifka et al., 1998; Bernasconi et al., 2002). Overall, kinetics of the antibody concentration in serum is defined by the two factors: a rapid increase of the titer after boosting is associated with the activity of short-lived plasma cells, whereas a population of long-lived plasma cells insensitive to the antigen maintains a level of high affinity antibodies for an extended period of time (Manz et al., 1998; Manz et al., 2005).

The role of inhibitory FcγRIIB in the regulation of proliferation and differentiation of B cells into plasma cells, antibody affinity maturation and plasma cell numbers has already been discussed in Section 2.4. Given all findings, one can suggest that long-lived plasma cells produce antibodies with immunosuppressive properties that can inhibit the activation and differentiation of B cells through FcγRIIB. First, anti-inflammatory antibodies can serve to arrest naïve B cells, i.e., to suppress the activation of the primary immune response upon the secondary contact with the antigen. This inhibition prevents secretion of low-affinity antibodies, thus directing the immune response along the way of a rapid and effective secondary (memory) response, which allows production of high-affinity antibodies. It is unlikely that suppression of the primary response requires high titers of immunosuppressive antibodies. Second, after a pool of long-lived plasma cells has already formed, inhibitory properties of the antibodies which they produce make it possible to restrict the activation of antigen-specific memory B cells and overproduction of antibodies in the case of the next antigen stimulus. However, this process should take place only against the background of a high level of corresponding antibodies. This is why the anti-D polyclonal immunoglobulin prepared from the plasma of repeatedly immunized donors with high-titer anti-D contains antibodies that, in the first place, are capable of suppressing effectively the primary immune response.

In contrast, short-lived plasma cells which are generated at the stage of accelerating the immune response should not produce antibodies capable of interacting with FcγRIIB and inhibiting proliferation of B cells until a pool of long-lived plasma cells and that of memory B cells have formed. Obviously, it is this regularity that we face when receiving anti-D producers by viral transformation of lymphocytes. As mentioned above, when we tried to receive anti-D IgGs having the same pattern of interaction with FcγR as polyclonal antibodies, we found that only rare monoclonal anti-D antibodies had the capability of utilizing the low-affinity FcγRs. The Epstein-Barr virus, a B-lymphotropic human herpesvirus, infects B cells, including memory B cells, by using CD21 as a receptor (Cooper et al., 1988) and drives them out of the resting state to become activated proliferating lymphoblasts that produce and secrete Ig of any isotype (Miyawaki et al., 1988; Rickinson & Lane, 2000; Thorley-Lawson, 2001). The Epstein-Barr virus infection deregulates multiple differentiation factors and processes in B cells, promoting their growth and differentiation towards plasma cells (Miyawaki et al., 1991; Siemer et al., 2008). However, the process of differentiation fails to proceed to the terminal stage, to the plasma cell, thereby yielding cell lines with an immature "lymphoblastoid" phenotype; all virus-transformed cell lines that we obtained were CD19 +, CD20 +, CD38 +, $Ig^{membrane}$ +. It seems that this is the answer to the question why monoclonal antibodies with the properties of polyclonal antibodies can be so rarely received: because serum polyclonal antibodies and monoclonal antibodies are produced by different B cell subsets, namely, serum anti-Ds by long-lived plasma cells, and monoclonal anti-Ds by B-lymphoblasts. Low affinity for FcγRIIIA of anti-D antibodies produced by virus-transformed peripheral B cells of an immune donor, and a high affinity of polyclonal antibodies from the same donor indicate that the effector activity of the antibodies produced by different subpopulations of B lymphocytes is different (no data suggesting that the Epstein-Barr virus in itself may alter the pattern of glycosylation are available).

The question of when a pool of the future long-lived plasma cells is generated and what factors are responsible for this branch point in the B cell differentiation still remains unanswered. Does this choice happen at the level of the memory B cell or does any B cell, once occurring in the right environment, trigger this program? Perhaps, the frequency of the clones secreting a monoclonal anti-D with the properties of polyclonal antibodies reflects the frequency of "pre-long-lived" plasma cells in the peripheral blood when migrating after the antigen boosting.
The way of regulating the immunomodulatory properties of antibodies may include some variations in their glycosylation that is defined by a set of glycosyltransferases expressing in the cells of different stages of the B cell ontogeny, in particular, in short-lived plasma cells and long-lived plasma cells. It is well known that the molar ratio of each glycoform of IgG from the sera of healthy individuals is quite constant (Kobata, 1990). It was suggested that a ratio of different clones of B cells which are equipped with different sets of glycosyltransferases is relatively constant in healthy individuals (Kobata, 1990; 2008). In light of the hypothesis proposed here, the constant ratio of IgG olygosaccharides from the sera may be explained by the programmed different patterns of IgG glycosylation in B cells at different developmental stages. The ratio of all the types of cells in the organism is approximately constant, which implies a stable ratio of IgG glycoforms. Moreover, B cell clones do not produce a monoclonal IgG with a unique sugar moiety, but with a wide range of olygosaccharides whose ratio is close to that of IgG glycoforms of a normal serum (Table 3).The question of whether glycosylation can be intended for regulation of the immunity is currently being discussed in the literature. For example, IgGs have been shown to acquire anti-inflammatory properties upon Fc sialylation (Kaneco et al., 2006); however, it is non-specific mechanisms that are likely to underlie their anti-inflammatory effect (Medzhitov & Janeway, 2002; Anthony & Ravetch, 2010). The anti-D response may serve as a model of how the antigen-specific feedback regulation works.

9. Conclusion

The two observations that had led to the application of anti-D antibodies for preventing D sensitization were: 1) a lower probability of D sensitization of an Rh-negative mother after the delivery of the ABO incompatible infant, and 2) the antigen-specific immunosuppressive effect of the antibodies injected simultaneously with the corresponding antigen. Paradoxically, none of these mechanisms is likely to play a crucial part in the anti-D immunoglobulin action. 1) Red cells coated with natural antibodies against A and B blood groups may be preferentially caught in the liver, where they are less likely to stimulate an immune response against the Rh antigens, whereas D+ red cells coated with anti-D antibodies are withdrawn through the spleen, i.e., through the organ of an active immune response. In addition, a fast clearance of the antigen from circulation did not appear to be a sufficient condition for preventing immunization. 2) Classical AMIS at which antibodies are abundant and saturate all antigen determinants may be accounted for by the antigen camouflage. However, this mechanism is inadequate in the case of the anti-D immune suppression since binding only a small portion of D sites is known to be sufficient for the immunosuppressive effect of the injected antibodies. Overall, the mechanism for an antibody-mediated suppression of the anti-D immune response by down-regulation of the specific B cells seems most relevant.

One can assume that anti-D antibodies secreted by long-lived plasma cells should have immunosuppressive properties to provide down-regulation of the immune response. When a pool of long-lived plasma cells has been formed, and the organism is sure to have a reliable protection by a sustainable production of high affinity antibodies, the immunosuppressive antibodies that have reached a threshold concentration begin to suppress the maturation of naïve and memory B cells following administration of the antigen. These protective measures are needed to prevent secretion of low-affinity antibodies of the primary response after repeated immunizations and avoid overproduction of the plasma cells of this specificity as the number of niches for long-lived plasma cells in the bone marrow is limited. A likely distinctive characteristic of antibodies with immunosuppressive properties is a unique pattern of glycosylation that provides opportunities for the interaction with low-affinity receptors. Thus, immunosuppressive anti-Ds are capable of binding both to an inhibitory FcγRIIB and an activating FcγRIIIA, which provides an effective clearance of sensitized D+ red cells. The proposed hypothesis explains the mechanism of a high efficiency of the polyclonal anti-D immunoglobulin derived from the sera of immune donors with a high titer of anti-D antibodies in the prevention of the primary anti-D response, as well as their low efficiency in the case of the secondary response.

The situation is different at the initial, accelerating, stage of the immune response when the antibodies produced by short-lived plasma cells should not suppress the immune response but instead enhance it. Apparently, we observed these antibodies when transforming the B cells derived from peripheral blood by the Epstein-Barr virus. The virus infects CD21+ B cells, thus evoking in them the process of differentiation towards plasma cells; however, a phenotype of the lymphoblastoid lines derived indicates a non-terminated process of differentiation. Analysis of a huge set of anti-D monoclonal antibodies has shown that the lymphoblastoid lines derived from peripheral B cells of large numbers of donors only rarely secrete antibodies that are able to interact with low-affinity receptors in contrast to the polyclonal antibodies simultaneously collected from the same donors.

Nevertheless, viral transformation sometimes makes it possible to obtain the lines secreting anti-D monoclonal antibodies with the properties of polyclonal antibodies. Further detailed analysis of their biochemical structure will, undoubtedly, provide information about peculiarities of their composition that make them different from inactive ones. We have found no differences in the primary nucleotide sequences of genes encoding for Fc fragments of active and non-active anti-Ds, which indicates the effect of posttranslational modifications on the functional properties of antibodies. It is known that the mode of glycosylation is associated with the level of affinity of the antibody Fc fragment for FcγRIIIA. We have also shown that the FcγR binding activity of antibodies can be significantly modified through their expression in different producer lines, and, furthermore, it is possible to transform any non-active anti-D into a highly active one *in vitro*. However, it is important to note that a structure of sugar should not be foreign, or, otherwise, antibodies may evoke stimulation rather than immunosuppression of the immune response. Such adjuvant-like effect was observed when we treated volunteers with monoclonal anti-Ds produced by human-mouse heterohybridomas.

Nevertheless, the answer to the question raised in the headline of this paper should, undoubtedly, be positive. Thus, the development of a relevant producer cell line that maintains the "right" glycosylation of antibodies is the most important challenge at present. It is already clear that traditional producers such as mouse myelomas or CHO cells are unlikely to become a source of efficient anti-D preparations. A human myeloma with defective fucosylation could be potentially attractive for the production of not only anti-D but also other therapeutic antibodies. Another approach may utilize a genetic engineering tuning of any lymphoblastoid cell line secreting anti-D IgG. This process should involve immortalization of the cell line, for example, with the help of hTERT (human telomerase reverse transcriptase) and regulation of the expression of glycosyltransferases, which is presently possible. The development of a monoclonal anti-D product not only will make it possible to replace a serum anti-D but will also serve a model for inducing an antibody-mediated immunosuppression at autoimmune diseases. The history of attempts to create a biotechnological anti-D immunoglobulin that would replace serum preparations is, on the one hand, the way of disappointments and failures; on the other hand, it is an example of how our approaches to solve this complex and fascinating task with so many unknowns have been evolving while new information becomes available in this area.

10. Acknowledgment

The research was financially supported by Russian Foundation for Basic Research, Hematolog Ltd, Masterclone Ltd.

I thank collaborators and co-authors of my papers concerning monoclonal anti-D for the prevention of the haemolytic disease of the newborn.

I wish to thank Helen Yunina for help in manuscript revision and editing.

11. References

Amigorena S, Bonnerot C, Drake JR, Choquet D, Hunziker W, Guillet JG, Webster P, Sautes C, Mellman I, Fridman WH. (1992). Cytoplasmic domain heterogeneity and functions of IgG Fc receptors in B lymphocytes. *Science,* 256(5065):1808-12.

Anthony RM, Ravetch JV. (2010). A novel role for the IgG Fc glycan: the anti-inflammatory activity of sialylated IgG Fcs. *Journal of Clinical Immunology,* 30 Suppl 1:S9-14.

Armstrong-Fisher SS, Sweeney GM, Greiss MA, Urbaniak SJ. (1995). Functional assessment of therapeutic anti-D immunoglobulin using Fc-mediated assays. *Transfusion Medicine,* 5(1):21-9.

Aschermann S., Lux A., Baerenwaldt A., Biburger M. and Nimmerjahn F. (2010). The other side of immunoglobulin G: suppressor of inflammation. *Clinical and Experimental Immunology,* 160(2):161-7.

Bayry J, Pashov A, Donkova V, Delignat S, Vassilev T, Stahl D, Bellon B, Kazatchkine MD, Lacroix-Desmazes S, Kaveri SV. (2002). Immunomodulation of autoimmunity by intravenous immunoglobulin through interaction with immune networks. *Vox Sanguinis, 83* Suppl 1:49-52.

von Behring E, Wernicke E.(1892). Über Immunisierung und Heilung von Versuchstieren bei der Diphterie. *Z Hyg Infektionskrankheit,* 12:10–44.

Béliard R. (2006). Monoclonal anti-D antibodies to prevent alloimmunization: lessons from clinical trials. *Transfusion Clinigue et Biologique,* 3(1-2):58-64.

Bernasconi NL, Traggiai E, Lanzavecchia A. (2002). Maintenance of serological memory by polyclonal activation of human memory B cells. *Science,* 298(5601):2199-202.

Bichler J, Spycher MO, Amstutz HP, Andresen I, Gaede K, Miescher S. (2004). Pharmacokinetics and safety of recombinant anti-RhD in healthy RhD-negative male volunteers. *Transfusion Medicine,* 14(2):165-71.

Blancher A, Socha WW, Roubinet F, Rowe AW, Broly H, Byrne P, Holuigue M, Bouzidi A, Huart JJ, Ruffié J. (1993). Human monoclonal anti-D-induced clearance of human D-positive red cells in a chimpanzee model. *Vox Sanguinis,* 65(1):47-54.

Bowman JM. (1988). The prevention of Rh immunization. *Transfusion Medicine Reviews,* 2(3):129-50.

Bowman J. (2003). Thirty-five years of Rh prophylaxis. *Transfusion,* 43(12):1661-6.

Branch DR, Shabani F, Lund N, Denomme GA. (2006). Antenatal administration of Rh-immune globulin causes significant increases in the immunomodulatory cytokines transforming growth factor-beta and prostaglandin E2. *Transfusion,* 46(8):1316-22.

Cartron G, Dacheux L, Salles G, Solal-Celigny P, Bardos P, Colombat P, Watier H. (2002). Therapeutic activity of humanized anti-CD20 monoclonal antibody and polymorphism in IgG Fc receptor FcgammaRIIIa gene. *Blood,* 99(3):754-8.

Clarke CA, Donohoe WT, McConnell RB, Woodrow JC, Finn R, Krevans JR, Kulke W, Lehane D, Sheppard PM. (1963). Further experimental studies on the prevention of Rh haemolytic disease. *British Medical Journal,* 1(5336):979-84.

Clarkson SB, Kimberly RP, Valinsky JE, Witmer MD, Bussel JB, Nachman RL, Unkeless JC. (1986). Blockade of clearance of immune complexes by an anti-Fc gamma receptor monoclonal antibody. *Journal of Experimental Medicine,* 164(2):474-89.

Clynes R, Maizes JS, Guinamard R, Ono M, Takai T, Ravetch JV. (1999). Modulation of immune complex-induced inflammation in vivo by the coordinate expression of activation and inhibitory Fc receptors. *Journal of Experimental Medicine,* 189(1):179-85.

Clynes RA, Towers TL, Presta LG, Ravetch JV. (2000). Inhibitory Fc receptors modulate in vivo cytotoxicity against tumor targets. *Nature Medicine,* 6(4):443-6.

Contreras M. (1998). The prevention of Rh haemolytic disease of the fetus and newborn--general background. *British Journal of Obstetrics and Gynaecology,* 105 Suppl 18:7-10.

Cooper NR, Moore MD, Nemerow GR. (1988). Immunobiology of CR2, the B lymphocyte receptor for Epstein-Barr virus and the C3d complement fragment. *Annual Review of Immunology,* 6:85-113.

Crispin M, Bowden TA, Coles CH, Harlos K, Aricescu AR, Harvey DJ, Stuart DI, Jones EY. (2009). Carbohydrate and domain architecture of an immature antibody glycoform exhibiting enhanced effector functions. *Journal of Molecular Biology,* 387(5):1061-6.

Daëron M. (1997). Fc receptor biology. *Annual Review of* Immunology, 15:203-34.

Deriugina EI, Olovnikova NI, Lemeneva LN, Belkina EV, Udalov GA, Chertkov IL. (1991). Monoclonal antibodies to Rho(D)-antigen of the Rhesus system. Obtaining the EBV-transformed B-lymphoblastoid human cell lines secreting IgG-anti-D antibodies. *Gematology and Transfusiology,* 36(8):11-6. Russian.

Ducrot T, Beliard R, Glacet A, Klein P, Harbonnier S, Benmostefa N, Bourel D. (1996). Use of the DAF assay to assess the functional properties of polyclonal and monoclonal RhD antibodies. *Vox Sanguinis,* 71(1):30-6.

Engelfriet CP, Overbeeke MA, Dooren MC, Ouwehand WH, von dem Borne AE. (1994). Bioassays to determine the clinical significance of red cell alloantibodies based on

Fc receptor-induced destruction of red cells sensitized by IgG. *Transfusion,* 34(7):617-26.

Ernst LK, Metes D, Herberman RB, Morel PA. (2002). Allelic polymorphisms in the FcgammaRIIC gene can influence its function on normal human natural killer cells. *Journal of Molecular Medicine,* 80(4):248-57.

Fournier EM, Sibéril S, Costes A, Varin A, Fridman WH, Teillaud JL, Sautès-Fridman C. (2008). Activation of Human Peripheral IgM+ B Cells Is Transiently Inhibited by BCR-Independent Aggregation of FcgammaRIIB. *The Journal of Immunology,* 181(8):5350-9.

Freda VJ, Gorman JG, Pollack W. (1964). Successful Prevention of Experimental RH Sensitization in Man with an anti-RH gamma2-globulin antibody preparation: a preliminary report. *Transfusion,* 4:26-32.

Furukawa K, Kobata A. (1991). IgG galactosylation--its biological significance and pathology. *Molecular Immunology,* 28(12):1333-40.

Goodrick J, Kumpel B, Pamphilon D, Fraser I, Chapman G, Dawes B, Anstee D. (1994). Plasma half-lives and bioavailability of human monoclonal Rh D antibodies BRAD-3 and BRAD-5 following intramuscular injection into Rh D-negative volunteers. *Clinical and Experimental Immunology,* 98(1):17-20.

Gorman JG, Freda VJ, Pollack WJ, Robertson JG. (1966). Protection from immunization in Rh-incompatible pregnancies: a progress report. *Bulletin of the New York Academy of Medicine,* 42(6):458-73.

Griffiths HL, Kumpel BM, Elson CJ, Hadley AG. (1994). The functional activity of human monocytes passively sensitized with monoclonal anti-D suggests a novel role for Fc gamma RI in the immune destruction of blood cells. *Immunology,* 83(3):370-7.

de Haas M, Vossebeld PJ, von dem Borne AE, Roos D. (1995). Fc gamma receptors of phagocytes. *The Journal of Laboratory and Clinical Medicine,* 126(4):330-41.

Hadley AG, Zupanska B, Kumpel BM, Pilkington C, Griffiths HL, Leader KA, Jones J, Booker DJ, Stamps R, Sokol RJ. (1995). The glycosylation of red cell autoantibodies affects their functional activity in vitro. *British Journal of Haematology,* 91(3):587-94.

Heyman B, Wigzell H. (1984). Immunoregulation by monoclonal sheep erythrocyte specific IgG antibodies: Suppression is correlated to level of antigen binding and not to isotype. *The Journal of Immunology,* 132(3):1136-43.

Heyman B. (1999). Antibody feedback suppression: towards a unifying concept? *Immunology Letter,* 68(1):41-5.

Heyman B. (2000). Regulation of antibody responses via antibodies, complement, and Fc receptors. *Annual Review of Immunology,* 18:709-37.

Heyman B. (2003). Feedback regulation by IgG antibodies. *Immunology Letters,* 88(2):157-61.

Hjelm F., F. Carlsson, A. Getahun & B. Heyman. (2006). Antibody-Mediated Regulation of the Immune Response. *Scandinavian Journal of Immunology,* 64(3):177-84.

Hossler P, Khattak SF, Li ZJ. (2009). Optimal and consistent protein glycosylation in mammalian cell culture. *Glycobiology,*19(9):936-49.

Igarashi K, Ochiai K, Muto A. (2007). Architecture and dynamics of the transcription factor network that regulates B-to-plasma cell differentiation. *The Journal of Biochemistry,* 141(6):783-9.

Isakov N. (1997). ITIMs and ITAMs. The Yin and Yang of antigen and Fc receptor-linked signaling machinery. *Immunologic Research,* 16(1):85-100.

Jones D, Kroos N, Anema R, van Montfort B, Vooys A, van der Kraats S, van der Helm E, Smits S, Schouten J, Brouwer K, Lagerwerf F, van Berkel P, Opstelten DJ, Logtenberg T, Bout A. (2003). High-level expression of recombinant IgG in the human cell line per.c6. *Biotechnology Progress,*19(1):163-8.

Kanda Y, Yamane-Ohnuki N, Sakai N, Yamano K, Nakano R, Inoue M, Misaka H, Iida S, Wakitani M, Konno Y, Yano K, Shitara K, Hosoi S, Satoh M. (2006). Comparison of cell lines for stable production of fucose-negative antibodies with enhanced ADCC. *Biotechnology and Bioengineering,* 94(4):680-8.

Kaneko Y, Nimmerjahn F, Ravetch JV. (2006). Anti-inflammatory activity of immunoglobulin G resulting from Fc sialylation. *Science,* 313(5787):670-3.

Karlsson MC, Wernersson S, Diaz de Stahl T, Gustavsson S, Heyman B. (1999). Efficient IgG-mediated suppression of primary antibody responses in Fcgamma receptor-deficient mice. *Proceedings of the National Academy of Sciences U S A,* 96(5):2244-2249.

Karlsson MC, De Stahl TD, Heyman B. (2001). IgE-mediated suppression of primary antibody responses in vivo. *Scandinavian Journal of Immunology,* 53(4):381-5.

Kobata A. (1990). Function and pathology of the sugar chains of human immunoglobulin G. *Glycobiology,* 1(1):5-8.

Kobata A. (2008). The N-linked sugar chains of human immunoglobulin G: their unique pattern, and their functional roles. *Biochimica et Biophysica Acta,* 1780(3):472-8.

Koskimies S. (1980). Human lymphoblastoid cell line producing specific antibody against Rh-antigen D. *Scandinavian Journal of Immunology,* 11(1):73-7.

Kumpel BM, Leader KA, Merry AH, Hadley AG, Poole GD, Blancher A, Goossens D, Hughes-Jones NC, Bradley BA. (1989). Heterogeneity in the ability of IgG1 monoclonal anti-D to promote lymphocyte-mediated red cell lysis. *European Journal of Immunology,* 19(12):2283-8.

Kumpel BM, Rademacher TW, Rook GA, Williams PJ, Wilson IB. (1994). Galactosylation of human IgG monoclonal anti-D produced by EBV-transformed B-lymphoblastoid cell lines is dependent on culture method and affects Fc receptor-mediated functional activity. *Human Antibodies and Hybridomas,* 5(3-4):143-51.

Kumpel BM, Goodrick MJ, Pamphilon DH, Fraser ID, Poole GD, Morse C, Standen GR, Chapman GE, Thomas DP, Anstee DJ. (1995). Human Rh D monoclonal antibodies (BRAD-3 and BRAD-5) cause accelerated clearance of Rh D+ red blood cells and suppression of Rh D immunization in Rh D- volunteers. *Blood,* 86(5):1701-9.

Kumpel BM, Beliard R, Brossard Y, Edelman L, de Haas M, Jackson DJ, Kooyman P, Ligthart PC, Monchâtre E, Overbeeke MA, Puillandre P, de Romeuf C, Wilkes AM. (2002a). Section 1C: Assessment of the functional activity and IgG Fc receptor utilisation of 64 IgG Rh monoclonal antibodies. Coordinator's report. *Transfusion Clinique et Biologique,* 9(1):45-53.

Kumpel BM. (2002 b). On the mechanism of tolerance to the Rh D antigen mediated by passive anti-D (Rh D prophylaxis). *Immunology Letters,* 82(1-2):67-73.

Kumpel BM. (2006). On the immunologic basis of Rh immune globulin (anti-D) prophylaxis. *Transfusion,* 46(9):1652-6.

Kumpel BM. (2007). Efficacy of RhD monoclonal antibodies in clinical trials as replacement therapy for prophylactic anti-D immunoglobulin: more questions than answers. *Vox Sanguinis,* 93(2):99-111.

Kumpel BM. (2008). Lessons learnt from many years of experience using anti-D in humans for prevention of RhD immunization and haemolytic disease of the fetus and newborn. *Clinical and Experimantal Immunology,*154(1):1-5.

Lazar GA, Dang W, Karki S, Vafa O, Peng JS, Hyun L, Chan C, Chung HS, Eivazi A, Yoder SC, Vielmetter J, Carmichael DF, Hayes RJ, Dahiyat BI. (2006). Engineered antibody Fc variants with enhanced effector function. *Proceedings of the National Academy of Sciences U S A,* 103(11):4005-10.

Levin P. (1943). Serological factors as possible causes of spontaneous abortions. *Journal of Heredity,* 34: 71-80

Mackay M, Stanevsky A, Wang T, Aranow C, Li M, Koenig S, Ravetch JV, Diamond B. (2006). Selective dysregulation of the FcgammaIIB receptor on memory B cells in SLE. *Journal of Experimental Medicine,* 203(9):2157– 64.

Manz RA, Löhning M, Cassese G, Thiel A, Radbruch A. (1998). Survival of long-lived plasma cells is independent of antigen. *International Immunology,* 10(11):1703-11.

Manz RA, Hauser AE, Hiepe F, Radbruch A. (2005). Maintenance of serum antibody levels. *Annual Review of* Immunology, 23:367-86.

Medzhitov R & Janeway CA Jr. (2002). Decoding the patterns of self and nonself by the innate immune system. *Science,* 296(5566):298-300.

Miescher S, Spycher MO, Amstutz H, De Haas M, Kleijer M, Kalus UJ, Radtke H, Hubsch A, Andresen I, Martin RM, Bichler J. (2004). A single recombinant anti-RhD IgG prevents RhD immunization: association of RhD-positive red blood cell clearance rate with polymorphisms in the FcgammaRIIA and FcgammaIIIA genes. *Blood,* 103(11):4028-35.

Miyawaki T, Kubagawa H, Butler JL, Cooper MD. (1988). Ig isotypes produced by EBV-transformed B cells as a function of age and tissue distribution. *Journal of Immunology,* 140(11):3887-92.

Miyawaki T, Butler JL, Radbruch A, Gartland GL, Cooper MD. (1991). Isotype commitment of human B cells that are transformed by Epstein-Barr virus. *Europian Journal of Immunology,* 21(1):215-20.

Mollison PL, Crome P, Hughes-Jones NC, Rochna E. (1965). Rate of removal from the circulation of red cells sensitised with different amounts of antibody. *British Journal of Haematology,* 11:461-470.

Mollison PL. (1984). Some aspects of Rh hemolytic disease and its prevention. In: G. Garratty, Editor, Arlington VA: *Hemolytic disease of the newborn.* American Association of Blood Banks.

Nashi E, Wang Y. and Diamond B. (2010). The Role of B Cells in Lupus Pathogenesis. *International Journal of Biochemistry & Cell Biology,* 42(4): 543–550.

Nicholas R & Sinclair SC. (1969). Regulation of the immune response. I. Reduction in ability of specific antibody to inhibit long-lasting IgG immunological priming after removal of the Fc fragment. *Journal of Experimental Medicine,* 129(6):1183-201.

Niwa R, Hatanaka S, Shoji-Hosaka E, Sakurada M, Kobayashi Y, Uehara A, Yokoi H, Nakamura K, Shitara K. (2004). Enhancement of the antibody-dependent cellular cytotoxicity of low-fucose IgG1 Is independent of FcgammaRIIIa functional polymorphism. *Clinical Cancer Research,* 10(18 Pt 1):6248-55.

Niwa R, Sakurada M, Kobayashi Y, Uehara A, Matsushima K, Ueda R, Nakamura K, Shitara K.(2005). Enhanced natural killer cell binding and activation by low-fucose IgG1 antibody results in potent antibody-dependent cellular cytotoxicity induction at lower antigen density. *Clinical Cancer Research,* 11(6):2327-36.

Nose M & Wigzell H. (1983). Biological significance of carbohydrate chains on monoclonal antibodies. *Proceedings of the National Academy of Sciences U S A,* 80(21):6632-6.

Odendahl M, Mei H, Hoyer BF, Jacobi AM, Hansen A, Muehlinghaus G, Berek C, Hiepe F, Manz R, Radbruch A, Dörner T. (2005). Generation of migratory antigen-specific plasma blasts and mobilization of resident plasma cells in a secondary immune response. *Blood,* 105(4):1614-21.

Olovnikova NI, Belkina EV, Drize NI, Lemeneva LN, Miterev GIu, Nikolaeva TL, Chertkov IL. (2000). Fast clearance of the rhesus-positive erythrocytes by monoclonal anti-rhesus antibodies--an insufficient condition for effective prophylaxis of rhesus-sensitization. *Bulletin of Experimental Biology and Medicine,* 129(1):77-81.

Olovnikova NI, Belkina EV, Nikolaeva TL, Miterev GY, Chertkov IL. (2006). Lymphocyte antibody-dependent cytotoxicity test for evaluation of clinical role of monoclonal anti-D-antibodies for prevention of rhesus sensitization. *Bulletin of Experimental Biology and Medicine,* 141(1):57-61.

Olovnikova NI, Ershler MA, Belkina EV, Nikolaeva TL, Miterev GY. (2009). Effect of producer cell line on functional activity of anti-D monoclonal antibodies destined for prevention of rhesus sensitization. *Bulletin of Experimental Biology and Medicine,* 147(4):448-52.

Omtvedt LA, Royle L, Husby G, Sletten K, Radcliffe CM, Harvey DJ, Dwek RA, Rudd PM. (2006). Glycan analysis of monoclonal antibodies secreted in deposition disorders indicates that subsets of plasma cells differentially process IgG glycans. *Arthritis and Rheumatism,* 54(11):3433-40.

Ono, M., S. Bolland, P. Tempst, and J.V. Ravetch. (1996). Role of the inositol phosphatase SHIP in negative regulation of the immune system by the receptor Fc(gamma)RIIB. *Nature,* 383(6597):263-6.

Petri IB, Lórincz A, Berek I. (1984). Detection of Fc-receptor-blocking antibodies in anti-Rh(D) hyperimmune gammaglobulin. *Lancet,* 2(8417-8418):1378-9.

Phillips, N.E. & D.C. Parker. (1984). Cross-linking of B lymphocyte Fc gamma receptors and membrane immunoglobulin inhibits anti-immunoglobulin-induced blastogenesis. *Journal of Immunology,*132(2):627-32.

Pollack W. (1984). Mechanisms of Rh Immune Suppression by Rh Immune Globulin. In: G. Garratty, Editor, Arlington VA: *Hemolytic disease of the newborn.* American Association of Blood Banks.

Prokopec KE, Rhodiner M, Matt P, Lindqvist U, Kleinau S. (2010). Down regulation of Fc and complement receptors on B cells in rheumatoid arthritis. *Clinical Immunology,* 137(3):322-9.

Radaev S & Sun P. (2001). Recognition of IgG by Fcgamma receptor. The role of Fc glycosylation and the binding of peptide inhibitors. *The Journal of Biological Chemistry,* 276(19):16478-83.

Rademacher TW. (1993). Glycosylation as a factor affecting product consistency. *Biologicals,* 21(2):103-4.

Raju TS. (2008). Terminal sugars of Fc glycans influence antibody effector functions of IgGs. *Current Opinion in Immunology,* 20(4):471-8.

Ravetch JV & Kinet JP. (1991). Fc receptors. *Annual Review of Immunology,* 9:457-92.

Rickinson AB & Lane PJ. (2000) Epstein-Barr virus: Co-opting B-cell memory and migration. *Current Biology*, 10(3):R120-3.

Scallon BJ, Tam SH, McCarthy SG, Cai AN, Raju TS. (2007). Higher levels of sialylated Fc glycans in immunoglobulin G molecules can adversely impact functionality. *Molecular Immunology*, 44(7):1524-34.

Shields RL, Lai J, Keck R, O'Connell LY, Hong K, Meng YG, Weikert SH, Presta LG. (2002). Lack of fucose on human IgG1 N-linked oligosaccharide improves binding to human Fcgamma RIII and antibody-dependent cellular toxicity. *The Journal of Biological Chemistry*, 277(30):26733-40.

Shinkawa T, Nakamura K, Yamane N, Shoji-Hosaka E, Kanda Y, Sakurada M, Uchida K, Anazawa H, Satoh M, Yamasaki M, Hanai N, Shitara K. (2003). The absence of fucose but not the presence of galactose or bisecting N-acetylglucosamine of human IgG1 complex-type oligosaccharides shows the critical role of enhancing antibody-dependent cellular cytotoxicity. *The Journal of Biological Chemistry*, 278(5):3466-73.

Sibéril S, de Romeuf C, Bihoreau N, Fernandez N, Meterreau JL, Regenman A, Nony E, Gaucher C, Glacet A, Jorieux S, Klein P, Hogarth MP, Fridman WH, Bourel D, Béliard R, Teillaud JL. (2006). Selection of a human anti-RhD monoclonal antibody for therapeutic use: Impact of IgG glycosylation on activating and inhibitory FcγR functions. *Clinical Immunology*, 118(2-3):170-9.

Sibéril S, Dutertre CA, Fridman WH, Teillaud JL. (2007). FcgammaR: The key to optimize therapeutic antibodies? *Critical Reviews in Oncology/ Hematology*, 62(1):26-33.

Siemer D, Kurth J, Lang S, Lehnerdt G, Stanelle J, Küppers R. (2008). EBV transformation overrides gene expression patterns of B cell differentiation stages. *Molecular Immunology*, 45(11):3133-41.

de Silva M, Contreras M, Mollison PL. (1985). Failure of passively administered anti-Rh to prevent secondary response. *Vox Sanguinis*, 48(3):178-80.

Simon HU, Späth PJ. (2003). IVIG - mechanisms of action. *Allergy*, 58(7):543-52.

Slifka MK, Antia R, Whitmire JK, Ahmed R. (1998). Humoral immunity due to long-lived plasma cells. *Immunity*, 8(3):363-72.

Smith KG, Hewitson TD, Nossal GJ, Tarlinton DM. (1996). The phenotype and fate of the antibodyforming cells of the splenic foci. *The European Journal of Immunology*, 26(2):444-8.

Stasi R. (2010). Rozrolimupab, symphobodies against rhesus D, for the potential prevention of hemolytic disease of the newborn and the treatment of idiopathic thrombocytopenic purpura. *Current Opinion in Molecular Therapeutics*, 12(6):734-40.

Stern K, Goodman HS, Berger M. (1961). Experimental Isoimmunization to Hemoantigens in Man. *Journal of Immunology*, 87:189-198.

Takai T, Ono M, Hikida M, Ohmori H, Ravetch JV. (1996). Augmented humoral and anaphylactic responses in Fc gamma RII-deficient mice. *Nature*, 379(6563):346-9.

Tandai M, Endo T, Sasaki S, Masuho Y, Kochibe N, Kobata A. (1991). Structural study of the sugar moieties of monoclonal antibodies secreted by human-mouse hybridoma. *Archives of Biochemistry and Biophysics*, 291(2):339-48.

Thomson A, Contreras M, Gorick B, Kumpel B, Chapman GE, Lane RS, Teesdale P, Hughes-Jones NC, Mollison PL. (1990). Clearance of Rh D-positive red cells with monoclonal anti-D. *Lancet*, 336(8724):1147-50.

Thorley-Lawson DA. (2001). Epstein-Barr virus: exploiting the immune system. *Nature Reviews. Immunology,* 1(1):75-82.
Tovey LA, Robinson AE. (1975). Reduced severity of Rh-haemolytic disease after anti-D immunoglobulin. *British Medical Journal,* 4(5992):320-2.
Uhr JW & Möller G. (1968). Regulatory effect of antibody on the immune response. *Advances in Immunology,* 8:81–127.
Urbain R, Teillaud JL, Prost JF. (2009). EMABling antibodies: from feto-maternal allo-immunisation prophylaxis to chronic lymphocytic leukaemia therapy. *Medecine Sciences (Paris),* 25(12):1141-4.
Urbaniak SJ. (1979a). ADCC (K-cell) lysis of human erythrocytes sensitized with rhesus alloantibodies. II. Investigation into the mechanism of lysis. *British Journal of Haematology,* 42(2):315-25.
Urbaniak SJ. (1979b). ADCC (K-cell) lysis of human erythrocytes sensitized with rhesus alloantibodies. I. Investigation of in vitro culture variables. *British Journal of Haematology,* 42(2):303-14.
Venkatesh J, Kawabata D, Kim S, Xu X, Chinnasamy P, Paul E, Diamond B, Grimaldi CM. (2009). Selective regulation of autoreactive B cells by FcgammaRIIB. *Journal of Autoimmunity,* 32(3-4):149-57.
Walker MR, Lund J, Thompson KM, Jefferis R. (1989). Aglycosylation of human IgG1 and IgG3 monoclonal antibodies can eliminate recognition by human cells expressing Fc gamma RI and/or Fc gamma RII receptors. *Biochemical Journal,* 259(2):347-53.
Weng WK & Levy R. (2003). Two immunoglobulin G fragment C receptor polymorphisms independently predict response to rituximab in patients with follicular lymphoma. *Journal of Clinical Oncology,* 21(21):3940-7.
Woodrow JC, Clarke CA, Donohow WT, Finn R, McConnell RB, Sheppard PM, Lehane D, Roberts FM, Gimlette TM. (1975). Mechanism of Rh prophylaxis: an experimental study on specificity of immunosuppression. *British Medical Journal,* 2(5962):57-9.
Xiang Z, Cutler AJ, Brownlie RJ, Fairfax K, Lawlor KE, Severinson E, Walker EU, Manz RA, Tarlinton DM, Smith KG. (2007). FcgammaRIIb controls bone marrow plasma cell persistence and apoptosis. *Nature Immunology,* 8(4):419-29.
Yamane-Ohnuki N, Kinoshita S, Inoue-Urakubo M, Kusunoki M, Iida S, Nakano R, Wakitani M, Niwa R, Sakurada M, Uchida K, Shitara K, Satoh M. (2004). Establishment of FUT8 knockout Chinese hamster ovary cells: an ideal host cell line for producing completely defucosylated antibodies with enhanced antibody-dependent cellular cytotoxicity. *Biotechnology and Bioengineering,* 87(5):614-22.
Zhou Q, Shankara S, Roy A, Qiu H, Estes S, McVie-Wylie A, Culm-Merdek K, Park A, Pan C, Edmunds T. (2008). Development of a simple and rapid method for producing non-fucosylated oligomannose containing antibodies with increased effector function. *Biotechnology and Bioengineering,* 99(3):652-65.

6

Immunotropic Properties of GABA-ergic Agents in Suppression

N. Tyurenkov[1] and M. A. Samotrueva[2,3]
[1]*The Volgograd State Medical University,*
[2]*The Astrakhan State Medical Academy,*
[3]*The Astrakhan State University*
Russia

1. Introduction

Vigorous development of immunology and immunopharmacology is closely interrelated with formation of new scientific "branches"of neuroimmunology and neuroimmunopathology which predetermines the hypotheses of mutual regulation-interaction of the nervous and immune systems, of the significance of neuroimmune mechanisms in the regulation of most physiological functions and development of pathophysiological processes (Alford L., 2007; Irwin M.R., 2008; Freund G.G., 2009). The formulated hypotheses that immunologic mechanisms are involved in the pathogenesis of the CNS diseases (stroke, multiple sclerosis, chronic fatigue syndrome, epilepsy, etc.), their systematization within the scope of special neuroimmunipathology have laid the groundwork for a vigorous pharmacological search of agents for eliminating neuroimmune disturbances (Kryzhanovsky G.N. et al., 2003; Fleshner M., Laudenslager M.L., 2004; Alexandrovsky Y.A., Chekhonin V.P., 2005; Samotrueva M.A. et al., 2009).
In light of this problem and considering the abundant factual material testifying to the involvement of GABAergic system in immunomodulation, substances which are GABA analogues become of particular interest (Devoyno L.V., Iliuchenok R.U., 1993; Korneva E.A., 2003). Thus, in this experimental work we studied the immunotropic properties of the known representatives of group of GABAergic agents such as phenotropil (N-carbamoyl-methyl-4-phenyl-2-pyrrolidone), phenibut (hydrochloride of γ-amino and β-phenylbutyric acids) and baclofen (γ-amino-para-chloro-β-phenylbutyric acid). Having a wide range of psychotropic effects these drugs improve cognitive activity, decrease emotional tension and anxiety, normalize sleep; diminish asthenic manifestations, vasovegetative symptoms, etc. (Arushanian E. B., 2004). In this work aiming to widen the activity range of the above-mentioned drugs as well as to search for drugs capable of eliminating immune imbalance which is often in causal relationship with the CNS pathologies we studied the immunomodulating activity of gamma-aminobutyric acid (GABA) derivatives using an experimental immunosuppression model and determined the most effective doses and regimens.

2. Materials and methods

The study was performed on 544 CBA-line mice both male and female aged 3-4 months weighing 20-25g. The animals were kept in standard vivarium conditions – in plastic cages on a sawdust bedding at a room temperature of +18-22°. They were fed twice a day with natural foods in the amount corresponding to daily doses (P 50258-92 State Standard) had a free access to water. The lighting in the daytime (12 hours) was combined (natural and luminescent). The animals were kept according to the guidelines on laboratory practice for preclinical trials in the RF (3 51000.3-96 and 51000.4-96 State Standards) and the Order of the Health Care Ministry of the RF № 267 of 19.06.2003 'On the Approval of the Guidelines on Laboratory Practice' (GLP) as well as in conformity with the International recommendations of the European Convention for the Protection of Vertebrae Animals Used for Experimental and Scientific Purposes, 1997.

By the moment when the experiments were held the animals had adapted to the human factor, acclimatized and were in good health (no changes in behaviour, appetite, circadian cycle, condition of fur and visible mucosas were detected). All the experiments were carried out in the spring-autumn period (without abrupt changes of weather conditions) within one and the same time interval (from 11.00 till 19.00) to avoid the influence daily biorhythms on the investigation results. The rodents were euthanized by means of fast cervical dislocation.

The pathology of the immune system was simulated by a single intraperitoneal introduction of cyclophosphamide (CPA) in a dose of 150 mg/kg 1 hour after the immunization with sheep erythrocytes (SE) (Arkadyev V.G. et al., 2003). The investigated substances were introduced 1 hour after the immunodepressant ("Biochimik", Russia).

The model of cyclophosphamide (CPA) immunosuppression was used to estimate the immunocorrective properties of phenotropil, phenibut and baclofen in a "dose-effect" respect, when administered intraperitoneally as a single dose and introduced during a peroral course of treatment; to study the immunopreventive and/or immunotherapeutic aspects of the action of the drugs when administered at different times in relation to CPA immunosuppression introduction ("time-effect").

2.1 Immunopharmacological tests

The immune status of the animals was evaluated on the basis of standard immunopharmacological tests: delayed hypersensitivity reaction (DHR) involving the reaction index definition, passive hemagglutination reaction (PHAR) involving the antibody titre definition, latex test to study the phagocytic activity of peripheral blood neutrophils as well as a leukogram, to define the weight and cellularity of immunocompetent organs (thymus, spleen) (Khaitov R.M. et al., 2005).

The DHR was used to evaluate a cellular link of the primary immune response to sheep erythrocytes (SE). The animals of all groups were immunized by receiving a single hypodermic SE injection (a sensibilizing injection) ($2x10^8$) in the interscapular area. The antigen booster dose was introduced on the 5th day ($1x10^8$ SE) in 0,02 ml of physiological saline into a hind leg paw - "experimental" leg (the booster injection). The equivalent amount of physiological saline was introduced into the contralateral leg - "control" leg. The reaction was estimated 24 hours later by euthanizing the animals by fast cervical dislocation, after which both legs were cut off at the level of an ankle-joint and weighed using analytical balances. The reaction index (DHRI) was calculated using the formula: $RI = (M_{ex} - M_c)/M_c \times 100\%$, where RI is a reaction index, M_{ex} is an "experimental" leg weight; M_c is "control" leg weight.

PHAR was used to estimate the humoral link of the primary immune response to SE. The animals were immunized once intraperitoneally in a dose of $5x10^8$ in the amount of 500 mcl 1-2 hours after the introduction of the investigated substance. 7 days later the animals were withdrawn from the experiment by administering serum. To inactivate the complement the serum was heated for 30 min at a temperature of 56°C. The hemagglutination reaction was carried out in 96-well plates in the amount of 500 mcl of a diluent (0.5% solution of bovine serum albumin (BSA), solved in physiological saline) in which the investigated serums were successively diluted twice. After the dilution of the serums 25 mcl of 1% SE suspension was introduced into each well. The preliminary analysis of the PHAR results was done after one hour of incubation at a temperature of 37C°, the plates were placed into a refrigerator and kept at a temperature of +4°C. The reaction was finally evaluated 18 hours later. The antibody titre (the maximal serum dilution in which SE agglutination was registered) was indicated using average compound indices.

To estimate *the phagocytic activity of neutrophils* the animals' heparinized blood was used. A suspension of latex particles of 1.3-1.5 μm size ("MinMedBioprom", Russia) was prepared in advance. The original latex suspension was three times washed with a 0.9% NaCl solution at 3000 rpm for 10 minutes. The sediment was resuspended in medium 199, the number of particles was calculated in a Goryaev's chamber and brought to the ultimate concentration of 150000 in 1mcl. 24-48 hours after the introduction of the investigated substances (in the control group it was physiological saline) the animals were withdrawn from the experiment and their blood samples were taken. 50 mcl of the latex work solution was mixed with 50 mcl of heparinized blood and placed into a temperature-regulated chamber at a temperature of 37°C. The test-tubes were shaken by hand every ten minutes and then centrifuged. Smears were taken from the sediment, they were dried and fixed in Nikiforov's mixture consisting of equal parts of absolute ethyl alcohol and ether (10 min). The next day they were stained by the Romanovsky-Giemsa method (20-30 min). After this the smears were washed with water and dried in the air. The stained smears were examined under a microscope in an immerse system. The number of leucocytes and neutrophils with latex and without it was calculated in a smear. At the same time the number of latex particles in neutrophils was counted. The phagocytic activity of neutrophils was evaluated on the basis of the following indices: phagocytic index (% of phagocytosis) - the number of neutrophils with latex in 100; phagocytic count = the number of latex particles/100.

The total leukocyte count was calculated in a Goryaev's chamber. 0.4 ml of a diluent (3-5% of acetic acid dyed with methylene blue (acetic acid lyses erythrocytes, methylene blue stains leukocyte nuclei)) and 0.02 ml of blood was placed in a test-tube. Leukocytes were counted in 100 large squares. The total leukocyte count was calculated using the formula: $X = A \times 50$, where X is the number of leukocytes in 1mcl of blood, A is the number of leukocytes calculated in a Goryaev's chamber.

A blood *leukogram* was calculated in blood smears stained by the Romanovsky-Giemsa method. The count of neutrophils (stab and segmented neutrophils), eosinophils, monocytes, and lymphocytes was calculated in a smear.

Lymphoproliferative processes in the immunocompetent organs were determined on the basis of the weight and cellularity of the thymus and spleen. After the animals were euthanized, the organs were extracted and weighed; cell suspensions were prepared in medium 199 with 50 mg/ml concentration for the spleen and 10 mg/ml for the thymus. They were filtrated, washed twice with medium 199 to remove adipose tissue particles (for 10 min at a rate of 1500 revolutions). After that they were resuspended in medium 199 to the original concentration in medium 199. To make calculations the suspensions of lymphoid organs were previously mixed in the ratio 1:1 with 3% acetic acid, dyed with methylene blue; the number of nucleated cells (NC) was counted in a Goryaev's chamber. The number of NC was indicated in absolute and relative (in relation to the weight of the lymphoid organ) values.

2.2 Experimental series and groups

A few sets of experiments were carried out: the 1st aimed to study the immunomodulating activity of GABA derivatives in a "dose-effect" respect; the 2nd st explored the immunopreventive and/or immunotherapeutic aspects of the effect of GABA derivatives when administered at different times in relation to CPA immunosuppression introduction ("time-effect"); the 3rd targeted to evaluate the activity of GABA derivatives when introduced during a peroral course of treatment; the 4th aimed to study the capability of the substances to eliminate leukogram disturbances and to restore lymphoproliferative and biochemical processes in the immunocompetent organs (thymus, spleen).

The animals in each set of experiments were divided into groups (n=8): control 1 was represented by mice receiving physiological saline as a placebo in the equivalent amount (similarly to the way and frequency of administration of the investigated substance in each set); control 2 included species with an immunopathology model, they also received physiological saline; experimental groups included animals with immunosuppression, which received GABA derivatives in accordance with the goal pursued in each set of experiments.

In the 1st and 3rd experimental sets CPA was introduced 1 hour after the immunization with SE to the animals of the control 2 group and experimental groups; in the 2nd set CPA was administered twice (simultaneously with the immunization and 24 hours after the immunization with SE).

3. Results and discussion

3.1 Immunosupression

All the conducted experimental sets proved the development of immunological insufficiency in the control 2 group mice: a reliable decrease by more than 50% in the DHR index, by more than 35% in the hemagglutin titre, by more than 40% in the neutrophil phagocytic activity as compared to the similar indicators in the control 1 group was observed. Moreover, depressed leucopoiesis manifesting itself both as a statistically relevant decrease of the total leukocyte count (by more than 20% with $p_1<0.05$) and a pronounced change in the cell ratio in the leukogram was registered in the animals exposed to CPA cytostatic drug. Particularly, a reliable decrease by more than 30 % in the count of leukocytes and segmented neutrophil leukocytes as compared to the background values in control 1 ($p_1<0.05$) and a total absence of eosinophils were observed in CPA immunosuppression. It should be noted that the number of stab neutrophils was more than 50% higher ($p_1<0.05$) in this group of mice. The study of lymphoproliferative and biochemical processes in the immunocompetent organs revealed involution of the thymus and spleen and a decreased cell count in them ($p_1<0.05$), as well as a reliable increase in the lipid peroxidation intensity associated with decreased catalase activity in the investigated organs ($p_1<0.05$).

3.2 The immunomodulating activity of GABA derivatives in a "dose-effect" respect

In the 1st experimental set the model CPA immunosuppression was used to study the activity of phenotropil, phenibut, and baclofen in the following doses: phenotropil - 25 mg/kg; 50 mg/kg; 100 mg/kg; phenibut -12.5 mg/kg; 25 mg/kg; 50 mg/kg; 100 mg/kg and baclofen - 2 mg/kg; 5 mg/kg; 10 mg/kg; 20 mg/kg (Samotrueva M.A. et al., 2010; Tyurenkov I.N. et al., 2008, 2009, 2010).

The conducted investigation demonstrated that a single intraperitoneal introduction of phenotropil in all studied doses promoted an over 50% restoration of the indices of cellular DHR and the level of antired-cell antibodies in PHAR as compared to the corresponding values in the animals with simulated immunopathology ($p_2<0.05$) (here and below p_1 and p_2 – are reliability degrees in the relatively intact animals and animals with immunosuppression correspondingly). Moreover, phenotropil introduced in doses of 25mg/kg and 50 mg/kg showed pronounced immunostimulating properties regarding DHR: the quantitative parameter of the local reaction was statistically reliably higher than that of control 1 ($p_1<0.05$). Phenotropil in a dose of 100 mg/kg had a less pronounced immunocorrective action in relation to the humoral and cellular immunity links: the indices of DHRI and the antibody titre were 30-40% higher than those in the immunosuppressed species ($p_2<0.05$). However, they did not exceed the values in the intact animals (fig. 1).

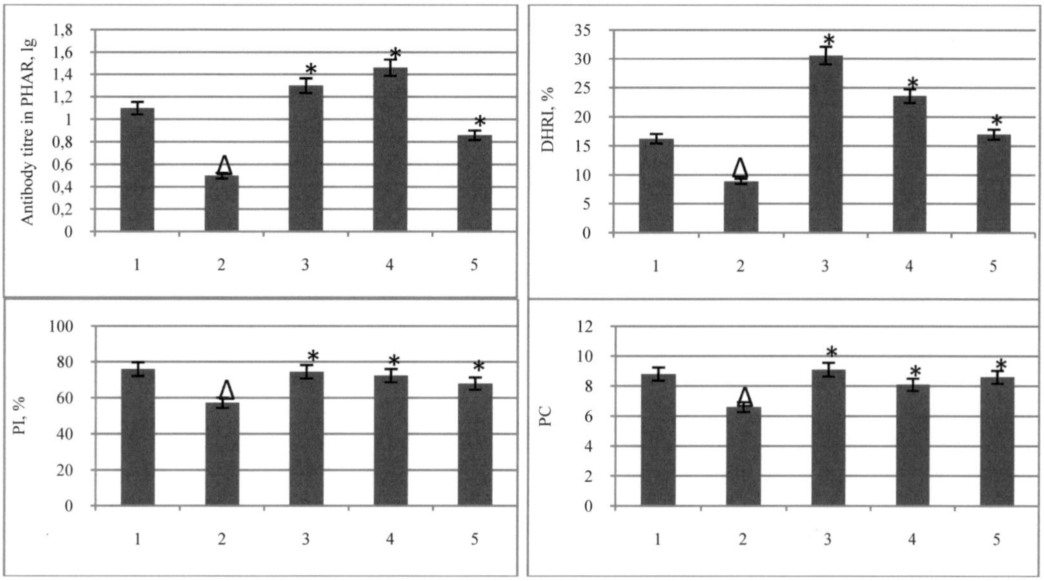

Experimental groups: 1 - control 1 (physiological saline); 2 - control 2 (CPA); 3 – phenotropil (25mg/kg) + CPA; 4 – phenotropil (50mg/kg) + CPA; 5 – phenotropil (100 mg/kg) + CPA
Notes: Δ and * – $p<0.05$ <– reliability of differences as compared to controls 1 and 2 correspondingly (Student's t-criterion with Bonferroni and Newman-Keuls' adjustment for multiple comparisons, single-factor analysis of variance involving the definition of Tukey-Kramer criterion and Scheffe's criterion)
In what follows: DHRI – delayed hypersensitivity reaction index, PHAR – passive hemagglutination reaction, PI – phagocytic index, PC – phagocytic count.

Fig. 1. Effect of phenotropil in different doses on PHAR, DHR development and the phagocytic activity of neutrophils in the immunosuppression conditions

The evaluation of phenotropil effect on the indices of the non-specific link of immunogenesis in the conditions of CPA-induced immunosuppression revealed that the drug eliminated the inhibiting action of the immunodepressant. A statistically reliable increase of PI (by more than 20%) when phenotropil was introduced in doses of 25 mg/kg ($p_2<0.05$) and 50 mg/kg ($p_2<0.001$) and PC (by more than 20%) in doses of 25 mg/kg ($p_2<0.05$) and 100 mg/kg ($p_2<0.05$) as compared to the immunosuppressed animals was registered. The administration of phenotropil in a dose of 25 mg/kg was associated with a restoration of the indices demonstrating the phagocytic activity of neutrophils almost to the "norm" (fig. 1).

Proceeding from the obtained results we selected the doses of 25 mg/kg and 50 mg/kg for a further study of phenotropil as an immunocorrective drug.

The administration of phenibut in doses of 25 mg/kg and 50 mg/kg was associated with a rise by more than 80% in the indices of both specific (the antibody titre in PHAR and the DHR index) and non-specific (PI and PC) immunoreactivity as compared to the similar values in the group of animals with simulated immunopathology (control 2) ($p_2<0.05$) and a rise by more than 20% as compared to control 1 ($p_1<0.05$) which proves the immunostimulating properties of phenibut in the specified doses (fig. 2).

A single intraperitoneal introduction of phenibut in a dose of 100 mg/kg promoted the elimination of CPA suppressor effect on the development of a primary immune response to SE: antibody titre in PHAR and DHRI reached the background values in the placebo control ($p_2<0.05$). No reliably significant change in phagocytosis indices induced by phenibut administration in a dose of 100 mg/kg was registered which proves that in this dose the drug has no corrective effect in respect to nonspecific resistance. A dose of 12.5mg/kg of the investigated substance appeared to be effective only with respect to the humoral link of pathogenesis: antibody titre in PHAR almost reached "the norm" values in control 1 ($p_2<0.05$) (fig. 2).

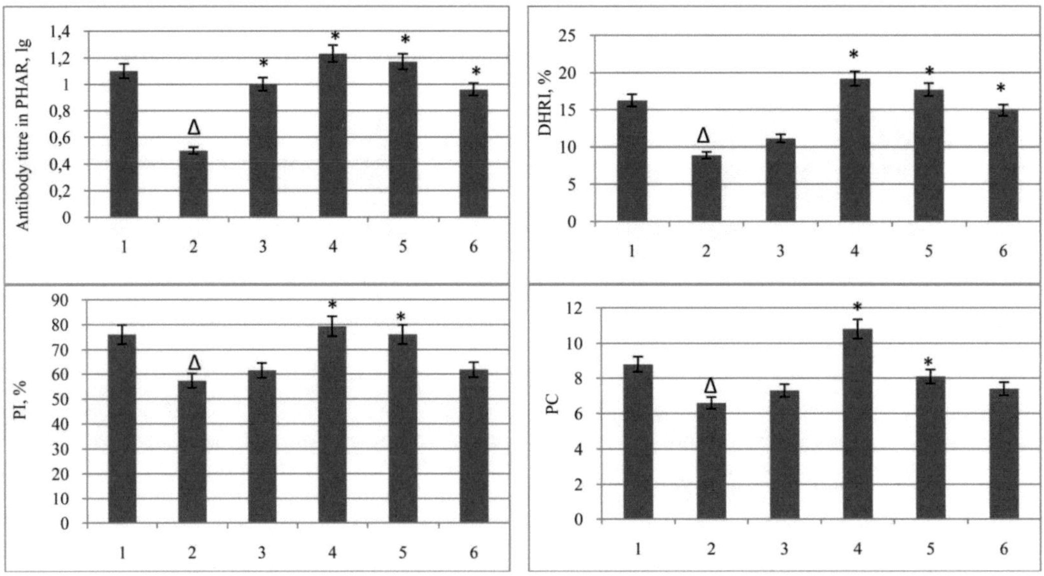

Experimental groups: 1 - control 1 (physiological saline); 2 - control 2 (CPA); 3 – phenibut (12.5 mg/kg) + CPA; 4 – phenibut (25 mg/kg) + CPA; 5 – phenibut (50 mg/kg) + CPA; 6 – phenibut (100 mg/kg) + CPA.

Notes: Δ and * – p<0.05 <– reliability of differences as compared to controls 1 and 2 correspondingly (Student's t-criterion with Bonferroni and Newman-Keuls' adjustment for multiple comparisons, single-factor analysis of variance involving the definition of Tukey-Kramer criterion and Scheffe's criterion)

Fig. 2. Effect of phenibut in different doses on PHAR, DHR development and the phagocytic activity of neutrophils in the immunosuppression conditions

Therefore, the most significant immunoreactivity changes in the animals with experimental immunosuppression were observed when phenibut was administered in doses of 25 mg/kg and 50 mg/kg which were recommended for a further study of the immunomodulating activity of phenibut.

The evaluation of the immunocorrective properties of baclofen using a CPA immunosuppression model revealed that the introduction of the drug in doses of 2 mg/kg, 5 mg/kg, and 10 mg/kg had a modulating effect on antibody formation ($p_2<0.05$). In addition, the most pronounced increase of the antibody titre in PHAR was registered in a dose of 10 mg/kg; the studied index was 2.5 times as high as that in the species with an immune pathology while the administration of baclofen in doses of 2 mg/kg and 5 mg/kg increased the index by no more than 60% ($p_2<0.05$). A dose of 20 mg/kg proved to be ineffective: the antibody titre in PHAR was similar to that in the animals with immunosuppression ($p_2<0.05$) (fig. 3).

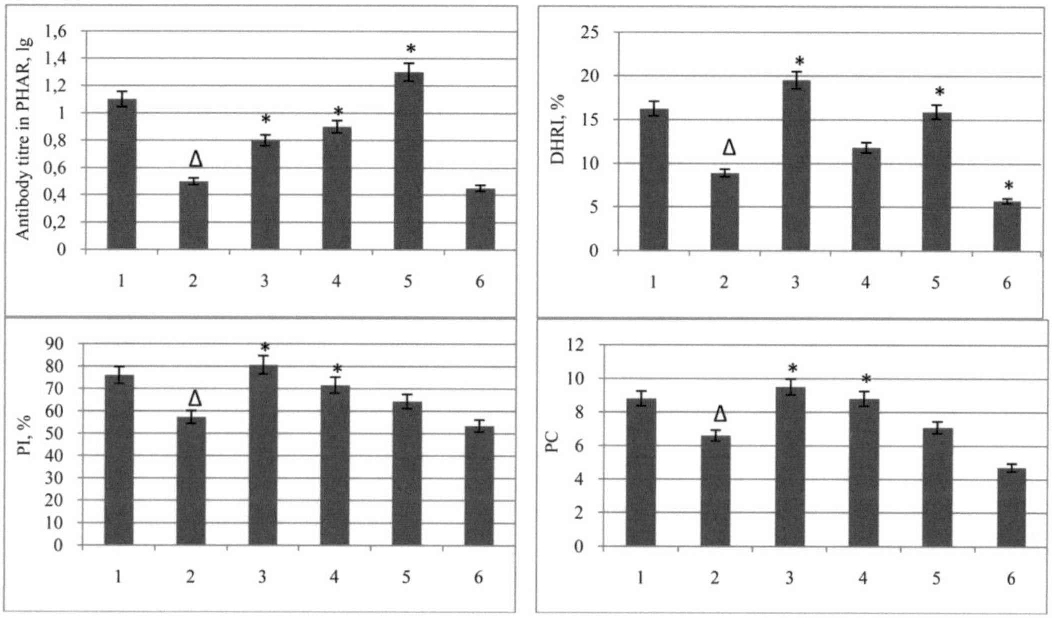

Experimental groups: 1 - control 1 (physiological saline); 2 - control 2 (CPA); 3 – baclofen (2 mg/kg) + CPA; 4 – baclofen (5 mg/kg) + CPA; 5 – baclofen (10 mg/kg) + CPA; 6 – baclofen (20 mg/kg) + CPA. Notes: Δ and * – $p<0.05$ – reliability of differences as compared to controls 1 and 2 correspondingly (Student's t-criterion with Bonferroni and Newman-Keuls' adjustment for multiple comparisons, single-factor analysis of variance involving the definition of Tukey-Kramer criterion and Scheffe's criterion)

Fig. 3. Effect of baclofen in different doses on PHAR, DHR development and the phagocytic activity of neutrophils in the immunosuppression conditions

As for the cellular link of immunogenesis baclofen was active in doses of 2 mg/kg, 5 mg/kg, and 10 mg/kg. The most significant changes in the DHRI were registered when the drug was administered in doses of 2 mg/kg and 10 mg/kg: the studied index exceeded that in the group of animals with an immune pathology by more than 80% at that. Moreover, baclofen in a dose of 2 mg/kg had a stimulating effect on a cellular immune response increasing the DHRI by 20% as compared to the intact animals. It should be noted that as a dose of

baclofen increased to 20 mg/kg, no corrective action of the drug on DHR development was observed while the CPA's immunoinhibiting effect intensified (CPA).
The results which demonstrate the effect of baclofen in different doses on the indices of the phagocytic activity of neutrophils are of particular interest. We found that regarding this index the drug had a dose-dependent effect: as a dose of baclofen increased from 2 mg/kg to 20 mg/kg its corrective action declined. Thus, when it was administered in a dose of 2 mg/kg phagocytosis activity increased by more than 35% as compared to the immunosuppressed animals ($p_2<0.05$); while in doses of 5 mg/kg and 10 mg/kg this index increased only by 10-20% ($p_2<0.05$); and in a dose of 20 mg/kg a slight increase of CPA immunosuppressive activity was registered (fig. 3). Therefore, proceeding from the analysis results a baclofen dose of 2 mg/kg was chosen for further research as the most active.

3.3 The immunopreventive and/or immunotherapeutic aspects of the effect of GABA derivatives

In the second set of experiments we explored the activity of phenotropil, phenibut, and baclofen using the CPA-induced immunosuppression model in a "time-effect" respect to reveal the immunopreventive and/or immunotherapeutic aspects of the action of the drugs (Samotrueva M.A. et al., 2009; Tyurenkov I.N. et al., 2010).

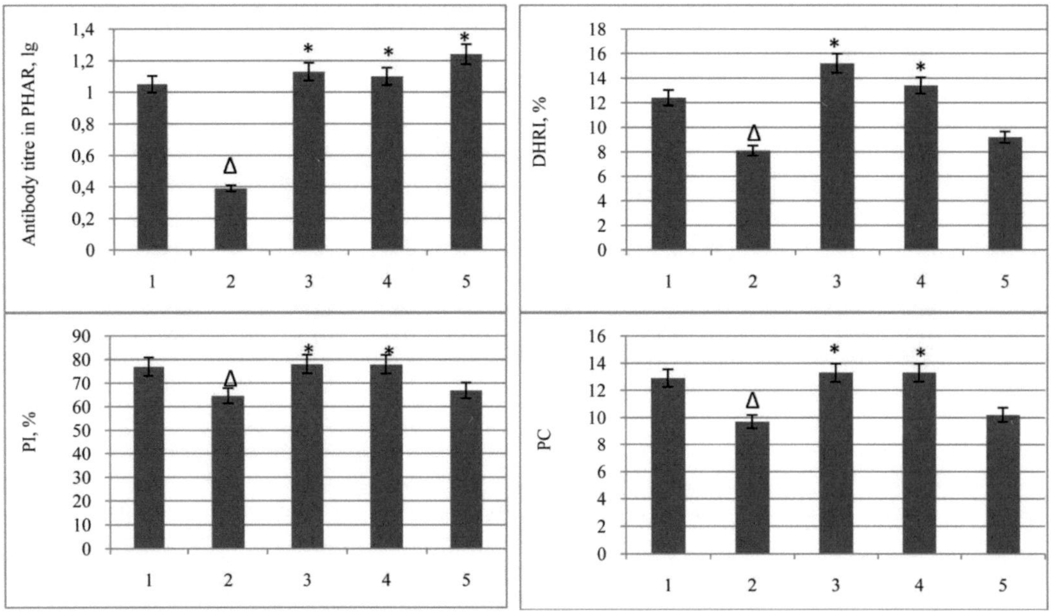

Experimental groups: 1 – control 1 (physiological saline); 2 – control 2 (CPA); 3 – phenotropil (preventive administration) + CPA; 4 – phenotropil (at immunosuppression induction) + CPA; 5 – phenotropil (therapeutic administration) + CPA
Designations: * – p<0.05 reliable difference of findings in experimental groups in comparison with control 2; Δ – p<0.05 reliable difference in comparison with control 1 (Student t-criterion with Bonferroni correction, Tukey-Kramer one-way ANOVA)

Fig. 4. Effect of phenotropil on the formation of DHR, PHAR and on phagocytic activity of neutrophils when administered at different times in relation to immunosuppression induction

The evaluation of the immunocorrective properties of phenotropil administered intraperitoneally for three times before antigen stimulation and/or immunosuppression induction revealed that the drug proved capable of preventing the disturbances of the cellular and humoral immunity links, as well as of the phagocytic activity of neutrophils induced by CPA. Thus, the DHR index and the level of antired-cell antibodies in the animals of the experimental group were more than 50% higher than the corresponding indices in the immunosuppressed species ($p_2<0.05$) approximating the immune response parameters in the control 1 group ($p_1<0.05$). The number of cells involved in the non-specific body defense (PI) and phagocytosis intensity (PC) in the animals receiving phenotropil before the immunosuppression induction was also restored ($p_2<0.05$) almost reaching the "norm" indices in control 1 (fig. 4).

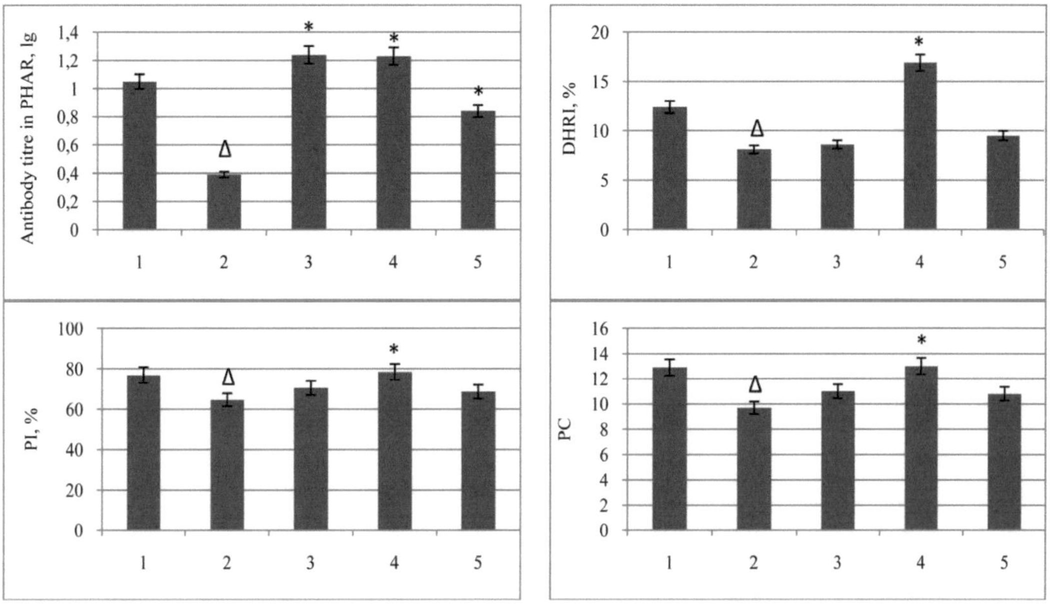

Experimental groups: 1 – control 1 (physiological saline); 2 – control 2 (CPA); 3 – phenibut (preventive administration) + CPA; 4 – phenibut (at immunosuppression induction) + CPA; 5 – phenibut (therapeutic administration) + CPA
Designations: * – p<0.05 reliable difference of findings in experimental groups in comparison with control 2; Δ – p<0.05 reliable difference in comparison with control 1 (Student t-criterion with Bonferroni correction, Tukey-Kramer one-way ANOVA)

Fig. 5. Effect of phenibut on the formation of DHR, PHAR and on phagocyric activity of neutrophils when administered at different times in relation to immunosuppression induction

The introduction of phenotropil after the immunization and/or immunosuppression induction contributed to the restoration of only the humoral link of immunogenesis: the level of serum antibodies in the experimental animals was more than 60% higher than that of the immunosuppressed species ($p_2<0.05$). No restoration of the cellular immunity link and phagocytic activity of neutrophils affected by phenotropil administered, when immunosuppression had already developed, was observed: DHR index, PI, and PC remained similar to the indices of the animals with an immune system pathology ($p_2<0.05$) (fig. 4).

Thus the therapeutic effect of phenotropil, once immunosuppression has been induced, is only manifested in relation to the humoral link of immune reactivity. However if the drug is administered prior to antigen stimulation and / or immunosuppression induction, this allows avoidance of immunological insufficiency development manifested by suppression of the activity of all links of immunogenesis, which indicates that phenotropil displays a therapeutic immunocorrective action.

Studying the time-effect aspect of the properties of phenibut demonstrated that the drug displays an ability to eliminate the immunosuppressive effect of CPA upon its administration during the induction phase of immunogeneis (that is, on the first day of antigen stimulation), and simultaneously with induction of immunopathology: the indices of cellular and humoral immune response in mice exceeded similar indices more than twice ($p_2<0.05$) both in immunosuppressed animals and in intact ones (fig. 5).

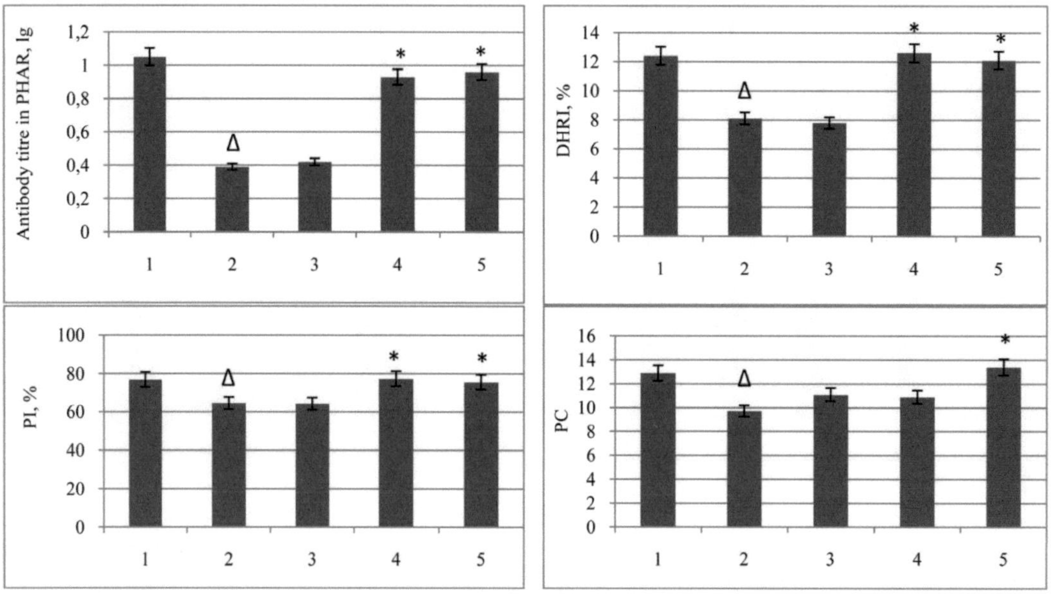

Experimental groups: 1 – control 1 (physiological saline); 2 – control 2 (CPA); 3 – baclofen (preventive administration) + CPA; 4 – baclofen (at immunosuppression induction) + CPA; 5 – baclofen (therapeutic administration) + CPA

Designations: * – $p<0.05$ reliable difference of findings in experimental groups in comparison with control 2; Δ – $p<0.05$ reliable difference in comparison with control 1 (Student t-criterion with Bonferroni correction, Tukey-Kramer one-way ANOVA)

Fig. 6. Effect of baclofen on the formation of DHR, PHAR and on phagocytic activity of neutrophils when administered at different times in relation to immunosuppression induction

As for humoral immunoreactivity, phenibut showed both an immunoprotective and immunotherapeutic effect: a reliable increase in the antibody level more than twice in comparison with control 2 ($p_2<0.05$) (fig. 5) upon preventive administration of the substance (three days prior to immunopathology induction) and upon its introduction to the productive phase of immunogenesis (three days after immunization and immunopathology induction). Phagocytic count and phagocytic index, parameters of nonspecific resistance, were also sensitive to the corrective effect of phenibut, but the effect of the drug was only manifest upon its administration on the day of the antigen and cytostatic exposure; at that time the indices of phagocytosis were virtually the same as in intact animals ($p_2<0.05$).

Thus the obtained results permit a conclusion that phenibut is capable of preventing the development of disturbances in all the components of the immune system under study, but this only occurs upon its administration on the day of immunization and of exposure to an immunopathology inductor.

An assessment of baclofen impact on the immunity status of animals with immunosuppression by cyclophosphamide upon administration at different times in relation to immunization and pathology simulation showed that the drug was only capable of displaying an immunocorrective effect either upon simultaneous administration with an immunodepressant agent or after the onset of a lesion. In the before-mentioned groups of animals the DHR index, antibody titer and the number of neutrophils participating in phagocytosis exceeded reliably the same parameters in animals with an immunity disorder ($p_2<0.05$) achieving background values of immune response in control 1 (fig. 6).

Thus the findings obtained in the course of studying the temporal dependence of immunocorrective effects of baclofen indicate that the drug exerts an immunotherapeutic effect while administration of baclofen for prevention of immunity disturbances in conditions of CPA-induced immunosuppression turned out to be ineffective.

3.4 The immunomodulating activity of GABA derivatives when introduced during a peroral course of treatment

The third series of experiments was devoted to studying the extent of immunomodulating effects of phenotropil, phenibut and baclofen upon their peroral administration over a 14-day course of therapy.

In conditions of immunosuppression, peroral administration of phenotropil and phenibut in a course led to a restoration of cellular immunoreactivity: the index of delayed-type hypersensitivity exceeded the corresponding values in control 2 ($p_2<0.05$) twice achieving the values displayed by intact animals. Baclofen showed no effect in relation to the studied parameter (fig. 7).

An estimation of the effect of substances of these experimental series on the humoral link of immunogenesis showed that phenotropil displayed the most effect in conditions of immunosuppression exerting a stimulating effect on the process of sheep erythrocyte-specific antibody formation. Thus the hemagglutinin titer in the reaction of passive hemagglutination exceeded that of control 2 animals 3.8 times ($p_2<0.05$) and 1.6 times - that of intact animals ($p_2<0.05$). Administration of phenibut also promoted a more than two-fold elevation of the level of anti-erythrocytic antibodies in comparison with the animals receiving the CPA immunodepressant ($p_2<0.05$). As for baclofen, it showed no activity in relation to the humoral link of immunogenesis in conditions of immunosuppression (fig. 7).

The nonspecific link of immunogenesis was also sensitive to the corrective effect of the substances under study. Thus phenotropil, phenibut and baclofen caused an intensification of phagocytosis (of phagocytic index and phagocytic number as well) in comparison with these parameters in immunosuppressed animals, and the intensity of phagocytosis virtually achieved the background values in control 1 ($p_2<0.05$) (fig. 7).

Therefore, the findings of the study of the effect of substances on the values of immune response upon peroral administration for 14 days indicated that the most activity upon administration in a course was shown by phenotropil and phenibut; these drugs eliminated the CPA-induced suppression of the cellular, humoral and nonspecific links of the immunity.

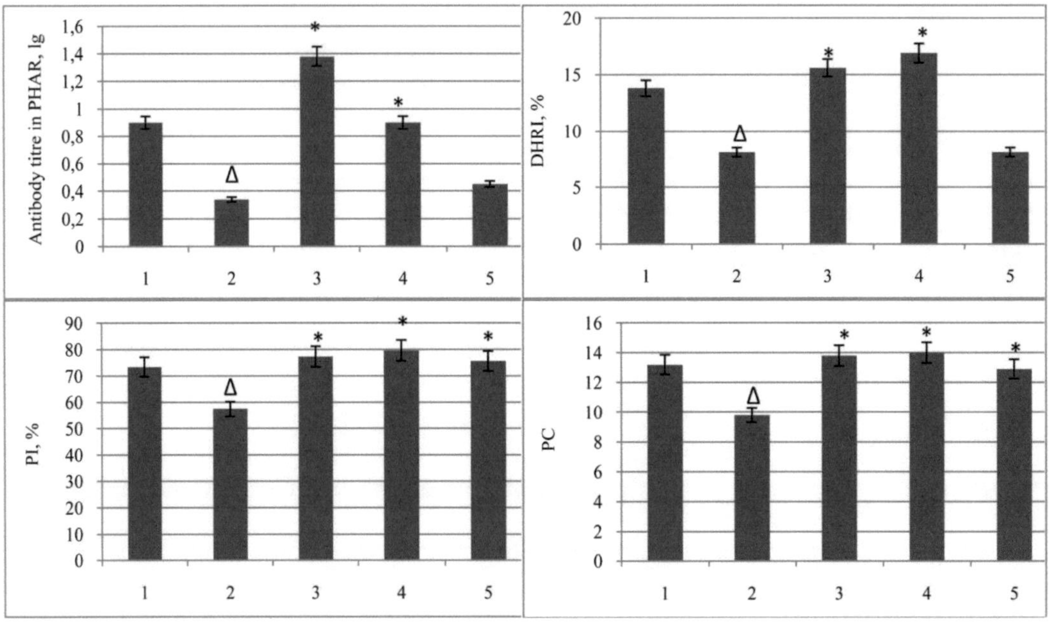

Experimental groups: 1 – control 1 (physiological saline); 2 – control 2 (CPA); 3 – phenotropil (25 mg/kg) + CPA; 4 – phenibut (25 mg/kg) + CPA; 5 – baclofen (2 mg/kg) + CPA

Designations: Δ – p<0.05 reliable difference in comparison with control 1 (Student t-criterion with Bonferroni correction and Newman-Keuls test for multiple comparisons); * – p<0.05 reliable difference in comparison with control 2 (Student t-criterion with Bonferroni correction and Newman-Keuls test for multiple comparisons)

Fig. 7. Effect of GABA derivatives after a 14-day peroral administration on the formation of PHAR, DHR and on phagocyric activity of neutrophils in peripheral blood of animals with CPA - induced immunosuppression

3.5 Influence of GABA derivatives on leukopoiesis and on lymphoproliferative and biochemical processes in the immunocompetent organs in conditions of immunosuppression

In the fourth series of experiments we studied the effect of phenotropil, phenibut and baclofen on leukopoiesis and on lymphoprolifertaive processes in immunocompetent organs (thymus, the spleen) in conditions of immunosuppression. In these series the

substances under study were introduced intraperitoneally for five days in the most active doses (first administration two days prior to CPA). Animals' blood sampling was done on the next day after the last administration of the substances under study (Samotrueva M.A. et al., 2008; Tyurenkov I.N. et al., 2009; Samotrueva M.A. et al., 2011).
An assessment of the effect of drugs under study on the total number and qualitative composition of leukocytes in peripheral blood showed that under the impact of CPA the administration of phenotropil resulted in an increase of the total leukocyte number up to background values of control 1($p_2<0.05$). Neither phenibut nor baclofen caused any significant change in the total leukocyte number in comparison with the group of immunosuppressed animals ($p>0.05$) (tab. 1).

Experimental groups	Total leukocyte number, x 10^9/L
Control 1 (physiological saline)	10.8 ± 0.7
Control 2 (CPA, 150 mg/kg)	8.3 ± 0.7 Δ
Phenibut (25 mg/kg) + CPA (150 mg/kg)	8.9 ± 0.3
Phenotropil (25 mg/kg) + CPA (150 mg/kg)	10.4 ± 0.4*
Baclofen (2 mg/kg) + CPA (150 mg/kg)	9.6 ± 1.1

The degree of credibility Δ – $p<0.05$ – in relation to control 1 and * – $p<0.05$ – in relation to control 2 (Student t-criterion with Bonferroni correction for multiple comparisons)

Table 1. Effect of GABA derivatives on total leukocyte count in animals with CPA -induced immunosuppression

In animals with CPA -induced immunological insufficiency a restoration of leukocyte population composition was only noted under the impact of phenotropil administration when a relative number of leukocytes was noted to increase; the content of lymphoid cells in peripheral blood of mice of experimental groups considerably exceeded this parameter in control 2 animals ($p_2<0.05$). Administration of baclofen was accompanied by an elevation of the number of mature segmented neutrophils ($p_2<0.05$), while the level of lymphocytes remained within the range of values typical of immunosuppressed animals ($p>0.05$). No significant changes in the leukogram were noted under the impact of phenibut ($p>0.05$) (fig. 8).
Thus phenotropil displayed the most activity in relation to the leukogram parameters by promoting a restoration of leukopoiesis processes which was manifested in an elimination of the inhibiting effect of CPA on the lymphoid hematopoietic lineage.
The results of studying the effects of phenotropil, phenibut and baclofen on lymphoproliferative and biochemical processes in immunocompetent organs in conditions of CPA -induced immunosuppression indicate that the drugs produce a corrective effect on the morphometric parameters which was evident from the increase in thymus and spleen weight, a restoration of their cellular composition ($p_2<0.05$) (fig. 9-11).

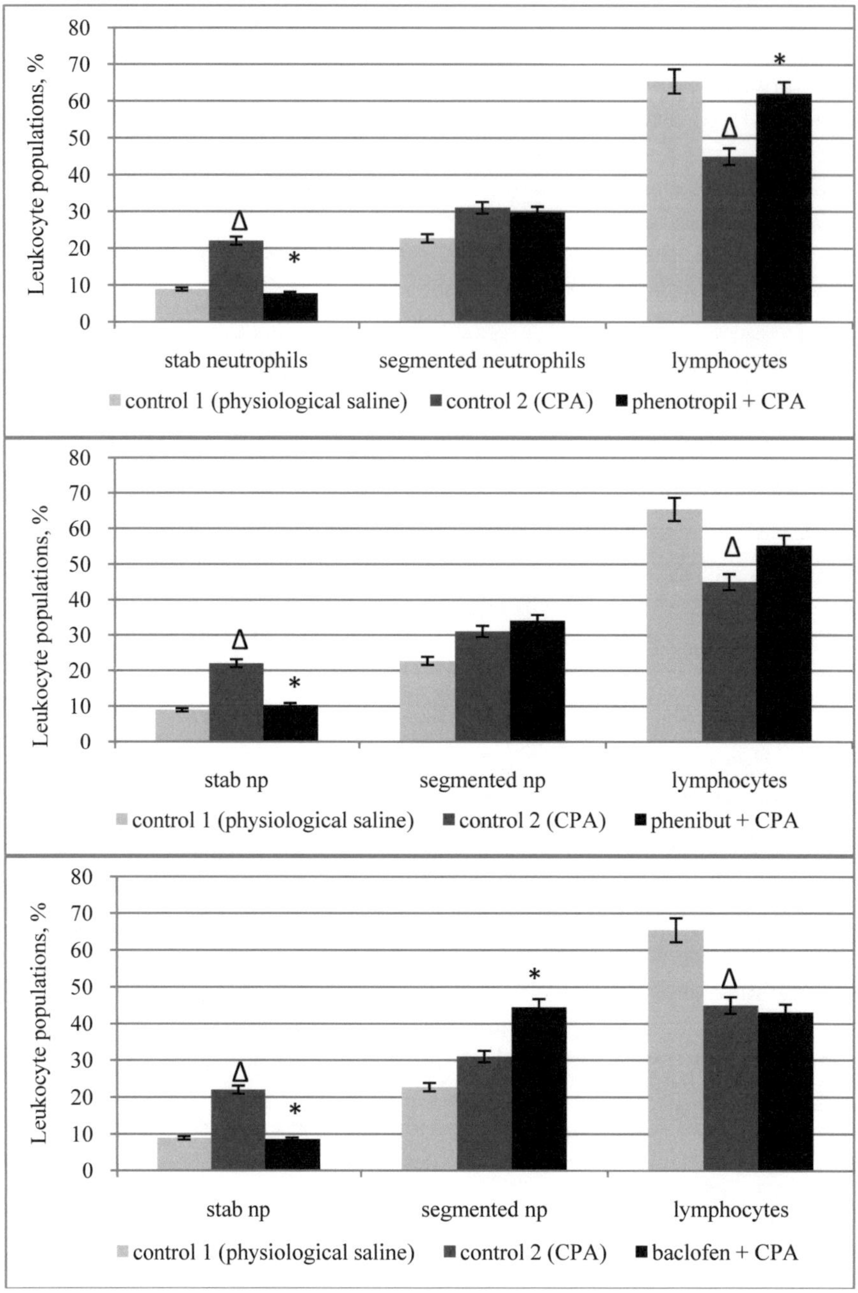

Designations: Δ – p<0.05 reliable difference in comparison with control 1 (Student t-criterion with Bonferroni correction and Newman-Keuls test for multiple comparisons); * – p<0.05 reliable difference in comparison with control 2 (Student t-criterion with Bonferroni correction and Newman-Keuls test for multiple comparisons)

Fig. 8. Effect of GABA derivatives on various leukocyte populations in the leukogram in animals with CPA -induced immunosupression

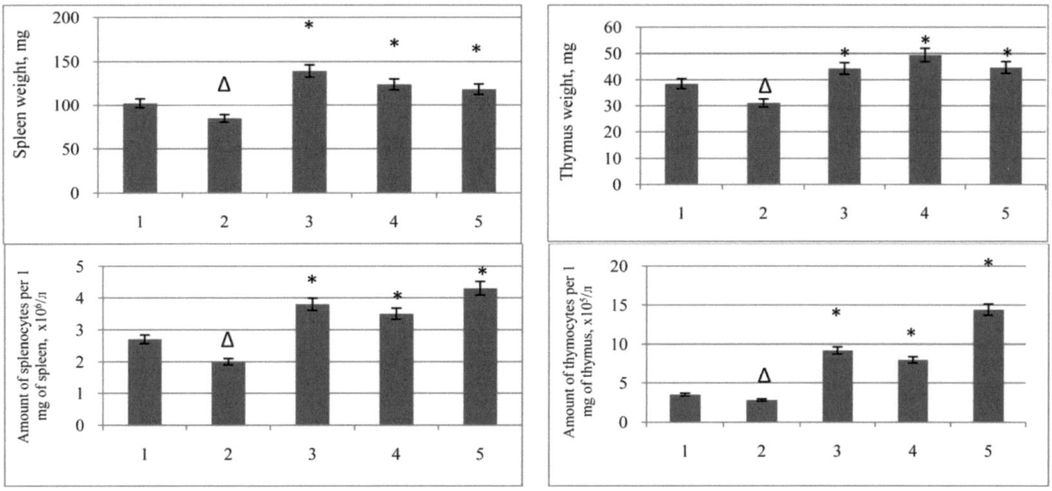

Experimental groups: 1 - control 1 (physiological saline); 2 - control 2 (CPA + physiological saline); 3 - phenotropil (25 mg/kg) + CPA; 4 - phenibut (25 mg/kg) + CPA; 5 - baclofen (2 mg/kg) + CPA
Designations: Δ - $p<0.05$ reliable difference in comparison with control 1 (Student t-criterion with Bonferroni correction and Newman-Keuls test for multiple comparisons); * - $p<0.05$ reliable difference in comparison with control 2 (Student t-criterion with Bonferroni correction and Newman-Keuls test for multiple comparisons)

Fig. 9. Effect of GABA derivatives on the weight and cellularity of immunocompetent organs in animals with CPA-induced immunosuppression

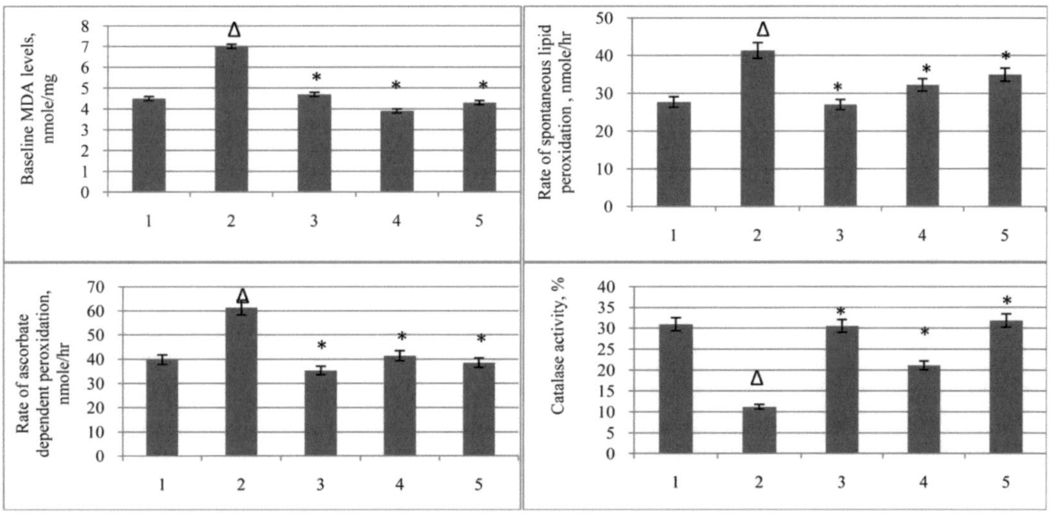

Experimental groups: 1 - control 1 (physiological saline); 2 - control 2 (CPA); 3 - phenotropil (25 mg/kg) + CPA; 4 - phenibut (25 mg/kg) + CPA; 5 - baclofen (2 mg/kg) + CPA
Designations: Δ - $p<0.05$ reliable difference in comparison with control 1 (Student t-criterion with Bonferroni correction and Newman-Keuls test for multiple comparisons); * - $p<0.05$ reliable difference in comparison with control 2 (Student t-criterion with Bonferroni correction and Newman-Keuls test for multiple comparisons)

Fig. 10. Effect of GABA derivatives on lipid peroxidation and catalase activity in the spleen of animals with CPA -induced immunosuppression

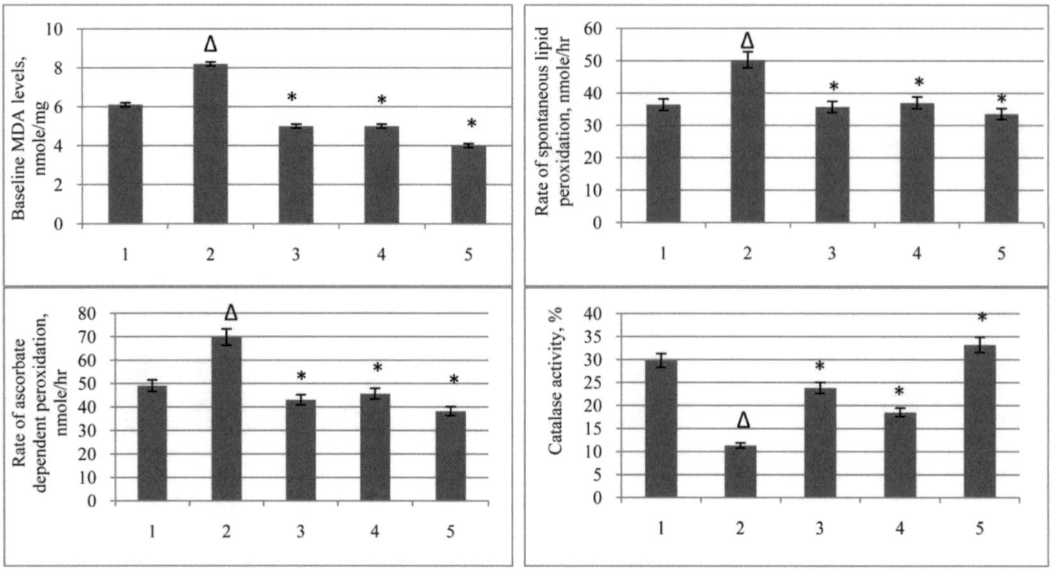

Experimental groups: 1 – control 1 (physiological saline); 2 – control 2 (CPA); 3 – phenotropil (25 mg/kg) + CPA; 4 – phenibut (25 mg/kg) + CPA; 5 – baclofen (2 mg/kg) + CPA

Designations: Δ – $p<0.05$ reliable difference in comparison with control 1 (Student t-criterion with Bonferroni correction and Newman-Keuls test for multiple comparisons); * – $p<0.05$ reliable difference in comparison with control 2 (Student t-criterion with Bonferroni correction and Newman-Keuls test for multiple comparisons)

Fig. 11. Effect of GABA derivatives on lipid peroxidation and catalase activity in the thymus of animals with CPA-induced immunosuppression

4. Conclusion

We would like to highlight the importance and urgency of the problem under discussion. Immune imbalance underlies the pathogenesis of CNS diseases (depression, disorder of cerebral circulation, epilepsy, multiple sclerosis, Alzheimer's disease, schizophrenia, etc.), and one of the causes of these conditions is dysregulation of GABA-ergic system as one of the key factors of neuro-immune interactions. An analysis of our own data and those from literature permits a conclusion that a realization of immunoactive properties of GABA-ergic substances is mediated by both central and direct impact on the corresponding receptors of effector cells in the immune system. The pronounced immunomodulating effect of phenotropil, phenibut and baclofen that we showed in CPA-induced immunosuppression widens the range of their possible administration not only in CNS diseases that are often accompanied by immune status disturbances, but also in the immune system diseases accompanied by suppression of certain immunogenesis links.

1. GABA derivatives – phenotropil, phenibut and baclofen – reduce the manifestations of immunosuppression induced by CPA administration.
2. Phenotropil at a dose of 25 mg/kg, 50 mg/kg and baclofen at a dose of 2 mg/kg produce the most pronounced immunomodulating effect in conditions of CPA-induced immunosuppression.
3. Immunotropic effects of phenotropil and phenibut are most pronounced upon their preventive administration prior to CPA-induced immunosuppression, while the effect

of baclofen is most pronounced upon its therapeutic administration when the immune system disease is already in progress.

4. All the substances studied in this work can restore lymphorpoliferative processes and normalize the parameters of lipid peroxisation in the immunicompetent organs (thymus and spleen); while only phenotropil was able to eliminate the disturbances of leukopoietic processes due to immunosuppression.
5. The immunomodulating effect of phenotropil, phenibut and baclofen established in our study as well as their neurotropic effects established by many researchers, allow an inclusion of GABA derivatives into a new class of neuroimmunomodulating agents.

5. References

[1] Alexandrovsky U.A., Chekhonin V.P. Clinical immunology of borderline mental disorders. - Moscow: GEOTAR-Media, 2005. -256 p.

[2] Alford L. Findings of interest from immunology and psychoneuroimmunology // Man. Ther. - 2007. - Vol. 12. - N 2. - P. 176-80.

[3] Arkadyev V.G., Makarenko A.N., Mironiuk U. M. Experimental reproduction of medium and severe immmunosuppression with cyclophosphane administration // Vestnik KNU. Biology series. - 2003. - Vol. 39. - P. 51-52.

[4] Arushanian E.B. Medicamentous amelioration of cognitive brain function. - Stavropol: SGMA Publishers, 2004. - 401 p.

[5] Devoyno L.V., Iliuchenok R.U. Neuromediator systems in psychoneuromodulation: dopamine, serotonin, GABA, neuropeptides. - Novosibirsk, ZE RIS, 1993. - 273 p.

[6] Fleshner M., Laudenslager M.L. Psychoneuroimmunology: then and now // Behav. Cogn. Neurosci Rev. - 2004. - N 3. - P. 114-130.

[7] Freund G.G. Psychoneuroimmunology // Preface Immunol. Allergy Clin. North. Am. - 2009. - Vol. 29. - N 2. - P. 15-16.

[8] Irwin M.R. Human psychoneuroimmunology: 20 years of discovery // Brain Behav. Immun. - 2008. - Vol. 22 (2). - P. 129-139.

[9] Khaitov R.M., Gushin I.S., Pinegin B.V. Methodological recommendations on studying immunotropic effects of pharmacological agents // Handbook of experimental preclinical study of new pharmacological agents / Ed. by R.U. Khabriev. - Moscow, 2005. - P. 501-514.

[10] Korneva E.A. Introduciton to immunophysiology. - St Petersburg: ELBI, 2003. - 48 p.

[11] Kryzhanovsky G.N., Magaeva S.V., Makarov S.V., Sepiashvili R.I. Neuroimmunopathology. - Moscow: Meditsina, 2003. - 438 p.

[12] Samotrueva M.A., Ovcharova A.N., Tyurenkov I.N. Evaluation of the immunocorrecting activity of phenibut // Vestnik novyh meditsinskih technologii. - 2008. - Vol. 15. - N 3. - P. 168-169.

[13] Samotrueva M.A., Ovcharova A.N., Tyurenkov I.N. Phenibut and its derivatives' influence on the cell section of the immune response in immunodeficiency // European Journal of Natural History. - 2008. - N 5. - P. 40-41.

[14] Samotrueva M.A., Tyurenkov I.N., Luzhnova S.A., Magomedov M.M., Kuleshevskaia N.R., Serezhnikova T.K. Experimental learning of dose-related influence of phenotropil on humoral link of immunogenesis // European Journal of Natural History. - 2010. - N 3. - P. 61-62.

[15] Samotrueva M.A., Tyurenkov I.N., Serezhnikova T.K., Grazhdantseva N.N., Khlebtsova E.B., Berestovitskaia V.M., Vassilieva O.S. Immunomodulating properties of phenotropil derivatives // Farmatsia. - 2011. - N 1. - P. 28-30.
[16] Samotrueva M.A., Tyurenkov I.N., Teply D.L., Luzhnova S.A., Magomedov M.M. Extent of immunocorrective effects of phenotropil upon its adminsitartion at different times in relation to immunosuppression induction // Meditsinskaia immunologia. - 2009. - N 6. - Vol. 11. - P 567-570.
[17] Samotryeva M.A., Teply D.L., Tyurenkov I.N. Ways to realization of neuro-immune-endocrine interactions // Estestvennye nauki. - 2009. - N 4. - Vol. 29. - P. 112-130.
[18] Tyurenkov I.N., Galimzianov H.M., Teply D.L., Samotrueva M.A., Luzhnova S.A. Experimental study of immunocorrective effects of phenotropil in the dose-effect aspect // Immunologia. - 2009. - N 5. - P. 302-305.
[19] Tyurenkov I.N., Samotrueva M.A. Comparative study of immunocorrective activity of phenibut and its organic salts in experimental immunodeficiency // Bull. Exp. Biol. Med. - 2009. - N 5. - P. 606-668.
[20] Tyurenkov I.N., Samotrueva M.A., Kuleshevskaia N.R., Serezhnikova T.K. Experimental substantiation of phenibut administration as a modulator of immune response // Farmatsia. - 2010. - N 4. - P. 42-44.
[21] Tyurenkov I.N., Samotrueva M.A., Ovcharova A.N. Baclofen influence on the cellular parts of immune reaction // Experimentalnaia i klinicheskaia farmakologia. - 2008. - N 3. - P. 43-45.

7

Immunodepression and Immunosuppression During Aging

Véronique Thomas-Vaslin, Adrien Six, Hang-Phuong Pham,
Cira Dansokho, Wahiba Chaara, Bruno Gouritin,
Bertrand Bellier and David Klatzmann
UPMC Univ Paris 06, UMR7211, Immunology, Immunopathology, Immunotherapy, Paris
CNRS UMR7211, Integrative Immunology: Differentiation, Diversity, Dynamics, Paris
France

1. Introduction

Much work has been done to understand isolated aspects of the immune system and effects of immunosuppression in young adults. However there has been little attempt to understand changes throughout the entire life-span of an organism, across organs, genetic backgrounds and at various scales of biological detail and to assess the effects of immunosuppression in old individuals.

The immune system plays a central role in a number of physiological phenomena to maintain the integrity of the individual, by a complex dynamic equilibrium involving immunity and inflammation, but also tolerance, in particular during the gestation. Disequilibrium can lead to pathological disorders such as auto-immune and infectious diseases, cancers and so on. With aging, there is a progressive alteration of the immune system and its responses, resulting in immuno senescence and **immunodepression**. Of importance thymic involution and infection contribute to aging of the immune system (Gress and Deeks 2009). This leads to less efficient lymphocyte production, activation and responsiveness, increased susceptibility to inflammatory responses and autoimmunity and decreased responses to infections, tumours and vaccinations, see reviews (2005; 2009; Aspinall and Goronzy 2010).

The most important feature of the immune system is to be able to respond to an almost infinite number of antigens and perform immune function to maintain the integrity of the individual. This activity depends on the availability of a **diverse repertoire** of lymphocytes, i.e. a collection of lymphocytes, each characterized by its antigen-specific receptor produced by random somatic rearrangements of V(D)J gene segments during lymphocyte differentiation. The selection constraints are important in particular for the initial construction of the immune system (in foetus/newborn), or for reconstitution in immunodeficient recipients (Ciupe, Devlin et al. 2009), but also during attrition with aging. In this line, recent studies regarding the question of lymphocyte diversity, selection and available niches have been discussed (Stirk, Molina-Paris et al. 2008; Ciupe, Devlin et al. 2009; Leitao, Freitas et al. 2009). Moreover, in old individual mice or humans, clonal expansions are often observed in CD8 T cells, probably as a result of chronic and repeated infections. This reduces the diversity of the repertoire (Ahmed, Lanzer et al. 2009), decreases the potential to drive an immune response and affects the CD4/CD8 ratio (LeMaoult, Messaoudi et al. 2000; Messaoudi, Lemaoult et al. 2004 ; Clambey, van Dyk et al. 2005; Goronzy and Weyand 2005; Pawelec, Akbar et al. 2005; Clambey, Kappler et al. 2007) reviewed in (Blackman and Woodland 2011). With age CD4 T cells have increased longevity (Tsukamoto, Clise-Dwyer et al. 2009) while under normal homeostatic conditions recent thymic migrant have to compete with already established mature naïve T cells (Houston, Higdon et al. 2011).

On the **life-scale**, lymphocyte and lymphoid organ emergence, cell selection and expansion during ontogeny are critical features of the immune system construction and determine its efficiency at the adult age. Thus, during life, homeostasis is maintained with a dynamic equilibrium between diversity and efficiency (naïf vs. effector/memory lymphocytes) with two periods of physiological relative immunodeficiency, early in ontogeny and in advanced old age. In females, the gestation also represents a relative immunodepressive period leading to embryo/foetus acceptance. During the life, dynamic equilibrium ensures complex interactions of highly diversified circulating lymphocytes, with high turnover, responsible for tolerance and immune protection of the organism, while controlling most pathogens. **Aging however induces complex and progressive alterations** that find their origins at **different biological scales**: organism, organ, cell populations, cells, molecules, genes. Table 1 summarizes some of these general observations.

Immune systems aging: multilevel scales

- Organism level
  - Increase susceptibilitty to infection, tumors, autoimmunity
  - Decreases vaccinale response and protection
- Organ level
  - Involution of primary lymphoid organs (bone marrow, thymus)
  - Desorganisation of thymic architecture
  - Alteration of germinal centers
- Cell population level
  - Decrease of precursor differentiation
  - Decrease of lymphoid repertoire diversity
  - Chronic or repeated stimulation of lymphoid cell by pathogen.
  - Accumulation of effector and memory cells
  - Decrease of naive /memory cell ratio
  - Decrease of CD4/ CD8 ratio
  - Increase of Treg cell numbers
- Cell level
  - Decrease of cell activation (defect of presentation or migration of APC, TLR Activation, Ag presentation)
  - Decrease of Antibody production
  - Decrease of IL-2 production
  - Alteration of stimulation signaling through the TCR
  - Accumulation of non functional senescent T cells
- Molecular level
  - Shortening of telomere in lymphoid naive and memory T cells
  - Alteration in lipid raft in lymphoid cells
  - Altered gene and protein expression
  - Altered apoptosis

Table 1. Aging alters immune functions at various biological levels. The levels can interfere with each other as depicted by the arrows.

Thymic involution is a primary sign of immunological aging at puberty and the reduced production of diverse naïve T cells is compensated for in the immune system by the proliferation of existing peripheral T cells. In very old humans and mice this leads to alteration in the T cell repertoire, appearance of oligoclonal expansions, restricting the lymphocyte repertoire (Messaoudi, Lemaoult et al. 2004; Clambey, van Dyk et al. 2005). Thymic involution is likely the result of alterations at different levels, aging being related to alteration of molecular process as somatic recombination of V-D-J gene, that seems related to deficiency in the RAG enzyme, leading to diminution of thymic export (Hale, Boursalian et al. 2006), and recent thymic emigrants (Boursalian, Golob et al. 2004). Direct alterations of thymocyte proliferation, differentiation process or environmental factors as alteration of the thymic epithelium also impact thymocyte differentiation (Thoman 1995; Yehuda, Friedman et al. 1998; Andrew and Aspinall 2001). In elderly humans, altered homeostasis also participates to decrease ratio of naive/memory and CD4/CD8 cells, with senescence of CD4 T cells (Ferrando-Martinez, Ruiz-Mateos et al.).

Moreover, **genetic & epigenetic mechanisms** (Yung and Julius 2008) participate to control or trigger aging alterations (Dorshkind, Montecino-Rodriguez et al. 2009). We need to improve our knowledge on (i) the effects of genetic variability and aging, on lymphocyte dynamics population, repertoire selection and related immunodepression and (ii) the effects of immunosuppressive treatment in aged mice. Murine models may give some indications to better understand similar perturbations in humans or the ways to study and model them.

In addition to aging that induces immunodepression, various clinical treatments used to control many diseases, induce **immunosuppression.** These treatments are designed to control unwanted immune responses, such as inflammation, autoimmunity, graft rejection, Graft Versus Host Disease (GVHD). Other treatments designed to fight cancer have the drawback to induce immunodepression since they target dividing (tumour) cells but they also kill the dividing cells from the immune system. The drawbacks of these treatments are their relative low specificity that impacts high dynamics biological system with high cell proliferation like lymphoid and haematopoietic systems. Aiming to understand the origins of immunodepression during aging or effects upon treatments but also the capacity of the immune system to regenerate should be coupled with the study of the immune system in homeostatic conditions. This requires specific investigation design related to system biology investigation and modelling.

These different levels of alteration with aging are related to the **immune system complexity** at inter- and intra-cell signalling, receptor diversity, clonotype selection and competition (Leitao, Freitas et al. 2009), fluid dissemination through the organism, homeostatic regulation and adaptation to a changing environment. In short, the immune system is a "complex system". In general, a complex system is comprised of a great number of heterogeneous entities, among which local interactions create multiple levels of collective structure and organization. Such systems require analysis at several spatial and temporal scales. Scientists are faced with radically new challenges when trying to observe, describe, control and develop original theories about these complex biological systems. We previously discussed concepts on the evaluation of multiscale systems dynamics, fluctuations, stability and resilience (Lavelle, Berry et al. 2008). In addition to looking to individual elements and isolated contexts, it is necessary to integrate information and devise more holistic approaches (Benoist, Germain et al. 2006; Cohn and Mata 2007). This is particularly true of the immune system (Cohen 2007). We recently delineated three challenges[1] to study the complexity of the immune systems: (i) the identification of lymphocyte populations, (ii) the reconstruction of their dynamics and repertoire selection process (iii) the mechanisms involved in the resilience or instabilities to perturbations, immune dysfunction in order to improve immuno-intervention strategies. It is obvious that the **fluctuations** related to aging that lead to progressive immunodepression or induced by therapeutic immunosuppression are both the consequence of the perturbations of the immune system and changes in the initial equilibrium state. Here, we moreover challenge the fact that immunosuppression during aging might increase the physiological immunodepression.

A number of studies aiming at providing a global analysis and **comprehensive modelling of immunological systems** have flourished around the world (Rangel, Angus et al. 2004; Braga-Neto and Marques 2006; Morel, Ta'asan et al. 2006; Petrovsky and Brusic 2006; Borghans and de Boer 2007; Chan and Kepler 2007; Efroni, Harel et al. 2007; Souza-e-Silva, Savino et al. 2009). We recently reported on methods and strategies to investigate lymphocyte dynamics and repertoires as well as the modelling concepts and formalism (Thomas-Vaslin & al. *in press*). Moreover scientists are faced with data storage and sharing. The SIDR initiative to store data with metadata and share them is under current development as illustrated in the "T cell and aging" project [2].

Interestingly, the **high turnover and division of lymphocytes was revealed by the initial use of immunosuppressive drugs**. In fact the early investigation of lymphoid cell dynamics and their precursors are related to the effects of perturbation induced by immunosuppression, as irradiation (Sprent, Anderson et al. 1974; Anderson, Olson et al. 1977; McLean and Michie 1995), following chemotherapy for cancer (Mackall, Fleisher et al. 1994) or other immunosuppressive drugs used to control the immune system. For example, Hydroyurea (HU) is a typical chemotherapy cytostatic treatment that non-specifically synchronizes all dividing cells and kills them. This drug particularly affects haematopoietic and lymphoid cells having high frequencies of cells in division and thus induces immunosuppressive effects. Experiments using HU allowed to reveal the reduced B cell functionality post-treatment in mice (Rusthoven and Phillips 1980). Such type of experiments and others like transfer experiment or labelling of dividing cells, were used to investigate population dynamics in the mouse and revealed the high turnover of B cells (Freitas, Rocha et al. 1982) reviewed in Freitas, Rocha et al. 1986). This high dynamic immune system display in fact internal activities observed in non-manipulated mice (Freitas, Pereira et al. 1989). We have also shown that the cellular environment determines the life-span of B cells by selection processes (Thomas-Vaslin and Freitas 1989). This drives clonal persistence of B cells through the variable region selection of the BCR (Thomas-Vaslin, Andrade et al. 1991), contributing to shape the B cell repertoire with aging (Andrade, Huetz et al. 1991). In T cells, similar HU immunosuppressive treatment revealed the short life expectancy, the continuous renewal and post thymic expansion of T cells (Rocha 1987). In fact, lymphocytes are under homeostatic control to regulate the growth and survival of T and B cells that occupy and compete for different "ecological niches" (Freitas and Rocha 2000). Several other methods have allowed to explore T cell dynamics by conditional ablation, using depleting antibodies (Qin, Wise et al. 1990; Waldmann and Cobbold 1998; Bourgeois and Stockinger 2006) chemical thymectomy (Bourgeois, Hao et al. 2008) or

[1] http://roadmap.csregistry.org/tiki-index.php?page=From%20molecules%20to%20organisms
[2] http://sidr-dr.inist.fr/fuge.jsp?idFuge=301796

lymphocyte proliferation in immunocompromised recipients. This highly dynamical system makes it very sensible and reactive to antigen stimulations, but also to immunosuppressive treatments.

Moreover **immunostimulatory and rejuvenation treatments** are explored to stimulate the immune system in aging or after immunosuppression (Dudakov, Goldberg et al. 2009; Lynch, Goldberg et al. 2009). Several factors like Keratinocyte growth factor, Growth hormone, cytokines like IL-7, IL-15 or IL2, steroid hormones are implicated in aging process. Immuno-stimulatory pathways and rejuvenation treatments are experimented to prevent or revert the immunodepression (Zuniga-Pflucker and van den Brink 2007; Dorshkind, Montecino-Rodriguez et al. 2009; Mackall, Fry et al. 2011). In particular, some hormones like Growth Hormone (GH) and Ghrelin stimulate thymic production, GH normalizing the T cell repertoire (Taub, Murphy et al. 2010).

2. Immunosuppression & aging: Some examples

Our comprehension of processes of immunodepression with aging or effect of immunosuppression requires the understanding of lymphocyte dynamics and the global description of lymphocyte populations. The Figure 1 depicts hypothetical T cell population subsets in the thymus and peripheral organs, with cell division, process of selection and death, differentiation from one population to another one.

The investigation and modelling of cell population dynamics is often based on knowledge obtained from young individuals that can be considered at steady for a short time period in absence of intentional immunisation. Alterations of the system and observation of the responses to perturbations is also a way to understand the systems properties. As stated before, modelling cell population dynamics is an active field of research in systems immunology and a plenty of model of T cell dynamics have been proposed (Mehr, Globerson et al. 1995; Mehr, Perelson et al. 1997; Efroni, Harel et al. 2007; Asquith, Borghans et al. 2009; Dowling and Hodgkin 2009; Souza-e-Silva, Savino et al. 2009). Our mathematical model of T cell dynamics is based on a conveyor-belt model of differentiation (Thomas-Vaslin, Altes et al. 2008) as summarised below in Figure 4.

Here, we (1) give some examples of the effects of aging on T cell population composition and repertoire, (2) show the additive effects of transient or chronic immunosuppression, (3) investigated the effects of rejuvenation treatments on T cells repertoire.

2.1 The physiological aging process & genetic influence

In order to quantify immunological alterations process through physiological aging we have studied the organ distribution, phenotype, repertoire and dynamics of T lymphocytes from young (2 months) to aged (25 months) mice. We have also evaluated the effect of genetic influences known to determine for example the CD4/CD8 ratio (Kraal, Weissman et al. 1983). Thus, two different mouse genetic backgrounds identified to provide various quality of repertoire selection and aging processes in non-manipulated lab mice C57BL/6 (B6) (H-2^b) and FVB (H-2^q) were used.

2.1.1 T cell populations and cell counts

Multicolour flow cytometry allows to define the phenotype of single cells and to identify thymocyte populations as $CD4^{lo}CD8^{lo}$ (DN), $CD4^{hi}$ $CD8^{hi}$ (DP) and mature T cell CD4 and

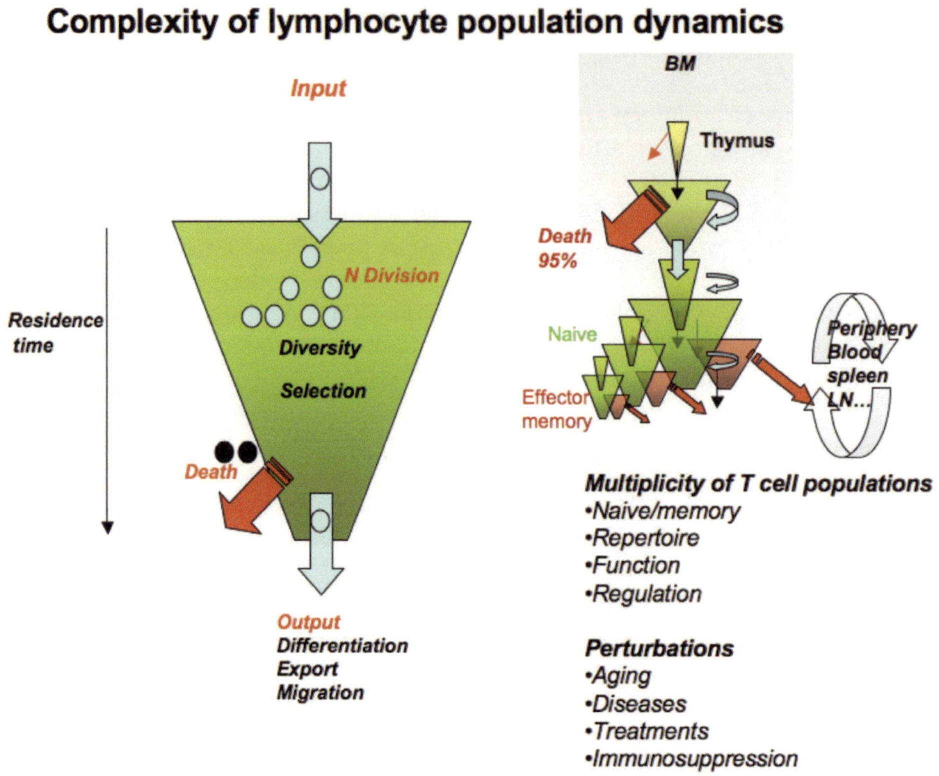

Fig. 1. Schematic hypothetical representation of T cell populations or compartments: a compartment could be considered as a green box, with input and output of cells. Inside a compartment, cells could be selected to proliferate or to die. In a central compartment such as the thymus, diversity of antigenic receptor is obtained by somatic gene rearrangements. Compartments could be multiplied according to tissue localisation, cell differentiation steps, cell function, receptor antigen repertoire expression… From a steady state equilibrium, perturbations can impact one particular or several compartments resizing them.

CD8 (Fig2A), representing the step of intrathymic T cell differentiation (see Fig. 4 below). From FACS we estimated cell percentages (Fig.2B) and numbers (Fig.2C). Similar identification of population in spleen and lymph nodes allows discriminating between CD4 or CD8 T cells and to estimate their percentages (Fig.2B) as well as the numbers of naïve T cells (with low CD44 expression) and antigen experienced cells (high CD44 expression) (Fig2.C).
In young mice, the CD4 and CD8 percentages are characteristic of each lymphoid tissue as thymus, spleen, lymph nodes (Fig.2B). The variability between individuals is low, and a typical CD4/CD8 ratio is displayed according to genetic characteristics and organs (decreasing from 3.2 in thymus to 1.4 in lymph nodes in B6 mice, while from 5.0 to 2.1 in FVB). In old mice, this typical pattern is altered with high variability from mouse to mouse, increased proportion of either CD4 or CD8 T cells that correspond to clonal expansions of peripheral $CD44^{hi}$ T cells. Thymic involution is accelerated in FVB mice compared to B6 (Fig.2C) with a 10 times decrease of thymocyte number between 2 months to 2 years. The acceleration of thymic involution in FVB might be related to alteration of thymic epithelial cell differentiation (Nabarra, Mulotte et al. 2001) that in turn could affect the early

differentiation of thymocytes. After thymic differentiation and selection, T lymphocytes reach peripheral organs as naïve CD44^{lo} T cells, where they can encounter antigens. In the spleen, the number of naïve T cells decreases with aging due to decreased thymic production, while those of CD44^{hi} T cells increased due to recruitment by antigenic stimulation. With aging the T cell population production is thus perturbed with less naïve production compensated in part by effector and memory T cell accumulation. Note that FVB young mice have twice the numbers of CD4 naïve T cells compared to B6, while other population looks quite similar, suggesting different selection processes and T cell population dynamics. With aging, alterations are higher in FVB due to the massive loss of naïve CD4 T cells while there is higher accumulation of CD8 CD44^{hi} T cells. Thus, FVB mice display an accelerated "immunological aging" compared to B6 mice.

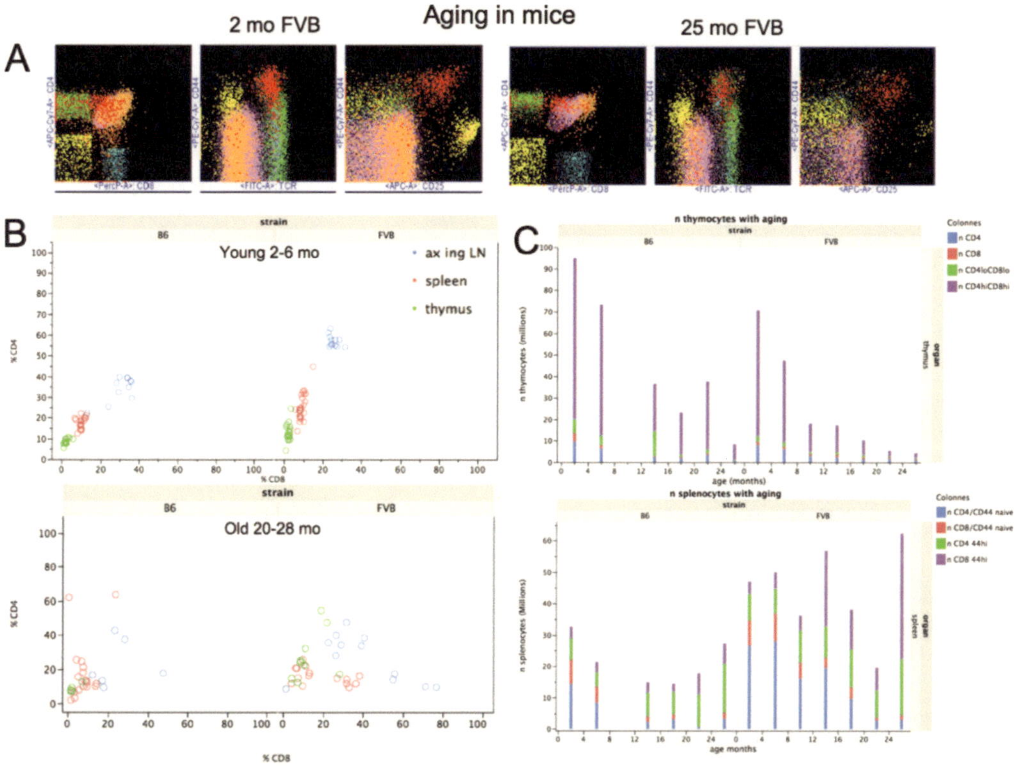

Fig. 2. Physiological aging in FVB and B6 mice: (A) Multicolour flow cytometry dot plot showing alterations of some cell populations in the thymus of 25 months old mouse compared to 2 months old mouse. (B) Percentages of CD4 and CD8 cells observed in thymus, spleen and lymph nodes from B6 or FVB in young or old mice. (C) Mean numbers of lymphocyte subpopulations in the thymus (upper part) and in the spleen (lower part) as a function of age. Graphs were done with JMP software.

2.1.2 T cell repertoire diversity

The diversity and variability of the TCR lymphocyte repertoire in young or old mice is an important point that is critical for the ability of an individual to respond to a huge variety of antigen. The potential diversity of T lymphocyte in mouse is estimated to 10^{15} while the size of splenic TCR repertoire is estimated to $2x10^6$ with a clonal size of 30-40 cells in young mice (Casrouge, Beaudoing et al. 2000). Although initially random rearrangement processes favour TCR diversity selection process, selection of particular TCR with germline encoded CDR1 and CDR2 sequence interacting with MHC also allows to control thymic selection (Scott-Browne, White et al. 2009; Jenkins, Chu et al. 2010). In B6, while there are Mammary tumour virus (Mtv) integrations in the genome, the absence of MHC II I-E expression avoids the superantigen presentation and prevents the deletion of some Vβ. Thus, in B6 mice the repertoire is very diversified compared to other strains that delete some Vβ related to superantigen recognition. FVB has a TCRβ chromosomal deletion of Vβ8 and 6 others Vβ (Osman, Hannibal et al. 1999).

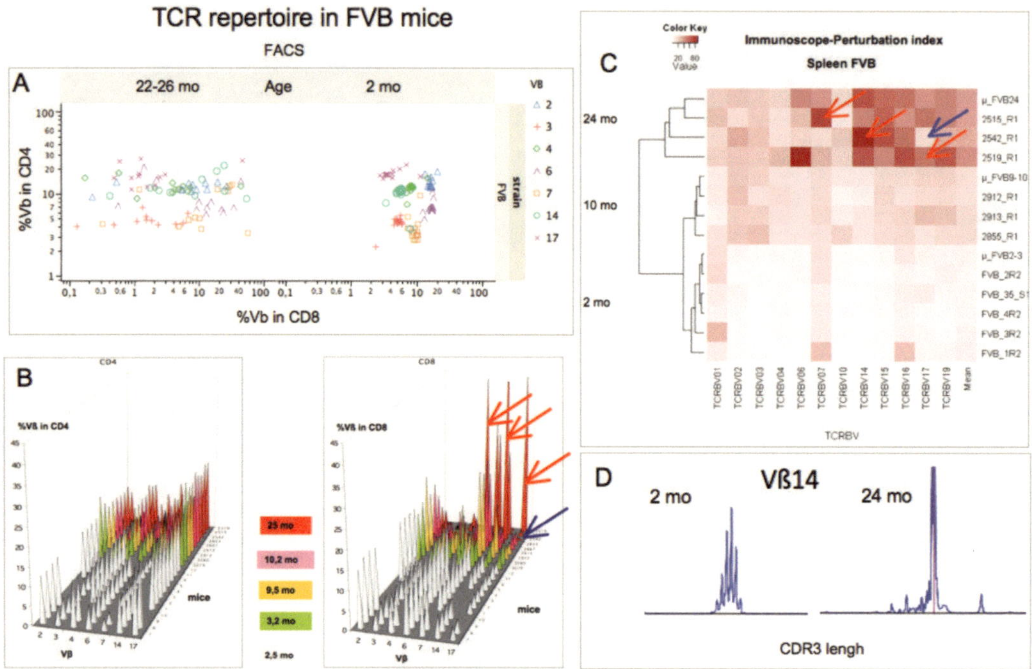

Fig. 3. Evolution of the TCR repertoire from FVB mice through ages in spleen. (A) Percentage of Vβ in CD4 versus CD8 T cells in 2 months and 22-26 months old FVB mice estimated by FACS. (B) Percentage of VB in CD4 or CD8 T cells in various group of age by FACS, (C) Estimation of a perturbation index, with a double hierarchical classification following Immunoscope analysis, as exemplified by a Vβ profile showing a Gaussian distribution of CDR3 length in young mice and an irregular profile with an oligoclonal expansion in 24 month old mice. The red arrows show clonal expansion in two-year old mice CD8 T cells. The blue arrow shows clonal deletion as revealed by FACS and Immunoscope in same mice

The TCR repertoire can be assessed either by FACS in individual CD4 or CD8 T cells with antibodies specific for each particular Vβ. Alternatively, Immunoscope analysis (Collette and Six 2002; Boudinot, Marriotti-Ferrandiz et al. 2008) allows measuring the variable length of the CDR3 region from the TCR involved in antigen recognition, for each Vβ family and to estimate the diversity for each Vβ. In young mice, we observed a very low variability in the TCR Vβ splenocyte repertoire, as shown for FVB mice in Figure 3. A typical signature of young FVB mice can be observed by FACS or immunoscope. In contrast, variability is observed in old mice, with occurrence of CD8 $CD44^{hi}$ clonal expansion. This is confirmed by measuring CDR3 length expression by Immunoscope, as observance of non-Gaussian peak distribution. Some Vβ clones also disappear in old mice. Thus, perturbations are important in old mice restricting the diversity of the repertoire, and consequently the possibility to respond to antigens. The T lymphocyte repertoire diversity shrinks due to clonal amplification and deletion as a consequence of the decrease of de novo thymic production and chronic antigenic stimulation by the environmental antigens (Kieper, Troy et al. 2005). The magnitude of these alterations depends on aging but also on genetic or epigenetic influences since in B6 mice the alterations seem less prominent (see Figure 8).

2.2 Immunosuppression: The effect of transient conditional depletion of dividing T cells on the immune system

The depletion of dividing T cells leads to immunosuppression. This could be the result of an immunotherapy to control the reactivity of the T cells involved in immune responses (allograft rejection, Graft versus host disease, autoimmunity, inflammatory diseases), or the consequences of anti-tumour chemotherapy targeting dividing tumour cells. Experimental T cell depletion can also be used to estimate the natural division, turnover of T cells and to evaluate the homeostatic capacity of the immune system to reconstitute. We previously studied the effects of transient conditional immunosuppression through the killing of dividing T cells by different methods.

2.2.1 Hydroxyurea

As reviewed above, Hydroxyurea a cytostatic agent targeting dividing cells, has allowed to investigate renewal rates and differentiation of T cells and B cells (Rocha, Freitas et al. 1983; Cumano, Vieira et al. 1986; Penit and Vasseur 1988 ; Penit, Vasseur et al. 1988). We have shown that HU treatment also induces "immune amnesia", i.e. this immunosuppressive treatments kills lymphocytes involved in the memory maintenance process and thus the treatment prevents secondary memory immune response (Bellier, Thomas-Vaslin et al. 2003). Moreover, we showed that the depletion of dividing cells induced by HU provokes an homeostatic perturbation that displace effector/regulatory T cells ratio, inducing dominant transplantation tolerance (Giraud, Barrou et al. 2008). Thus, depleting dividing cells is a way to manipulate the immune system and immune responses.

2.2.2 Pharmaco-genetic conditional immunosuppression

To restrict the effect of chemotherapy to lymphocytes, engineering a specific conditional pharmaco-genetic immunosuppression in mice expressing the HSV1-TK suicide (TK) gene has allowed to achieve the ablation of B and T cell lineages (Heyman, Borrelli et al. 1989). To achieve specific T cell depletion we engineered mice expressing the suicide gene (TK+) under a CD4 enhancer and promoter: upon a nucleoside analogue as ganciclovir (GCV) treatment in these TK^{+} transgenic mice, only the CD4 and CD8 T cells that are in division are killed, while all other body cells can continue to divide.

Transient depletion of dividing T cells to evaluate T cells dynamics

Using the TK/GCV strategy, we have shown the effect of transient (1 week) dividing T cells depletion followed by an homeostatic recovery of the various T cell subsets in the thymus and spleen of young adult mice. The mathematical modelling of these experimental data, showing depletion and repletion of T cells compartment led us to evaluate the impact of dividing cell depletion treatment on T cells, the time necessary to return to pre-treatment values. Moreover, it allows to estimate parameters values at the steady state describing the continuous T cell differentiation, fluxes, cell division in the thymus and spleen of young adult mice (Thomas-Vaslin, Altes et al. 2008). Figure 4 depicts the results of this model in young FVB mice and estimation of T cell composition in old mice from our experimental data.

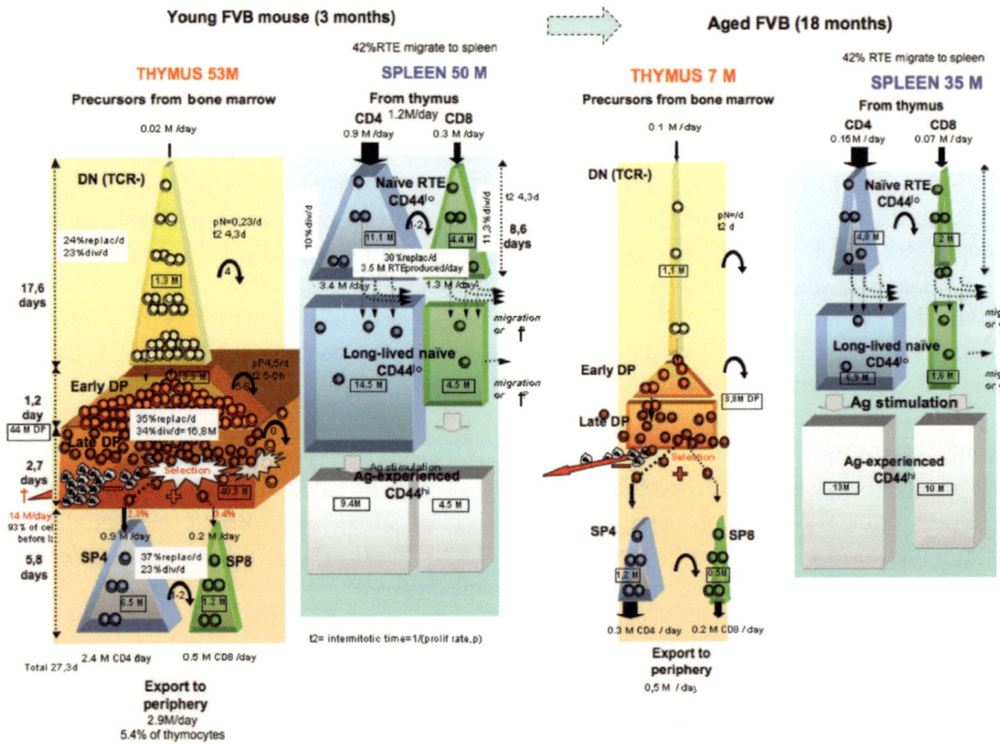

Fig. 4. T cell dynamics at steady state in young (3 months old) or middle aged (18 months old) FVB mice. The coloured boxes represent the cell populations (white boxes indicate Millions cells) differentiating from bone marrow precursors entering the thymus, the number of cell cycle (curved arrows), the time (days) for thymic differentiation (left shaded arrows) with transit through Double Negative CD4-CD8- (DN), Double Positive CD4+CD8+ (DP) submitted to selection process, and finally single positive CD4+CD8- or CD4-CD8+ (SP) stage. Then, recent thymic emigrants (RTE) enter the spleen, divide and fill the Long-Lived naïve compartment. Antigenic stimulations trigger naïve cells to differentiate in antigen-experimented T cells (details on the model are in Thomas-Vaslin, Altes et al. 2008). In old mice, the thymus was involuted, thus the naïve T cell is considerably reduced while the population of Ag-experiment T cells had increased following chronic antigenic challenges.

Transient depletion of dividing T cells induces the lack of immunological memory maintenance

We have also studied the effects of a time controlled specific T cell depletion in immune mice, using the TK/GCV pharmacogenetic control and shown the lack of secondary immune response following such a treatment, confirming the effects observed with HU treatment (Bellier, Thomas-Vaslin et al. 2003).

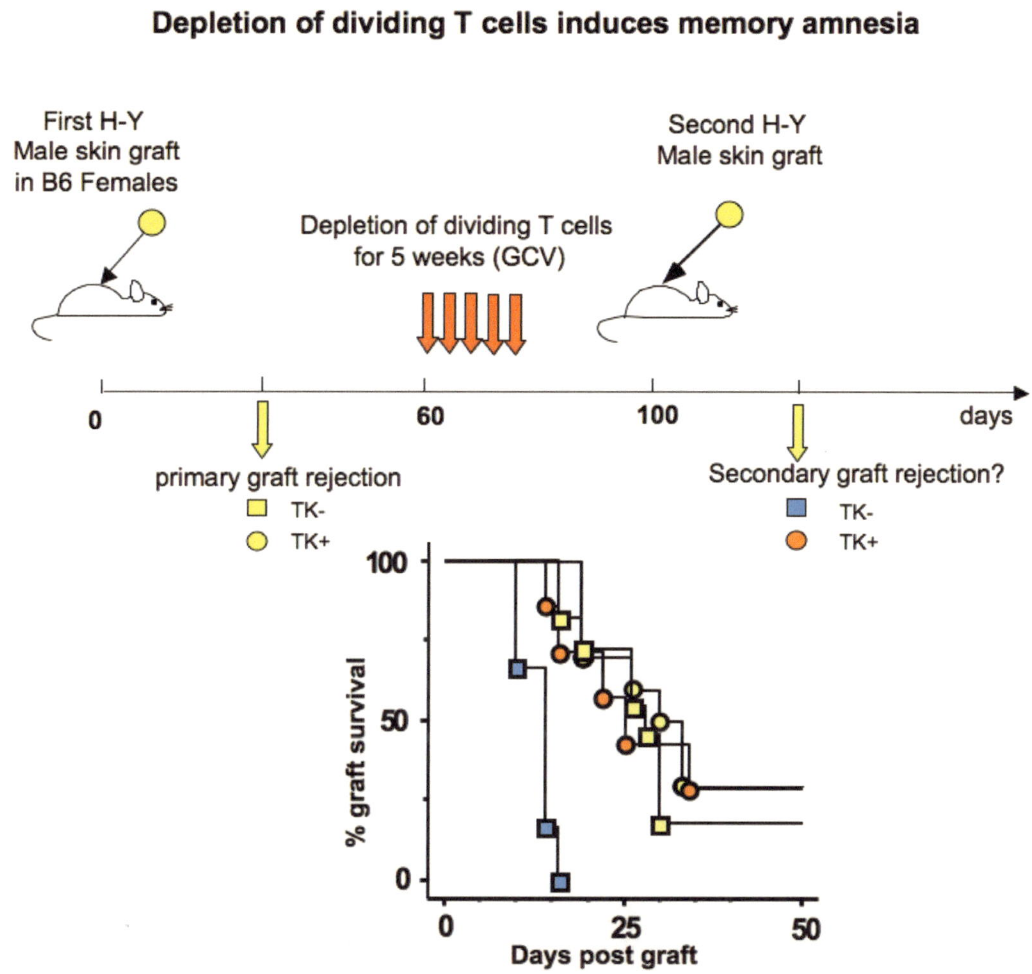

Fig. 5. Effect of immunosuppression on the immunological memory maintenance: B6 female mice were sensitized on day 0 to male skin antigen through a male skin graft. Female mice rejected this first male graft in about 30 days with a typical primary rejection kinetics (yellow symbols). After establishment of immune memory, the dividing T cells were depleted for 2 to 5 weeks. After cessation of treatment a second skin graft is performed and the kinetics of rejection is observed: in mice where the depletion of dividing T cells is inefficient (TK-GCV+) all skin grafts are rapidly rejected in less than 20 days, with a typical acceleration compatible with a second set kinetics (blue symbols). In mice where the depletion of dividing cells is efficient (TK+GCV+, orange symbols) the grafts are rejected with a primary set kinetics.

Figure 5 depicts an example of T cell immune memory failure in the case of sensitisation with an allogeneic skin graft. Similar lack of memory responses were observed after the viral infection of mice with the lymphocytic choriomeningitis virus (LCMV). This demonstrates that immunological memory is maintained by a pool of T cells in constant division, which is sensible to some immunosuppressive treatments. This effect could be a drawback of immunosuppressant that might disturb the beneficial immune memory induced by vaccination. However, it also suggests that such immunosuppressive treatment could be used to target dividing cells responsible of undesirable memory T cell response (as in allograft sensitized recipient).

Specific transient depletion of dividing T cells to control immunopathological T cell responses

Used in pathological situations, the conditional pharmacogenetic immunosuppression induced by the TK/GCV system allows to (i) transiently control LCMV infection (Boyer, Cohen et al. 2000). (ii) control GVHD (Cohen, Boyer et al. 1997; Cohen, Boyer et al. 1999; Cohen, Boyer et al. 1999; Cohen, Saron et al. 2000; Cohen, Boyer et al. 2001). Clinical protocol associated with injection of regulatory T cells expressing the TK gene as a safety gene to control GVHD are under assessment (Guillot-Delost, Cherai et al. 2008). Applied upon an allograft this treatment allows delayed rejection (skin graft) or tolerance of the graft (vascularized heart allograft) (Braunberger, Cohen et al. 2000; Braunberger, Raynal-Raschilas et al. 2000; Thomas-Vaslin, Bellier et al. 2000). In fact, we further showed that the depletion treatment (either HU or TK/GCV) induces disequilibrium favouring regulatory T cells (Treg) responsible for dominant tolerance able to control islet pancreatic allografts rejection (Giraud, Barrou et al. 2008). While aging by itself leads to multilevel alterations and finally immunodepression at biological level, little is know about the additive effect of clinical immunosuppression during aging. Observations that allograft rejection is decreased in old recipient lead to recommendations that older recipient may require less immunosuppression than young patients to control allograft rejection and to treat autoimmunity or inflammation diseases (Bradley 2002).

Effect of transient depletion of dividing T cells according to age

We have compared the kinetics of T cells in mice during and after a transient depletion of dividing T cells according to the age of the mice. In young adult mice, the immunosuppressive treatment applied during two weeks initially induces the depletion of naïve T ($CD44^{lo}$) cells in FVB mice and in both naïve and effector/memory ($CD44^{hi}$) T cell in B6 mice (Figure 6).

Then, homeostatic recovery occurs within two months and both strains recovered initial T lymphocyte counts. In contrast, in aged mice the two weeks ganciclovir treatment induces in FVB a continuous decrease of naïve T cells counts while effector/memory T cells accumulate. In B6 mice the GCV treatment induces less perturbation probably because the thymic involution is less prominent than in FVB at the same age. Thus reconstitution of naïve T cells can occur post treatment, while accumulation of effector/memory T cells is limited.

The use of conditional pharmacogenetic immunosuppression has allowed proposing the model depicted in Figure 4 from mathematical modelling. Visual computer modelling of T cell population dynamics is currently under progress (McEwan, Bersini et al. 2011; McEwan, Bersini et al. 2011) to develop our comprehension of cell fluxes between cell compartment and organs, cell division. This modelling should allow quantifying parameter values in young to aged mice at steady state, but also simulating some treatments, to confirm our experimental observations and hypothesis.

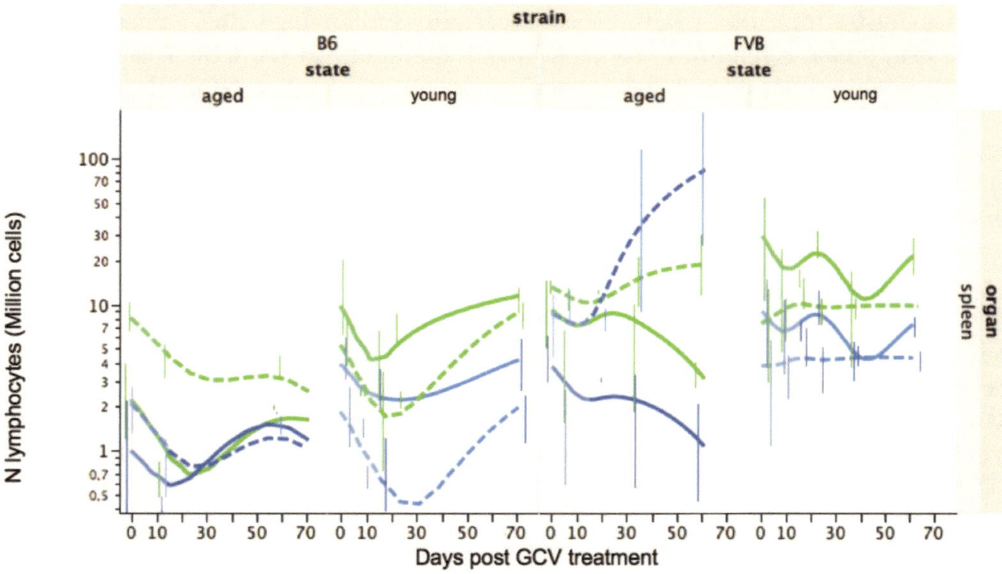

Fig. 6. Effect of transient pharmacogenetic immunosuppression in the spleen of transgenic B6 or FVB mice expressing the HSV1-TK suicide gene in the T cell lineage. Ganciclovir treatment is applied for 14 days (grey area) in young (2 months old) or aged (18 months old) mice. Box plot and spline curves show the numbers of CD4 CD44^{lo} (continuous green line), CD8 CD44^{lo} (continuous blue line), CD4CD44^{hi} (dashed green line) CD8CD44^{hi} (dashed blue line) T cells.

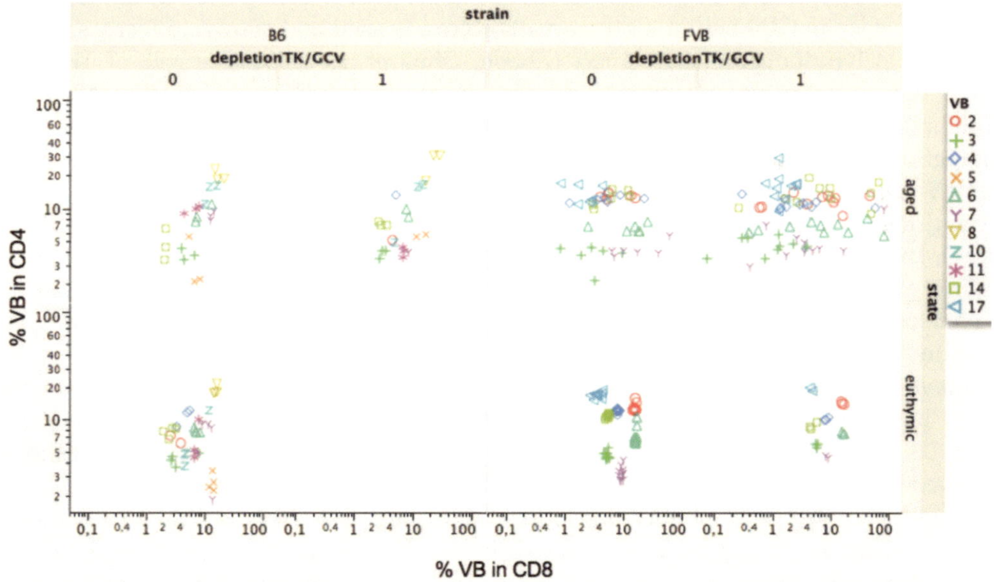

Fig. 7. Vß TCR repertoire by FACS of spleen cells, showing the percentage of each Vß in CD4 vs CD8 T cells, in controls TK-GCV^{+}, TK^{+}GCV^{-} and TK-GCV^{-} mice (TK/GCV depletion= 0) and in depletion sensitive TK^{+}GCV^{+} mice (TK/GCV depletion =1).

The analysis of the TCR Vß repertoire following the pharmacogenetic immunosuppression (Figure 7) revealed major alterations in the CD8 T cells from aged FVB mice with either oligoclonal expansion (representing up to 60 millions of cells) or partial clonal deletion (manuscript in preparation). In contrast, in B6 mice the alterations following treatment are more limited although detectable. Again the slower "immunological aging" of B6 mice seems to preserve homeostatic recovery and the T cell repertoire diversity.

2.3 Prevention of aging and immunodepression

IL-2 has been shown to have a dual role in CD8 memory maintenance, being able to inhibit the proliferation of CD8 memory T cells (Dai, Konieczny et al. 2000) via down regulation of the γc chain expression of its receptor, increasing apoptotic cell death (Li, Demirci et al. 2001). The growth of very large CD8 T cell clones observed in old mice was attributed to cytokine deregulation, IL-15 being stimulatory, while IL-2 is inhibitory (Ku, Kappler et al. 2001). IL-2 is a cytokine that acts centrally and peripherally to increase CD4 naïve T cell numbers (Foussat, Bouchet-Delbos et al. 2004). There is a defect of IL-2 production by CD4 T cells from aged mice, reducing their expansion capacity (Haynes, Linton et al. 1999). IL-2 is also necessary to maintain $CD4^{+}CD25^{+}$ regulatory T cells that control CD4 T cell homeostasis (Almeida, Legrand et al. 2002). $CD4^{+}CD25^{+}$ regulatory T cells are involved in IL-2 mediated inhibition of memory CD8 T cells, reducing their division (Murakami, Sakamoto et al. 2002).

Regulatory T cells were shown to accumulate with aging contributing to decrease immune responses. However the augmentation of suppressive function is not due to $CD4^{+}CD25^{+}Foxp3^{+}$ T cells but to $CD4^{+}CD25^{-}$ Foxp3+ T cells that appear with aging (Nishioka, Shimizu et al. 2006). Since a lack of IL-2 secretion is reported in old individuals, with deficiency in CD4 help, IL-2 treatments were assessed and shown to increase Treg cell numbers in lymphopenic individuals (Zhang, Chua et al. 2005). The role of Treg in the prevention of repertoire alteration was also shown in the case of lymphopenia induced proliferation (Winstead, Reilly et al.). Treg also modulate the effector function of CD8 by competing for IL-2 (McNally, Hill et al. 2011). IL-2 also has positive effect to control T cell homeostasis in autoimmunity (Humrich, Morbach et al.). In NOD type-1 diabetic mice, IL-2 can prevent or reverse autoimmunity, by stimulation of Tregs (Grinberg-Bleyer, Baeyens et al.). In infectious diseases, HIV infected patient IL-2 treatment induces an increase of thymic export (Carcelain, Saint-Mezard et al. 2003) and induces a peripheral CD4 T cell expansion by limiting CD4 proliferation and increasing CD4CD25+ subset (Sereti, Anthony et al. 2004).

To prevent the effects of aging homeostatic deregulation and TCR repertoire alterations, we tested the effect of IL-2 or transfer of regulatory T cells (CD4+CD25+) injected in middle-aged B6 mice (15-month old) (Figure 8). Both treatments prevent clonal alterations as revealed by FACS analysis of TCRVB repertoire at the age of 24-28 months. Non-treated B6 mice developed by 24-28 months oligoclonal expansions essentially in CD4 T cells and loose CD8 T cell clones. IL-2 treated mice have lower CD4 clonal expansions, that are absent in Treg treated mice and repertoire looks "younger". Both treatments limited the decrease of CD8 cell clones. Note that at variance with FVB mice, in B6 mice the aging of the repertoire is delayed, and that oligoclonal expansions concern mostly CD4 T cells in B6 but CD8 T cells in FVB.

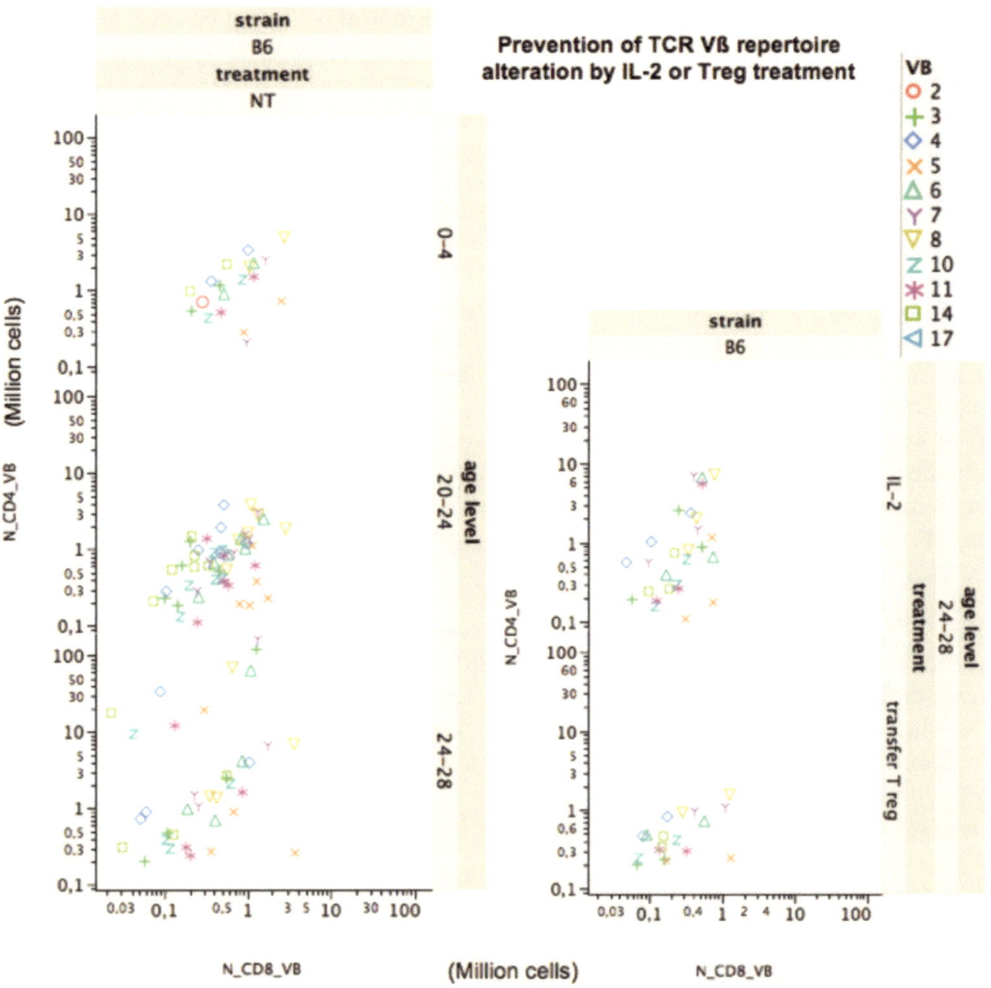

Fig. 8. Vß TCR repertoire by FACS of spleen cells from B6 mice, showing the number of each Vß in CD4 vs. CD8 T cells, in non treated B6 mice according to age, and in B6 mice that received an IL-2 treatment or an injection of regulatory T cells (CD25+) at the age of 15 months and are analysed at the age of 24-28 months.

3. Conclusions

We pointed out that the different initial T cell numbers available according to age and genetic background determines the kinetics of depletion and recovery in B6 and FVB mice. This suggests that the T cell dynamics and turnover differs according to genetic influence. FVB mice have an accelerated immunological aging, with accelerated thymic involution and finally accumulation of CD8 clonal T cell expansions by 22 months. The transient depletion of dividing T cells temporarily disturb the dynamic T cell equilibrium of young mice of both genetic background, with a return to steady-state values and no alteration in repertoire diversity. However, in middle-aged mice the effect of the transient depletion can be more dramatic: in FVB mice it leads to accelerated occurrence of CD8 T cell clones. In B6 mice, the long term consequences of treatment are less important, most likely because the thymus is more productive at the same age. However, we also observed that a preventive treatment by serial injection of IL-2 or a single injection of Treg cells in middle aged mice can successfully prevent the natural occurrence of repertoire alterations.

Our work allows us to observe the physiological aging that impacts on the quality and quantity of T cells in the central and peripheral organs as well as on the diversity of the repertoire. It indicates that some immunosuppressive treatments inducing a homeostatic disturbance of the immune systems might accelerate the aging of the T cell composition and reduce the TCR repertoire diversity, while some immunostimulatory treatment or regulatory T cells might prevent such alterations. As underlined before, several biological scales are involved in these processes and the variability observed between genetic background, ages of the same individual at the level of cell population, cells or TCR cellular or molecular repertoire have to be evaluated.

Use of systems immunology approaches as multidimensional statistical models (Pham, in preparation) and computer models (McEwan, in preparation) are novel approaches that will give a more thorough evaluation of complex T cell population dynamics to be able to simulate the physiological behaviour and effects of perturbations.

4. Acknowledgments

We thank the financial supports from INSERM ATC vieillissement, CNRS Programme Interdisciplinaire Longévité & Vieillissement, Emergence UPMC. PP is recipient of Ph.D. fellowship ED CDV, Ministry of Research. We thanks the Centre d'Experimentation Fonctionnelle Pitié-Salpétrière, Paris for the long term care of our old mice.

5. References

(2005). Aging and the immune system. Curr Opin Immunol 17: 455-.

(2009). Immune senescence special issue. Trends Immunol 30(7): 293-382.

Ahmed, M., K. G. Lanzer, et al. (2009). Clonal expansions and loss of receptor diversity in the naive CD8 T cell repertoire of aged mice. J Immunol 182(2): 784-92.

Almeida, A. R., N. Legrand, et al. (2002). Homeostasis of peripheral CD4+ T cells: IL-2R alpha and IL-2 shape a population of regulatory cells that controls CD4+ T cell numbers. J Immunol 169(9): 4850-60.

Anderson, R. E., G. B. Olson, et al. (1977). Radiosensitivity of T and B lymphocytes. IV. Effect of whole body irradiation upon various lymphoid tissues and numbers of recirculating lymphocytes. J Immunol 118(4): 1191-200.

Andrade, L., F. Huetz, et al. (1991). Biased VH gene expression in murine CD5 B cells results from age-dependent cellular selection. Eur J Immunol 21(9): 2017-23.

Andrew, D. and R. Aspinall (2001). Il-7 and not stem cell factor reverses both the increase in apoptosis and the decline in thymopoiesis seen in aged mice. J Immunol 166(3): 1524-30.

Aspinall, R. and J. J. Goronzy (2010). Immune senescence. Curr Opin Immunol 22(4): 497-9.

Asquith, B., J. A. Borghans, et al. (2009). Lymphocyte kinetics in health and disease. Trends Immunol 30(4): 182-9.

Bellier, B., V. Thomas-Vaslin, et al. (2003). Turning immunological memory into amnesia by depletion of dividing T cells. Proc Natl Acad Sci U S A 100(25): 15017-15022.

Benoist, C., R. N. Germain, et al. (2006). A plaidoyer for 'systems immunology'. Immunol Rev 210: 229-34.

Blackman, M. A. and D. L. Woodland (2011). The narrowing of the CD8 T cell repertoire in old age. Curr Opin Immunol 23: 1-6.

Borghans, J. A. and R. J. de Boer (2007). Quantification of T-cell dynamics: from telomeres to DNA labeling. Immunol Rev 216: 35-47.

Boudinot, P., M. E. Marriotti-Ferrandiz, et al. (2008). New perspectives for large-scale repertoire analysis of immune receptors. Mol Immunol 45(9): 2437-45.

Bourgeois, C., Z. Hao, et al. (2008). Ablation of thymic export causes accelerated decay of naive CD4 T cells in the periphery because of activation by environmental antigen. Proc Natl Acad Sci U S A 105(25): 8691-6.

Bourgeois, C. and B. Stockinger (2006). CD25+CD4+ regulatory T cells and memory T cells prevent lymphopenia-induced proliferation of naive T cells in transient states of lymphopenia. J Immunol 177(7): 4558-66.

Boursalian, T. E., J. Golob, et al. (2004). Continued maturation of thymic emigrants in the periphery. Nat Immunol 5(4): 418-25.

Boyer, O., J. L. Cohen, et al. (2000). Transient control of a virus-induced immunopathology by genetic immunosuppression. Gene Ther 7(18): 1536-42.

Bradley, B. A. (2002). Rejection and recipient age. Transpl Immunol 10(2-3): 125-32.

Braga-Neto, U. M. and E. T. Marques, Jr. (2006). From functional genomics to functional immunomics: new challenges, old problems, big rewards. PLoS Comput Biol 2(7): e81.

Braunberger, E., J. L. Cohen, et al. (2000). T-Cell suicide gene therapy for organ transplantation: induction of long-lasting tolerance to allogeneic heart without generalized immunosuppression. Mol Ther 2(6): 596-601.

Braunberger, E., N. Raynal-Raschilas, et al. (2000). Tolerance induced without immunosuppression in a T-lymphocyte suicide-gene therapy cardiac allograft model in mice. J Thorac Cardiovasc Surg 119(1): 46-51.

Carcelain, G., P. Saint-Mezard, et al. (2003). IL-2 therapy and thymic production of naive CD4 T cells in HIV-infected patients with severe CD4 lymphopenia. Aids 17(6): 841-50.

Casrouge, A., E. Beaudoing, et al. (2000). Size estimate of the alpha beta TCR repertoire of naive mouse splenocytes. J Immunol 164(11): 5782-7.

Chan, C. and T. B. Kepler (2007). Computational immunology--from bench to virtual reality. Ann Acad Med Singapore 36(2): 123-7.

Ciupe, S. M., B. H. Devlin, et al. (2009). The dynamics of T-cell receptor repertoire diversity following thymus transplantation for DiGeorge anomaly. PLoS Comput Biol 5(6): e1000396.

Clambey, E. T., J. W. Kappler, et al. (2007). CD8 T cell clonal expansions & aging: a heterogeneous phenomenon with a common outcome. Exp Gerontol 42(5): 407-11.

Clambey, E. T., L. F. van Dyk, et al. (2005). Non-malignant clonal expansions of CD8+ memory T cells in aged individuals. Immunol Rev 205: 170-89.

Cohen, I. R. (2007). Modeling immune behavior for experimentalists. Immunol Rev 216: 232-6.

Cohen, J. L., O. Boyer, et al. (1999). Would suicide gene therapy solve the T-cell dilemma of allogeneic bone marrow transplantation ? Immunol Today 20(4): 172-176.

Cohen, J. L., O. Boyer, et al. (2001). Suicide gene therapy of graft-versus-host disease: immune reconstitution with transplanted mature T cells. Blood 98(7): 2071-6.

Cohen, J. L., O. Boyer, et al. (1997). Prevention of graft-versus-host disease in mice using a suicide gene expressed in T lymphocytes. Blood 89(12): 4636-45.

Cohen, J. L., O. Boyer, et al. (1999). Suicide gene-mediated modulation of graft-versus-host disease [In Process Citation]. Leuk Lymphoma 34(5-6): 473-80.

Cohen, J. L., M. F. Saron, et al. (2000). Preservation of graft-versus-infection effects after suicide gene therapy for prevention of graft-versus-host disease. Hum Gene Ther 11(18): 2473-81.

Cohn, M. and J. Mata (2007). Quantitative modeling of immune response. Imm. Rev. 216: 1-236.

Collette, A. and A. Six (2002). ISEApeaks: an Excel platform for GeneScan and Immunoscope data retrieval, management and analysis. Bioinformatics 18(2): 329-30.

Cumano, A., P. Vieira, et al. (1986). Effects of hydroxyurea in vivo treatment on the antibody response in mice. Ann Inst Pasteur Immunol 137D(3): 355-67.

Dai, Z., B. T. Konieczny, et al. (2000). The dual role of IL-2 in the generation and maintenance of CD8+ memory T cells. J Immunol 165(6): 3031-6.

Dorshkind, K., E. Montecino-Rodriguez, et al. (2009). The ageing immune system: is it ever too old to become young again? Nat Rev Immunol 9(1): 57-62.

Dowling, M. R. and P. D. Hodgkin (2009). Modelling naive T-cell homeostasis: consequences of heritable cellular lifespan during ageing. Immunol Cell Biol 87(6): 445-56.

Dudakov, J. A., G. L. Goldberg, et al. (2009). Sex steroid ablation enhances hematopoietic recovery following cytotoxic antineoplastic therapy in aged mice. J Immunol 183(11): 7084-94.

Efroni, S., D. Harel, et al. (2007). Emergent dynamics of thymocyte development and lineage determination. PLoS Comput Biol 3(1): e13.

Ferrando-Martinez, S., E. Ruiz-Mateos, et al. Age-related deregulation of naive T cell homeostasis in elderly humans. Age (Dordr) 33(2): 197-207.

Foussat, A., L. Bouchet-Delbos, et al. (2004). Effects of exogenous IL-2 administration on the homeostasis of CD4+ T lymphocytes. J Clin Immunol 24(5): 503-14.

Freitas, A., P. Pereira, et al. (1989). B cell activities in normal unmanipulated mice. Contrib Microbiol Immunol 11: 1-26.

Freitas, A. A. and B. Rocha (2000). Population biology of lymphocytes: the flight for survival. Annu Rev Immunol 18: 83-111.

Freitas, A. A., B. Rocha, et al. (1986). Lymphocyte population kinetics in the mouse. Immunol. Rev. 91: 5.

Freitas, A. A., B. Rocha, et al. (1982). Population dynamics of B lymphocytes and their precursors: demonstration of high turnover in the central and peripheral lymphoid organs. J. Immunol. 128: 54-60.

Giraud, S., B. Barrou, et al. (2008). Transient Depletion of Dividing T Lymphocytes in Mice Induces the Emergence of Regulatory T Cells and Dominant Tolerance to Islet Allografts. Am J Transplant 8: 1-12.

Goronzy, J. J. and C. M. Weyand (2005). T cell development and receptor diversity during aging. Curr Opin Immunol 17(5): 468-75.
Gress, R. E. and S. G. Deeks (2009). Reduced thymus activity and infection prematurely age the immune system. J Clin Invest 119(10): 2884-7.
Grinberg-Bleyer, Y., A. Baeyens, et al. IL-2 reverses established type 1 diabetes in NOD mice by a local effect on pancreatic regulatory T cells. J Exp Med 207(9): 1871-8.
Guillot-Delost, M., M. Cherai, et al. (2008). Clinical-grade preparation of human natural regulatory T-cells encoding the thymidine kinase suicide gene as a safety gene. J Gene Med 10(8): 834-46.
Hale, J. S., T. E. Boursalian, et al. (2006). Thymic output in aged mice. Proc Natl Acad Sci U S A 103(22): 8447-52.
Haynes, L., P. J. Linton, et al. (1999). Interleukin 2, but not other common gamma chain-binding cytokines, can reverse the defect in generation of CD4 effector T cells from naive T cells of aged mice. J Exp Med 190(7): 1013-24.
Heyman, R. A., E. Borrelli, et al. (1989). Thymidine kinase obliteration: creation of transgenic mice with controlled immune deficiency. Proc Natl Acad Sci U S A 86(8): 2698-702.
Houston, E. G., Jr., L. E. Higdon, et al. (2011). Recent thymic emigrants are preferentially incorporated only into the depleted T-cell pool. Proc Natl Acad Sci U S A 108(13): 5366-71.
Humrich, J. Y., H. Morbach, et al. Homeostatic imbalance of regulatory and effector T cells due to IL-2 deprivation amplifies murine lupus. Proc Natl Acad Sci U S A 107(1): 204-9.
Jenkins, M. K., H. H. Chu, et al. (2010). On the composition of the preimmune repertoire of T cells specific for Peptide-major histocompatibility complex ligands. Annu Rev Immunol 28: 275-94.
Kieper, W. C., A. Troy, et al. (2005). Recent immune status determines the source of antigens that drive homeostatic T cell expansion. J Immunol 174(6): 3158-63.
Kraal, G., I. L. Weissman, et al. (1983). Genetic control of T-cell subset representation in inbred mice. Immunogenetics 18(6): 585-92.
Ku, C. C., J. Kappler, et al. (2001). The growth of the very large CD8+ T cell clones in older mice is controlled by cytokines. J Immunol 166(4): 2186-93.
Lavelle, C., H. Berry, et al. (2008). From molecules to organisms: towards multiscale integrated models of biological systems. Theoretical Biology Insights 1: 13-22.
Leitao, C., A. A. Freitas, et al. (2009). The role of TCR specificity and clonal competition during reconstruction of the peripheral T cell pool. J Immunol 182(9): 5232-9.
LeMaoult, J., I. Messaoudi, et al. (2000). Age-related dysregulation in CD8 T cell homeostasis: kinetics of a diversity loss. J Immunol 165(5): 2367-73.
Li, X. C., G. Demirci, et al. (2001). IL-15 and IL-2: a matter of life and death for T cells in vivo. Nat Med 7(1): 114-8.
Lynch, H. E., G. L. Goldberg, et al. (2009). Thymic involution and immune reconstitution. Trends Immunol 30(7): 366-73.
Mackall, C. L., T. A. Fleisher, et al. (1994). Lymphocyte depletion during treatment with intensive chemotherapy for cancer. Blood 84(7): 2221-8.
Mackall, C. L., T. J. Fry, et al. (2011). Harnessing the biology of IL-7 for therapeutic application. Nat Rev Immunol 11(5): 330-42.

McEwan, C. H., H. Bersini, et al. (2011). A computational technique to scale mathematical models towards complex heterogeneous systems COSMOS workshop ECAL 2011 Conference, Paris, Luniver Press.

McEwan, C. H., H. Bersini, et al. (2011). Refitting Harel statecharts for systemic mathematical models in computational immunology. 10th International Conference on

Artificial Immune Systems (ICARIS), Cambridge.

McLean, A. R. and C. A. Michie (1995). In vivo estimates of division and death rates of human T lymphocytes. Proc Natl Acad Sci U S A 92(9): 3707-11.

McNally, A., G. R. Hill, et al. (2011). CD4+CD25+ regulatory T cells control CD8+ T-cell effector differentiation by modulating IL-2 homeostasis. Proc Natl Acad Sci U S A 108(18): 7529-34.

Mehr, R., A. Globerson, et al. (1995). Modeling positive and negative selection and differentiation processes in the thymus. J Theor Biol 175(1): 103-26.

Mehr, R., A. S. Perelson, et al. (1997). Regulatory feedback pathways in the thymus. Immunol Today 18(12): 581-5.

Messaoudi, I., J. Lemaoult, et al. (2004). Age-related CD8 T cell clonal expansions constrict CD8 T cell repertoire and have the potential to impair immune defense. J Exp Med 200(10): 1347-58.

Morel, P. A., S. Ta'asan, et al. (2006). New insights into mathematical modeling of the immune system. Immunol Res 36(1-3): 157-65.

Murakami, M., A. Sakamoto, et al. (2002). CD25+CD4+ T cells contribute to the control of memory CD8+ T cells. Proc Natl Acad Sci U S A 99(13): 8832-7.

Nabarra, B., M. Mulotte, et al. (2001). Ultrastructural study of the FVB/N mouse thymus: presence of an immature epithelial cell in the medulla and premature involution. Dev Comp Immunol 25(3): 231-43.

Nishioka, T., J. Shimizu, et al. (2006). CD4+CD25+Foxp3+ T cells and CD4+CD25-Foxp3+ T cells in aged mice. J Immunol 176(11): 6586-93.

Osman, G. E., M. C. Hannibal, et al. (1999). FVB/N (H2(q)) mouse is resistant to arthritis induction and exhibits a genomic deletion of T-cell receptor V beta gene segments. Immunogenetics 49(10): 851-9.

Pawelec, G., A. Akbar, et al. (2005). Human immunosenescence: is it infectious? Immunol Rev 205: 257-68.

Penit, C. and F. Vasseur (1988). Sequential events in thymocyte differentiation and thymus regeneration revealed by a combination of bromodeoxyuridine DNA labeling and antimitotic drug treatment. J Immunol 140(10): 3315-23.

Penit, C., F. Vasseur, et al. (1988). In vivo dynamics of CD4-8- thymocytes. Proliferation, renewal and differentiation of different cell subsets studied by DNA biosynthetic labeling and surface antigen detection. Eur J Immunol 18(9): 1343-50.

Petrovsky, N. and V. Brusic (2006). Bioinformatics for study of autoimmunity. Autoimmunity 39(8): 635-43.

Qin, S., M. Wise, et al. (1990). Induction of tolerance in peripheral T cells with monoclonal antibodies. Eur. J. Immunol. 20: 2737-2745.

Rangel, C., J. Angus, et al. (2004). Modeling T-cell activation using gene expression profiling and state-space models. Bioinformatics 20(9): 1361-72.

Rocha, B., A. A. Freitas, et al. (1983). Population dynamics of T lymphocytes. Renewal rate and expansion in the peripheral lymphoid organs. J Immunol 131(5): 2158-64.
Rocha, B. B. (1987). Population kinetics of precursors of IL 2-producing peripheral T lymphocytes: evidence for short life expectancy, continuous renewal, and post-thymic expansion. J Immunol 139(2): 365-72.
Rusthoven, J. J. and R. A. Phillips (1980). Hydroxyurea kills B cell precursors and markedly reduces functional B cell activity in mouse bone marrow. J. Immunol. 124: 781-786.
Scott-Browne, J. P., J. White, et al. (2009). Germline-encoded amino acids in the alphabeta T-cell receptor control thymic selection. Nature 458(7241): 1043-6.
Sereti, I., K. B. Anthony, et al. (2004). IL-2-induced CD4+ T-cell expansion in HIV-infected patients is associated with long-term decreases in T-cell proliferation. Blood 104(3): 775-80.
Souza-e-Silva, H., W. Savino, et al. (2009). A cellular automata-based mathematical model for thymocyte development. PLoS One 4(12): e8233.
Sprent, J., R. E. Anderson, et al. (1974). Radiosensitivity of T and B lymphocytes. II. Effect of irradiation on response of T cells to alloantigens. Eur J Immunol 4(3): 204-10.
Stirk, E. R., C. Molina-Paris, et al. (2008). Stochastic niche structure and diversity maintenance in the T cell repertoire. J Theor Biol 255(2): 237-49.
Taub, D. D., W. J. Murphy, et al. (2010). Rejuvenation of the aging thymus: growth hormone-mediated and ghrelin-mediated signaling pathways. Curr Opin Pharmacol 10(4): 408-24.
Thoman, M. L. (1995). The pattern of T lymphocyte differentiation is altered during thymic involution. Mech Ageing Dev 82(2-3): 155-70.
Thomas-Vaslin, V., H. K. Altes, et al. (2008). Comprehensive assessment and mathematical modeling of T cell population dynamics and homeostasis. J Immunol 180(4): 2240-50.
Thomas-Vaslin, V., L. Andrade, et al. (1991). Clonal persistence of B lymphocytes in normal mice is determined by variable region-dependent selection. Eur J Immunol 21(9): 2239-46.
Thomas-Vaslin, V., B. Bellier, et al. (2000). Prolonged allograft survival through conditional and specific ablation of alloreactive T cells expressing a suicide gene [see comments]. Transplantation 69(10): 2154-61.
Thomas-Vaslin, V. and A. A. Freitas (1989). Lymphocyte population kinetics during the development of the immune system. B cell persistence and life-span can be determined by the host environment. Int Immunol 1(3): 237-46.
Thomas-Vaslin, V., A. Six, B. Bellier and D. Klatzmann (in press). Lymphocyte Dynamics and Repertoire, Biological Methods. Encyclopedia of Systems Biology. W. O. Dubitzky W., Kwang-Hyun C., Hiroki Y. (eds), Springer, Heidelberg New York.
Thomas-Vaslin, V., A. Six, B. Bellier and D. Klatzmann (in press). Lymphocytes dynamics repertoires, modeling. Encyclopedia of Systems Biology. W. O. Dubitzky W., Kwang-Hyun C., Hiroki Y. (eds), Springer, Heidelberg New York.
Tsukamoto, H., K. Clise-Dwyer, et al. (2009). Age-associated increase in lifespan of naive CD4 T cells contributes to T-cell homeostasis but facilitates development of functional defects. Proc Natl Acad Sci U S A 106(43): 18333-8.
Waldmann, H. and S. Cobbold (1998). How do monoclonal antibodies induce tolerance? A role for infectious tolerance? Annu Rev Immunol 16: 619-44.

Winstead, C. J., C. S. Reilly, et al. (2010). CD4+CD25+Foxp3+ regulatory T cells optimize diversity of the conventional T cell repertoire during reconstitution from lymphopenia. J Immunol 184(9): 4749-60.

Yehuda, A. B., G. Friedman, et al. (1998). Checkpoints in thymocytopoiesis in aging: expression of the recombination activating genes RAG-1 and RAG-2. Mech Ageing Dev 102(2-3): 239-47.

Yung, R. L. and A. Julius (2008). Epigenetics, aging, and autoimmunity. Autoimmunity 41(4): 329-35.

Zhang, H., K. S. Chua, et al. (2005). Lymphopenia and interleukin-2 therapy alter homeostasis of CD4+CD25+ regulatory T cells. Nat Med 11(11): 1238-43.

Zuniga-Pflucker, J. C. and M. R. van den Brink (2007). Giving T cells a chance to come back. Semin Immunol 19(5): 279.

8

Chronic Immune Response Hypothesis for Chronic Fatigue Syndrome: Experimental Results and Literature Overview

E. V. Svirshchevskaya
Shemyakin &Ovchinnikov Institute of Bioorganic Chemistry RAS, Moscow
Russian Federation

1. Introduction

Chronic fatigue is characterized by severe disabling fatigue associated with physical, mental, and immunological disturbances. Chronic fatigue lasting for more than 6 months is known as chronic fatigue syndrome (CFS). This condition has been known for at least two centuries under the names "neurasthenia", "post-viral fatigue", "myalgic encephalomyelitis" or "chronic mononucleosis". The estimated worldwide prevalence of CFS is about 1% and this number can be under estimated due to mild character of the symptoms which can be explained by normal reasons. No physical examination signs are specific to CFS; no diagnostic tests identify this syndrome; no definitive treatment for it exists. Pathophysiology of CFS is analyzed from various points of view among which a relation to chronic infections or/and hypothalamic-pituitary adrenal (HPA) axis disturbances seem to be the most important ones. Up to now there are no convincing evidences found to support any of the proposed hypothesis trying to explain its pathogenesis. The current concept is that chronic fatigue condition is multi-factorial where an unidentified infective agent causes an aberrant ongoing immune response which fails to be switched-off [Lorusso L et al, 2009]. Here we put forward a new hypothesis that this "unidentified" infective agent is mycobacteria, and protective response controlling mycobacterial infection exhausts immunity and total reserves of body leading to chronic fatigue [Roth J et al, 2011].

CFS is a long-lasting condition. Among 265 patients with established CFS diagnosis studied by Tirelli U et al. [1994] many patients reported profound fatigue, lasting from 6 months to 10 years, among them 102 (38%) patients had to stop their working activities for a period of time ranging from 3 months to 2 years. CFS affects all racial-ethnic groups and more often females than males [Dinos S et al, 2009]. The prevalence of women is estimated from 6 to 1 [Capelli E et al, 2010] to no difference [Ravindran MK et al, 2011]. CFS is rarely found in childhood and adolescence however often affects young adults from 20 to 40 years old.

The diagnosis of CFS is based on clinical criteria and depends on exclusion of other physical and psychiatric diseases. Besides significant, unexplained fatigue lasting more than 6 months, at least 4 of 8-11 additional symptoms should be present: 4-5 of immunological nature such as sore throat or lymph nodes; joint or muscle pain; irritable bowel syndrome; and 4-6 neurological ones: headaches, problems with concentration or memory; dizziness, impaired co-ordination, sleep disturbances; post-exertional exhaustion [Sharpe MC et al, 1991].

2. A review of literature

2.1 Immunological findings

A possible involvement of the immune system is supported by the observation that the onset of CFS is often preceded by virus infections and a 'flu-like' illness. Among immune disfunctions the decrease either in number or functional activity of natural killer (NK) cells, especially in the number or activation status of CD56+ cells was found by many groups [Brenu EW et al, 2011; Fletcher MA, et al, 2010; Brenu EW et al, 2010; Mihaylova I. et al, 2007; Maher KJ et al, 2005, Nas K, 2011]. Lorusso L. at al [2009] reported an increased number of CD8+ cytotoxic T lymphocytes; CD38 and HLA-DR activation markers and a decrease in CD11b expression associated with an increased expression of CD28+ T subsets. The reduction in CD16+ and CD57+/CD56+ NK lymphocytes along with an expansion of CD8+/CD56+ and CD16-/CD56+ NK subsets were found in the CFS group by [Tirelli et al, 1994]. Other works also found an increase in CD8+ T-cell numbers [Robertson MJ et al, 2005] while Barker E et al [1994] found no significant differences in the absolute numbers of circulating total T cells (CD3+) and of total helper/inducer (CD4+) or suppressor/cytotoxic (CD8+) T cells.

Some papers report a post-vaccination or post-infection onset of CFS. Exogenous insults, such as Lyme disease, infectious mononucleosis, Epstein-Barr virus, enteroviruses, parvovirus, gastric and other infections, vaccinations, exposure to toxins, some stressful life events can lead to CFS [Devanur LD et al, 2006, Ortega-Hernandez OD et al., 2009]. However a working group of the Canadian Laboratory Center for Disease Control that examined the suspected association between CFS and vaccinations did not find relation of CFS to vaccination [Appel S at al, 2007].

2.2 Immune cells activation

Cell associated adhesion molecules and the level of their soluble forms can be used as activation markers. CD56+ NK cells from CFS subjects were found to express an increased amount of cell adhesion molecules CD11b, CD11c, CD54; and activation antigen CD38 [Tirelli et al, 1994]. CD4+ T lymphocytes from CFS patients displayed an increased expression of the intercellular adhesion molecule-1 (ICAM-1/CD54). The total number of circulating (CD19+) B lymphocytes was higher in CFS patients than in controls [Tirelli U et al, 1994].

Another marker of activation is the production of pro-inflammatory cytokines. Brenu EW et al have studied Th1 and Th2 cytokine profile of CD4+T cells. Compared to healthy individuals, CFS patients displayed significantly increased levels of IL-10, IFN-γ, and TNF-α [Brenu EW et al, 2010]. An alteration in cytokine profile was found by many other groups [Patarca R, 2001; Carlo-Stella N et al, 2006; Tomoda A et al, 2005].

2.3 Genomics of CFS

Starting from 2005, a microarray analysis was applied to determine gene expression profiles of CFS patients. The results published differ significantly between research groups [Kaushik N et al, 2005; Fang H et al, 2006; Carmel L et al, 2006; Frampton D et al, 2011]. For example, upregulated expression of ABCD4, PRKCL1, MRPL23, CD2BP2, GSN, NTE, POLR2G, PEX16, EIF2B4, EIF4G1, ANAPC11, PDCD2, KHSRP, BRMS1, and GABARAPL1 was found by Kaushik N et al [2005]. A completely different gene set (PTPRR, DEFB1, FLJ, HSFY1, EST, HPRT1, GUCA1B, CACNG2, ESR2, MOG, DFFA, ACBD6 and 12 others) was identified by

Fang H et al [2006]. The most recent publication attempted and failed to predict the diagnosis basing on genomic data [Frampton D et al, 2011]. Thus, genes involved in CFS still to be found more accurately. However, most authors conclude that genes responsible for immune cell activation and perturbation of neuronal and mitochondrial functions are involved.

2.4 Treatment of CFS patients

In recent decades, many therapies for CFS have been examined including: psychological "cognitive behaviour therapy", gradual physical exercise, pharmacological therapies, which included antibiotics and anti-depressant drugs [Avellaneda FA et al, 2009]. Mild improvements were found in adolescent groups after cognitive behaviour therapy [Smith M et al, 2003]. Other approached were not effective [Alegre de Miquel C et al, 2005; Vermeulen&Scholte, 2004; Staud R, 2007, Romani A et al, 2008]. We want to emphasize that antidepressant medication has been found to have no beneficial effect on improving the symptoms of CFS showing that CFS does not have a dominant psychological aetiology as it was considered for many years [Friedberg & Jason 2001, Chambers et al. 2006].

2.5 Chronic immune response hypothesis

It can be hypothesized that CFS, at least at its early stages and at least in some CFS patients, results from immune system exhaustion induced by an excessive immune response against widely spread pathogens such as *M.tuberculosis* or *Herpes virus. Mycobacterium tuberculosis* (MBT) is the most successful pathogen of mankind and remains a leading cause of death due to a bacterial pathogen. It is estimated that every third person on the planet is infected with MBT. Yet 90-95% of those who are infected with MBT remain otherwise healthy. These people are classified as "latently infected". Mouse studies have shown that susceptibility or resistance to tuberculosis (TB) depends on genetic factors [Kondratieva et al, 2010]. It is also the case for humans. Epidemiological evidence points to a major role of human genetic factors in the development of TB. Numerous genetic studies were conducted with variable results. Some HLA class II alleles and variants of the natural resistance-associated macrophage protein 1 (NRAMP1) gene are most likely involved [Abel&Casanova, 2010, Stein CM, 2011].

We hypothesize that human population can be divided on genetic basis into three TB groups: i) resistant; ii) susceptible; and iii) intermediate ones. The susceptible group in low pathogen environment is a reservoir from which active TB cases emerge (reactivation TB). Resistant group can control MBT without any signs of infection or immune system activation. While the last one - intermediate group, is resistant to TB for the expanse of immune system exhaust leading to chronic fatigue as one possibility. Rheumatoid arthritis is a disease where cross reactivity to MBT and self heat shock proteins is considered as one of disease onset mechanisms [Adebajo AO et al, 1995]. The risk of tuberculosis is increased 2- to 10-fold in RA patients [Baronnet L et al, 2011]. Cases of joint/bone tuberculosis are reported [Yagi O et al, 2007]. Among pulmonary TB patients 72% show severe to moderate level of anxiety and depression according to Hospital Anxiety and Depression Scale (HADS) [Aamir&Aisha, 2010]. Sore throat or laryngopharyngitis can also be found in TB [Raza&Rahat, 2010; Huon et al, 2009]. The coincidence of major CFS signs and TB infection can be continued.

2.6 Biomarkers predictive of susceptibility and resistance to TB

Recently whole-blood microarray gene expression analyses were performed in TB patients and in latently as well as uninfected healthy controls to define biomarkers predictive of susceptibility and resistance [Maertzdorf J et al. 2011]. Fc gamma receptor 1B was identified as the most differentially expressed gene, and, in combination with four other markers, produced a high degree of accuracy in discriminating TB patients and latently infected donors. Elevated expression of innate immune-related genes in active TB and higher expression of particular gene clusters involved in apoptosis and natural killer cell activity in latently infected donors are likely to be the major distinctive factors determining failure or success in controlling TB. As it was shown above, a decrease in NK cell numbers or their functional activity is the major immune disturbances found in CFS patients. Could it be a connection to TB?

3. Experimental data

3.1 Methods

3.1.1 Individuals

We have collected retrospectively cases of 14 individuals who came as donors among other volunteers who took part in different clinical trials hold by our laboratory during 2003-2008 [Popova I et al, 2008; Svirshchevskaya E et al, 2008; Ertneeva I et al, 2008; Skripkina P et al, 2008]. These 14 patients were selected on the basis of their deviated immune status. They were asked to fill in two questionnaires: Multidimensional Fatigue Inventory (MFI) and Zung depression scale [Smets EM et al, 1995; Zung, 1971]. For comparison the questionnaires were also filled in by 18 donors with normal parameters of immune cells. MFI and Zung scores demonstrated an increased level of depression and fatigue in 10 out of 14 persons with deviated immune status. The rest 4 had immunodeficiency and chronic infections. All 14 were suggested to take part in a trial aimed to verify our hypothesis. Each patient signed the voluntary consent to take part in the trial. Immunological data of healthy donors were used as a control.

3.1.2 Flow cytometry analysis for surface markers

Peripheral blood lymphocytes (PBL) were isolated on density gradient and washed three times in phosphate buffered saline (PBS). For the fluorescence-activated cell sorter (FACS) analysis cells were transferred to FACS buffer (PBS, 1% bovine serum albumin, 0.05% NaN_3). Three-color flow cytometry was performed using FACScan instrument, CellQuest software (BD Biosciences) and the following antibodies: CD3-PE, CD19-FITC, CD4-FITC, CD8-PE, CD16-FITC, CD56-PE, HLA-DR-FITC (all from Sorbent, Moscow). Live events (5,000–10,000) were acquired with propidium iodide exclusion of dead cells.

3.1.3 Treatment

Volunteers with signs of chronic fatigue were suggested the treatment with isoniazid, 300 mg per day during 30 days. Immune status was estimated before and after treatment at days 0, 30, and 90.

4. Results

4.1 Abnormal immune status in some healthy volunteers

PBL were collected from 102 volunteers involved in 4 clinical trials (antiviral drug Panavir, itraconazole generic Rumicoz, topic steroid cream Akriderm, anti-histamine generic Klarotadin) conducted in our laboratory during 2003-2008. Invited volunteers were medical students, health workers, graduate and Ph.D. students, friends and colleagues. Among them 8 persons took part in all four trials. So we were able to analyze the average parameters of immune cells for the whole population (Table 1) and variations with time for 8 persons (Fig.1). Among 8 volunteers 6 have normal CD4/CD8 ratio during all period of testing (Fig.1). Patient #5 showed a significant increase in this parameter while patient #8 demonstrated immunodeficiency at 3d and 4th testing. Patient #5, a young girl, suffered from seasonal allergy. Patient #8 was asymptomatic.

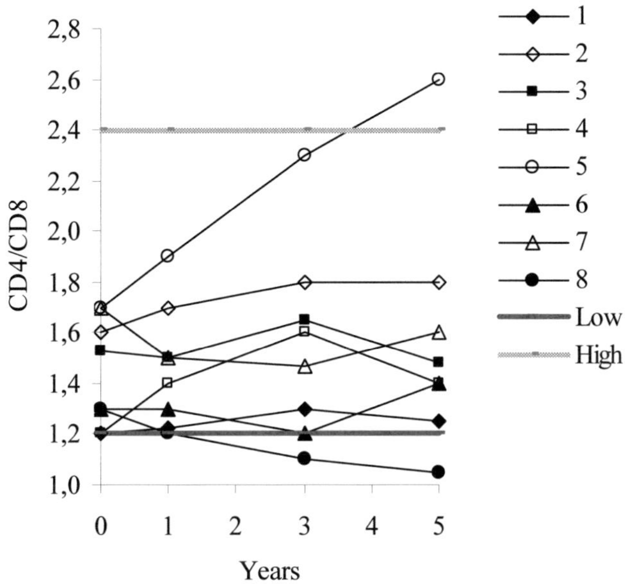

Fig. 1. Change in CD4/CD8 ratio in healthy volunteers with time. The percentage of CD4 and CD8 cells were estimated by cytofluorimetry. Normal range is shown as '"low-high" zone

CD		**Trials**			**Average**
	Panavir n=27	**Rumicoz n=25**	**Akriderm n=28**	**Klarotadin n=22**	**n=102**
CD3	72.5±7.2	70.8±5.2	75.1±4.3	74.3±8.2	**73.1**
CD4	39.0±5.3	37.6±8.1	38.3±5.8	39.2±7.3	**38.5**
CD8	23.9±4.9	25.1±6.2	29.3±4.6	26.3±5.4	**26.2**
CD16	12.2±4.5	10.6±4.6	12.9±3.5	12.8±6.6	**12.1**
CD56	14.5±5.5	11.3±5.5	13.1±5.6	10.0±4.3	**12.2**
CD19	9.0±6.2	7.5±3.2	10.1±5.3	8.7±6.3	**8.8**
HLA-DR	14.7±7.0	12.8±7.7	13.3±7.7	12.5±5.0	**13.3**
CD4/CD8	1.57±0.55	1.55±0.63	1.31±0.43	1.49±0.49	**1.47**
CD4/CD16	3.08±0.75	3.68±0.57	2.97±0.68	3.06±0.44	**3.18**
CD4/CD56	3.76±0.68	2.69±0.89	3.39±0.55	2.99±0.60	**3.15**

Table 1. Phenotype of lymphocytes in healthy donors

Among total group of donors we have found two types of immune deviations: decrease in CD4/CD8 ratios (≤1.2) or NK cell numbers (<5%) was found in 12 persons (12%) and a significant increase in CD4/CD8 (≥3) or NK numbers (>20%) was found in 11 volunteers (11%).

4.2 Clinical characteristics of fatigue group patients

All 23 individuals with deviated immune status were suggested to take part in the experimental trial. Fourteen persons agreed, while 9 refused. We asked 14 volunteers to fill in two questionnaires: Multidimensional Fatigue Inventory (MFI) and Zung depression scale. MFI estimates general fatigue, physical fatigue, mental fatigue, reduced motivation and reduced activity. Zung depression scale estimates the level of emotional depression. The summary of MFI for our patients varied from 15 to 35 with two cases 50 and 55. The summary of Zung scale was from 14 to 40. According to the work of Fang et al [2006] patients with MFI>54 and Zung scale >44 are considered as having CFS. With one exception all our patients cannot be classified as having CFS. Thus, we supposed that we worked with a group of patients with chronic fatigue induced by immune deviations. Most patients have various clinical symptoms shown in Table 2.

	Fatigue grade	Clinical symptoms	History of tuberculosis	Age
1	Severe, > 3 mo	none	10 year ago	52
2	Severe, > 12 mo	Prostatitis, herpes, sore throat, couth, phlegm	TB in family	24
3	Severe, > 5 mo	depression	none	24
4	Mild, > 3 mo	Sinusitis, pharyngitis, abnormalities with sleep	TB in family	47
5	Mild, > 6 mo	Depression, non refreshing sleep	none	55
6	Severe, > 12 mo	Depression, anxiety, non refreshing sleep, flu-like symptoms, often infections	none	56
7	Mild, > 3 mo	flu-like symptoms, often infections	none	22
8	Severe, > 12 mo	Depression, often infections, herpes	none	55
9	Mild or no	Reumathoid arthritis, hepatopathology, anxiety	25 years ago	67
10	Mild, > 6 mo	Depression, often infections, osteoarthrosis	none	52
11	Mild, > 12 mo	Lung inflammation	none	64
12	Mild, >12 mo	None	TB in family	53
13	Mild, > 3 mo	None	none	50
14	Mild, > 3 mo	Asthma	none	55

Table 2. Clinical characteristics of patients

4.3 Immunological characteristics of fatigue group patients

Blood from all patients was collected before the treatment and total numbers and percentages of T, B and NK subsets were analyzed. The results are shown in Tables 3-4. All these patients have different disturbances in immune parameters: either a deviation in CD4,

CD8 subsets or in CD16, CD56 cells. So, we divided the patients into two groups basing on CD4/CD8 ratio. Group 1 included patients with CD4/CD8≤1.2 and was designated "immunodeficiency group" (IDG) (Table 3). Group 2 included patients with ≥2.1 and was designated as "hyperstatus group" (HSG) (Table 4). We also included CD4/CD16 and CD4/CD56 ratios for comparison. Table 5 shows in the same way as Tables 3-4 summary from Table 1 for healthy controls. The statistical difference between IDG and HSG is significant for the CD4, CD8 percentage and their ratios only because we have selected patients using CD4/CD8 criteria for division. If we do the same using CD16 differences (low group <12, high group >12) we will also get significant difference, in this case for CD16, CD56 percentage and ratios (Tables 6 and 7).

	CD4	CD8	CD16	CD56	CD4/CD8	CD4/CD16	CD4/CD56
1	32	29	30	12	1.1	1.1	2.7
3	32	35	8.5	7.2	0.9	3.8	4.4
4	40	33	8.2	6.8	1.2	4.9	5.9
6	38	39	11	9.3	1.0	3.5	4.1
7	30	38	14	6.3	0.8	2.1	4.8
13	38	35	15	18	1.1	2.5	2.1
AV	**36**	**35**	**14**	**10**	**1.0**	**3.0**	**3.9**
SD	**4.2**	**3.4**	**7.4**	**4.2**	**0.2**	**1.2**	**1.3**

AV -Average meaning
SD - Standard deviation

Table 3. Immunological characteristics of fatigue patients with CD4/CD8 immunodeficiency

	CD4	CD8	CD16	CD56	CD4/CD8	CD4/CD16	CD4/CD56
2	38	18	28	6.1	2.1	1.4	6.2
5	61	20	16	18	3.1	3.8	3.4
8	58	12	8.0	5.9	4.8	7.3	9.8
9	65	8.9	11	4.1	7.4	5.9	16
10	58	10	18	16	5.8	3.2	3.6
11	40	12	10	14	3.3	4.0	2.9
12	61	23	4.4	5.3	2.7	14	12
14	38	11	6.9	5.1	3.5	5.5	7.5
AV	**52**	**14**	13	9,3	**4.1**	**5.6**	**7.6**
SD	**11.6**	**5.2**	**7.6**	**5.7**	**1.8**	**3.8**	**4.6**
t-test	**0.00**	**0.00**	0.34	0.37	**0.00**	**0.05**	**0.03**

t-test - probability estimated by Student' t-test between data shown in Tables 3 and 4.

Table 4. Immunological characteristics of fatigue patients with CD4/CD8 hyperstatus

There was no correlation between T and NK cell deviations. There results show that there are two non-related mechanisms of immune disturbances in these patients. Heterogeneity in immune parameters of fatigue patients can at least partially explain why no significant difference in comparison with healthy subjects was found by previously published studies. As our patients cannot be diagnosed strictly as CFS patients, we may only hypothesize that either immune abnormalities in CFS patients are overseen or they can be less pronounced during disease progression.

	CD4	CD8	CD16	CD56	CD4/CD8	CD4/CD16	CD4/CD56
AV	39	26	12	12	1.47	3.18	3.15
SD	5.0	4.5	4.9	4.3	0.52	0.77	0.60

Table 5. Immunological pattern of the control group (n=102)

	CD4	CD8	CD16	CD56	CD4/CD8	CD4/CD16	CD4/CD56
3	32	35	8.5	7.2	0.9	3.8	4.4
4	40	33	8.2	6.8	1.2	4.9	5.9
6	38	39	11	9.3	1.0	3.5	4.1
8	58	12	8	5.9	4.8	7.3	9.8
9	65	8.8	11	4.1	7.4	5.9	15.9
12	61	23	4.4	5.3	2.7	13.9	11.5
14	38	11	6.9	5.1	3.5	5.5	7.5
AV	**47**	**23**	**8.3**	**6.2**	**3.1**	**6.4**	**8.4**
SD	**12**	**11**	**7.5**	**5.1**	**1.8**	**1.1**	**1.4**

Table 6. Immunological characteristics of fatigue patients with NK immunodeficiency

	CD4	CD8	CD16	CD56	CD4/CD8	CD4/CD16	CD4/CD56
1	32	29	30	12	1.1	1.1	2.7
2	38	18	28	6.1	2.1	1.4	6.2
5	61	20	16	18	3.1	3.8	3.4
7	30	38	14	6.3	0.8	2.1	4.8
11	40	12	10	14	3.3	4.0	2.9
10	58	10	18	16	5.8	3.2	3.6
13	38	35	15	18	1.1	2.5	2.1
AV	**43**	**25**	**20**	**13**	**2.3**	**2.4**	**3.8**
SD	**13**	**13**	**2.3**	**1.7**	**2.4**	**3.5**	**4.3**
t-test	0.30	0.31	**0.00**	**0.02**	0.26	**0.01**	**0.03**

t-test – probability estimated by Student' t-test between data shown in Tables 6 and 7.

Table 7. Immunological characteristics of fatigue patients with NK hyperstatus

4.4 Clinical effect of izoniazid treatment on fatigue

Three patients reported nausea during first 2-5 days. No other side effects of this treatment were reported. Among 14 patients one (#7) discontinued the treatment. All patients were asked to fill in again MFI and Zung questionnaire (ZQ). Patients with severe forms of fatigue (##1, 2, 3, 8) found that they started feeling "better and more energetic" after 2-3 weeks of treatment. Their MFI and ZQ scores were significantly improved. Patient 6 described the effect as "relaxing" and "sleep impoving". Other patients self-rated the effect as neutral however the MFI and ZQ scores on average were better for 8 of 9 patients.

Clinical symptoms of other associated pathologies (prostatitis, sore throat, couth, phlegm, flu-like symptoms) subsided to the end of treatment in those patients who had them at the time of the trial. We monitored 8 of 14 patients for 1 year. Two months post-treatment all of them felt significantly better than before with no signs of fatigue. At 6 mo post treatment 2 persons who earlier suffered severe fatigue, again had sings of it and were recommended the second course. The results were the same: quick elimination of fatigue symptoms and slow improvement in somatic symptoms.

4.5 Immunological effects of izoniazid treatment

We analyzed parameters of lymphocytes in treated patients before the treatment and at days 30 and 90. The results are shown in Fig.2. All parameters of immune status were better than before the treatment showing that the therapy was effective.

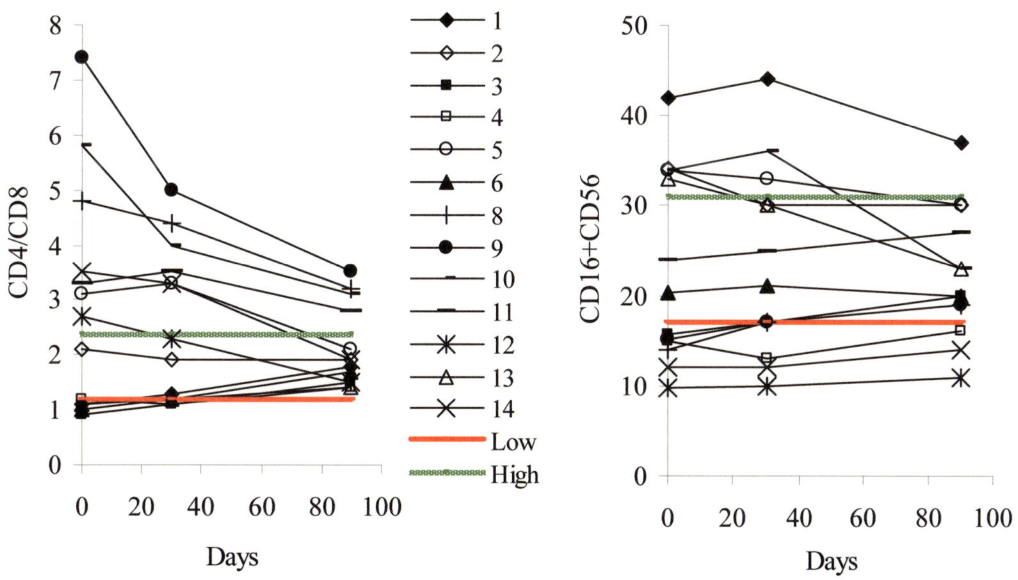

Fig. 2. Changes in CD4/CD8 ratio (left panel) or number of CD16+CD56 NK cells (right panel) before and after izoniazid treatment of patients with chronic fatigue.
Normal range is shown as '"low-high" zone

5. Discussion

MTB, the causative agent of tuberculosis remains a major threat to global health as the leading cause of death due to a bacterial pathogen. Every third person on the planet is infected with MBT. However, only 10% among infected individuals develop TB while others remain otherwise healthy. These people are classified as "latently infected," but remain a reservoir of MBT. Latent TB has traditionally been defined as infection with MBT in foci within granuloma that remain in nonreplicating state but retain their ability to induce TB when a disruption of the immune response occurs. However, recent experimental data support a dynamic model of latent TB where endogenous reactivation as well as damage response occur constantly in immunocompetent individuals [Cardona PJ, 2009, Ahmad S, 2011]. This model suggests that some type of macrophages (foamy macrophages) phagocytose extracellular nonreplicating MBT; however, the bacilli do not grow in the intracellular environment of activated macrophages but are also not killed due to the nonreplicating state of the bacilli. The nonreplicating bacilli-loaded foamy macrophages drain from lung granuloma towards the bronchial tree and return to a different region of lungs and begin the infection process at a new location once again [See review Ahmad S, 2011]. It can be speculated that activated foamy macrophages can enter not only the lungs but also other organs as TB is known in many forms of localization [Horsburgh&Rubin, 2011; Russell, 2011; Dorhoi et al, 2011, Galimi R, 2011]. These new locations of MBT can attract immune cells inducing all the symptoms characteristic for CFS patients.

Here we put forward a new hypothesis that at least in some patients chronic fatigue can be induced by ongoing immune response against MBT. We have chosen patients from a large cohort of individuals basing on two criteria: i) they have signs of fatigue and depression; and ii) their immune status was deviated from a normal one. Selected patients have various medical problems (prostatitis, herpes, sore throat, couth, phlegm, sinusitis, pharyngitis, mild reumathoid arthritis). The aims of the trial were: i) to estimate whether anti-tuberculosis treatment can help in resolving fatigue and depression; and ii) if the treatment affects immune status of the patients. The results were encouraging as most patients felt a decrease in fatigue symptoms. This effect was not long-lasting as in severe cases 6 mo later some patients again complained the signs of fatigue. The remittance of the disease can again be explained in terms of "chronic interaction between MBT and immune cells". Izoniazid treatment hypothetically removed some active foci inducing a following decrease in immune response. However, new locations of MBT were formed with time due to a genetic susceptibility to TB. This means that anti-tuberculosis treatment could possible be needed for a longer time or for repeated courses during several years.

We have also shown that parameters of immunity were improved after anti-tuberculosis treatment. These results showed that immune status can be used as a parameter to monitor. In our trial only persons with deviated immunity were included. Possibly among CFS patients also individuals with immune disturbances can be considered as candidates for izoniazid therapy.

Finally I want to emphasize that the effect of izoniazid on fatigue could be a by-stander to MBT infection and be connected to some other targets in brains of immune system. However, new studies are required to clarify this matter.

6. Acknowledgments

This publication was made possible in part by RAS Fundamental Research Program "Molecular and Cellular Biology".

7. References

Aamir S, Aisha. Co-morbid anxiety and depression among pulmonary tuberculosis patients. J Coll Physicians Surg Pak. 2010 Oct;20(10):703-4.

Abel L, Casanova JL. [Human genetics of tuberculosis]. Bull Acad Natl Med. 2010 Jun;194(6):943-50; discussion 951-2. French.

Adebajo AO, Williams DG, Hazleman BL, Maini RN. Antibodies to the 65 kDa mycobacterial stress protein in west Africans with rheumatoid arthritis, tuberculosis and malaria. Br J Rheumatol. 1995 Apr;34(4):352-4.

Ahmad S. Pathogenesis, immunology, and diagnosis of latent Mycobacterium tuberculosis infection. Clin Dev Immunol. 2011;2011:814943.

Alegre de Miquel C, Pereda C, Nishishinya M, Rivera J: Pharmocology interventions in fibromyalgia. A sistematic Review. MedClin (Barc) 2005, 125:784-7.

Appel S, Chapman J, Shoenfeld Y. Infection and vaccination in chronic fatigue syndrome: myth or reality? Autoimmunity. 2007 Feb;40(1):48-53.

Avellaneda Fernández A, Pérez Martín A, Izquierdo Martínez M, Arruti Bustillo M, Barbado Hernández FJ, de la Cruz Labrado J, Díaz-Delgado Peñas R, Gutiérrez

Barker E, Fujimura SF, Fadem MB, Landay AL, Levy JA. Immunologic abnormalities associated with chronic fatigue syndrome. Clin Infect Dis. 1994 Jan;18 Suppl 1:S136-41.

Baronnet L, Barnetche T, Kahn V, Lacoin C, Richez C, Schaeverbeke T. Incidence of tuberculosis in patients with rheumatoid arthritis. A systematic literature review. Joint Bone Spine. 2011 May;78(3):279-84.

Brenu EW, Staines DR, Baskurt OK, Ashton KJ, Ramos SB, Christy RM, Marshall-Gradisnik SM. Immune and hemorheological changes in chronic fatigue syndrome. J Transl Med. 2010 Jan 11;8:1.

Brenu EW, van Driel ML, Staines DR, Ashton KJ, Ramos SB, Keane J, Klimas NG, Marshall-Gradisnik SM. Immunological abnormalities as potential biomarkers in Chronic Fatigue Syndrome/Myalgic Encephalomyelitis. J Transl Med. 2011 May 28;9:81.

Capelli E, Zola R, Lorusso L, Venturini L, Sardi F, Ricevuti G. Chronic fatigue syndrome/myalgic encephalomyelitis: an update. Int J Immunopathol Pharmacol. 2010 Oct-Dec;23(4):981-9.

Cardona P-J, A dynamic reinfection hypothesis of latent tuberculosis infection. Infection, 2 vol. 37, no. 2, pp. 80–86, 2009.

Carlo-Stella N, Badulli C, De Silvestri A, Bazzichi L, Martinetti M, Lorusso L, et al. A first study of cytokine genomic polymorphisms in CFS: positive association of TNF-857 and IFN γ874 rare alleles. Clin Exp Rheumathol 2006;24:179–82.

Carmel L, Efroni S, White PD, Aslakson E, Vollmer-Conna U, Rajeevan MS. Gene expression profile of empirically delineated classes of unexplained chronic fatigue. Pharmacogenomics. 2006 Apr;7(3):375-86. PubMed PMID: 16610948.

Chambers D, Bagnall AM, Hempel S, Forbes C. Interventions for the treatment, management and rehabilitation of patients with chronic fatigue syndrome/myalgic encephalomyelitis: an updated systematic review. J R Soc Med. 2006 Oct;99(10):506-20.

Devanur LD, Kerr JR. Chronic fatigue syndrome. J Clin Virol. 2006 Nov;37(3):139-50.

Dinos S, Khoshaba B, Ashby D, White PD, Nazroo J, Wessely S, Bhui KS. A systematic review of chronic fatigue, its syndromes and ethnicity: prevalence, severity, co-morbidity and coping. Int J Epidemiol. 2009 Dec;38(6):1554-70

Dorhoi A, Reece ST, Kaufmann SH. For better or for worse: the immune response against Mycobacterium tuberculosis balances pathology and protection. Immunol Rev. 2011 Mar;240(1):235-51. doi: 10.1111/j.1600-065X.2010.00994.x.

Ertneeva I,Y., Matushevskaya E.V., Svirshchevskaya E.V. Clinical and immunological parameters of atopic dermatitis patients treated with Acriderm preparations. Clinical dermatovenereologic. 2008, 5, 39-44 (In Russian).

Fang H, Xie Q, Boneva R, Fostel J, Perkins R, Tory W. Gene expression profile exploration of a large dataset on chronic fatigue syndrome. Pharmacogenomics 2006;7:429–40.

Fletcher MA, Zeng XR, Maher K, Levis S, Hurwitz B, Antoni M, Broderick G, Klimas NG. Biomarkers in chronic fatigue syndrome: evaluation of natural killer cell function and dipeptidyl peptidase IV/CD26. PLoS One. 2010 May 25;5(5):e10817.

Frampton D, Kerr J, Harrison TJ, Kellam P. Assessment of a 44 gene classifier for the evaluation of chronic fatigue syndrome from peripheral blood mononuclear cell gene expression. PLoS One. 2011 Mar 30;6(3):e16872.

Friedberg F, Jason LA. Chronic fatigue syndrome and fibromyalgia: clinical assessment and treatment. J Clin Psychol. 2001 Apr;57(4):433-55.

Galimi R. Extrapulmonary tuberculosis: tuberculous meningitis new developments. Eur Rev Med Pharmacol Sci. 2011 Apr;15(4):365-86.

Horsburgh CR Jr, Rubin EJ. Clinical practice. Latent tuberculosis infection in the United States. N Engl J Med. 2011 Apr 14;364(15):1441-8.

Huon LK, Huang SH, Wang PC, Chen LC. Clinical photograph. Laryngopharyngeal tuberculosis masquerading as chronic laryngopharyngitis. Otolaryngol Head Neck Surg. 2009 Oct;141(4):537-8.

Kaushik N, Fear D, Richards SC, McDermott CR, Nuwaysir EF, Kellam P, Harrison TJ, Wilkinson RJ, Tyrrell DA, Holgate ST, Kerr JR. Gene expression in peripheral blood mononuclear cells from patients with chronic fatigue syndrome. J Clin Pathol. 2005 Aug;58(8):826-32.

Kondratieva E, Logunova N, Majorov K, Averbakh M, Apt A. Host genetics in granuloma formation: human-like lung pathology in mice with reciprocal genetic susceptibility to M. tuberculosis and M. avium. PLoS One. 2010 May 6;5(5): e10515.

Lorusso L, Mikhaylova SV, Capelli E, Ferrari D, Ngonga GK, Ricevuti G. Immunological aspects of chronic fatigue syndrome. Autoimmun Rev. 2009 8(4):287-91.

Maher KJ, Klimas NG, Fletcher MA. Chronic fatigue syndrome is associated with diminished intracellular perforin. Clin Exp Immunol. 2005 Dec;142(3):505-11.

Mihaylova I, DeRuyter M, Rummens JL, Bosmans E, Maes M. Decreased expression of CD69 in chronic fatigue syndrome in relation to inflammatory markers: evidence for a severe disorder in the early activation of T lymphocytes and natural killer cells. Neuro Endocrinol Lett. 2007 Aug;28(4):477-83.

Nas K, Cevik R, Batum S, Sarac AJ, Acar S, Kalkanli S. Immunologic and psychosocial status in chronic fatigue syndrome. Bratisl Lek Listy. 2011;112(4): 208-12.

Ortega-Hernandez OD, Shoenfeld Y. Infection, vaccination, and autoantibodies in chronic fatigue syndrome, cause or coincidence? Ann N Y Acad Sci. 2009 Sep;1173:600-9

Patarca R. Cytokines and chronic fatigue syndrome. Ann N Y Acad Sci 2001;933: 185–200

Popova I.S., Matushevskaya E.V., Svirshchevskaya E.V. Double blinded randomized placebo-controlled trial of safety and efficacy of klarotadine in atopic dermatitis patients. Russian J.Immunology. 2003, 8, 1, 99-104.

Ravindran MK, Zheng Y, Timbol C, Merck SJ, Baraniuk JN. Migraine headaches in chronic fatigue syndrome (CFS): comparison of two prospective cross-sectional studies. BMC Neurol. 2011 Mar 5;11:30.

Raza SN, Rahat ZM. Horner's syndrome as a co-presentation of tuberculous retropharyngeal abscess. J Coll Physicians Surg Pak. 2010 Apr;20(4):279-81.

Rivas E, Palacín Delgado C, Rivera Redondo J, Ramón Giménez JR. Chronic fatigue syndrome: aetiology, diagnosis and treatment. BMC Psychiatry. 2009 Oct 23;9 Suppl 1:S1.

Robertson MJ, Schacterle RS, Mackin GA, Wilson SN, Bloomingdale KL, Ritz J, et al. Lymphocyte subset differences in patients with chronic fatigue syndrome, multiple sclerosis and major depression. Clin Exp Immunol 2005;141:326–33.

Romani A. The treatment of fatigue. Neurol Sci. 2008 Sep;29 Suppl 2:S247-9.

Roth J, Szulc AL, Danoff A. Energy, evolution, and human diseases: an overview. Am J Clin Nutr. 2011; 93(4):875S-83.

Russell DG. Mycobacterium tuberculosis and the intimate discourse of a chronic infection. Immunol Rev. 2011 Mar;240(1):252-68. doi:10.1111/j.1600-065X.2010.00984.x.

Sharpe MC, Archard LC, Banatvala JE, et al. A report-chronic fatigue syndrome: guidelines for research. J R Soc Med 1991; 84:118-21.

Skripkina P.A., Matushevskaya E.V., Grigoriev V.S., Svirshchevskaya E.V. Immunomodulating and antiviral therapy of atopic dermatitis. Russian Journal of dermatovenereological diseases. 2008, 2, 30-37 ((In Russian).

Smets EM, Garssen B, Bonke B, De Haes JC. The Multidimensional Fatigue Inventory (MFI) psychometric qualities of an instrument to assess fatigue. J Psychosom Res. 1995 Apr;39(3):315-25.

Smith M, Martin-Hertz S, Womack W, Marsigan J: Comparativestudy of anxiety, depression, somatization, functional disability and disease attribution in adolescents with chronic fatigue or migraine. Pediatrics 2003, 111:376-381.

Staud R: Treatment of fibromyalgia and its symptoms. Expert Opin Pharmacother 2007, 8(11):1629-42.

Stein CM. Genetic epidemiology of tuberculosis susceptibility: impact of study design. PLoS Pathog. 2011 Jan 20;7(1):e1001189.

Svirshchevskaya E.V., Airapetyan N.R., Matushevskaya E.V., Karpenkova S.V., Skripkina P.A., Grigoriev V.S. Immune status of nail onichomicosis patients. Russian Journal of dermatovenereological diseases. 2008, 2, 43-48 (In Russian).

Tirelli U, Marotta G, Improta S, Pinto A. Immunological abnormalities in patients with chronic fatigue syndrome. Scand J Immunol. 1994;40(6):601-8.

Tomoda A, Joudoi T, Rabab el-M, MatsumotoT, Park TH, Miike T. Cytokine production and modulation: comparison of patients with chronic fatigue syndrome and normal controls. Psychiatry Res 2005;134:101–4.

Vermeulen R, Scholte H: Exploratory open label, randomized study of acetyl- and propionylcarnitine in chronic fatigue syndrome. Psychosom Med 2004, 66:276-282.

Yagi O, Kawabe Y, Nagayama N, Shimada M, Kawashima M, Kaneko Y, Ariga H, Ohshima N, Matsui Y, Suzuki J, Masuda K, Tamura A, Nagai H, Akagawa S, Machida K, Kurashima A, Nakajima Y, Yotsumoto H. [Bone and joint tuberculosis concurrent with tuberculosis of other organs]. Kekkaku. 2007 Jun;82(6):523-9. Japanese.

Zung WW. A rating instrument for anxiety disorders. Psychosomatics. 1971 Nov-Dec;12(6):371-9.

9

T Cell Suppression in Burn and Septic Injuries

Nadeem Fazal
*Pharmaceutical Sciences, College of Pharmacy / DH 206,
Chicago State University, Chicago, IL
USA*

1. Introduction

The mechanism responsible for initiating and controlling burn-induced immunosuppression remains unknown. Accumulating experimental and clinical data indicates that burn injury promotes suppressed immune function, predisposing the host to infectious complications (Moss NM, 1988). Skin plays an indispensable first line of defense against microorganisms; the disruption of this primary barrier in burn injury leaves patients greatly susceptible to invasion by pathogens and increases their morbidity and mortality. Severely burn-injured patients exhibit classical signs of suppressed immune function such as loss of delayed-type hypersensitivity responses, prolonged skin allograft survival and reduced T-cell proliferation to polyclonal and antigen-specific stimulation (Ninnemann JL, 1994, Lederer, JA, 1999, Faist E, 1996). The disturbances in T-cell mediated responses include low T-helper 1 (Th-1) type cytokine production and reduced Th-1 type antibody isotype secretion (Kelly, JL, 1999). There is a rising incidence of nosocomial infections accompanied by burn-induced adaptive immunosuppression (Baker, CC, 1979, Angele MK, 2002). This shift of adaptive immune response towards a counter-inflammatory phenotype takes place in the presence of proinflammatory innate immune response (Harris, BH, 1995). An estimated 40, 000 adults are admitted to hospitals in USA with burns each year (Salinas J et al, 2008, White CE, 2008). Severe burn-injury stimulates a massive release of cytokines into the bloodstream leading to shock, immune dysfunction, and multiorgan failure. Serum levels of interleukin (IL)-8, tumor necrosis factor-α, IL-6, and granulocyte-macrophage colony stimulatory factor (GM-CSF) peak within first week postburn. In addition to shock, this rush of cytokines triggers a hypercatabolic state, with muscle wasting and immunosuppression. Eventually, this immunosuppression follows multiorgan dysfunction, sepsis and heralds death.

2. SIRS-CARS (Figures 1-5)

This paradigm is currently accepted by the investigators in the field of burn, shock and trauma. Extensive tissue destruction following burn-injury predisposes patients to consequences of different and dysregulated inflammatory immune responses (Saffle, JR, 1993, Baue, AE, 1998, Still, JM, 1993). Following the initial resuscitation period, patients develop systemic inflammatory response syndrome (SIRS), which leads to multiple organ dysfunction syndrome (MODS) which is associated with high mortality. If the patients do not develop early MODS and survive SIRS they characterize suppressed immunity and resistance to infection, which is termed as compensatory anti-inflammatory response syndrome (CARS). Baue et al, 1998 supports the theory that interactions between the innate

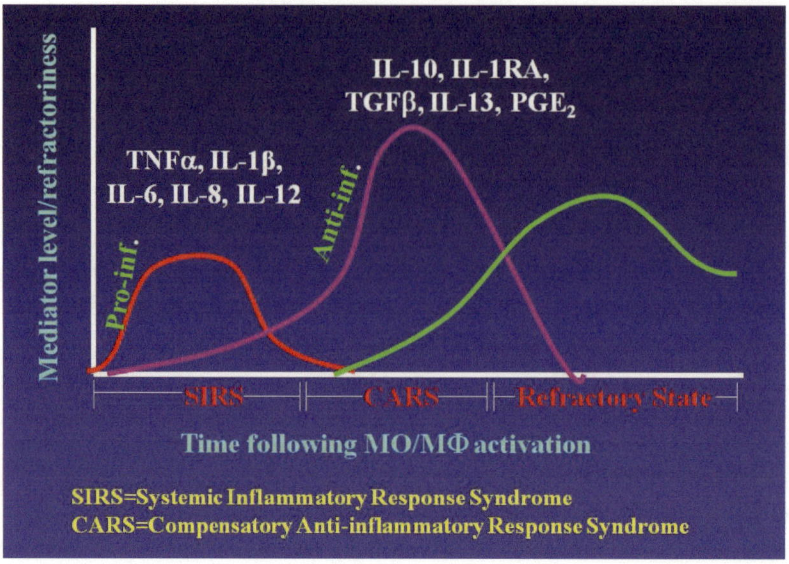

Fig. 1. A schematic drawing of mediators released during different phases of immune response following burn injury. X-axis show levels of mediators released against time (y-axis) following monocyte/macrophages activation. Mediators released during the early pro-inflammatory phase (Systemic inflammatory response syndrome (SIRS) are TNFα, IL-1, IL-6, IL-8 and IL-12 followed by anti-inflammatory phase where IL-10, IL-1RA, TGFβ, IL-13, PGE2 are released. Mixed antagonistic response syndrome (MARS) with both pro-and anti-inflammatory components has not been in literature since year 2000. At the meantime a refractory state is also initiated which continues even after compensatory anti-inflammatory response syndrome (CARS) is over.

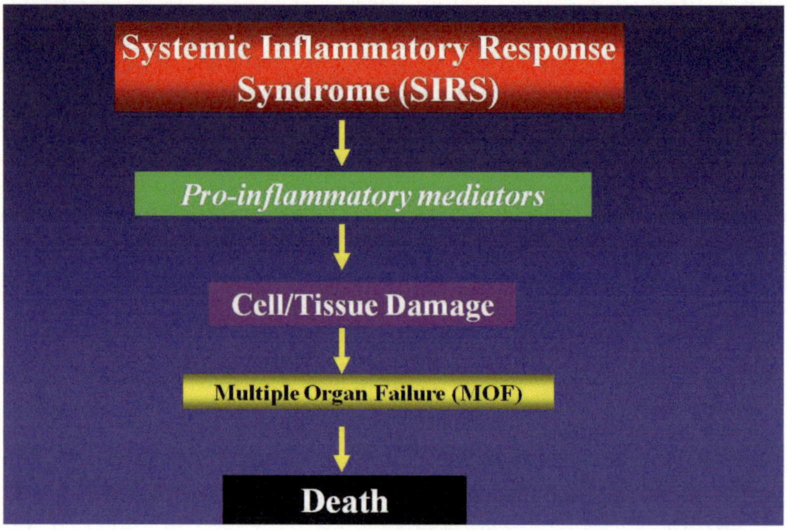

Fig. 2. Systemic inflammatory response syndrome (SIRS) leading to release of pro-inflammatory mediators; leading to cell/tissue damage; leading to multiple organ failure; leading to death.

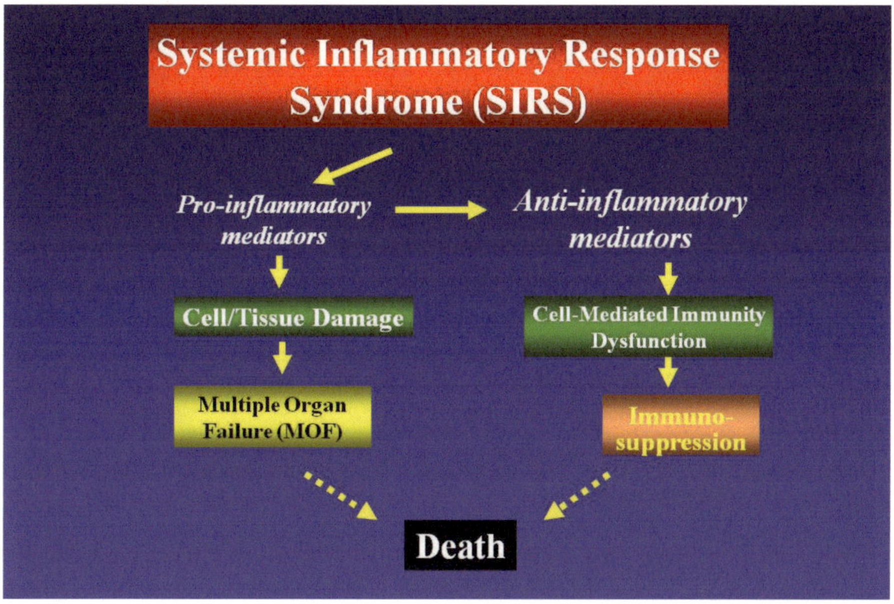

Fig. 3. A schematic drawing of cascade of events (first scenario) where both pro-inflammatory as well as anti-inflammatory immune responses are initiated, eventually leading to mortality. In this scenario anti-inflammatory mediators cause dysfunction of cell-mediated immunity (CMI) leading to death via immunosuppression.

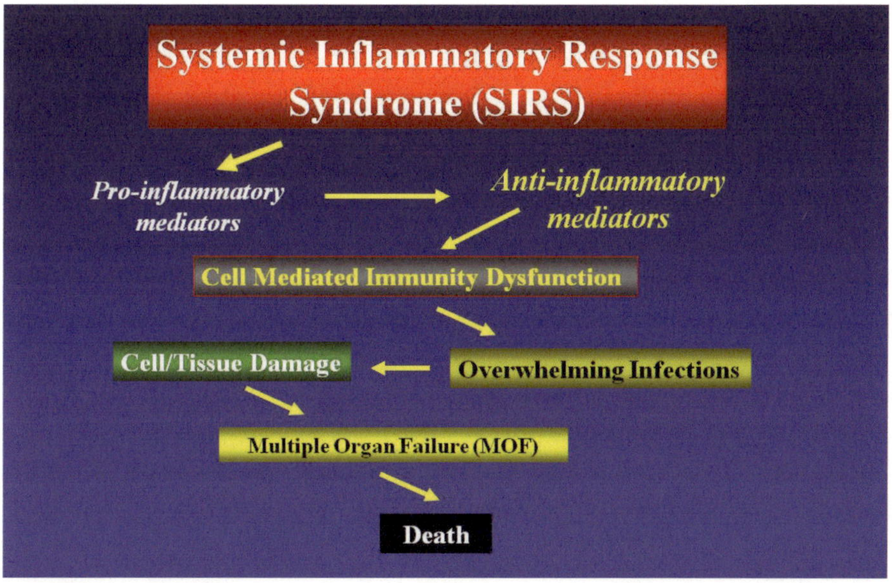

Fig. 4. A schematic drawing of cascade of events (second scenario) when SIRS is complicated by overwhelming infections following dysregulated cell-mediated immunity, leading to mortality. In this case dysfunction of cell-mediated immunity leads a way to overwhelming infections and then classical pathway of cell and tissue damage responsible for multiple organ failure (MOF) paves the way to mortality.

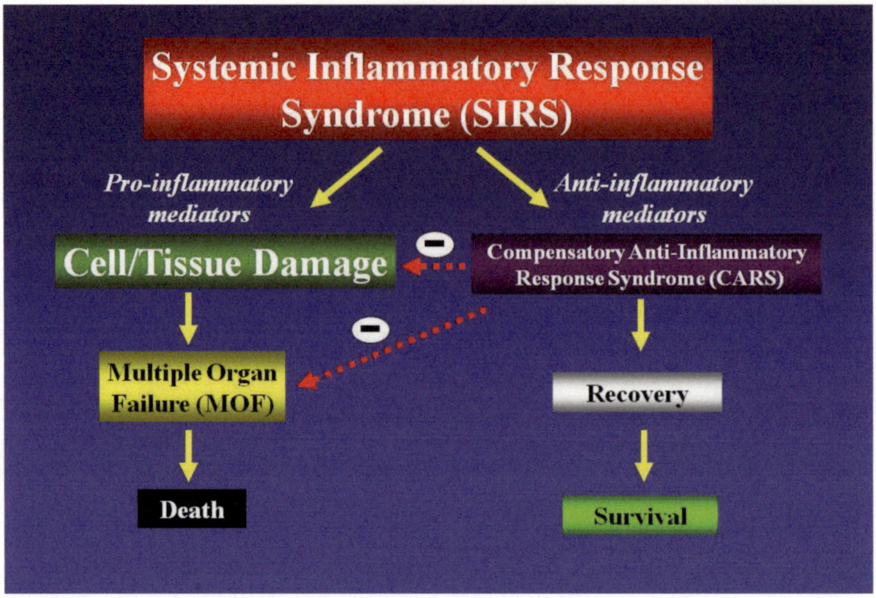

Fig. 5. A schematic outcome of compensatory anti-inflammatory response syndrome (CARS) in a beneficial outcome of recovery leading to survival (third scenario). In this alternative sequence of events anti-inflammatory mediators set the stage up for a compensatory anti-inflammatory response syndrome (CARS) which down regulates cell and tissue damage and halts multiple organ failure thus positively influence the outcome of (SIRS) towards a recovery phase.

and adaptive immune systems are important in the induction of CARS and SIRS. Burn-induced immune dysregulation is a continuously changing process and evolves over time and goes into a refractory state.

3. Locally released inflammatory mediators (Figure 6-7)

Pro-inflammatory cascade of cytokine released immediately after injury is a harbinger of subsequent immune dysfunction, sepsis and multiple organ failure (Meakins, JL, 1990). The cells of innate immune system including macrophages, fibroblasts, natural killer (NK) cells, activated T-cells release pro-inflammatory cytokines i.e., interleukin-1 (IL-1), tumor necrosis factor–α (TNF-α), IL-6, transforming growth factor–β (TGF-β), reactive nitrogen intermediates (RNI), prostaglandin E2 (PGE2) (Ogle, CK, 1994). These cytokines and other mediators are triggered by both non-infectious and infectious stimuli (Figures 6 and 7). The inflammatory SIRS response is known to be caused by stimuli other than sepsis in contrast to CARS that follows invasive infection. Marano MA, 1990 and Gamelli RL, 1995 documented increased systemic levels of these inflammatory mediators following burn injury altering the functional capacity of their parent cells. This elevated production of inflammatory mediators has thus been implicated for post-burn sepsis (Schwacha MG, 1998, Yang L, 1992, O'Riordain, MG, 1992). Locally released inflammatory mediators, i.e, C3a, C5a, PG, LT, O_2^-, NO, TNFα, IL1, IL6, IL8, IL10, TGFβ act on different circulating cells (leukocytes/platelets) and other tissues (endothelium, epithelium and parenchymal cells) and neuro-endocrine axis to enhance different effector responses.

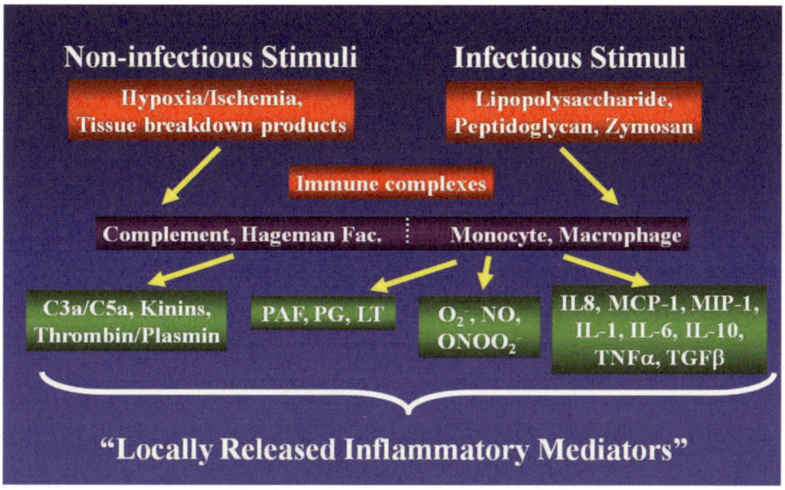

Fig. 6. Locally released inflammatory mediators triggered by both non-infectious vs. infectious stimuli. A list of humoral and cell-derived factors is given which will determine the potential outcome of burn-injury associated tissue damage. In the first sequence of events non-infectious stimuli cause hypoxia/ischemia type of injury and release of tissue breakdown products, mostly initiating a humoral response and a list of modulators causing inflammation. In the event of infectious stimuli LPS, Peptidoglycan activate predominantly a cellular immune response, again triggering release of a list of cytokines and chemokines. These include but do not limit to release of platelet-activating factor (PAF), prostaglandin (PG), lymphotoxin (LT), reactive oxygen species (ROS), reactive nitrogen species (RNI), monocyte chemotactic protein-1 (MCP-1), and macrophage inflammatory protein-1 (MIP-1).

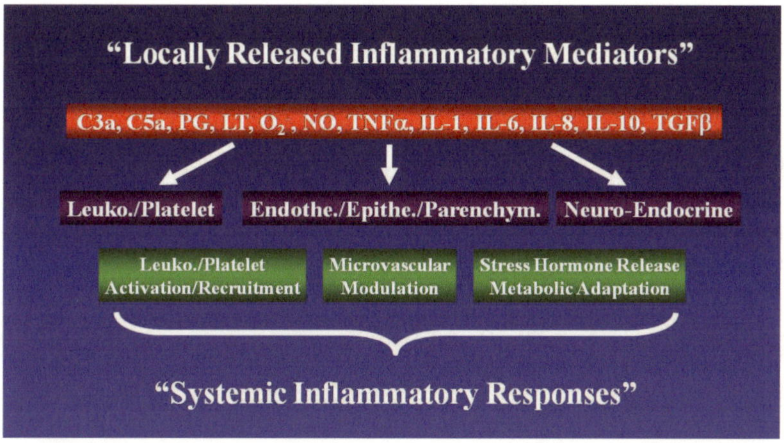

Fig. 7. Locally released inflammatory mediators act on different circulating cells (leukocytes/platelets) and other tissues (endothelium, epithelium and parenchymal cells) and neuro-endocrine axis to enhance different effector responses. Leucocytes and platelets are activated and are recruited to the site of injury. Microvascular changes are brought about by both humoral and cell-mediated factors acting on endothelium, epithelium and parencyhmal cells, and finally, via neuroendocrine axis stress hormones (i.e, cortisol) are released which affect metabolism.

4. Systemically released mediators (Figure 8)

Endogenous mediators related to burn injury include a list, i.e., C-reactive proteins, serum amyloid A, procalcitonin, C3 complement and haptaglobin, etc. These circulating mediators influence endothelial, epithelial and other types of cells. These inflammatory mediators act as double-edged swords (Figure 8).

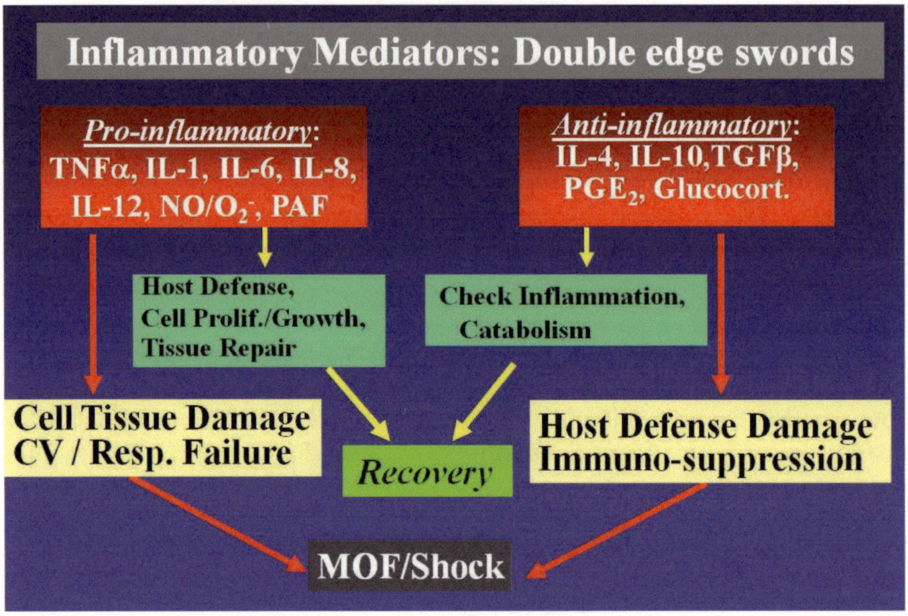

Fig. 8. Inflammatory mediators act like double-edged swords. Cascade of events could either lead to recovery or causing cell tissue damage and/or immunosuppression culminating in multiple organ failure and shock. Pro-inflammatory mediators help in host defense and positively influence cell proliferation/growth and enhance tissue repair-all processes leading to recovery, whereas anti-inflammatory mediators assist in controlling inflammation and limit catabolism thus helping recovery. On the flipside, pro-inflammatory mediators may also culminate in cell/tissue damage, cardiovascular/respiratory failure, and likewise anti-inflammatory mediators decrease host defense via initiating immunosuppression. Thus it acts like a double-edged sword- complementing further multiple organ failure and shock.

5. Pro-inflammatory and anti-inflammatory immune responses (Figures 9-16)

In the midst of burn-injury immune responses pro-inflammatory and anti-inflammatory immune responses elicit different responses. The most notable of pro-inflammatory responses include leukocytosis, enhanced adherence, fever, hypermetablism, activation of HPA axis and acute phase protein response in the liver. Anti-inflammatory immune responses serve to deactivate leukocyte activation, myelosuppression, abrogate hypermetabolism, and suppress tissue repair and most importantly immunosuppression of cell-mediated adaptive immunity. Figures 9-16 explain the dual hit immune response and the details of burn-induced cascade of effector responses leading to infection, sepsis and later complications.

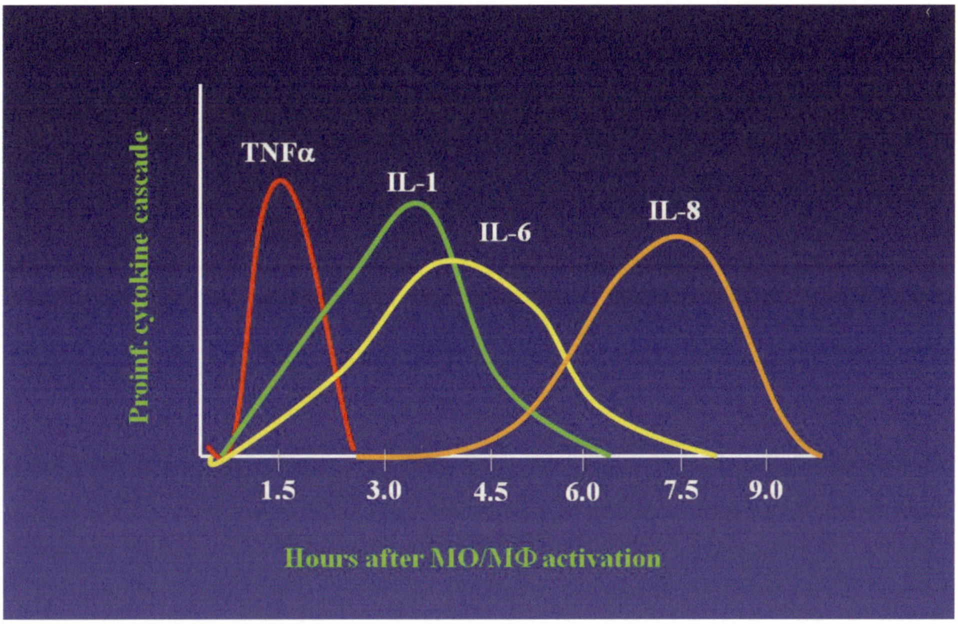

Fig. 9. Timeline of release of pro-inflammatory cytokine cascade in term of hours following their release from activated monocytes and/or macrophages. The first cytokine to appear and peak within hours is TNFα. IL-1 and IL-6 are also initiated but peak when TNFα levels begin to fall down. IL-1 peaks at higher levels than IL-6 and finally IL-8 is among the last to appear in this sequence of cascade of inflammatory cytokines.

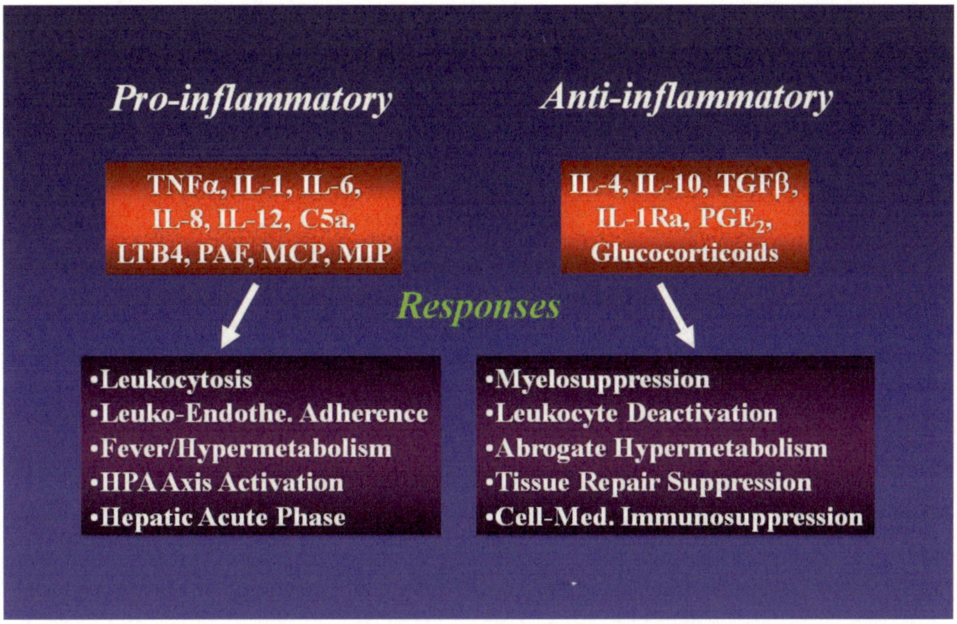

Fig. 10. Pro- and/or anti-inflammatory immune responses are initiated by the respective pro- or anti-inflammatory cytokines leading to two different outcomes as given in this figure.

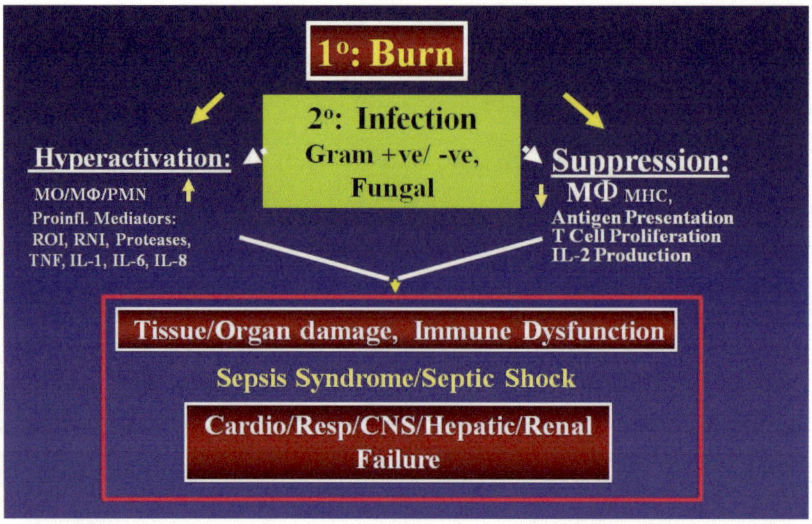

Fig. 11. A two-hit model: Primary hit (burn) when compounded by secondary hit (infection) operates through hyperactivation response (monocytes, macrophages and neutrophil)-mediated or immunosuppression (macrophages, antigen-presenting cells, T cells)-mediated-leading to tissue damage and immune dysfunction. This unregulated immune responses leads to sepsis syndrome/septic shock and multiple organ failure.

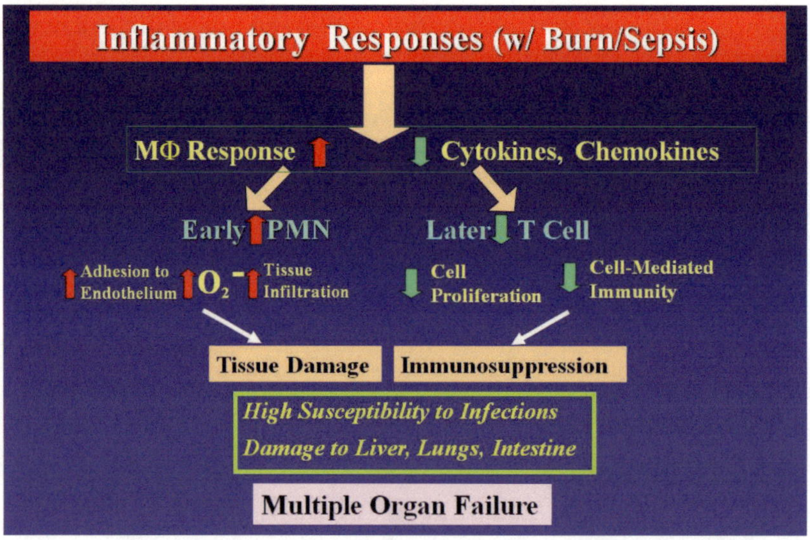

Fig. 12. This figure shows the timeline of burn with sepsis immune response. There is early neutrophil-mediated exaggerated or excessive immune response followed by T-cell mediated immunosuppression. Early PMN-responsible increases adhesion of neutrophils to endothelium, increased tissue infiltration, and increased oxygen radical burst. This heightened PMN response then causes tissue damage to liver, lungs, and intestine, especially compromised intestinal barrier leads to bacterial translocation. A later T cell-mediated response causing immunosuppression (decreased cell proliferation and cell-mediated immunity). These early PMN and late T-cell cause multiple organ failure.

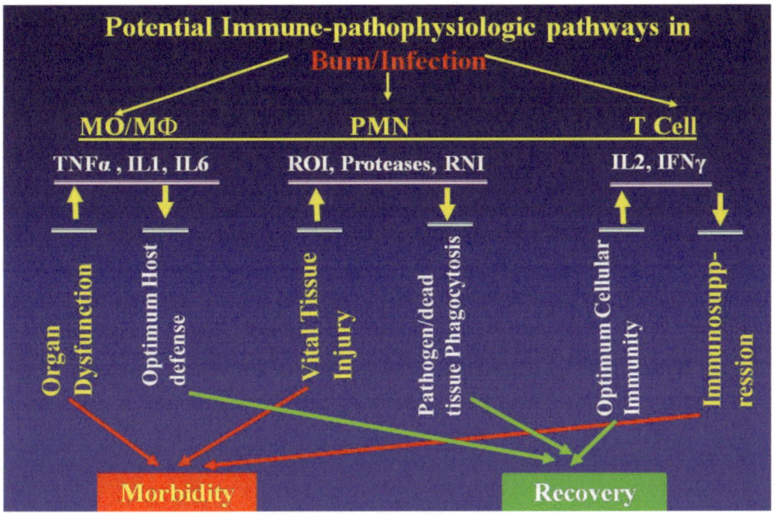

Fig. 13. Sequence of potential immune-pathologic pathways following burn/infection. Organ dysfunction, vital tissue injury and immunosuppression lead to morbidity. Optimal host defense, enhanced phagocytosis/infection control and an optimum cellular immunity leads to recovery. Three probable cells of innate and adaptive immunity are involved in a mixture of positive (recovery) or negative (morbidity) outcome; Firstly, Monocytes and macrophages get activated and release pro-inflammatory cytokines, which have a positive (optimal host defense)-leading to recovery or negative (organ dysfunction)-leading to morbidity. Secondly, PMN release reactive oxygen intermediates (ROI), reactive nitrogen intermediates (RNI), proteases which have a positive (phagocytosis of pathogens)-leading to recovery or a negative (tissue injury to vital organs)-leading to morbidity. Thirdly, T cell-mediated events; positive (optimum cellular immunity)-leading to recovery or negative (immunosuppression)-leading to morbidity.

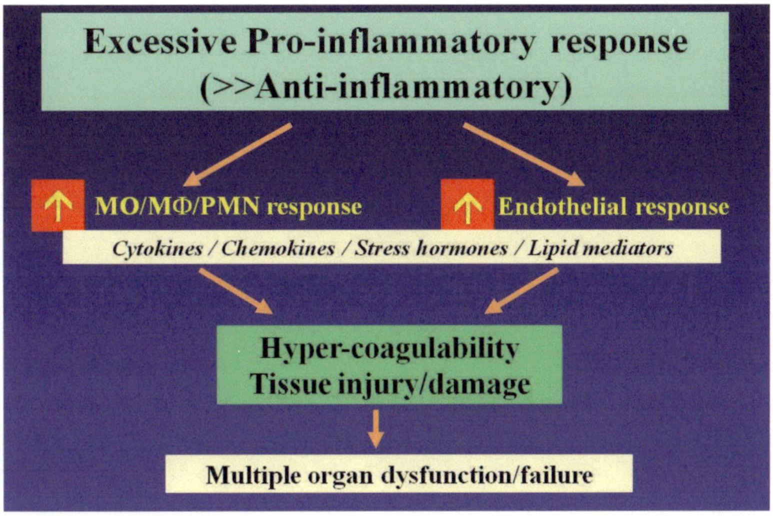

Fig. 14. A possible scenario when pro-inflammatory immune response is stronger than anti-inflammatory immune response.

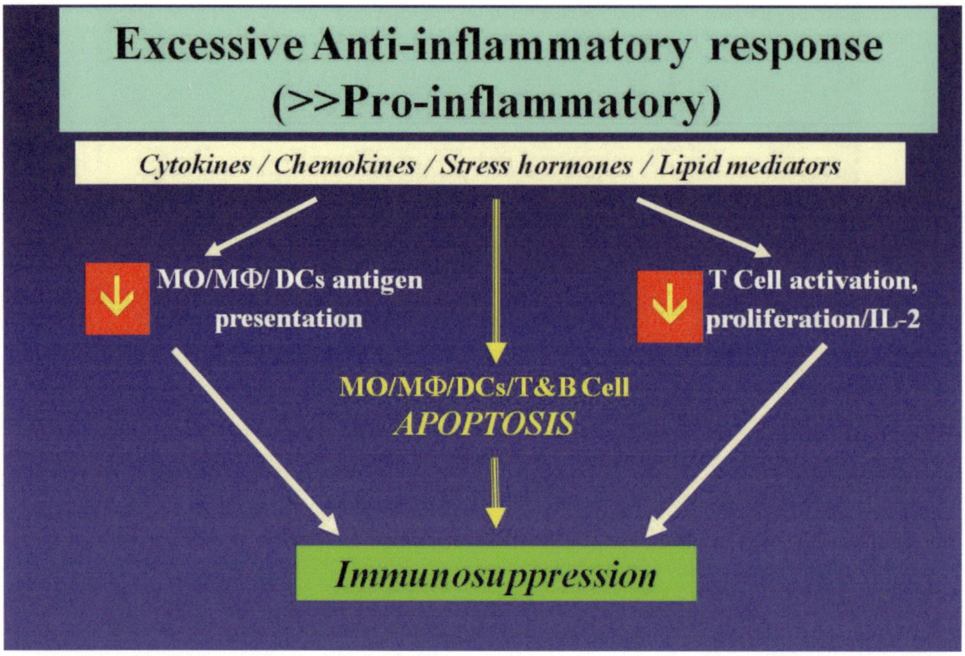

Fig. 15. A possible scenario when anti-inflammatory immune response is stronger than pro-inflammatory immune response.

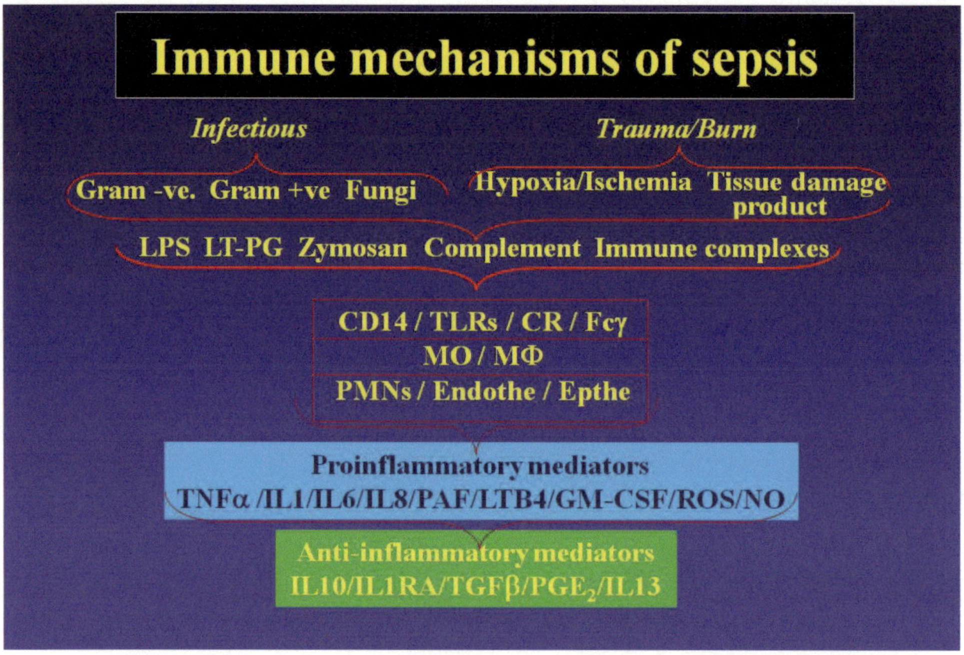

Fig. 16. A flow diagram of immune mechanisms of sepsis involving infectious only, or trauma/burn injury, detailing the list of possible immunomodulators that affect the final outcome leading to immunosuppression.

6. Role of lymphocyte subsets in burn injury and sepsis

The known roles of lymphocyte subsets i.e., natural killer (NK) cells, natural killer T (NKT), gamma-delta (γδ) T cells, and naturally occurring regulatory T cells (Treg) cells in the context of burn and septic injury have recently emerged (Schneider DF, 2007). Jobin et al, 2000 showed that in serum of human burn patient's concentration of sIL-2Ra correlated with intake of fat in diet and inhibition of in vitro NK-cell activity by recombinant sIL-2Ra. Primary mechanisms of NK cell cytotoxicity is known to be via perforin, granzymes, TNF-α, and Fas/FasL. The data obtained from human studies is although inconsistent; and known to be modulated by stress hormones, number of circulating NK cells, presence of IL-4 and IL-10, catalase enzyme, etc. In sepsis, antigen-presenting cells (APCs; macrophages and dendritic cells) recognize antigens or endotoxin and secrete IL-12, which activates NK cells to produce copious amounts of IFN-γ and TNF-α (Medzhitov R, 1998). Burn-induced T cell immunosuppression in a mouse scald burn model along with delayed-type hypersensitivity (DTH) required both CD1d expressing antigen-presenting cells and NK cells (Faunce et al, 2003, Palmer et al, 2006). The role of gamma-delta (γδ) in early burn injury has been elaborated by Schwacha MG 2003, et al, 2000), and has been found to contribute in wound healing, inflammation, and overall survival. However, in other burn studies γδ T cells contributed to neutrophil-mediated tissue damage of lung and small intestine (Toth B et al, 2004, Wu X, 2004). Hence beneficial and harmful effects of γδ T cells are unclear and conflicting, although some researchers have proposed a bimodal response, where they act as proinflammatory in early phases of infection and regulatory in the later phases. CD4+CD25+ regulatory T cells (Treg), overall anti-inflammatory cells are known to comprise 5-12% of CD4+ T cells both in lymphoid and circulatory compartments. In burn model Treg were found to decrease inflammatory cytokine release a week after burn and infectious challenge (Murphy et al, 2005). In a similar burn model Treg were found to inhibit TGF-β and CD4+ proliferation in a cell-to-cell contact (Ni Choileain N, et al, 2006). In contrast a study of polymicrobial cecal-ligation-puncture (CLP) peritonitis model Tregs were found to have protective effects (Heuer JG et al, 2005). The mechanisms by which these small lymphocyte subsets regulate or control remains subject of future studies but final effector responses are modulated through cascade of cytokines, like IFN-γ, IL-4, IL-6, IL-10 and TGF-β.

7. Role of antigen presenting cells and T cells

To date, their involvement as critical regulatory molecules responsible for T cell suppression in burn and septic injuries continues to be a subject of extensive studies as evident from reports from several laboratories (Schneider DF, 2007). Recent studies have provided evidence that alterations in costimulatory signaling between APCs (antigen presenting cells) and CD4+ T cells play key roles in disturbing T cell activation and effector responses. For example, altered expression and functions of costimulatory molecules on APCs, CD80/86, CD40, ICOSL, and/or alterations in their interactions with the complementary molecules on T cells, CD28, CTLA-4, CD40L, ICOS can adversely affect T cell activation and responses (Alegre ML, 2001, Okazaki T., 2002, Grohmann U, 2002). Such derangements in APC and T cell interactions may also contribute to burn/sepsis-related down-regulation of CD4+ T cells. Of APCs, dendritic cells (DC) are recognized to be unique not only in effectively activating naïve T cells but also in adversely affecting their functioning. Recent studies have emphasized the role of induction of indoleamine 2, 3-dioxygenase (IDO) in DCs inhibiting growth and survival of T cells interacting with such DCs (Grohmann U, 2002, Uyttenhove, C, 2003, Mellor, AL, 2003). A derangement in DCs' CD40 interaction with T cell CD40L has also been implicated in T cell functional inhibition (Bingaman, AW, 2001, Straw, AD, 2003). The end effect(s) of alerted co-stimulatory signaling between APCs and CD4+ T cells could be derangements in cell signaling pathways leading to anergy, apoptosis and/or a regulatory T cell (T_{reg}) mediated suppression of CD4+ T cells (Tang, Q, 2003). Our previous studies have assessed individual effects of burn and sepsis as well as of superimposition of sepsis on burn in rats on CD4+ T cell dysfunction and intestinal dysfunction, and animal mortality (Fazal et al, 2000-2010). While burn or sepsis produced low mortality, the combined injury resulted in exacerbation of mortality. The focus in these studies on burn and/or sepsis affords us an opportunity to assess potential sub-lethal versus lethal implications of combined T cell and APC dysfunction. A lack of functional adaptive and innate immunity would lead to high mortality. These studies indicated also that while burn or sepsis suppressed IL-2 production/proliferation without a substantial increase in apoptosis in MLN CD4+T cells, burn-plus-sepsis caused not only suppressed IL-2 production/proliferation but also a substantial increase in apoptosis in CD4+T cells. Our findings also support potential disturbances in interactions between T cells' and APCs' co-stimulatory receptors/ligands contributing to CD4+T cell deficits in burn and/or sepsis injured animals. We hypothesized that CD4+T cell functional inhibition/apoptosis with burn and/sepsis injuries resulted from altered co-stimulatory signaling between the T cell and APC. Recent studies, while indicating immature DC to adversely affect naive T cells have also shown inappropriately activated T cells to adversely affect APCs including DCs and macrophages. Both the DC effects on T cells and the T cell effects on APCs are best understood to be exerted through altered co-stimulatory signaling between T cells and DCs/APCs. These recent findings would seem to support the concept that burn and/or sepsis-related T cell dysfunction may also emanate from DCs defectively activating naïve T cells, and that functionally incompetent T cells in turn adversely affect tissue DCs and macrophages. Such interdependent disturbances in T cell and DC/APC functions can contribute to not only impaired cell mediated immunity but also concurrent increased risk of bacterial infections, and thereby further increase risks for morbidity and mortality in burn and/or sepsis injured hosts.

8. Immune deficits after thermal injury and septic complications

A number of laboratory and clinical studies have shown that extensive thermal injury induces a state of immune-insufficiency, and that the immune-refractoriness predisposes the injured host to critical morbidity and mortality (Toliver-Kinsky, TE, 2002, Kobayashi, M. 2002). The principal outcome of such immune-insufficiency is an increased susceptibility of injured host to opportunistic pathogens causing high risk of death. Both clinical and laboratory studies have shown that immune-insufficiency with burns is characterized by monocyte/macrophage hypoactivity and/or depressed adaptive cell-mediated immunity associated with T lymphocyte functional deficits (Ravindranath, T, 2001). Despite rather extensive studies of T cell functional deficits in animal models of burn injury and in patients (Barret, JP, 2003); the mechanisms of such deficits and a potential role of these deficits in the lethal outcome following burns particularly with the septic complications have remained unknown.

9. Gastrointestinal mucosal immune defense in burn/septic injuries (Figures 17-18)

The intestinal mucosal compartment is presumably the most active regional lymphocyte defense system in the body. It serves as an important first line of defense against pathogenic/non-pathogenic antigens such as those found in ingested food and those derived from the commensal gut bacteria. An early pathophysiologic event following burn as well as sepsis injury, of certain critical magnitude, is a disturbance in intestinal microvascular dynamics which adversely affects the mucosal barrier integrity. Such a loss of barrier integrity has a high probability of grossly increasing the antigen load particularly that derived from the commensal bacteria and potentially aggravating the mucosal lymphocyte defense. There is also the likelihood that the resulting inadequacy of the lymphocytes could exacerbate pathogenic injury to host tissues and organs exacerbating host morbidity and mortality. Thus, by virtue of their location, intestine associated lymphocytes constitute a vulnerable immune defense system, which could be investigated to elucidate the mechanism(s) of immune dysfunction contributing to host morbidity and mortality after burn-plus-sepsis. T lymphocytes are found in the GI tract in the mucosal epithelial layer (intraepithelial T cells), Peyer's patches, and lamina propria. While the intraepithelial T cells are primarily CD8+ cells, the majority of T cells in the lamina propria are CD4+ cells. Peyer's patches contain predominantly B cells and a relatively small population of CD4+ T cells; their lymphoid follicles resemble those in spleens and other lymph nodes. The CD4+T cells in lamina propria are the activated ($CD45RC^{low}$) cells, and have been shown to be derived from the mesenteric lymph nodes (MLN) (Ramirez, F, 2000,

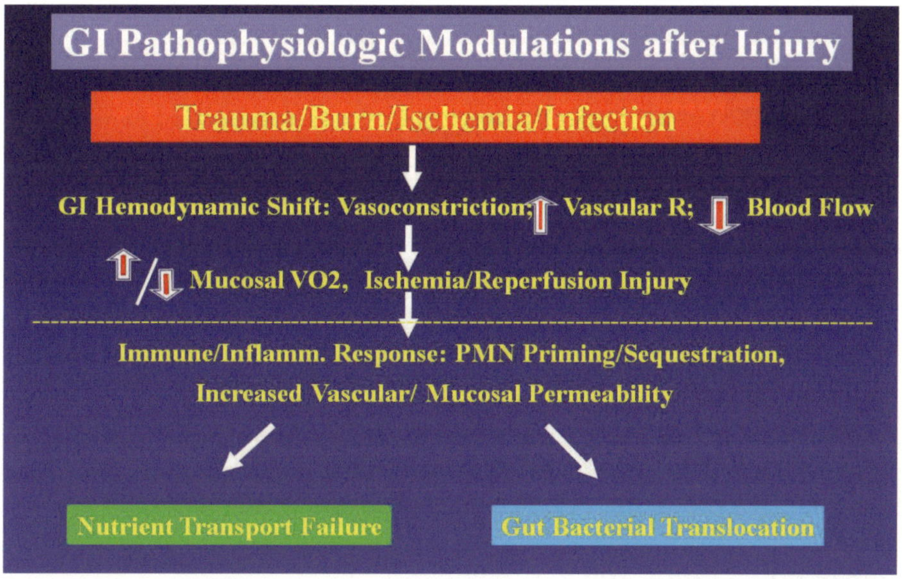

Fig. 17. Pathophysiological gastrointestinal modulations following injury caused by Trauma/Burn/Ischemia/Infection. There are changes in splanchnic blood vessels and mucosal beds mimicking ischemia/reperfusion injury. This leads to chemotaxis of activated neutrophils, increased vascular and mucosal permeability. These vascular and mucosal barrier interruptions cause nutrient transport failure and translocation of bacteria across the gut barrier.

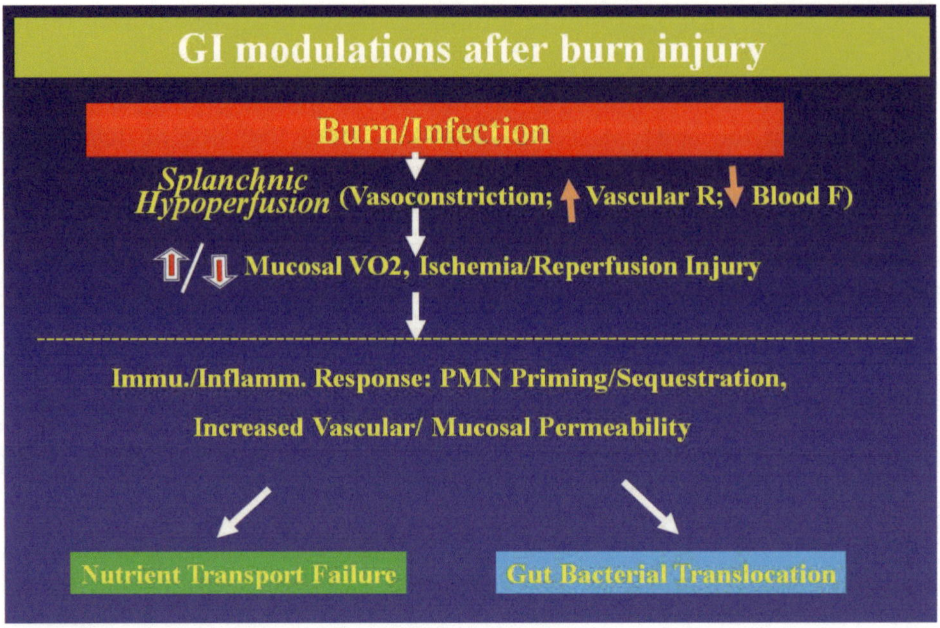

Fig. 18. Gastrointestinal modulations following exclusive burn injury and/or burn/infection. There are changes in splanchnic blood vessels and mucosal beds mimicking ischemia/reperfusion injury. This leads to chemotaxis of activated neutrophils, increased vascular and mucosal permeability. These vascular and mucosal barrier interruptions cause nutrient transport failure and translocation of bacteria across the gut barrier.

Bode U, 2002). The CD4+T cells probably recognized and activated by the antigens presenting cells (APCs) in the MLN (Homann, D, 1999). T cells activated in MLN circulate to intestine as well as other lymphoid tissues including spleen. Previous studies in rats have also shown that activated CD4+T cells originating from MLN recirculate to the intestinal lymphoid tissues and MLN, where they proliferate; their proliferation on restimulation is highest in MLN. The proliferation of CD4+ cells in the MLN was also higher than that of CD8+ cells. Whereas MLN contained both naïve T cells (CD45RC ^{high}) and activated/memory cells (CD45RC ^{low}), lamina propria and PP have been shown to contain mostly activated T cells. Recent studies in rodents including rat have emphasized the importance of dendritic cells (DCs) as exclusive antigen presenters and activators of naïve T cells in the draining lymph nodes (Turnbull, E, 2001). Moreover, in the intestine of rat, DCs play a prominent role in presenting self tissue antigen, such as derived from apoptotic intestinal epithelial cells, to presumably induce tolerance in the lymph node T cells. In rats, such tolerogenic DCs appear to be CD4-, while immunogenic DCs are CD4+ cells.

10. Roles of proliferation and apoptosis in T cell homeostasis/dyshomeostasis (Figures 19-20)

While proliferation and subsequent differentiation of T cells is essential for antigen-specific defense against pathogens, T cell apoptosis is an essential cell death process for the maintenance of T cell homeostasis. Apoptosis is required also for the deletion of overactivated/autoreactive cells and thereby provides for a control of an excessive immune response (Banz, A. 2002). IL-2 is recognized as a T cell growth factor, but it serves other functions as well (Wells, AD, 1999). T cells, following their interaction with antigen presenting cells, produce IL-2, and express high affinity (~10^{-11} M) IL-2 receptor (IL-2Rαβγ). IL-2 acts on the T cells in an autocrine and/or paracrine manner to trigger intracellular signaling through JAK/STAT and PI-3K/Ras pathways, and thereby increase cell concentrations of cell cycle proteins, cyclin D/E, which in turn associate and activate cyclin-dependent kinases (Laliberte, J, 1998, Sakaida, H, 1998). These kinases are known to phosphorylate proteins responsible for the progression of the cell cycle from G1 to the S phase. Thus, IL-2 promotes T cell proliferation. IL-2 also increases production of IFN-γ (responsible for stimulation of macrophages) and IL-4 (responsible for developing Th2 CD4+Tcells, promoting production of antibodies by B cells, and blocking stimulation of macrophages) (Jain, J, 1995). IL-2 also modulates T cell apoptosis. T cells (CD4+ and CD8+) undergo apoptosis via a "passive" and an "active" mechanism. Active apoptosis of T cells occurs after antigen activated T cells, which are producing IL-2 and through IL-2 stimulus are proliferating, are restimulated through TCR. Active T cell apoptosis (antigen/activation-induced cell death, AICD) caused by restimulation restrains T cell expansion due to persistent stimulation of T cells (Zheng, L, 1995). Although recent studies support the concept that IL-2 is a key regulator of AICD, they have not elucidated mechanism in AICD (Boldin, MP, 1995, 1996). Unlike the initial T cell activation which is dependent on TCR and costimulatory CD28 receptor activation, AICD is promoted by TCR signal without the activation of CD28 (Lenardo, M, 1999). The initial event in AICD is expression on the activated T cell surface of FasL/TNF and interactions (in an autocrine or paracrine manner) with constitutively expressed Fas receptor (CD95) (and/or TNF-receptor gene superfamily members, e.g. TNFR-1 and TNFR-2). Such interactions lead to aggregation of cytoplasmic "death domain" of Fas; the components of this complex are: 1) adapter protein, FADD/mort-1, and 2) pro-Caspase8 (Zhang, J, 1998). A subsequent step in AICD release of active Caspase 8 may initiate lethal proteolytic events and activation of caspases including Caspase 3. Caspase 3 has been considered as a primary initiator of DNA fragmentation (Lenardo, M, 1999). Unlike the Fas-FasL mediated apoptosis, TNFR-1 interaction with TNF can signal either apoptosis or cell survival. The antiapoptotic process involves activation of NFκB, which transcriptionally upregulates anti-apoptotic proteins. Recent studies have indicated also that while Fas preferentially controls the death of CD4+ cells, TNFR-1 plays a major role in CD8+T cell death. Passive T cell apoptosis presumably occurs after cessation of antigen interaction with T cells and of IL-2 production. Passive apoptosis involves activation of the mitochondrial apoptotic pathway initiated by a shift in mitochondrial inner membrane permeability causing dissipation of mitochondrial membrane potential, $\delta\psi_{mw}$, and release of cytochrome c from mitochondria. Cytochrome c complexes with the protein, Apaf-1, and the complex serve to activate Caspase 9, which eventually causes activation of Caspase 3 and apoptosis (Clement, MV, 1994, Adachi, S. 1997). Under physiological conditions, AICD would be initiated with antigen restimulation of T cells, and passive apoptosis involving mitochondrial pathway occurs after cessation of IL-2 production. In cases of inadequate activation of AICD, a mechanism seems to exist that allows for an amplification of AICD via activation of the mitochondrial pathway even in the presence of optimum level of IL-2. It is conceivable that in burn/sepsis injury conditions, with suppressed level of IL-2 production by inadequately activated T cells, apoptosis might be occurring via both AICD and mitochondrial pathways (Luo, X, 1998). Previous studies have supported the concept of AICD potentiation via

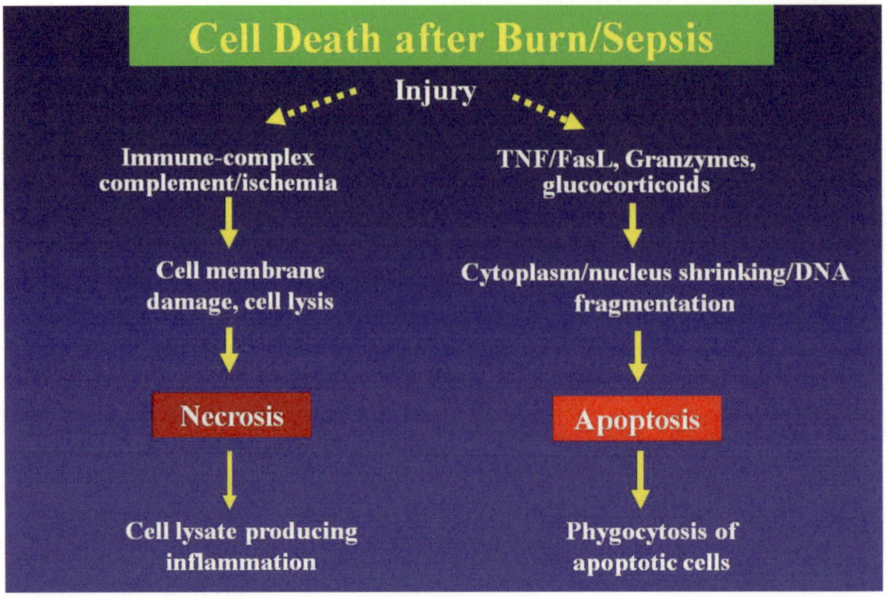

Fig. 19. The mode of cell death following burn- and sepsis-injury. One cascade of events leads to necrosis-mediated inflammation, while another line of events leads to apoptosis. In burn and sepsis injury when humoral factors complicated by immune-complex deposition and ischemia lead to damaged cell membrane and lysis lead to necrosis and inflammation is caused by cell lysate. On the other side TNF/FasL, granzymes and glucocorticoids leading to apoptotic changes in the cytoplasm and DNA fragmentation.

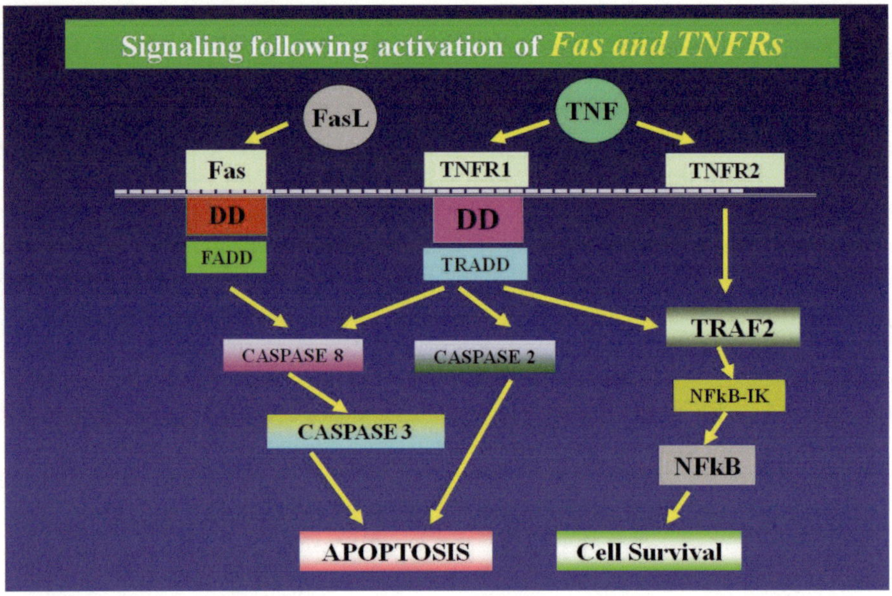

Fig. 20. A schema of signaling pathways following burn injury-mediated FasL and TNF-receptors mediated cell death. Fas and TNF-R1-meditated signaling events lead to apoptosis, while TNF-R2 leads to cell survival.

mitochondrial path subsequent to an over expression of pro-Caspase 3. Other mechanisms of augmentation of apoptosis in T cells with burn/sepsis injury may include that mediated by glucocorticoids and/or reactive oxygen species (ROS), both of which are known to be generated/released in the burn/sepsis conditions (Fukuzuka, K, 2000, Chao, DT, 1995). The glucocorticoids and ROS initiated apoptosis in T cells relies on the mitochondrial pathway (Rathmell, JC, 1999). Although apoptosis via various above-discussed mechanisms is accompanied by activation of the caspase cascade, there is recent evidence that T cells undergo apoptosis independently of the activation of caspases, in vitro. Such caspase-independent cell death primarily involves the activation of the mitochondrial pathway without the involvement of death domain receptors. It is marked, like the caspase-dependent apoptosis, by the loss of $\delta\psi_{mw}$ as well as PS (phosphatidyl serine) translocation from inner plasma membrane leaflet to the outer leaflet but, unlike the caspase-dependent apoptosis, not marked by DNA fragmentation (Rathmell, JC, 1999). Cell death regulatory proteins of Bcl-2 family play a major role in modulating T cell passive apoptosis. Whereas Bcl-2 itself and its homologues, Bcl-xL, Mcl-1 and A1 block apoptosis, others in the family such as Bax, Bak, Bad and Bid are known to promote T cell apoptosis. Bcl-2/Bcl-xL inhibit(s) release of cytochrome c from mitochondria, prevent (s) cytochrome c binding to Apaf-1 and pro-caspase 9, and thereby blocking mitochondrial pathway of apoptosis (Rathmell, JC, 1999). A possible mechanism by which Bad promotes apoptosis after IL-2 withdrawal could be its dephosphorylation and release from its chaperone, in the cytoplasm, followed by its binding to Bcl-2 and thus preventing Bcl-2 from blocking apoptosis (Rathmell, JC, 1999). Bcl-2's antiapoptotic action could also abrogate if Bax or Bak are highly expressed. Activation of Caspase 8 following Fas/FasL interaction can lead to cleavage of cytosolic Bid, and the cleaved product has been implicated in the mitochondrial amplification of apoptosis (Rathmell, JC, 1999).

11. Roles of interactions between APCs and T cells through co-stimulatory ligands and receptors

A variety of receptor-ligand interactions take place between APCs (namely, macrophages, dendritic cells, B cells) and the T cells after antigen presented by APC is recognized by TCR. While some such interactions are 'adhesive' and provide for firm cell-cell positioning, others transduce cell-cell signals that modulate functional responses by T cells and APCs. APC ligands, CD80/86 (B7-1/B7-2), interacting with the CD28 receptor on T cells and causing augmentation of TCR-CD3-initiated T cell proliferation and cytokine production, is a classic example of a co-stimulatory signal transmission from APC to T cells (Wekerle, T, 2001, Zhang, J, 1998). The importance of CD28 co-stimulation is underscored by the observation that in its complete absence, the TCR-mediated cell activation, in vitro, results in T cell anergy typified by inadequate IL-2 production and proliferation, and accompanied by apoptosis. CD28 signaling appears to be involved in both T cell priming and in generation of effector functions in primed T cells; it is, however, critical in T cell priming. Its role in T cell differentiation into effector cells is less clear. While CD28 may promote both Th1 and Th2 responses, it may generate a more exuberant Th2 responses (IL-4 production) than Th1 type (IFN-γ production) (Tang Q, 2003). Recent studies have identified a CD28-related molecule, ICOS (inducible co-stimulator) as a TCR inducible T cell receptor that binds to APC ligand, ICOSL (inducible co-stimulator ligand), a B7 related molecule (B7h) (Lohning, M, 2003,

Okazaki, T, 2002, Villegas, EN, 2002). Like CD28/B7-1&2 interactions, ICOS/ICOSL upregulate T cell proliferation and cytokine production. Unlike CD28, ICOS signaling may be more important in effector cell (Th2 responses) than in CD4+ T cell priming. Unlike CD28 and ICOS, the T cell receptor, CTLA-4 (cytotoxic T lymphocyte associated protein-4), or the recent identified PD-1 (program death-1), both also homologues of CD28, seemingly transmit to T cells inhibitory signals that suppress proliferation and cytokine production in activated cells (Coyle, AJ, 2001). CTLA-4 also interacts with APC's CD80/86 molecules. It, however, binds to these ligands with greater affinity (~20X greater) than CD28 (Egen, JG, 2002), which accounts for the abrogation of the co-stimulatory effects of CD28 in the face of expression of CTLA-4 on activated T cells. CTLA-4 not only interferes with IL-2 production but also causes arrest of T cell cycle in the G1 phase (Alegre ML, 2001). Unlike CD28, which is constitutively expressed and stable, CTLA-4 is induced in activated cells, is relatively unstable, and has a much shorter half life (Egen JG, 2002). The CD40 ligand (CD40L), a member of TNF family, is expressed on activated T cells; its counterpart CD40, a member of TNF-receptor family, is expressed on APCs (Wesa A, 2002). Interactions between T cells' CD40L and B cells' CD40 are important in humoral immunity (Grammer, AC, 2002). In addition, CD40 and CD40L interactions between T cells and other APCs (macrophages, DCs) lead to APCs' upregulation of CD80/86 molecules, and production of IL-12 which is a potent cytokine for generation of Th1 type of T cell responses (Coyle AJ, 2001). T cells' response subsequent to CD40L ligation by anti-CD40 was an early/short-term priming of TCR followed by cytokine production and proliferation, and a later induction of T cell unresponsiveness with upregulation of cytokines, TGFβ and IL-10, and cell cycle disruption (Blair PJ, 2000). The inhibitory effects of CD40L ligation in activated T cells are not clearly understood. Several previous studies produced blockade of CD80/86 ligands by treatment of experimental animals with a soluble CTLA-4-Ig fusion protein, or of blockade in experimental animals of CD40L that prevents CD40 mediated induction of CD80/86 ligands, have shown a resulting a resulting hyporesponsiveness of T cells allowing for acceptance of allotransplanted solid organs by these animals (Honey KS, 1999). Recent investigations have indicated that T cell unresponsiveness produced by CTLA-4-Ig treatment of animals, receiving solid organ transplantation, may not necessarily be due to CD80/86 blockade affecting CD28 co-stimulation but that it could be due to CTLA-4-Ig acting as a CTLA-4 mimic that binds and activates CD80/86 molecules on dendritic cells (Grohmann U, 2002). Such activation apparently leads to activation of dendritic cell intracellular enzyme, indoleamine 2, 3-dioxygenase (IDO), which causes breakdown of tryptophan, and accumulation of the breakdown product kynurenine. Since tryptophan is required in the microenvironment of the T cells for their proliferation and their possible survival, and kynurenine could inhibit T cell proliferation, and promote their apoptosis (Grohmann U, 2002, Uyttenhove, C, 2003, Mellor, AL, 2003), the CTLA-4-Ig mediated induction of IDO could effectively disturb T cell expansion. This action of CTLA-4-Ig on the dendritic cells appears to be mediated by induction of IFNγ, and IFNγ-mediated transcriptional upregulation of IDO. IFNγ presumably acted on DCs in an autocrine/paracrine manner, and activated STAT-1/NF-κB/p38MAPK signaling pathway. As can be surmised from above discussion, studies now support the concept that APC/T cell receptor-ligand molecules allow for a bi-directional transmission of signals between APCs and T cells; CD80/86/CTLA-4 and CD40L/CD40 appear to be operating in this manner. Potential disturbances in CD80/86/CTLA-4 and CD40L/CD40 interactions may play role(s) in the T cell hyporesponsiveness in burn/sepsis injury conditions.

12. Signaling through receptor systems in T cells

T cell activation is initiated by triggering TCR with its natural ligand, antigen-MHC complex. The proximal signaling events that follow are activations of Src kinases, Lck, Fyn, and Lyn, associated with the membrane lipid rafts. Activated Src kinases then phosphorylate tyrosine residues in ITAMs (motifs present in the cytoplasmic signaling domains of the TCR-CD3 complex) which become the docking sites for the SH2 domains of the syk kinase, ZAP-70 (Weiss, A, 1994, Chu D, 1998, Weil R, 1994). ZAP-70 is also phosphorylated by the Src kinases. Active ZAP-70 phosphorylate the adapter protein LAT present in the lipid rafts. Phosphorylated LAT is able to recruit several other phosphorylated key molecules, including enzymes and non-enzyme adapter proteins, to its tyrosine-based motifs (Finco, TS, 1998, Zhang W, 1998). Such molecules are: 1) Grb2 (associated with SOS) which Ras (Downward, J. 1996, Henning, SW, 1998), and 2) SLP-76 (associated with Gad). SLP-76 recruits a Tec kinase which activates PLCγ. PLCγ enzymatically cleaves membrane inositol-4, 5 bisphosphate leading to formation of inositol-1, 4, 5 triphosphate (IP-3) and diacylglycerol (DAG) (Berridge, MJ, 1998). Ras couples to distal effector signaling pathways including the activation of MAPKs (Erk, JNK, and p38 MAPK). Erk plays an essential role in the activation of transcription factors, c-Fos and c-myc; c-Fos is involved in the transcriptional regulation of activated protein-1 (AP-1) response element in the IL-2 promoter (Gupta, S, 1994, Rincon, M, 2000). JNK is also involved in the activation of IL-2 promoter but a lesser extent than Erk (Su B, 1994). p38 MAPK is involved in the activation of IFNγ gene expression, as well as playing a role in the induction of T cell apoptosis (Gupta, S, 1994). IP-3, generated after the action of PLCγ, causes release of Ca^{2+} from endoplasmic reticulum storage site. Once the stored Ca^{2+} is depleted from the endoplasmic reticulum, depletion triggers extracellular Ca^{2+} influx through a plasma membrane capacitative Ca^{2+} entry channel (Berridge, MJ, 1998), sustaining high Ca^{2+} concentration required for IL-2 promoter activation by calcineurin, a Ca^{2+}-calmodulin dependent serine phosphatase. Calcineurin dephosphorylates NFAT which translocates to the nucleus and binds in the IL-2 promoter region (Baksh, S., 2000, Penninger, JM, 1999). DAG activates certain isoforms of PKC, also dependent on Ca^{2+}, namely, PKC and certain novel isoforms, PKCδ, ε, ν, and θ, that are not dependent on Ca^{2+} (Mellor H, 1998). In T cells, PKCθ is the only isoform that is recruited to the membrane and is involved in the activation of NFκB (Monks CR, 1997). Src and Syk kinases are thus involved in the activation of distal pathways: 1) Grb2/p21ras/MAPKs, 2) PLCγ/Ca^{2+}/calcineurin, and 3) DAG/PKCθ/NFκB pathways; Src/Syk tyrosine kinases additionally activate phosphatidylinositol 3-kinase (PI-3K) which leads activation of a 4th Vav/Rac-1/PKCθ/Akt/NFκB pathway. PI-3K is recruited through its regulatory SH-2 domain to LAT, and phosphorylates the D-3 position of inositol phosphate (IP) in the membrane. Phosphorylated IPs interact with PH domains of PLCγ, Tec kinase, Vav in the lipid rafts (Viola A, 1999). Vav is a GEF for Rac-1, which activates JNK and cytoskeletal assembly; Vav also recruits PKCθ (Herndon, TM, 2001). PI-3K also activates serine-threonine kinase, Akt (PKB) (Ward, SG, 1996, Bruyns, E, 1998). Both Akt and PKCθ activate NFκB (Alessi, DR, 1998). Nascent NFκB/Rel family proteins, present as dimers, are held in the cytoplasm by IκB. Degradation of IκB by proteasome (dependent on ubiquitination) occurs phosphorylation of IκB by IκB kinase complex (IKK) (DiDonato, JA, 1997, Regnier, CH. 1997), and allows for liberation of NFκB dimmers allows which them translocate to the nucleus, and bind DNA to transcriptionally upregulate various genes. Co-stimulatory receptor CD28's cytoplasmic tail PR motifs are also involved in the recruitment and activation of Srk kinases, Fyn and Lck, and Tec kinases leading to acticvation of PI-3K, Grb2, and JNK (Su B, 1994, Harhaj, EW, 1998). Although several studies have attempted to evaluate the roles of PI-3K and Grb2 after CD28 costimulation on IL-2 production and proliferation, no definitive information has yet come forth from them (Chan, TO, 1999, Parry, RV, 1997). However, PI-3K activation with co-stimulation has been implicated in the activation of Akt followed by that of NFκB resulting in an upregulation of the anti-apoptotic protein Bcl-xL (Chao, DT, 1995, Boise, LH, 1995). Akt regulation with CD28 costimulation has been shown to possibly induce IL-2 and IFNγ production without affecting IL-4 and IL-5 but remains questionable. Thus, although CD28 costimulation is known to prevent T cell anergy through its effect on IL-2 production and cell cycle progression, the signaling mechanisms of this effect have remained elusive. CD28 stimulation probably exerts its effect on IL-2 mRNA upregulation and proliferation by enhancing tyrosine phosphorylation of TCR, and by decreasing threshold for naïve T cell activation through the assembly of signaling components in the "immunological synapse" housing the TCR/CD3-MHC-peptide/CD28/CD80, 86/SrcKs/PKCθ molecular complex at the T cell and APC interface. Like CD28, CTLA-4 contains in its cytoplasmic tail tyrosine and PR regions. An unphosphorylated tyrosine residue allows for an association between CTLA-4 cytoplasmic domain and the AP50 (medium chain subunit of the clathrin adapter, AP-2) resulting in clathrin-dependent endocytosis of CTLA-4, and thus control over its cell surface retention. After TCR stimulation, the cytoplasmic tyrosine(s) are phosphorylated by Src kinases Lck/Fyn that promotes CTLA-4's surface retention. Crosslinking of CTLA-4 reduces TCR-dependent activation of MAPKs, Erk and JNK, as well as of NFκB, NFAT, and AP-1. Ligation of CTLA-4 during TCR stimulation results in decreased T cell cytokine production and arrest of the cell cycle (Coyle AJ, 2001, Sharpe, AH, 2002). Although an association of SH-2 motif containing tyrosine phosphatase (SHP-2) with CTLA-4's cytoplasmic tyrosine residue is not established, an indirect association of CTLA-4 with SHP-2 might result in dephosphorylation of the CD3 complex and inactivation of TCR signaling mechanism (Walunas, TL, 1996, Marengere, LE, 1996). The available research reports of T cell signaling pathways provide a more extensive characterization of TCR-related signaling than that triggered by co-stimulatory or inhibitory T cell/APC surface molecules. However, it is clear there are redundancies in the pathways activated by the TCR-related and co-stimulatory signals.

13. Conclusion (Figure 21-23)

Attempts to clinically improve immunosuppression following burn and/or sepsis has been largely unsuccessful. Immune dysfunction that normally occurs in such a massive burn injury condition affects both innate and adaptive immune responses, including humoral and especially cell-mediated responses. T-cell or antigen-presenting cell malfunctions occur late. Infection, sepsis, and multiple organ failure take weeks to months to evolve following burn injury. Most of the experimental animal models of burn injury target early adaptive immune response and fail to give the true picture of ensuing immunosuppression. Effective therapy requiring modifying signaling pathways distal to CD3 ligation have been proposed by some while others propose nuclear factor-KB and downstream mediators as potential targets for treating burn-induced immunosuppression.

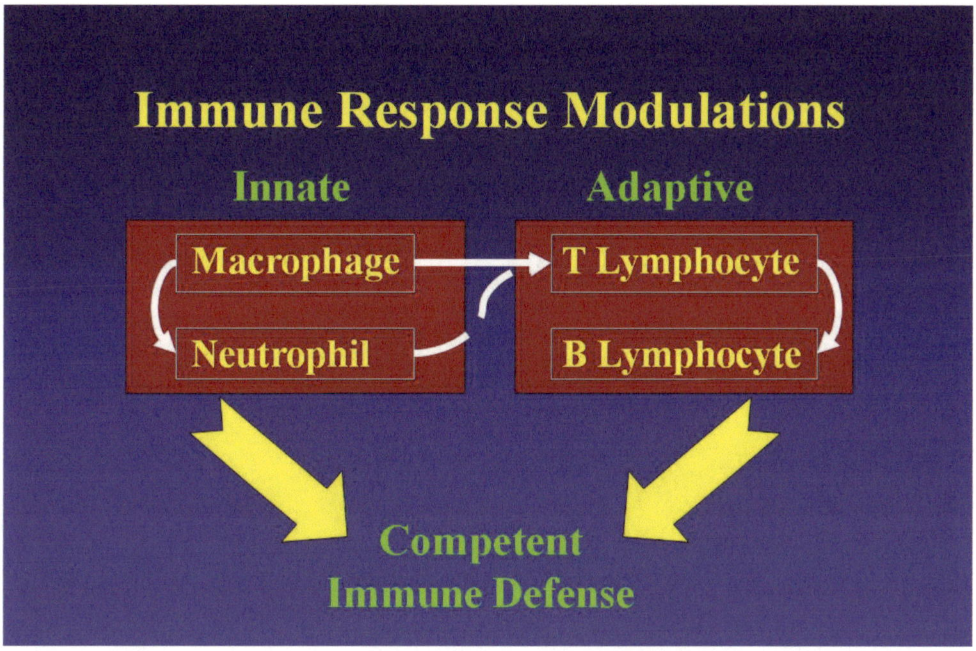

Fig. 21. A summary of events where both inname and adaptive immune response orchestrate complex interaction of cells and their released products to mount a competent immune defense.

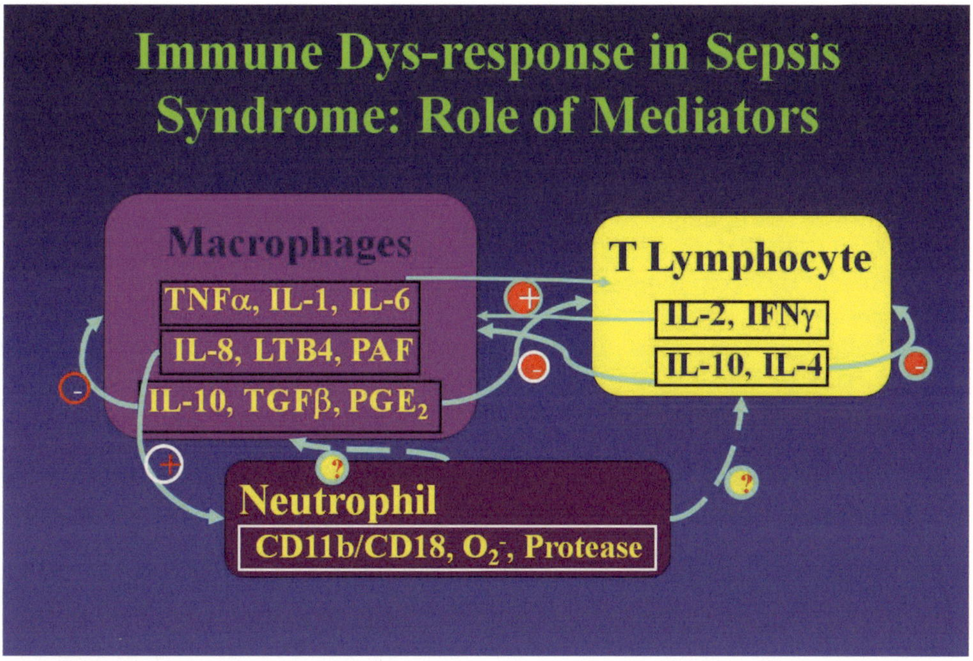

Fig. 22. A flow diagram of possible cellular and humoral factor interactions that occurs in a dysregulated immune response in sepsis.

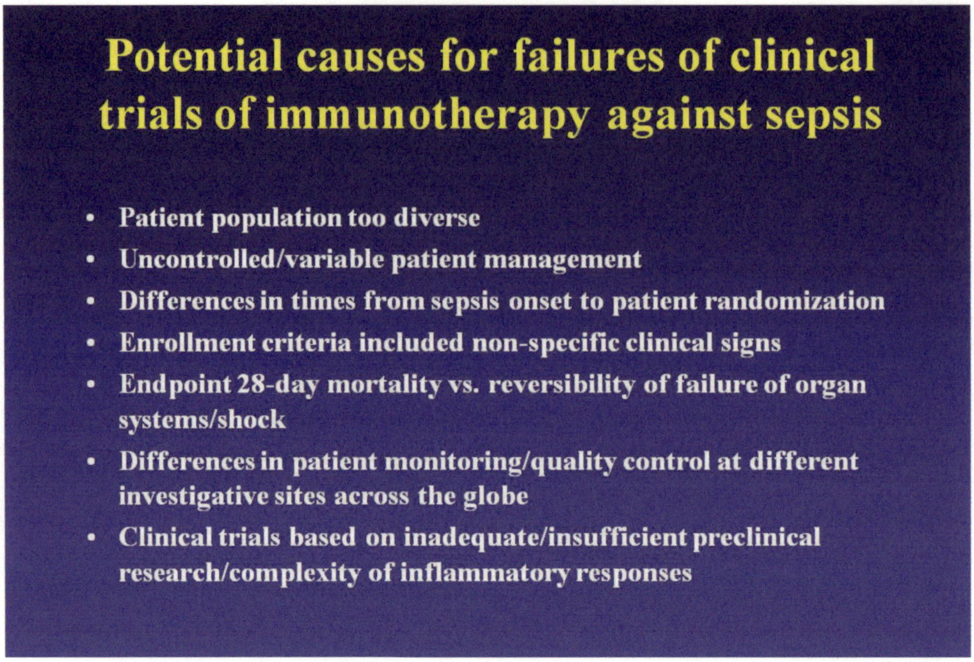

Fig. 23. A list of potential causes accounting for a failed immunotherapy against clinical sepsis.

14. References

Adachi, S., A. R. Cross, B. M. Babior, and R. A. Gottlieb. 1997. Bcl-2 and the outer mitochondrial membrane in the inactivation of cytochrome c during Fas-mediated apoptosis. *J Biol Chem* 272:21878.

Alegre, M. L., K. A. Frauwirth, and C. B. Thompson. 2001. T-cell regulation by CD28 and CTLA-4. *Nat Rev Immunol* 1:220.

Angele MK, Faist E. 2002. Clinical review: immunodepression in the surgical patient and increased susceptibility to infection. *Crit Care*. Aug; 6 (4):298-305.

Ayala, A., C. S. Chung, G. Y. Song, and I. H. Chaudry. 2001. IL-10 mediation of activation-induced TH1 cell apoptosis and lymphoid dysfunction in polymicrobial sepsis. *Cytokine* 14:37.

Baker CC, Miller CL, Trunkey DD. 1979. Predicting fatal sepsis in burn patients. *J Trauma*; 19 (9):641-8.

Baksh, S., and S. J. Burakoff. 2000. The role of calcineurin in lymphocyte activation. *Semin Immunol* 12:405.

Banz, A., C. Pontoux, and M. Papiernik. 2002. Modulation of Fas-dependent apoptosis: a dynamic process controlling both the persistence and death of CD4 regulatory T cells and effector T cells. *J Immunol* 169:750.

Barret, J. P., and D. N. Herndon. 2003. Modulation of inflammatory and catabolic responses in severely burned children by early burn wound excision in the first 24 hours. *Arch Surg* 138:127.

Baue AE, Durham R, Faist E. 1998. Systemic inflammatory response syndrome (SIRS), multiple organ dysfunction syndrome (MODS), multiple organ failure (MOF): are we winning the battle? *Shock*. Aug;10(2):79-89.

Berridge, M. J., M. D. Bootman, and P. Lipp. 1998. Calcium--a life and death signal. *Nature* 395:645.

Bingaman, A. W., J. Ha, M. M. Durham, S. Y. Waitze, C. Tucker-Burden, S. R. Cowan, T. C. Pearson, and C. P. Larsen. 2001. Analysis of the CD40 and CD28 pathways on alloimmune responses by CD4+ T cells in vivo. *Transplantation* 72:1286.

Blair, P. J., J. L. Riley, D. M. Harlan, R. Abe, D. K. Tadaki, S. C. Hoffmann, L. White, T. Francomano, S. J. Perfetto, A. D. Kirk, and C. H. June. 2000. CD40 ligand (CD154) triggers a short-term CD4 (+) T cell activation response that results in secretion of immunomodulatory cytokines and apoptosis. *J Exp Med* 191:651.

Bode, U., A. Sahle, G. Sparmann, F. Weidner, and J. Westermann. 2002. The fate of effector T cells in vivo is determined during activation and differs for CD4+ and CD8+ cells. *J Immunol* 169:6085.

Boehme, S. A., and M. J. Lenardo. 1993. Propriocidal apoptosis of mature T lymphocytes occurs at S phase of the cell cycle. *Eur J Immunol* 23:1552.

Boise, L. H., A. J. Minn, P. J. Noel, C. H. June, M. A. Accavitti, T. Lindsten, and C. B. Thompson. 1995. CD28 costimulation can promote T cell survival by enhancing the expression of Bcl-XL. *Immunity* 3:87.

Boldin, M. P., E. E. Varfolomeev, Z. Pancer, I. L. Mett, J. H. Camonis, and D. Wallach. 1995. A novel protein that interacts with the death domain of Fas/APO1 contains a sequence motif related to the death domain. *J Biol Chem* 270:7795.

Boldin, M. P., T. M. Goncharov, Y. V. Goltsev, and D. Wallach. 1996. Involvement of MACH, a novel MORT1/FADD-interacting protease, in Fas/APO-1- and TNF receptor-induced cell death. *Cell* 85:803.

Chan, T. O., S. E. Rittenhouse, and P. N. Tsichlis. 1999. AKT/PKB and other D3 phosphoinositide-regulated kinases: kinase activation by phosphoinositide-dependent phosphorylation. *Annu Rev Biochem* 68:965.

Chao, D. T., G. P. Linette, L. H. Boise, L. S. White, C. B. Thompson, and S. J. Korsmeyer. 1995. Bcl-XL and Bcl-2 repress a common pathway of cell death. *J Exp Med* 182:821.

Chu, D. H., C. T. Morita, and A. Weiss. 1998. The Syk family of protein tyrosine kinases in T-cell activation and development. *Immunol Rev* 165:167.

Chung, C. S., G. Y. Song, W. Wang, I. H. Chaudry, and A. Ayala. 2000. Septic mucosal intraepithelial lymphoid immune suppression: role for nitric oxide not interleukin-10 or transforming growth factor-beta. *J Trauma* 48:807.

Clement, M. V, and I. Stamenkovic. 1994. Fas and tumor necrosis factor receptor-mediated cell death: similarities and distinctions. *J Exp Med 180:557.*

Coyle, A. J., and J. C. Gutierrez-Ramos. 2001. The expanding B7 superfamily: increasing complexity in costimulatory signals regulating T cell function. *Nat Immunol 2:203.*

DiDonato, J. A., M. Hayakawa, D. M. Rothwarf, E. Zandi, and M. Karin. 1997. A cytokine-responsive IkappaB kinase that activates the transcription factor NF-kappaB. *Nature* 388:548.

Downward, J. 1996. Control of ras activation. *Cancer Surv* 27:87.

Egen, J. G., and J. P. Allison. 2002. Cytotoxic T lymphocyte antigen-4 accumulation in the immunological synapse is regulated by TCR signal strength. *Immunity 16:23.*

Faist E, Schinkel C, Zimmer S. 1996. Update on the mechanisms of immune suppression of injury and immune modulation. *World J Surg*. May; 20(4):454-9.

Faunce DE, Gamelli RL, Choudhry MA, Kovacs EJ. 2003. A role for CD1d-restricted NKT cells in injury-associated T cell suppression. *J Leukoc Biol*. Jun; 73 (6):747-55.

Fazal, N, Al-Ghoul WM. 2007. Thermal injury-plus-sepsis contributes to a substantial deletion of intestinal mesenteric lymph node CD4 T cell via apoptosis. *Int J Biol Sci*. Sep 12; 3(6):393-401.

Fazal, N, Raziuddin, S, Khan, M, Al-Ghoul, WA. 2006. Antigen presenting cells (APCs) from thermally injured and/or septic rats modulate CD4+ T cell responses of naïve rat. *Biochim Biophys Acta*. ; 1762(1): 46-53.

Fazal, N., Choudhry, M.A., Sayeed, M.M., 2005. Inhibition of T cell MAPKs (Erk 1/2, p38) with thermal injury is related to downregulation of Ca2+ signaling. *Biochim Biophys Acta*. Jun 30; 1741(1-2): 113-9.

Fazal N, Al-Ghoul WM, Schmidt MJ, Choudhry MA, Sayeed MM. 2002. Lyn- and ERK-mediated vs. Ca2+ -mediated neutrophil O2- responses with thermal injury. *Am J Physiol Cell Physiol*; 283(5): C1469-79

Fazal N, Al Ghoul WM, Choudhry MA, and Sayeed MM. 2001. PAF receptor antagonist modulates neutrophil responses with thermal injury, in vivo. *Am J Physiol*. 281:C1310-7.

Fazal, N., Shamim, M., Choudhry, M. A., Ravindranath, T and Sayeed, M.M., 2000. CINC blockade prevents neutrophil Ca2+ signaling upregulation and gut bacterial translocation in burn-injured rats. *Biochim Biophys Acta*; 15; 1535(1): 50-9.

Fazal, N., Shamim, M., Khan, S. S., Gamelli, R.L., and Sayeed, M.M., 2000. Neutrophil depletion in rats reduces burn-injury induced intestinal bacterial translocation. *Critical Care Medicine*; 28(5): 1550-56.

Finco, T. S., T. Kadlecek, W. Zhang, L. E. Samelson, and A. Weiss. 1998. LAT is required for TCR-mediated activation of PLCgamma1 and the Ras pathway. *Immunity* 9:617.

Fukuzuka, K., C. K. Edwards, 3rd, M. Clare-Salzler, E. M. Copeland, 3rd, L. L. Moldawer, and D. W. Mozingo. 2000. Glucocorticoid-induced, caspase-dependent organ apoptosis early after burn injury. *Am J Physiol Regul Integr Comp Physiol* 278:R1005.

Gamelli RL, George M, Sharp-Pucci M, Dries DJ, Radisavljevic Z. 1995. Burn-induced nitric oxide release in humans. *J Trauma*. Nov; 39(5):869-77; discussion 877-8.

Gonzalo, J. A., J. Tian, T. Delaney, J. Corcoran, J. B. Rottman, J. Lora, A. Al-garawi, R. Kroczek, J. C. Gutierrez-Ramos, and A. J. Coyle. 2001. ICOS is critical for T helper cell-mediated lung mucosal inflammatory responses. *Nat Immunol* 2:597.

Grammer, A. C., and P. E. Lipsky. 2002. CD154-CD40 interactions mediate differentiation to plasma cells in healthy individuals and persons with systemic lupus erythematosus. *Arthritis Rheum* 46:1417.

Grohmann, U., C. Orabona, F. Fallarino, C. Vacca, F. Calcinaro, A. Falorni, P. Candeloro, M. L. Belladonna, R. Bianchi, M. C. Fioretti, and P. Puccetti. 2002. CTLA-4-Ig regulates tryptophan catabolism in vivo. *Nat Immunol* 3:1097.

Gupta, S., A. Weiss, G. Kumar, S. Wang, and A. Nel. 1994. The T-cell antigen receptor utilizes Lck, Raf-1, and MEK-1 for activating mitogen-activated protein kinase. Evidence for the existence of a second protein kinase C-dependent pathway in an Lck-negative Jurkat cell mutant. *J Biol Chem* 269:17349.

Harris BH, Gelfand JA. 1995. The immune response to trauma. *Semin Pediatr Surg*. May; 4 (2):77-82.

Henning, S. W., and D. A. Cantrell. 1998. GTPases in antigen receptor signalling. *Curr Opin Immunol* 10:322.

Harhaj, E. W., and S. C. Sun. 1998. IkappaB kinases serve as a target of CD28 signaling. *J Biol Chem* 273:25185.

Herndon, T. M., X. C. Shan, G. C. Tsokos, and R. L. Wange. 2001. ZAP-70 and SLP-76 regulate protein kinase C-theta and NF-kappa B activation in response to engagement of CD3 and CD28. *J Immunol* 166:5654.

Heuer JG, Zhang T, Zhao J, Ding C, Cramer M, Justen KL, Vonderfecht SL, Na S. 2005. Adoptive transfer of in vitro-stimulated CD4+CD25+ regulatory T cells increases bacterial clearance and improves survival in polymicrobial sepsis. *J Immunol*. Jun 1; 174(11):7141-6.

Homann, D., A. Holz, A. Bot, B. Coon, T. Wolfe, J. Petersen, T. P. Dyrberg, M. J. Grusby, and M. G. von Herrath. 1999. Autoreactive CD4+ T cells protect from autoimmune diabetes via bystander suppression using the IL-4/Stat6 pathway. *Immunity* 11:463.

Honey, K., S. P. Cobbold, and H. Waldmann. 1999. CD40 ligand blockade induces CD4+ T cell tolerance and linked suppression. *J Immunol* 163:4805.

Huang, F. P., C. F. Farquhar, N. A. Mabbott, M. E. Bruce, and G. G. MacPherson. 2002. Migrating intestinal dendritic cells transport PrP(Sc) from the gut. *J Gen Virol* 83:267.

Huang, F. P., N. Platt, M. Wykes, J. R. Major, T. J. Powell, C. D. Jenkins, and G. G. MacPherson. 2000. A discrete subpopulation of dendritic cells transports apoptotic intestinal epithelial cells to T cell areas of mesenteric lymph nodes. *J Exp Med* 191:435.

Jain, J., C. Loh, and A. Rao. 1995. Transcriptional regulation of the IL-2 gene. *Curr Opin Immunol* 7:333.

Jeschke, M. G., J. F. Low, M. Spies, R. Vita, H. K. Hawkins, D. N. Herndon, and R. E. Barrow. 2001. Cell proliferation, apoptosis, NF-kappaB expression, enzyme, protein, and weight changes in livers of burned rats. *Am J Physiol Gastrointest Liver Physiol* 280:G1314.

Jobin N, Garrel DR, Bernier J. 2000. Increased burn-induced immunosuppression in lipopolysaccharide-resistant mice. *Cell Immunol.* ; 200(2):65-75.

Ju, S. T., D. J. Panka, H. Cui, R. Ettinger, M. el-Khatib, D. H. Sherr, B. Z. Stanger, and A. Marshak-Rothstein. 1995. Fas (CD95)/FasL interactions required for programmed cell death after T-cell activation. *Nature* 373:444.

Kell, M. R., O. Shelley, J. A. Mannick, Z. Guo, and J. A. Lederer. 2000. A central role for CD95 (Fas) in T-cell reactivity after injury. *Surgery* 128:159.

Kelly JL, O'Suilleabhain CB, Soberg CC, Mannick JA, Lederer JA. 1999, Severe injury triggers antigen-specific T-helper cell dysfunction. *Shock*; 12(1):39-45.

Kelly, J. L., C. B. O'Suilleabhain, C. C. Soberg, J. A. Mannick, and J. A. Lederer. 1999. Severe injury triggers antigen-specific T-helper cell dysfunction. *Shock* 12:39.

Kobayashi, M., H. Takahashi, A. P. Sanford, D. N. Herndon, R. B. Pollard, and F. Suzuki. 2002. An increase in the susceptibility of burned patients to infectious complications due to impaired production of macrophage inflammatory protein 1 alpha. *J Immunol* 169:4460.

Kung, J. T., D. Beller, and S. T. Ju. 1998. Lymphokine regulation of activation-induced apoptosis in T cells of IL-2 and IL-2R beta knockout mice. *Cell Immunol* 185:158.

Laliberte, J., A. Yee, Y. Xiong, and B. S. Mitchell. 1998. Effects of guanine nucleotide depletion on cell cycle progression in human T lymphocytes. *Blood* 91:2896.

Lederer JA, Rodrick ML, Mannick JA. 1999. The effects of injury on the adaptive immune response. *Shock.* Mar; 11(3):153-9.

Lenardo, M., K. M. Chan, F. Hornung, H. McFarland, R. Siegel, J. Wang, and L. Zheng. 1999. Mature T lymphocyte apoptosis--immune regulation in a dynamic and unpredictable antigenic environment. *Annu Rev Immunol* 17:221.

Li, H., H. Zhu, C. J. Xu, and J. Yuan. 1998. Cleavage of BID by caspase 8 mediates the mitochondrial damage in the Fas pathway of apoptosis. *Cell* 94:491.

Li, P., D. Nijhawan, I. Budihardjo, S. M. Srinivasula, M. Ahmad, E. S. Alnemri, and X. Wang. 1997. Cytochrome c and dATP-dependent formation of Apaf-1/caspase-9 complex initiates an apoptotic protease cascade. *Cell* 91:479.

Li, X. C., Y. Li, I. Dodge, A. D. Wells, X. X. Zheng, L. A. Turka, and T. B. Strom. 1999. Induction of allograft tolerance in the absence of Fas-mediated apoptosis. *J Immunol* 163:2500.

Li, Y., X. C. Li, X. X. Zheng, A. D. Wells, L. A. Turka, and T. B. Strom. 1999. Blocking both signal 1 and signal 2 of T-cell activation prevents apoptosis of alloreactive T cells and induction of peripheral allograft tolerance. *Nat Med* 5:1298.

Liu, L. M., and G. G. MacPherson. 1995. Rat intestinal dendritic cells: immunostimulatory potency and phenotypic characterization. *Immunology* 85:88.

Liu, L., M. Zhang, C. Jenkins, and G. G. MacPherson. 1998. Dendritic cell heterogeneity in vivo: two functionally different dendritic cell populations in rat intestinal lymph can be distinguished by CD4 expression. *J Immunol* 161:1146.

Lohning, M., A. Hutloff, T. Kallinich, H. W. Mages, K. Bonhagen, A. Radbruch, E. Hamelmann, and R. A. Kroczek. 2003. Expression of ICOS in vivo defines CD4+ effector T cells with high inflammatory potential and a strong bias for secretion of interleukin 10. *J Exp Med* 197:181.

Luo, X., I. Budihardjo, H. Zou, C. Slaughter, and X. Wang. 1998. Bid, a Bcl2 interacting protein, mediates cytochrome c release from mitochondria in response to activation of cell surface death receptors. *Cell* 94:481.

Maloy, K. J., and F. Powrie. 2001. Regulatory T cells in the control of immune pathology. *Nat Immunol* 2:816.

Marano MA, Fong Y, Moldawer LL, Wei H, Calvano SE, Tracey KJ, Barie PS, Manogue K, Cerami A, Shires GT, et al. 1990. Serum cachectin/tumor necrosis factor in critically ill patients with burns correlates with infection and mortality. *Surg Gynecol Obstet.* Jan; 170(1):32-8.

Marengere, L. E., P. Waterhouse, G. S. Duncan, H. W. Mittrucker, G. S. Feng, and T. W. Mak. 1996. Regulation of T cell receptor signaling by tyrosine phosphatase SYP association with CTLA-4. *Science* 272:1170.

Martin, E., B. O'Sullivan, P. Low, and R. Thomas. 2003. Antigen-specific suppression of a primed immune response by dendritic cells mediated by regulatory T cells secreting interleukin-10. *Immunity* 18:155.

Meakins JL. 1990. Etiology of multiple organ failure. *J Trauma.* Dec; 30(12 Suppl):S165-8.

Medzhitov R, Janeway CA Jr. 1998. Innate immune recognition and control of adaptive immune responses.*Semin Immunol*. Oct; 10 (5):351-3.

Mellor, A. L., B. Baban, P. Chandler, B. Marshall, K. Jhaver, A. Hansen, P. A. Koni, M. Iwashima, and D. H. Munn. 2003. Cutting edge: induced indoleamine 2, 3 dioxygenase expression in dendritic cell subsets suppresses T cell clonal expansion. *J Immunol* 171:1652.

Mellor, H., and P. J. Parker. 1998. The extended protein kinase C superfamily. *Biochem J* 332 (Pt 2):281.

Mittrucker, H. W., M. Kursar, A. Kohler, D. Yanagihara, S. K. Yoshinaga, and S. H. Kaufmann. 2002. Inducible costimulator protein controls the protective T cell response against Listeria monocytogenes. *J Immunol* 169:5813.

Miyazaki, T., Z. J. Liu, A. Kawahara, Y. Minami, K. Yamada, Y. Tsujimoto, E. L. Barsoumian, R. M. Permutter, and T. Taniguchi. 1995. Three distinct IL-2 signaling pathways mediated by bcl-2, c-myc, and lck cooperate in hematopoietic cell proliferation. *Cell* 81:223.

Molloy RG, O'Riordain M, Holzheimer R, Nestor M, Collins K, Mannick JA, Rodrick ML. 1993. Mechanism of increased tumor necrosis factor production after thermal injury. Altered sensitivity to PGE2 and immunomodulation with indomethacin. *J Immunol*. Aug 15; 151(4):2142-9.

Monks, C. R., H. Kupfer, I. Tamir, A. Barlow, and A. Kupfer. 1997. Selective modulation of protein kinase C-theta during T-cell activation. *Nature* 385:83.

Moss NM, Gough DB, Jordan AL, Grbic JT, Wood JJ, Rodrick ML, Mannick JA. 1988. Temporal correlation of impaired immune response after thermal injury with susceptibility to infection in a murine model. *Surgery*. Nov; 104 (5):882-7.

Murphy TJ, Ni Choileain N, Zang Y, Mannick JA, Lederer JA. 2005. CD4+CD25+ regulatory T cells control innate immune reactivity after injury. *J Immunol*. Mar 1; 174(5):2957-63.

Muzio, M., A. M. Chinnaiyan, F. C. Kischkel, K. O'Rourke, A. Shevchenko, J. Ni, C. Scaffidi, J. D. Bretz, M. Zhang, R. Gentz, M. Mann, P. H. Krammer, M. E. Peter, and V. M. Dixit. 1996. FLICE, a novel FADD-homologous ICE/CED-3-like protease, is recruited to the CD95 (Fas/APO-1) death--inducing signaling complex. *Cell* 85:817.

Nagasawa, M., I. Melamed, A. Kupfer, E. W. Gelfand, and J. J. Lucas. 1997. Rapid nuclear translocation and increased activity of cyclin-dependent kinase 6 after T cell activation. *J Immunol* 158:5146.

Ni Choileain N, MacConmara M, Zang Y, Murphy TJ, Mannick JA, Lederer JA. 2006. Enhanced regulatory T cell activity is an element of the host response to injury. *J Immunol*. Jan 1; 176(1):225-36.

Ninnemann JL, Fisher JC, Frank HA. 1978. Prolonged survival of human skin allografts following thermal injury. *Transplantation*. Feb; 25(2):69-72.

Ogle CK, Mao JX, Wu JZ, Ogle JD, Alexander JW. 1994. The 1994 Lindberg Award. The production of tumor necrosis factor, interleukin-1, interleukin-6, and prostaglandin E2 by isolated enterocytes and gut macrophages: effect of lipopolysaccharide and thermal injury. *J Burn Care Rehabil*. Nov-Dec; 15 (6):470-7.

Okazaki, T., Y. Iwai, and T. Honjo. 2002. New regulatory co-receptors: inducible co-stimulator and PD-1. *Curr Opin Immunol* 14:779.

O'Riordain MG, Collins KH, Pilz M, Saporoschetz IB, Mannick JA, Rodrick ML. 1992. Modulation of macrophage hyperactivity improves survival in a burn-sepsis model. *Arch Surg*. Feb; 127(2):152-7; discussion 157-8.

Palmer JL, Tulley JM, Kovacs EJ, Gamelli RL, Taniguchi M, Faunce DE. 2006. Injury-induced suppression of effector T cell immunity requires CD1d-positive APCs and CD1d-restricted NKT cells. *J Immunol*. 2006 Jul 1; 177(1):92-9.

Parry RV, Reif K, Smith G, Sansom DM, Hemmings BA, Ward SG. Ligation of the T cell co-stimulatory receptor CD28 activates the serine-threonine protein kinase protein kinase B. *Eur J Immunol*; 27(10):2495-501.

Penninger, J. M., and G. R. Crabtree. 1999. The actin cytoskeleton and lymphocyte activation. *Cell* 96:9.

Ramirez, F., and D. Mason. 2000. Recirculatory and sessile CD4+ T lymphocytes differ on CD45RC expression. *J Immunol* 165:1816.

Rathmell, J. C., and C. B. Thompson. 1999. The central effectors of cell death in the immune system. *Annu Rev Immunol* 17:781.

Ravindranath, T., W. Al-Ghoul, S. Namak, N. Fazal, R. Durazo-Arvizu, M. Choudhry, and M. M. Sayeed. 2001. Effects of burn with and without Escherichia coli infection in rats on intestinal vs. splenic T-cell responses. *Crit Care Med* 29:2245.

Regnier, C. H., H. Y. Song, X. Gao, D. V. Goeddel, Z. Cao, and M. Rothe. 1997. Identification and characterization of an IkappaB kinase. *Cell* 90:373.

Renno, T., M. Hahne, and H. R. MacDonald. 1995. Proliferation is a prerequisite for bacterial superantigen-induced T cell apoptosis in vivo. *J Exp Med* 181:2283.

Riley, J. L., M. Mao, S. Kobayashi, M. Biery, J. Burchard, G. Cavet, B. P. Gregson, C. H. June, and P. S. Linsley. 2002. Modulation of TCR-induced transcriptional profiles by ligation of CD28, ICOS, and CTLA-4 receptors. *Proc Natl Acad Sci USA* 99:11790.

Rincon, M., D. Conze, L. Weiss, N. L. Diehl, K. A. Fortner, D. Yang, R. A. Flavell, H. Enslen, A. Whitmarsh, and R. J. Davis. 2000. Conference highlight: do T cells care about the mitogen-activated protein kinase signalling pathways? *Immunol Cell Biol* 78:166.

Saffle JR, Sullivan JJ, Tuohig GM, Larson CM. 1993; Multiple organ failure in patients with thermal injury. *Crit Care Med*; 21(11):1673-83.

Sakaida, H., S. Kawamata, T. Hattori, and T. Uchiyama. 1998. V3 loop of human immunodeficiency virus type 1 reduces cyclin E expression and induces G1 arrest in interleukin 2-dependent T cells. *AIDS Res Hum Retroviruses* 14:31.

Salinas J, Drew G, Gallagher J, Cancio LC, Wolf SE, Wade CE, Holcomb JB, Herndon DN, Kramer GC. 2008. Closed-loop and decision-assist resuscitation of burn patients. *J Trauma*; 64(4 Suppl):S321-32.

Schneider DF, Glenn CH, Faunce DE. 2007. Innate lymphocyte subsets and their immunoregulatory roles in burn injury and sepsis. *J Burn Care Res*. May-Jun; 28 (3):365-79.

Schwacha MG, Ayala A, Chaudry IH. 2000. Insights into the role of gammadelta T lymphocytes in the immunopathogenic response to thermal injury. *J Leukoc Biol*. May; 67(5):644-50.

Schwacha MG, Samy TS, Catania RA, Chaudry IH. 1998. Thermal injury alters macrophage responses to prostaglandin E2: contribution to the enhancement of inducible nitric oxide synthase activity. *J Leukoc Biol*. Dec; 64 (6):740-6.

Schwacha MG. 2003. Macrophages and post-burn immune dysfunction.*Burns*. Feb; 29(1):1-14.

Sharpe, A. H., and G. J. Freeman. 2002. The B7-CD28 superfamily. *Nat Rev Immunol* 2:116.

Steinman, R. M., and M. C. Nussenzweig. 2002. Avoiding horror autotoxicus: the importance of dendritic cells in peripheral T cell tolerance. *Proc Natl Acad Sci USA* 99:351.

Still JM Jr, Belcher K, Law EJ. 1993. Experience with polymicrobial sepsis in a regional burn unit. *Burns*. Oct;19 (5):434-6.

Straw, A. D., A. S. MacDonald, E. Y. Denkers, and E. J. Pearce. 2003. CD154 plays a central role in regulating dendritic cell activation during infections that induce Th1 or Th2 responses. *J Immunol* 170:727.

Su, B., E. Jacinto, M. Hibi, T. Kallunki, M. Karin, and Y. Ben-Neriah. 1994. JNK is involved in signal integration during costimulation of T lymphocytes. *Cell* 77:727.

Tang, Q., J. A. Smith, G. L. Szot, P. Zhou, M. L. Alegre, K. J. Henriksen, C. B. Thompson, and J. A. Bluestone. 2003. CD28/B7 regulation of anti-CD3-mediated immunosuppression in vivo. *J Immunol* 170:1510.

Toliver-Kinsky, T. E., T. K. Varma, C. Y. Lin, D. N. Herndon, and E. R. Sherwood. 2002. Interferon-gamma production is suppressed in thermally injured mice: decreased production of regulatory cytokines and corresponding receptors. *Shock* 18:322.

Toth B, Alexander M, Daniel T, Chaudry IH, Hubbard WJ, Schwacha MG. 2004. The role of gammadelta T cells in the regulation of neutrophil-mediated tissue damage after thermal injury. *J Leukoc Biol.* Sep; 76 (3):545-52. Epub 2004 Jun 14.

Turnbull, E., and G. MacPherson. 2001. Immunobiology of dendritic cells in the rat. *Immunol Rev* 184:58.

Uyttenhove, C., L. Pilotte, I. Theate, V. Stroobant, D. Colau, N. Parmentier, T. Boon, and B. J. Van Den Eynde. 2003. Evidence for a tumoral immune resistance mechanism based on tryptophan degradation by indoleamine 2, 3-dioxygenase. *Nat Med* 9:1269.

Varedi, M., M. G. Jeschke, E. W. Englander, D. N. Herndon, and R. E. Barrow. 2001. Serum TGF-beta in thermally injured rats. *Shock 16:380.*

Villegas, E. N., L. A. Lieberman, N. Mason, S. L. Blass, V. P. Zediak, R. Peach, T. Horan, S. Yoshinaga, and C. A. Hunter. 2002. A role for inducible costimulator protein in the CD28- independent mechanism of resistance to Toxoplasma gondii. *J Immunol* 169:937.

Viola, A., S. Schroeder, Y. Sakakibara, and A. Lanzavecchia. 1999. T lymphocyte costimulation mediated by reorganization of membrane microdomains. *Science* 283:680.

Walunas, T. L., C. Y. Bakker, and J. A. Bluestone. 1996. CTLA-4 ligation blocks CD28-dependent T cell activation. *J Exp Med* 183:2541.

Wang, J., E. Guan, G. Roderiquez, and M. A. Norcross. 2001. Synergistic induction of apoptosis in primary CD4 (+) T cells by macrophage-tropic HIV-1 and TGF-beta1. *J Immunol* 167:3360.

Wang, K., X. M. Yin, D. T. Chao, C. L. Milliman, and S. J. Korsmeyer. 1996. BID: a novel BH3 domain-only death agonist. *Genes Dev* 10:2859.

Wang, R., T. L. Ciardelli, and J. H. Russell. 1997. Partial signaling by cytokines: cytokine regulation of cell cycle and Fas-dependent, activation-induced death in CD4+ subsets. *Cell Immunol* 182:152.

Weil, R., and A. Veillette. 1994. Intramolecular and extramolecular mechanisms repress the catalytic function of p56lck in resting T-lymphocytes. *J Biol Chem* 269:22830.

Weiss, A., and D. R. Littman. 1994. Signal transduction by lymphocyte antigen receptors. *Cell* 76:263.

Wekerle, T., J. Kurtz, M. Sayegh, H. Ito, A. Wells, S. Bensinger, J. Shaffer, L. Turka, and M. Sykes. 2001. Peripheral deletion after bone marrow transplantation with costimulatory blockade has features of both activation-induced cell death and passive cell death. *J Immunol* 166:2311.

Wells, A. D., X. C. Li, Y. Li, M. C. Walsh, X. X. Zheng, Z. Wu, G. Nunez, A. Tang, M. Sayegh, W. W. Hancock, T. B. Strom, and L. A. Turka. 1999. Requirement for T-cell apoptosis in the induction of peripheral transplantation tolerance. *Nat Med* 5:1303.

Wesa, A., and A. Galy. 2002. Increased production of pro-inflammatory cytokines and enhanced T cell responses after activation of human dendritic cells with IL-1 and CD40 ligand. *BMC Immunol* 3:14.

White CE, Renz EM. 2008; Advances in surgical care: management of severe burn injury. *Crit Care Med*; 36 (7 Suppl):S318-24.

Wu X, Woodside KJ, Song J, Wolf SE. 2004. Burn-induced gut mucosal homeostasis in TCR delta receptor-deficient mice. *Shock*. Jan; 21 (1):52-7.

Yang L, Hsu B. 1992. The roles of macrophage (M phi) and PGE-2 in postburn immunosuppression. *Burns*. Apr; 18 (2):132-6.

Zhang, J., D. Cado, A. Chen, N. H. Kabra, and A. Winoto. 1998. Fas-mediated apoptosis and activation-induced T-cell proliferation are defective in mice lacking FADD/Mort1. *Nature* 392:296.

Zhang, W., R. P. Trible, and L. E. Samelson. 1998. LAT palmitoylation: it's essential role in membrane microdomain targeting and tyrosine phosphorylation during T cell activation. *Immunity* 9:239.

Zheng, L., G. Fisher, R. E. Miller, J. Peschon, D. H. Lynch, and M. J. Lenardo. 1995. Induction of apoptosis in mature T cells by tumour necrosis factor. *Nature* 377:348.

10

Immunosuppression in Helminth Infection

Maria Doligalska and Katarzyna Donskow-Łysoniewska
Department of Parasitology, University of Warsaw, Warsaw
Poland

1. Introduction

1.1 Parasitism

Parasitism is an antagonistic relationship between organisms of different species where the parasite benefits at the expense of the host. Helminths are long-living, multicellular parasites. There are two major phylla of helminths; Nematodes and Platyhelminthes. The nematodes contain the intestinal worms known as soil-transmitted helminths including hookworms, whipworms and the filarial worms that cause lymphatic filariasis and onchocerciasis. The Platyhelminthes, known as flatworms, include the flukes and the tapeworms. Both nematodes, flukes and tapeworms widely infect humans and animals (Hotez & Kamath, 2009). Most of the parasitic species causing weakness and disease survive in and explore the host as natural environment. Helminths can be found in a great variety of tissue niches, and although they cause very high morbidity, direct mortality of the host species remains low (Brooker, 2010). Human hookworm infection is a common soil-transmitted helminth infection that is caused by the nematode parasites *Necator americanus* and *Ancylostoma duodenale*. Hookworm infections are asymptomatic however substantially contributes to the incidence of anemia and malnutrition in developing nations (de Silva et. al 2003, WHO 2010).

Filarial diseases are rarely fatal and morbidity of human filariasis results mainly from the host reaction to microfilariae or developing adult worms in different areas of the body. Most of the filarial infected individuals have a subclinical condition associated with patent infection, and acute manifestations which are rarely life threatening. However, chronic manifestations, such as lymphedema (elephantiasis) and hydrocele, are debilitating (Keiser et al., 2002).

Schistosomes, the blood flukes reside in the mesenteric and vesical venules. They have a life span of many years and daily produce large numbers of eggs, which must traverse the gut or bladder tissues on their way to the lumens of the excretory organs. Many of the eggs remain in the host tissues, inducing immunologically mediated granulomatous inflammation and fibrosis (Warren, 1982). The relationship between the presence of schistosome infection and clinical morbidity revealed schistosomiasis-related disease and associated death (Van der Werf et al., 2003).

Worldwide, many cestode infestations occur with very low prevalence of infections and are asymptomatic. Nevertheless some of the more serious infestations result in symptoms from mass effects on vital organs, inflammatory responses, nutritional deficiencies, and the potential of fatal anaphylaxis (Del Brutto, 2005; Morar & Feldman, 2003; Ozturk et al., 2007).

1.2 The outcome of immunosuppression in population

However the immune system is the system responsible for protection against parasites, mlticellular helminths which actively destroy host tissue evolved in effective immune system; the aim of parasite-related suppression is to get the right environment for existence and survival. The number of larvae which successfully invade the host, the number of migrating parasites and the number of settled adult forms and their reproductive capacity depend on the activity of the host immune system. Immune recognition, effectiveness of immune reactivity and protective response are the mechanisms that affect parasite abundance and survival in the host. In response to the action of immune system, parasites induce a plethora of mechanisms which evade or manipulate host defence. All these reactions take place at the host–parasite interface and are regulated by gene products of both species. In the evolutionary sense both parasite products and host immune system are adjusted to their intimate relationship.

Genetic population studies shown that helminths have been a major selective force on a subset of interleukin receptor genes (IL genes) from which some genes, have been a target of balancing selection, a process that maintains genetic variability within a population (Fumagalli et al., 2009). Allele frequency, host behaviour and helminth distribution in population may influence of heritable factors both in patterns of infection and immunity (Ellis et al., 2007). It is reflected in the effect of helminths on individual host responses to other pathogens such as microparasites, which is considerable variable. In concurrent infections with multiple coinfecting species, parasites interact with one another through the host's immune system *via* mechanisms such as immune trade-offs and immunosuppression (Ezenwa & Jolles, 2011). A subset of immunomodulatory parasite species may have a key role in structuring other infections in natural vertebrate populations. Affecting expression of toll-like receptors (TLR) are important in initiating immunity; populations free from immunosuppressive parasites may exist at 'unnaturally' elevated levels of innate immune activation, leading to an increased risk of immunopathology (Jackson et al. 2009). The host immunocompetence may give some indications of the control of parasite infection and of the host mediation effect, through immunity, on the parasite community structure (Combes, 1997; Mouritsen & Poulin, 2005). Thus immunosuppression promotes over-dispersal of parasites and favours the most suitable genotype of the host for better propagation of the parasite. As intestinal mucins are an important component of innate defence even a single gene deficiency predisposes to infection with nematodes (Hasnain et al., 2010; McKay and Khan, 2003).

The distribution of parasites among different individuals in the host population, infected with the same helminth species is heterogeneous. A consequence of this is the aggregated distribution of helminth infection in endemic communities; a small proportion of hosts are rapidly, frequently, and/or heavily infected (May & Anderson, 1990). Such a pattern of distribution suggests that some individuals are predisposed to heavy infection and intensity of parasitic infections are also under genetic control (Iraqi et al., 2003, Stear & Wakelin, 1998). It is shown in humans as individual predisposition to infection, ethnic variation in susceptibility to disease and familial aggregation to infection (Quinnell, 2003). Genetic background determines both the favorable level of immune suppression necessary to sustain chronic infection as well as a highly active immune response to eradicate worms from the infected host. In lambs, naturally exposed to nematodes on pasture season, genetics acts mainly through the control of acquired anti-fecundity immune response (Stear et al., 1997). Moreover, as the consequence of anthropogenic changes in natural environment the evolution of different traits in parasites e.g. specificity, virulence, and polymorphism may be influenced by humans (Lebarbenchon et al., 2008).

1.3 The outcome of immunosuppression in the host

Helminths tend to settle in privileged localization in the host which is reflected in the distinct location of larvae and adults in the host. Helminths need a suitable and non-destructive localization to propagate and transmit their offspring. The state of immune unresponsiveness protects growing larvae during migration through the host tissue. Some nematode species larvae such as *Ascaris* and *Strongylus* undergo extensive migrations which begin and end in the same location, the intestine. Nematodes which migrate during development are usually bigger than their closest relatives that develop wholly within the gastrointestinal tract. Time to reproduction is the same, indicating that worms with a tissue phase during development grow faster in the intestine. Because fecundity is intimately linked with size in nematodes, this provides an explanation for the maintenance of tissue migration by natural selection (Read & Sharping, 1995). For example *Trichinella spiralis* infection results in depression of various parameters of immunity, including delayed type hypersensitivity and responses to bacterial lipopolysaccharide (Barriga, 1978; Beiting et al., 2007; Gerencer et al., 1992). The nematode is a source of macrophage inhibitory factor (TspMIF) and is able to subvert host immunoregulation; MIF has been cloned and characterized with respect to structural, enzymic and cytokine properties (Tan et al., 2001). The maintenance of an immunosuppressed state in the host may improve the fitness of the parasite.

Immunosuppression induced by helminths not only affects the parasite which already has infected the host, but also promotes infection with further infectious larvae. Parasite acquisition is density-dependent and the number of parasites successfully establishing in the host may over time increase with the parasite burden in the host. In long-lasting infections, immunosuppressive mechanisms prevent or limit parasite killing and expulsion; the ongoing infections do not elicit a strong host effector response; infection with one species predisposes for infection with other species and polyparasitism is common (Blaxter, 2003; Ellis & McManus, 2009; Keiser et al., 2002).

2. When immunosuppression is expressed

Immunosuppression may be recognized as; (i) the state when immune system is not specifically suppressed but is not active. That has been characterized for young or older individuals and also with genetic defects resulted in dysfunction of immune system or is artificially induced with immune suppressant for different reason; (ii) suppression activated during immune response which regulates inflammatory reactions and inhibits specific response to sustain the state of physiological homeostasis.

2.1 When the immunosuppression is used

The steady-state of immunosuppression develops as a naturally occurring regulatory pathway resulting in antigen-specific inhibition (von Boehmer, 1991) and the lack of immune response to antigen. Physiological immune homeostasis depends on a balance between the responses to infection or neoplasia and the reciprocal responses that prevent inflammation and autoimmune diseases. These phenomena lead to immunotolerance; the immunosuppressed host fails to responds to the presence of specific antigens or fails to respond to specific antigen. The outcome of these immune-compromising may be beneficial to the host, through limiting the immunopathology and also beneficial to the pathogen, through subversion of the protective immune responses of the host (Kingston & Mills, 2004). Helminths survive within the host because they may induce the state of physiological and immune compromise and may consequently evade immune attack and actively subvert the host immune response (Mitchell, 1991; Ogilive & Wilson, 1976).

The immune system does not function efficiently throughout the life of the host. Host individuals are more susceptible to infection when their immune system is less sensitive to antigenic signals and doesn't react as quickly or efficiently to infection (Matzinger, 1994). This immune suppression is related to the physiological state of the host and influences the pattern of infection in the population. Most parasitic species are propagated preferentially in young individuals when the immune system is not completely developed or educated (Roberts, 1999). Especially physiological immunosuppression associated with parturition and lactation and the immunological unresponsiveness of young ruminants allows parasites to increase transmission; these states are correlated with the unresponsiveness of lymphocytes to mitogens (Soulsby, 1987).

Neonatal exposure to antigens appears to develop immune tolerance (Billingham et al., 1956). From the neonate major environmentally associated changes in immune response phenotype occurred (Wilkie et al., 2011) and neonatal T cells were susceptible to induction of tolerance (Gammon et al., 1986). In such immune milieu morbidity is acceptable in the host population. From evolution, it is likely that immunosuppression in the meaning of unresponsiveness or selective mortality of the most sensitive individuals, protect the better (suitable) genotypes of the host which are able to tolerate surviving parasites.

Changes with age in the average intensity of *Ascaris* infection tend to be convex, rising in childhood and declining in adulthood (Bundy et al., 1987). Also piglets are more susceptible to *Trichuris suis* infection than adult pigs (Pedersen & Saeed, 2002). In contrast, hookworm frequently exhibits a steady rise in intensity of infection with age, peaking in adulthood (Hotez et al., 2008). Similarly, *Brugia malayi* infection establishes more rapidly in adults than in children (Terhell et al., 2001). Changes in cytokine phenotype, particularly CD4 T cells, contribute to age-associated switch from *Trichuris muris* resistance to susceptibility in mice (Humphreys & Grencis, 2002). As the parasite load gained through the life differs among parasite and host species, the establishment of infection may be therefore dependent not only on the host immune response but also on parasite–related factors which may actively modulate immune reactions.

The immune system is involved in creating a favorable environment in the tissue for the parasites. The compromise of immune responsiveness by the host endocrine system may support establishment, growth, reproduction and survival of helminths. The contribution of stress, host sex or age may also reflect neuroimmunoendocrine interactions. The gender-dependent immune regulation was identified; adult individuals of Senegalese population chronically infected with *Schistosoma haematobium* parasite presenting similar intensities of infection showed specific IgA response and production of TGF-β and IL-10 significantly higher in females compared to males. This specific profile was supposed to be associated with T helper type-3 (Th3) immune response. Nonimmunological factors like sexual hormones, were proposed to influence the chronicity of the infection (Remoué et al., 2001). Hormones are strongly involved in immune suppression observed in stress-fully conditions which predispose to greater and longer infection or make the host susceptible to infection (Hernandez-Bello et al., 2010). Increases in gastrointestinal nematode egg production in sheep with age were greatest among individuals that had experienced the highest degree of stress (Hayward et al., 2009).

2.2 When the immunosuppression is expressed

Immunosuppression may be reached by different mechanisms in response to a plethora of parasitic molecules and may be expressed at each point of infection; from the ongoing invasion to chronic prolonged infection (Robinson et al., 2010). When parasites enter host tissues, a balance between the host effector mechanisms and the defense by the parasite have to be established allowing the survival of a number of larvae that escape from the first immune attack, and as long as some parasites persist, are able to act as effectors to regulate immune responses. One of the possibilities to cope with host defence is to inhibit innate immunity. Helminth derived products are able to modulate the function of non-immune and immune cells (Perrigoue et al, 2008). T cell hyporesponsiveness to antigen-specific stimuli from the beginning of infection may support survival of the developing stages of the parasite (Schwartz, 2003; Taylor et al., 2009). Induced hyporesponsiveness of T cells as a defect in lymphocyte function may contribute to the failure of the immune system to eliminate filarial nematodes (W. Harnett & M.M. Harnett, 2008; W. Harnett & M.M. Harnett, 2006). In ruminants immunosuppression caused by parasites leads to reduced responsiveness of lymphocytes to mitogens (Soulsby, 1987).

Helminth infections induce regulatory T cells (Treg: Tr1, Th3) secreting IL-10 and transforming growth factor (TGF-β) (Doetze et al, 2000) as well as $CD4^+CD25^+$ Treg expressing the Foxp3 transcription factor in the host (Cervi et al.; 2009; Pacífico et al., 2009). These regulatory T cells can alter the course of inflammatory disorders by increased production of IL-10 and TGF-β, together with induction of $CD25^+CD4^+$ $Foxp3^+$ T cells (Correale & Farez, 2007). This also may represent a potential explanation regarding how exposure to a parasite could alter immune reactivity to unrelated stimuli.

Parasites release products whose molecular structure and specificity may be changed during infection and most parasite immune evasion mechanisms depend on a form of molecular recognition between parasite and host. Helminths especially in long lasting infection produce factors that interfere with the tissue of the host and for that many helminths-derived substances are considered as immune modulators (W. Harnett & M.M. Harnett, 2008; Harn et al., 2009; Imai & Fujita, 2004). Infection with helminths drives $CD4^+$ T cell biasing towards Th2-types and also induces the state of immunosuppression or anergy (Stadecker, 1992; Tawill et al., 2004).

From the beginning of infection down regulation of innate response may occur. Typically for helminthic infections, expanded populations of eosinophils, basophils, mast cells and macrophages appear (Anthony et al., 2007; Jenkins & Allen, 2010). Nitric oxide produced by activated macrophages, eosinophils and other myeloid cells, is involved in many signalling pathways and may mediate induction of immunosuppression (Stamler et al., 1992). Hookworm infection inducing NO production is associated with impaired function of antigen-presenting cells and depletion of lymphocyte subpopulations (Dondji et al., 2008); myeloid cells derived from helminth infected animals exhibit antiproliferative properties (Mylonas et al., 2000).

Myeloid suppressor cells displaying an alternative activation phenotype CD11b/GR-1 emerged gradually in progression of *Taenia crassiceps* infection and in the late stage of infection, the suppressive activity relied on arginase activity, which facilitated the production of reactive oxygen species including H_2O_2 and superoxide (Brys et al., 2005). These cells are potent to impair antigen-specific T cell responses (Terrazas et al., 2001). Helminth extracts activate various macrophage populations and the most active in regulation of immune response are alternatively activated macrophages (AAMΦ) (Herbert et al., 2004).

2.3 Immunosuppression for tissue repair

During helminth infections Th2 immune responses and parasitic-related products downregulate immunity; both of which minimize pathology in the host (Maizels & Yazdanbakhsh, 2003; Tawill et al., 2004).

Macrophages are frequently the most abundant cell type recruited to the site of helminth infection but their activation and role are strictly dependent on the stage of infection and localization of the parasite. In the construction of tissue homeostasis suppression of inflammation is propagated by AAMΦ as anti-inflammatory down-regulatory cells (Allen & Loke, 2001; Villanueva et al., 1994). These cells are sources of TGF-β and IL-10 (Mylonas et al., 2009; Loke et al., 2000) as well prostaglandins PGE2 (Rodriguez-Sosa et al., 2002) and the IL-1 receptor antagonist (Goerdt & Orfanos, 1999). AAMΦ are also involved in repairing tissue or wound healing followed migration of larvae through the host tissue (Gratchev et al., 2001; Munder et al., 1998). Activation of myeloid cells may represent not only the state of innate protection but also have been already activated by helminth products and represent suppressor or repair responses.

Metazoan parasites localized in the tissue require a supply of nutrients and the removal of waste products therefore angiogenesis may be a key mechanism for helminth survival and presumably depend on the host tissue. The multifactorial induction of parasitic helminth-associated neovascularization could arise through, either a host-, a parasite- or a host-/parasite-dependent, angiogenic switch (Dennis et al., 2011). It is possible that mechanisms that downregulate the inflammatory reaction and support wound healing are the main outcome of immunosuppression in the host tissue. Upon immunosuppression, the activation or efficacy of the immune response is reduced. Some portions of the immune system itself have immunosuppressive effects on other parts of the immune system, and immunosuppression may also occur as an adverse reaction to treatment of other conditions. It is really that helminths inducing inflammatory responses provoke opposite or reverse reactions of immune cells (Erb, 2009). Depending on the parasite stages and their localization a distinct local and systemic immune reaction may be observed in the host tissue (Löscher & Saathoff, 2008). The rapid and persistent release of tegument glycoconjugates play a key role in immune evasion and life-long inflammation seen in many neurocysticercosis patients (Alvarez et al., 2008). The production of pro-inflammatory cytokines is often required to control parasites but the same cytokines contribute to immunopathology. In the tissue, cytokines and prostaglandins or glucocorticoid hormones may differentially suppress an inflammatory response provoked by the parasite (Dhabhar, 2009; Noverr et al., 2003; Wiegers & Reul, 1998).

The immunosuppressive effect may be also maintained by other mechanisms such as induction of immunosuppressive B cells (Wilson et al., 2010) and regulatory function in helminth infection is also pointed for B cells. IL-10 and TGF-β are secreted form B cells during *Schistosoma mansoni* infection (Velupillai & Harn, 1994) or in mice infected with *Brugia pahangi* (Gillan et al., 2005).

2.4 The action of immunosuppressive factors

Immune non-responsiveness may also be the result of particular external processes such as deactivation of immune molecules or factors by helminthic products. Helminth parasites secrete considerable quantities of proteins and glycoproteins into the host environment, many of which are capable of modulating antiparasite immunity. Such molecules interfere with crucial stages in the immune response such as extravasations (blocked by parasite lectins and glycans through binding to endothelial selectins), chemokine attraction (hookworms release proteases capable of degrading eotaxin), release of host proteases (inhibited by helminth serpins), attack by reactive nitrogen and oxygen intermediates by eosinophils and other effector cells (inhibited by helminth antioxidants such as glutathione-S-transferase) (Falcone et al., 2004; Maizels et al., 2004).

Helminth parasites may also secrete cytokine homologues such as TGF-β and produce protease inhibitors that are capable of blocking peptide antigen presentation and of eliciting an IL-10 response from macrophages. Immune non-responsiveness may also be the result of deactivation of immune molecules or factors by helminthic products such as macrophage migration inhibitory factor (Vermeire et al., 2008). Lipid-like molecules of schistosomes such as lyso-PS can interact with dendritic cells to induce T regulatory phenotypes in naïve T cells (van der Kleij et al., 2002) and homologous molecules have been identified in *Ascaris.* Potent immunosuppressive effect of *Ascaris suum* extract components on the host immune system was related to their property of down-regulating the antigen presenting ability of dendritic cells *via* an IL-10-mediated mechanism (Silva et al., 2006). Filariae cystatin as immunoregulator exploits host signalling events to regulate cytokine production in macrophages (Klotz et al., 2011).

The efficiency of the innate response is crucial for invasion and survival of arriving larvae. Key attack points for selective immunoregulation conducted by parasites rely on (i) modulation of antigen recognition with changes in pathways of signal transduction; (ii) costimulation blockade; (iii) induction of regulatory cells; (iv) deviation to protective responses; (v) neutralization of proinflammatory cytokines; (vi) induction of anti-inflammatory cytokines and; (vii) modulation of leukocyte trafficking. Immunosuppressive action of parasites can be primarily directed to antigen-presenting cells (APC) and induction of suppressor/regulatory T cells and macrophages, with the common effect to selectively inhibition of local or systemic immune response.

2.5 How and when to get the immunosuppression

2.5.1 Innate and adaptive immune response

Innate immunity provides the first line of defence against invading pathogens. Excretory - secretory products released by helminths described as conserved molecular patterns associated with the pathogen (PAMP) may interact with the host pattern recognition receptor (PRRs) (Jackson et. al., 2009). Different carbohydrate moieties of helminths molecules are recognized by toll-like receptors (Medzhitov, 2007) and the C-type lectins receptors on dendritic cells and macrophages (Cambi et al., 2005). As a consequence of ligation, these DC will receive signals that are subsequently translated into different sets of Th1-, Th2-, or Treg-polarizing molecules. However, TLR ligation by helminth derived factors is recognized as a mechanism to limit of Th1 cytokine-mediated inflammation. Mature DC generated during helminth infection express relatively low levels of co-stimulatory molecules and proinflammatory cytokines promoting proliferation of CD4-positive T cells with Th2 phenotypes (MacDonald & Maizels, 2008; Semnani et al., 2008). Regulation of the host response starts from the recognition of the parasite; helminths products are able to stimulate partially activated dendritic cells with suppressed expression of TLRs and activate factors which promote Th2 and Treg phenotypes (Jackson et al., 2008). Some molecules which are released during tissue damage may interact with and induce anti-inflammatory effects (Ehlers & Ravetch, 2007).

Helminths strongly drive Th2-cell differentiation (Liu et al., 2005). Th2 related defence is involved in protective immune responses to helminths and is dominated by IL-4, IL5 and IL-

13 production (Finkelman et al., 2004). During Th2 related response, in addition to IL-4, IL-13, IL-5, IL-9, and IL-10 (Anthony et al., 2007). Th2 cells can make IL-25 and IL-33 (Fallon et al., 2006; Neill et al., 2010) which can further promote and/or regulate Th2 immune responses. IL-10 is differentially used by helminths to regulate immune response and as produced by different cells *in vivo* downregulates both Th1 and Th2 response (Hoffman et al., 2000; Taylor et al., 2006). Induction of type 2 immune responses may also be influenced by thymic stromal lymphopoietin (TSLP) synthesized by epithelial cells, and blocking IL-12 production can condition dendritic cells to promote Th2 cell development (Rimoldi et al., 2005). The innate cell sources of factors promoting Th2 and Treg response were only now proposed as a new innate type-2 immune effector leukocyte that were named the nuocyte. Nuocytes expand *in vivo* in response to the type-2-inducing cytokines IL-25 and IL-33, and represent the predominant early source of IL-13 during helminth infection with *Nippostrongylus brasiliensis* (Neill et al., 2010).

Apoptosis is mechanism which is involved in regulation of cell abundance during immune response. Cells induced to die release extramembrane phosphotidylserine which causes differentiation of immature dendritic cells to cells with a tolerogenic phenotype which favours anti-inflammatory responses (Steinman et al., 2000; Wallet et al., 2005). However, a plethora of helminths are able to modulate host apoptosis pathways to their own advantage. The involvement of apoptosis in immune regulation of the host immune function was proposed as one possible mechanism in creating the host–parasite relationship. The relative numbers of activated cells in both tissue and lymph nodes *via* the apoptotic pathway could determine pathology (Donskow-Schmelter & Doligalska, 2005). There is growing evidence that parasites can regulate apoptosis of T cells. Apoptosis can be triggered by diverse stimuli (Domen, 2001), including stimulation *via* T cells, Fas receptor, TNF receptors, glucocorticoids, removal of growth factors and enhanced expression of some proteases. In mice infected with microfilariae of the filariae nematode *B. malayi*, $CD4^+$ T cells showed high levels of apoptosis and displayed an antigen specific proliferative defect what is related to elevated macrophages activity (Jenson et al., 2002). Parasites may provoke apoptosis directly by secretion of active mediators or indirectly by producing an inflammatory milieu that promotes death of reactive T cells.

2.5.2 The regulation of immunosuppression by *Heligmosomoides polygyrus*

The *H. polygyrus* nematode is known to induce a dominant Th2 $CD4^+$ response and it provides an excellent example of downregulation of immune responsiveness. The adult worms had a potent immunosuppressive influence on the mouse host, but the histotropic L4 larvae provided the strongest signal for acquired immunity (Wahid & Behnke, 1992). In helminths, glycans provide a major contribution to the induction of Th2 development which is strongly skewed but the effectiveness of these responses for elimination or maintenance of the parasite is not fully elucidated. Additionally, in response to IL-4 and/or IL-13 producing cells, alternatively activated macrophages are activated, and express high levels of PRR. These population of cells produce high amounts of IL-10 and TGF-β but fail to generate NO (Gordon, 2003; Rodríguez-Sosa et al., 2002) and therefore may contribute to the general immune hyporesponsiveness observed in helminth-infected individuals (Leng et al., 2006; van Riet et al., 2007). Profoundly downregulatory cytokine TGF-β is critical to the immunosuppression induced by nematodes. Neutralization of these cytokines in human peripheral blood lymphocyte (PBL) cultures reversed antigen responsiveness toward filarial antigens (Cooper et a., 2001). Neutralization of TGF-β in BALB/c infected with *H. polygyrus* mice did not affect the Th2 related immune response (Doligalska et al., 2006). However adult worms might express ligands from the TGF-β superfamily- TGH-2 to bind to mammalian TGF-β receptors which may induce naïve T cells to adopt a regulatory T-cell phenotype; thereby promoting long-term survival of parasites (Peng et al., 2004).

Intestinal submucosa	Reference	**Mesenteric lymph node**	Reference
L3 Larvae			
Neutrophils↑	Morimoto et al., 2004	T cells proliferation↑	Doligalska et al., 2006
Eosinophils↑	Morimoto et al., 2004	CD4^{+} T cells apoptosis↓	Doligalska et al., 2006
AAMΦ↓	Morimoto et al., 2004		
Basophils↓	Anthony et al., 2006		
Mast cells↓	Morimoto et al., 2004		
CD4^{+} T cells↑	Morimoto et al., 2004		
CD8^{+} T cells↓	Liu et al., 2007		
B cells↓	Liu et al., 2007		
Cytokines & chemokines		*Cytokines & chemokines*	
IL-4↑, IL-13↑, IL-6↑	Donskow-Schmelter et al., 2008	IL-4↓, IL-6↓	Doligalska et al., 2007
IL-2↑, IL-12p70↑, IFN-γ↑	Donskow-Schmelter et al., 2008	IL-2↓, IL-12 p70↓, IFN-γ↓	Doligalska et al., 2007
TNF-α↑, IL-10↑, MCP-1↑	Donskow-Schmelter et al., 2008	TNF-α↑, IL-10 , MCP-1↑	Doligalska et al., 2007
		TGF-β↓	Doligalska et al., 2006
L4 Larvae			
AAMΦ↑	Kreider et al., 2007	T cells proliferation↓	Doligalska et al., 2006
CAMΦ↓	Donskow-Schmelter et al., 2008	CD4^{+} T cells apoptosis↓	Doligalska et al., 2006
CD4^{+} T cells↓	Kreider et al., 2007		
CD8^{+} T cells↓	Kreider et al., 2007		
Cytokines & chemokines		*Cytokines & chemokines*	
IL-4↓ , IL-13↓, IL-6↑	Donskow-Schmelter et al., 2008	IL-4↓, IL-6↓	Doligalska et al., 2007
IL-2↓, IL-12p70↑, IFN-γ↑	Donskow-Schmelter et al., 2008	IL-2↓, IL-12 p70↓, IFN-γ↓	Doligalska et al., 2007
TNF-α↑, IL-10↓, MCP-1↑	Donskow-Schmelter et al., 2008	TNF-α↑, IL-10↓, MCP-1↓	Doligalska et al., 2007
		TGF-β↑	Doligalska et al., 2006
Adult worms			
Eosinophils ↓	Doligalska et al., 2006	T cells proliferation↓	Donskow et al., 2011
AAMΦ ↑	Anthony et al., 2006	CD4^{+} T cells apoptosis ↓	Donskow et al., 2011
CD4^{+} T cells ↓	Doligalska et al., 2006	CD8^{+} T cells apoptosis↓	Donskow et al., 2011
CD8^{+} T cells↑	Metwali, 2008	CD4^{+}CD25^{hi} Treg apoptosis↓	Donskow et al., 2011
CD4^{+}CD25^{hi} Treg ↑	Metwali, 2008		
Cytokines & chemokines		*Cytokines & chemokines*	
IL-4↑, IL-13↓, IL-6↓	Donskow-Schmelter et al., 2008	IL-4↓, IL-6↑	Doligalska et al., 2007
IL-2↓, IL-12p70↑, IFN-γ↓	Donskow-Schmelter et al., 2008	IL-2↓, IL-12 p70↓, IFN-γ ↑	Doligalska et al., 2007
TNF-α↓, IL-10↑, MCP-1↓	Donskow-Schmelter et al., 2008	TNF-α↑, IL-10↑, MCP-1↑	Doligalska et al., 2007
IL-5↑	Doligalska et al., 2006	TGF-β↑	Doligalska et al., 2006
IL-17↓	Elliott et al., 2009	IL-17↓	Elliott et al., 2009

Table 1. Cellular and cytokines responses to *H. polygyrus* infection in BALB/c mice. *H. polygyrus* is trichostrongylid nematode parasite used as a model of human gastrointestinal nematode infection. Within 24 hrs of infection by gavage larvae, the stage L3, penetrate the submucosa of duodenum. The fourth larval molt takes place about 90-96 hrs after infection and larvae reside in for 8 days. Pre-adult stage re-enter the lumen of the intestine and mature to adult stages. *H. polygyrus* infection in BALB/c mice is widely used for studies of parasite immunomodulation. BALB/c mice moderately respond to *H. polygyrus* infection and the immunoresponsiveness of this strains is well documented (Donskow-Schmelter et al., 2008). The *H. polygyrus* causes chronic, asymptomatic infection. Primary exposure to L3 larvae results in an upregulation of the Th2 cytokine response, minimal damage in the tissue provoked by L4 larvae and significant reduction of inflammation by adult stages. AAMΦ, alternatively activated macrophage; CAMΦ, classically activated macrophage

The induced immunosuppressive mechanisms including apoptosis of activated cells is dependent on the host genotype (Donskow-Schmelter et al., 2007). The other immune response of fast FVB responder and slow C57Bl/6 responder mice during infection with *H. polygyrus* is associated with differences in apoptosis of $CD4^+$ T cells in mesenteric lymph nodes (MLN). The apoptosis of these lymphocytes at the beginning of infection, when the first immune signal is given by infective L3 larvae, might play an important role in the modulation of the response in C57Bl/6 slow responder (Donskow-Schmelter, et al., 2007) but not in fast responder mice.

The expression of host-protective immunity to *H. polygyrus* was dependent on the development of resistance to the immunomodulatory factors secreted by the worms (Behnke & Parish, 1979). The differences in sensitivity of T cells to apoptosis is provoked by distinct protein production by *H. polygyrus* worms in different strains of mice (Morgan et al., 2006). Calreticulin or other proteins produced by *H. polygyrus* (Morgan et al., 2006; Rzepecka et al., 2006) in slow responder mouse could be responsible for the observed apoptosis in C56Bl/6 mice. The recombinant form of human hookworm calreticulin can disturb the complement cascade and induce cell apoptosis *in vitro* (Kasper et al., 2001; Chow et al., 2000) thereby supporting chronic infection (Donskow-Schmelter et al., 2007).

Interestingly, in resistant strains immunosuppression during infection does not affect the outcome of parasite-induced apoptosis, but results from a hyporesponsiveness experienced by $CD4^+$ T cells during *H. polygyrus* infection (Doligalska et al., 2006). In the prepatent and chronic phase of infection, $CD4^+$ T cells that are leaving the MLN survive better, do not proliferate and already have a hyporesponsive or anergic phenotype induced by $CD4^+CD25hi$ T cells which increased in number (Donskow et al., 2011).

Chronic helminth infections are associated with a general hyporesponsiveness in which the activity of regulatory T cells can induce peripheral tolerance and constrain mucosal reactivity. However, little is known about particular helminth molecules that can induce Treg cells but characterization of some of them has started. The role of native and adaptive regulatory T cells and $CD8^+$ lymphocytes have been elucidated. The *H. polygyrus* downregulation of immune responsiveness, is attributable in part to the activity of host natural Treg cells with the $CD4^+CD25hi$ phenotype (Finney et al., 2007) and regulatory $CD8^+$ T cells (Metwali et al., 2006). The expansion of $CD4^+CD25hi$ Treg cells in mice MLN is a consequence of inhibited apoptosis of this subpopulation regulated by glucocorticoid during the infection (Donskow et al., 2011). *H. bakeri* antigen modulates CD4- positive T cell resistance to glucocorticoid induced apoptosis by inducing overexpression of Bcl-2 and FLICE-like inhibitory protein (FLIP). They are transcriptionally regulated by the transcription factor, nuclear factor kappa B (NF-κB) (Doligalska, unpublished data).

Additionally colonization with *H. polygyrus* induces a mucosal $CD8^+$ T cell that inhibits proliferation of CD4+ T cells and CD8+ T cells through a contact and transporter associated with antigen processing (TAP)-dependent mechanism (Metwali et al., 2006). These observations have far-reaching implications. Undoubted host parasite relationships are complex and there may be several mechanisms by which parasites could protect host from inflammation.

Helminths and their hosts need to achieve a state of homeostatic balance in which regulatory mechanisms operate for the survival of both the parasite and the host. Molecular signalling and cross-talk between cells of the endocrine, neuronal or immune systems and secreted factors such as hormones, neuropeptides, cytokines and chemokines influence the course of infection and severity of disease. Neural pathways regulate immune response at regional, local and systemic levels through neurotransmitters and neuropeptides, and may have variable effects on immune cell activation and cytokine production. In turn, cytokines and chemokines produced both at peripheral inflammatory sites and/or locally in the CNS can modulate neural tissue function and hormonal secretion by endocrine glands (Delgado et al., 2004; Escobedo et al., 2005; Hernandez-Bello et al, 2010). One consequence of the invasion of nematode larvae is inflammation and tissue damage which provokes immunosuppression and analgesia. An increased number of neuronal opioid receptors on neurons is necessary for analgesic effects of opioids and their expression on immune effector cells allows immunomodulatory effects.

H. polygyrus is a strictly intestinal nematode and displays no systemic migration during its development in the host. L3 larvae briefly inhabit the duodenal wall and during this period the inflammation provoked by the larvae is regulated by opioids (Donskow-Schmelter et al., 2008). The endogenous opioid peptides have a wide array of immunomodulatory effects on the immune system, directly through MOR opioid receptor of macrophages and indirectly through the hypothalamic-pituitary-adrenal (HPA) axis. The administration of naltrexone (NLX), an oral antagonist of opioid receptors which completely blocks the effects of opioid agonists in mice infected with L4 larvae, caused a dramatic increase in classically activated macrophages (CAMΦ) activity; NO and cytokine production and migration. Additionally, as end-effectors of the HPA axis, endogenous glucocorticoids play an important role in the suppression of immunity by induction of $CD4^{+}CD25^{+}$ Treg lymphocytes. The opioid action is strictly determined by tissue damage; adult worms in the intestinal lumen inhibit inflammation without opioid receptor-linked mechanism activation (Donskow-Schmelter et al., 2008).

2.5.3 "Therapeutic helminths"

Nematode suppress the immunity generated by infection and also affect systemic responses to other non-nematode antigens (Barthlott et al., 2003). For this reason there has been a dramatic increase in the prevalence of immune-mediated diseases in areas where previously common exposure to helminths is now rare. These observations suggest that the parasites produce a natural governor that helps to prevent autoimmune disease such as inflammatory bowel disease (IBD), asthma, autoimmune diabetes (type I) or multiple sclerosis (Yazdanbakhsh et al., 2001). Laboratory and clinical studies confirm that nematodes can both prevent disease onset and reverse ongoing diseases.

The development of immunologically well-defined laboratory models of nematode infection helps to understand the immunological basis of effector mechanisms operating during these and other infections. Infected mice develop immunological characteristics which are very similar to those observed in m infection in man. *H. polygyrus* infection in mice is a laboratory model which generates new information in the wider fields of allergic and autoimmune inflammatory disorders.

Nematode infection of humans and animals induce immune responses which are characterized by the production of Th2 associated cytokines IL-4, IL-5, IL-10, IL-13 and Treg associated cytokines IL-10 and TGF-β. This type of response generally down regulates the Th1 immune responses and persists for the duration of the infection. *H. polygyrus* infection suppresses asthma in a murine model by induction of $CD4^{+}CD25^{+}Foxp3^{+}$ regulatory T cells and IL-10 production (Wilson et. al., 2005). In ovalbumin (OVA) induced asthmatic mice infected with *H. polygyrus* reduced Th2 responses and eosinophil responses by down-regulation of eotaxin concentration, reduced CCR3 chemokine receptor expression on eosinophils and decreased chemotactic activity of these cells toward eotaxin (Rzepecka et al., 2006). The suppression of OVA-induced inflammation by *Nippostrngylus brasiliensis* is additional strictly mediated by IL-10 (Wohlleben et al., 2004). IL-10 which is a component of the natural host response to infection with enteric helminth parasites could be the key for therapeutic benefit.

T. spiralis, Trichuris trichiura and *H. polygyrus* infection protects animals from IBD (Eliott et. Al., 2007), but the complex pathways activated by nematodes to regulate the host's immune system, especially during *colitis,* is unknown. The combined induction of both Th2 (Setiawan et al., 2007) and Treg cells (Eliott et al., 2005) provoked by concurrent infection with *H. polygyrus* only partly explain the beneficial effects in mice with *colitis*. The inflammatory infiltrate in *colitis* is both Th1- and Th2-mediated. Therefore, additional parasite-induced mechanisms reduce inflammation.

Such regulatory cells can control self-reactive T cells and are functionally important in limiting inflammation in various animal models of IBD. In addition, *H. polygyrus* suppression of *colitis* requires $CD8^+$ T cells, suggesting that such these population of T cells may be important for this protection (Metwali et al., 2006). Furthermore, a resistance of *Schistosoma mansoni* infected mice to *dextran* sulfate sodium (DSS) induced *colitis* is macrophage dependent but not mediated by alternatively activated macrophages in the colon (Smith et al., 2007). *H. polygyrus* reduced established *colitis* by proopiomelanocortin-alpha (Pomc-a) and MOR opioid pathway (Donskow, unpublished data).

Recently treatment with living helminths such as *T. suis* or *N. americanus,* was initiated to control Cohn's disease, ulcerative colitis and asthma in human (Ruyssers et al., 2008). The opportunity to reveal novel ways to manipulate the human immune system to treat autoimmune inflammatory diseases by utilization of the natural response of the host to infection is exciting. In order that they may survive for long periods in an adverse and aggressive environment, nematodes secrete several soluble factors that interact with host cells. Some of these molecules may modify host-cell homeostasis and increase the susceptibility to infection and oncogenic factors. Undoubtedly, host parasite relationships are complex and there may be several mechanisms by which parasites induce immunosuppression and modulate host cells. Therapeutic helminth infection of humans needs to be closely examined for potential adverse side effects. For this reason the complex pathways that nematodes activate to regulate the host's immune system need further investigation.

3. Conclusions

Helminth infections are widely distributed. The extended survival of parasitic worms suggests that they are successful in an evolutionary sense. It is because they survive in and explore the host as natural environment. Helminths are often long lived and support tolerogenic reactions in host tissue rather than devastating immune reactions; they may induce the state of physiological and immune compromise and may consequently evade immune attack and actively subvert the host immune response. The immunosuppressive reactions provoked by different stages of the parasite in different periods of the host life span are embroiled in the host-parasite relationship and in this sense sustain the state of physiological homeostasis.

Helminths seeking for survive themselves using a plethora of mechanisms have been a major selective force for the host population and may influence of heritable factors both in patterns of infection and host immunity. The state of immune unresponsiveness in the host protects growing larvae during migration through the tissue and allow for non-destructive localization of adults to propagate and transmit their offspring. The maintenance of an immunosuppressed state in the host may improve the fitness of the parasite, promotes infection with further infectious larvae. Infection with one species predisposes also for infection with other species. As the parasite load gained through the life differs among parasite and host species, the establishment of infection may be therefore dependent not only on the host immune response but also on parasite-related factors which may actively modulate immune reactions. Immunosuppression may be reached by different mechanisms in response to a plethora of parasitic molecules and may be expressed at each point of infection. Helminths especially in long lasting infection produce factors that directly interfere with the tissue of the host and for that many helminths-derived substances are considered as immune modulators.

The efficiency of the innate response is crucial for invasion and survival of arriving larvae. Key attack points for selective immunoregulation conducted by parasites rely on: modulation of antigen recognition with changes in pathways of signal transduction; costimulation blockade; induction of regulatory cells; deviation to protective responses, neutralization of proinflammatory cytokines, induction of anti-inflammatory cytokines and modulation of leukocyte trafficking. Immunosuppressive action of parasites can be primarily directed to antigen-presenting cells (APC) and induction of suppressor/regulatory T cells and macrophages with the common effect to selectively inhibition of local or systemic immune response. The development of immunologically well-defined laboratory models of nematode infection helps to understand the immunological basis of effector mechanisms operating during hyperactive or auto-destructive disorders. *Heligmosomoides bakeri* related mechanisms involved in suppression of immune response in mice as representing for regulation of the host immune response are proposed. Helminths and their hosts need to achieve a state of homeostatic balance in which immunosuppressive and regulatory mechanisms operate for the survival of both the parasite and the host.

4. Acknowledgment

This research was supported through the Polish Ministry of Science and Higher Education (NN 303 819140 and NN 303 357233). We thank Professor M.J. Stear for help with the English.

5. References

Allen, J.E. & Loke, P. (2001). Divergent roles for macrophages in lymphatic filariasis. *Parasite Immunology,* Vol.23, No.7, (July 2001), pp. 345-352, ISSN 0141-9838

Alvarez, J.I.; Rivera, J. & Teale, J.M. (2008). Differential release and phagocytosis of tegument glycoconjugates in neurocysticercosis: implications for immune evasion strategies. *PLoS Neglected Tropical Diseases,* Vol.2, Issue 4, (April 2008), pp. e218, ISSN 1935-2727

Anthony, R.M.; Rutitzky, L.I.; Urban J.F.Jr.; Stadecker, M.J. & Gause, W.C. (2007). Protective immune mechanisms in helminth infection. *Nature Reviews Immunology,* Vol.7, Issue 12, (December 2007), pp. 975-987, ISSN 1474-1733

Anthony, R.M.; Urban, J.F.Jr.; Alem, F.; Hamed, H.A.; Rozo, C.T.; Boucher, J-L.; van Rooijen, N. & Gause, W.C. (2006). Memory TH2 cells induce alternatively activated macrophages to mediate protection against nematode parasites. *Nature Medicine,* Vol.12, No.8, (August 2006), pp. 955–960, ISSN 1078-8956

Barriga, O.O. (1978). Depression of cell-mediated immunity following inoculation of *Trichinella spiralis* extract in the mouse. *Immunology,* Vol.34, Issue 1, (January 1978), pp. 167-173, ISSN 0019-2805

Barthlott, T.; Kassiotis, G. & Stockinger, B. (2003). T cell regulation as a side effect of homeostasis and competition. *The Journal of Experimental Medicine,* Vol.197, No.4, (February 2003), pp. 451-460, ISSN 0022-1007

Behnke, J.M. & Robinson, M. (1985). Genetic control of immunity to *Nematospiroides dubius:* a 9-day anthelmintic abbreviated immunizing regime which separates weak and strong responder strains of mice. *Parasite Immunology,* Vol. 7, Issue 3, (May 1985), pp. 235-253, ISSN 0141-9838

Beiting, D.P.; Gagliardo, L.F.; Hesse, M.; Bliss, S.K.; Meskill, D. & Appleton, J.A. (2007). Coordinated control of immunity to muscle stage *Trichinella spiralis* by IL-10, regulatory T cells, and TGF-β. *The Journal of Immunology,* Vol.178, No.2, (January 2007), pp. 1039-1047, ISSN 0022-1767

Billingham, R. E.; Brent, L. & Medawar, B.P. (1956). Quantitative studies of tissue transplantation immunity. III. Acutely acquired tolerance. *Philosophical Transactions of the Royal Society of London. Series B, Biological Sciences, Vol.239, No.666, (March 1956), pp. 357-414, ISSN 0080-4622*

Blaxter, M.L. (2003). Nematoda: Genes, genomes and the evolution of parasitism. *Advances in Parasitology,* Vol.54, pp. 101-195, ISSN 0065-308X

Brooker, S. (2010). Estimating the global distribution and disease burden of intestinal nematode infections: Adding up the numbers - A review. *International Journal for Parasitology,* Vol.40, Issue 10, (August 2010), pp. 1137-1144, ISSN 0020-7519

Brys, L.; Beschin, A.; Raes, G.; Ghassabeh, G.H.; Noel, W.; Brandt, J.; Brombacher, F. & De Baetselier, P. (2005). Reactive oxygen species and 12/15-lipoxygenase contribute to the antiproliferative capacity of alternatively activated myeloid cells elicited during helminth infection. *The Journal of Immunology,* Vol.174, No.10, (May 2005), pp. 6095-6104, ISSN 0022-1767

Bundy, D.A.P.; Cooper, E.S.; Thompson, D.E.; Didier, J.M. & Simmons, I. (1987). Epidemiology and population dynamics of *Ascaris lumbricoides* and *Trichuris trichiura* infection in the same communit. *Transactions of the Royal Society of Tropical Medicine and Hygiene,* Vol.81, Issue 6, (November-December 1987), pp. 987-993, ISSN 00359203

Cambi, A.; Koopman, M. & Figdor, C.G. (2005). How C-type lectins detect pathogene. *Cellular Microbiology,* Vol.7, Issue 4, (April 2005), pp. 481-488, ISSN 1462-5814

Capron, A. & Dessaint, J.P. (1992). Immunologic aspects of *Schistosomiasis. Annual Review of Medicine,* Vol.43, (February 1992), pp. 209-218, ISSN 0066-4219

Cervi, L.; Serradell, M.C.; Guasconi, L. & Masih, D.T. (2009). New insights into the modulation of immune response by *Fasciola hepatica* excretory-secretory products. *Current Immunology Reviews,* Vol.5, No.4, (November 2009), pp. 277-284, ISSN 1573-3955

Combes, C. (1997). Fitness of parasites: Pathology and selection. *International Journal for Parasitology,* Vol.27, Issue 1, (January 1997), pp. 1-10, ISSN 0020-7519

Cooper, P.J.; Mancero, T.; Espinel, M.; Sandoval, C.; Lokato, R.; Guderian, R.H. & Nutman, T.B. (2001). Early human infection with *Onchocerca volvulus* is associated with an enhanced parasite-specific cellular immune response. *The Journal of Infectious Diseases,* Vol.183, Issue 11, (June 2001), pp. 1662-1668, ISSN 0022-1899

Correale, J. MD & Farez, M. MD. (2007). Association between parasite infection and immune responses in multiple sclerosis. *Annals of Neurology,* Vol.61, Issue 2, (February 2007), pp. 97-108, ISSN 0364-5134

Del Brutto, O.H. (2005). Neurocysticercosis. *Seminars in Neurology,* Vol.25, Issue 3, (September 2005), pp. 243-251, ISSN 0271-8235

Delgado, M.; Pozo, D. & Ganea, D. (2004). The significance of vasoactive intestinal peptide in immunomodulation. *Pharmacological Reviews,* Vol.56, No.2, (June 2004), pp. 249-290, ISSN 0031-699

Dennis, R.D.; Schubert, U. & Bauer, C. (2011). Angiogenesis and parasitic helminth-associated neovascularization. *Parasitology,* Vol.138, Issue 4, (April 2011), pp. 426-439, ISSN 1469-8161

de Silva, N.R.; Brooker, S.; Hotez, P.J.; Montresor, A.; Engels, D. & Savioli, L. (2003). Soil-transmitted helminth infections: updating the global picture. *Trends in Parasitology,* Vol.19, No.12, (December 2003), pp. 547-551, ISSN 1471-4922

Dhabhar, F.S. (2009). Enhancing versus suppressive effects of stress on immune function: implications for immunoprotection and immunopathology. *Neuroimmunomodulation,* Vol.16, No.5, (June 2009), pp. 300–317, ISSN 1021-7401

Doetze, A.; Satoguina, J.; Burchard, G.; Rau, T.; Loliger, C.; Fleischer, B. & Hoerauf, A. (2000). Antigen-specific cellular hyporesponsiveness in a chronic human helminth infection is mediated by Th3/Tr1-type cytokines IL-10 and transforming growth factor-beta but not by a Th1 to Th2 shift. *International Immunology,* Vol.12, Issue 5, (May 2003), pp. 623-630, ISSN 0953-8178

Doligalska, M., Donskow-Schmelter, K.; Rzepecka, J. & Drela, N. (2007). Reduced apoptosis in BALB/c mice infected with *Heligmosomoides polygyrus. Parasite Immunology,* Vol.29, No.6, (June 2007), pp. 283-291, ISSN 0141-9838

Domen, J. (2001). The role of apoptosis in regulating hematopoietic stem cell numbers. *Apoptosis,* Vol.6, No.4, (August 2001), pp. 239–252, ISSN 1360-8185

Dondji, B.; Bungiro, R.D.; Harrison, L.M.; Vermeire, J.J.; Bifulco, C.; McMahon-Pratt, D. & Cappello, M. (2008). Role for nitric oxide in hookworm-associated immune suppression. *Infection and Immunity,* Vol.76, No.6, (June 2008), pp. 2560-2567, ISSN 0019-9567

Donskow-Schmelter, K. & Doligalska, M. (2005). Apoptosis, a protective mechanism for pathogens and their hosts. *Wiadomości Parazytologiczne,* Vol. 51, No.4, pp. 271-280, ISSN 0043-5163

Donskow, K.; Drela, N. & Doligalska, M. (2011). *Heligmosomoides bakeri* antigen rescues CD4 positive T cells from glucocorticoid-induced apoptosis by Bcl-2 protein expression. *Parasite Immunology,* Vol.33, Issue 3, (March 2011), pp.158–169, ISSN 0141-9838

Donskow-Schmelter, K.; Doligalska, M.; Rzepecka, J. & Jedlina-Panasiuk, L. (2007). *Heligmosomoides polygyrus*: Decreased apoptosis in fast responder FVB mice during infection. *Experimental Parasitology,* Vol.117, Issue 2, (October 2007), pp. 149-156, ISSN 0014-4894

Donskow-Schmelter, K.; Laskowska, M. & Doligalska, M. (2008). *Heligmosomoides polygyrus:* Opioid peptides are involved in immune regulation of histotropic phase of infection. *Experimental Parasitology,* Vol.118, Issue 3, (March 2008), pp. 338-344, ISSN 0014-4894

Ehlers, M. & Ravetch, J.V. (2007). Opposing effects of Toll-like receptor stimulation induced autoimmunity or tolerance. *Trends in Immunology,* Vol.28, Issue 2, (February 2007), pp. 74-79, ISSN 1471-4906

Elliott, D. E., A. Metwali, J. Leung, T. Setiawan, A. M. Blum, M. N. Ince, L. E. Bazzone, M. J. Stadecker, J. F. Urban, Jr, J. V. Weinstock. (2008). Colonization with *Heligmosomoides polygyrus* suppresses mucosal IL-17 production. *Journal of Immunology.* Vol.181, Issue 4 (August 15) pp. 2414-2419, ISSN 0022-1767

Elliott, D.E.; Summers, R.W. & Weinstock, J.V. (2007). Helminths as a governors of immune mediated inflammation. *International Journal for Parasitology,*Vol. 37, Issue 5, (April 2007), pp. 457-464, ISSN 0020-7519

Ellis, M.K. & McManus, D.P. (2009). Familial aggregation of human helminth infection in the Poyang lake area of China with a focus on genetic susceptibility to schistosomiasis japonica and associated markers of disease. *Parasitology,* Vol.136, Issue 7, (June 2009), pp. 699-712, ISSN 1469-8161

Ellis, M.K.; Raso, G.; Li, Y.S.; Rong, Z.; Chen, H.G. & McManus, D.P. (2007). Familial aggregation of human susceptibility to co- and multiple helminth infections in a population from Poyang Lake region China. *Intrenational Journal for Parasitilogy,* Vol.37, Issue 10, (August 2007), pp. 1153-1161, ISSN 0020-7519

Erb, K.J. (2009). Can helminths or helminth-derived products be used in humans to prevent or treat allergic diseases? *Trends in Immunology,* Vol.30, Issue 2, (January 2009), pp. 275-282, ISSN 1471-4906

Escobedo, G.; Roberts, C.W.; Carrero J.C. & Morales-Montor, J. (2005). Parasite regulation by host hormones:an old mechanism of host exploitation? *Trends in Parasitology,* Vol.21, Issue 12, (December 2005), pp. 588-593, ISSN 1471-4922

Ezenwa, V.O. & Jolles, A.E. (2011). From host immunity to pathogen invasion: The effects of helminth coinfection on the dynamics of microparasites. *Integrative Comparitive Biology,* DOI: 10.1093/icb/icr058, ISSN: 1540-7063

Falcone, F.; Loukas, A.; Quinnell, R.J. & Pritchard, D.I. (2004). The innate allergenicity of helminth parasites. *Clinical Reviews in Allergy and Immunology,* Vol.26, No.1, (February 2004), pp. 61-72, ISSN 1080-0549

Fallon, P.G.; Ballantyne, S.J.; Mangan, N.E.; Barlow, J.L.; Dasvarma, A.; Hewet, D.R.; McIlqorm, A.; Jolin, H.E. & McKenzie, A.N. (2006). Identification of an interleukin (IL-25)-dependent cell population that provides Il-4,vIL-5 and Il-13 at the onset of helminth explusion. *Journal of Experimental Medicine,* Vol.203, No.4, (April 2006), pp. 1105-1116, ISSN 0022-1007

Finkelman, F.D.; Shea-Donohue, T.; Morris, S.C.; Gildea, L.; Strait, R.; Madden, K.B.; Schopf, L. & Urban, J.F.Jr. (2004). Interleukin 4 and interleukin 13-mediated host protection against intestinal nematode parasites. *Immunological Reviews,* Vol.201, (October 2004), pp. 139-155, ISSN 0105-2896

Finney, C.A.M.; Taylor, M.D.; Wilson, M.S. & Maizels, R.M. (2007). Expansion and activation of CD4+CD25+ regulatory T cells in *Heligmosomoides polygyrus* infection. *European Journal of Immunology,* Vol.37, No.7, (July 2007), pp. 1874-1886, ISSN 0014-2980

Fumagalli, M.; Pozzoli, U.; Cagliani, R.; Comi, G.P. & Riva, M. (2009). Parasites represent a major selective force for interleukin genes and shape the genetic predisposition to autoimmune conditions. *The Journal of Experimental Medicine,* Vol.206, No.6, (May 2009), pp. 1395-1408, ISSN 0022-1007

Gammon, G.; Dunn, K.; Shastri, N.; Oki, A.; Wilbur, S. & Sercarz, E.E. (1986). Neonatal T cell tolerance to minimal immunogenic peptides is caused by clonal inactivation. *Nature,* Vol. 319, Issue 6052, (January 1986), pp. 413-415, ISSN 0028-0836

Gerencer, M.; Marinculic, A.; Rapic, D.; Frankovic, M. & Valpotic, I. (1992). Immunosuppression of in vivo and in vitro lymphocyte responses in swine induced by *Trichinella spiralis* or excretory-secretory antigens of the parasite. *Veterinary Parasitology,* Vol.44, Issue 3-4, (October 1992), pp. 263-273, ISSN 0304-4017

Gillan, V.; Lawrence, R.A. & Devaney, E. (2005). B cells play a regulatory role in mice infected with the L3 of *Brugia pahangi. Intrenational Immunology,* Vol.17, No.4, (February 2005), pp. 373-382, ISSN 0953-8178

Goerdt, S. & Orfanos, C. E. (1999). Other functions, other genes:alternative activation of antigen-presenting cells. *Immunity,* Vol.10, No.2, (February 1999), pp. 137-142, ISSN 1074-7613

Gordon, S. (2003). Alternative activation of macrophages. *Nature Reviews Immunology,* Vol.3, Issue 1, (January 2003), pp. 23-35, ISSN 1474-1733

Gratchev, A.; Guillot, P.; Hakiy, N.; Politz, O.; Orfanos, C.E.; Schledzewski, K. & Goerdt, S. (2001). Alternatively activated macrophages differentially express fibronectin and its splice variants and the extracellular matrix protein βIGH3. *Scandinavian Journal of Immunology,* Vol.53, No.4, (April 2001), pp. 386-392, ISSN 0300-9475

Harn, D.A.; McDonald, J.; Atochina, O. & Da'dara, A.A. (2009). Modulation of host immune responses by helminths glycans. *Immunological Reviews,* Vol.230, No.1, (July 2009), pp. 247-257, ISSN 0105-2896

Harnett, W. & Harnett, M.M. (2006). What causes lymphocyte hyporesponsiveness during filarial nematode infection? *Trends in Parasitology,* Vol.22, Issue 3, (March 2006), pp. 105-110, ISSN 1471-4922

Harnett, W. & Harnett, M.M. (2008). Therapeutic immunomodulators from nematode parasites. *Expert Reviews in Molecular Medicine,* Vol.10, (June 2008), pp. e18, ISSN 1462-3994

Harnett, W. & Harnett, M.M. (2008). Lymphocyte hyporesponsiveness during filarial nematode infection. *Parasite Immunology,* Vol.30, Issue 9, (September 2008), pp. 447-53, ISSN 0141-9838

Hasnain, S.Z.; Wang, H.; Ghia, J.E.; Haq, N.; Deng, Y.; Velcich, A.; Grencis, R.K.; Thornton, D.J. & Khan, W.I. (2010). Mucin gene deficiency in mice impairs host resistance to an enteric parasitic infection. *Gastroenterology,* Vol.138, Issue 5, (May 2010), pp. 1763-1771.e5, ISSN 1528-0012

Hayward, A.D.; Wilson, A.J.; Pilkington, J.G.; Pemberton, J.M. & Kruuk, L.E.B. (2009). Ageing in a variable habitat: environmental stress affects senescence in parasite resistance in St Kilda Soay sheep. *Proceedings of the Royal Society B: Biological Sciences,* Vol.276, Issue 1672, (October 2009), pp. 3477-3485, ISSN 0962-8452

Herbert, D.R.; Holscher, C.; Mohrs, M.; Arendse, B.; Schwegmann, A.; Radwanska, M.; Leeto, M.; Kirsch, R.; Hall, P.; Mossmann, H.; Claussen, B.; Forster, I. & Brombacher, F. (2004). Alternative macrophage activation is essential for survival during schistosomiasis and downmodulates T helper I response and immunopathology. *Immunity,* Vol.20, Issue 5, (May 2004), pp. 623-635, ISSN 1074-7613

Hernandez-Bello, R.; Escobedo, G.; Guzman C.; Ibarra-Coronado, E.G.; Lopez-Griego, L. & Morales-Montor, J. (2010). Immunoendocrine host-parasite interactions during helminths infections: from the basic knowledge to its possible therapeutic applications. *Parasite Immunology,* Vol.32, Issue 9-10, (September/October 2010), pp. 633-643, ISSN 0141-9838

Hoffmann, K.F.; Cheever, A.W. & Wynn, T.A. (2000). IL-10 and the dangers of immune polarization: excessive type 1 and 2 cytokine response induced distinct forms of lethal immunopathology in murine schistosomiasis. *The Journal of Immunology,* Vol.164, No.12, (June 2000), pp. 6406-6416, ISSN 0022-1767

Hotez, P.J.; Brindley, P.J.; Bethony, J.M.; King, C.H.; Pearce, E.J. & Jacobson, J. (2008). Helminth infections: the great neglected tropical diseases. *Journal of Clinical Investigation,* Vol.118, Issue 4, (April 2008), pp. 1311-1321, ISSN 0021-9738

Hotez, P.J. & Kamath, A. (2009). Neglected tropical diseases in Sub-Saharan Africa: review of their prevalence, distribution and disease burden. *PLoS Neglected Tropical Disease,* Vol. 3, No.8, (August 2009), pp. e412, ISSN 1935-2727

Humphreys†, N.E. & Grencis, R.K. (2002). Effects of ageing on the immunoregulation of parasitic infection. *Infection and Immunity,* Vol.70, No.9, (September 2002), pp. 5148-5157, ISSN 0019-9567

Imai, S. & Fujita, K. (2004). Molecules of parasites as immunomodulatory drugs. *Current Topics in Medicinal Chemistry,* Vol.4, Issue 5, pp. 539-552, ISSN 1568-0266

Iraqi, F.A.; Behnke, J.M.; Menge, D.M.; Lowe, A.; Teale, A.J.; Gibson, J.P.; Baker, L.R. & Wakelin, D. (2003). Chromosomal regions controlling resistance to gastro-intestinal nematode infections in mice. *Mammalian Genome,* Vol.14, No.3, (March 2003), pp. 184-191, ISSN 0938-8990

Jackson, J.A.; Friberg, I.M.; Bolch, L.; Lowe, A.; Ralli, C.; Harris, P.D.; Behnke, J.M. & Bradley, J.E. (2009). Immunomodulatory parasites and toll-like receptor-mediated tumour necrosis factor alpha responsiveness in wild mammals. *BMC Biology,* Vol.7, (April 2009), pp. 16, ISSN 1741-7007

Jackson, J.A.; Friberg, I.M.; Little, S. & Bradley, J.E. (2009). Review series on helminths, immune modulation and the hygiene hypothesis: Immunity against helminthes and immunological phenomena in modern human populations: coevolutinary legacies. *Immunology,* Vol.126, No.1, (January 2009), pp. 18-27, ISSN 0019-2805

Jenkins, S.J. & Allen, J.E. (2010). Similarity and diversity in macrophage activation by nematodes, trematodes, and cestodes. *Journal Biomedicine and Biotechnology,* 2010;2010:262609, ISSN 1110-7243

Jenson, J.S.; O'Connor, R.; Osborne, J. & Devaney E. (2002). Infection with *Brugia* microfilariae induces apoptosis of T cells: a mechanism of immune unresponsiveness in filariasis. *European Journal of Immunology,* Vol.32, Issue 3, (March 2002), pp. 858-867, ISSN 0014-2980

Keiser, J.; N'Goran, E.K.; Traoré, M.; Lohourignon, K.L.; Singer, B.H.; Lengeler, C.; Tanner, M. & Utzinger, J. (2002). Polyparasitism with *Schistosoma mansoni*, geohelminths, and intestinal protozoa in rural Côte d'Ivoire. *The Journal of Parasitology,* Vol.88, No.3, (June 2002), pp. 461-466, ISSN 0022-3395

Keiser, P.B. & Nutman, T.B. (2002). Update on lymphatic filarial infections. *Current Infections Disease Reports,* Vol.4, No.1, pp. 65-69, ISSN 1523-3847

Kingston, H. & Mills, G. (2004). Regulatory T cells: friend or foe in immunity to infection? *Nature Reviews Immunology,* Vol.4, Issue 11, (November 2004), pp. 841-855, ISSN 1474-1733

Klotz, C.; Ziegler, T.; Figueiredo, A.S.; Rausch, S.; Hepworth, M.R.; Obsivac, N.; Sers, C.; Lang, R.; Hammerstein, P.; Lucius, R. & Hartmann, S. (2011). A helminth immunomodulator exploits host signaling events to regulate cytokine production in macrophages. *PLoS Pathogens,* Vol.7, Issue 1, (January 2011), pp. e1001248, ISSN 1553-7366

Kreider, T.; Anthony, R.M.; Urban, J.F., Jr. & Gause, W. C. (2007). Alternatively activated macrophages in helminth infections. *Current Opinion in Immunology.* Vol.19, Issue 4, (August 2007), pp. 448-453, ISSN 0952-7915

Lebarbenchon, C.; Brown, S.P.; Poulin, R.; Gauthier-Clerc, M. & Thomas, F. (2008). Evolution of pathogens in a man-made world. *Molecular Ecology,* Vol.17, No.1, (January 2008), pp. 475–484, ISSN 0962-1083

Leng, Q.; Bentwich, Z. & Borkow, G. (2006). Increased TGF-β, Cbl-b and CTLA-4 levels and immunosuppression in association with chronic immune activation. *International Immunology*, Vol.18, No.5, (November 2005), pp. 637-644, ISSN 0953-8178

Liu, Z.; Liu, Q.; Hamed, H.; Anthony, R.M.; Foster, A.; Finkelman, F.D.; Urban, J.F.Jr. & Gause, W.C. (2005). IL-2 and autocrine IL-4 drive the in vivo development of antigen-specific Th2 T cells elicited by nematode parasites. *Journal of Immunology,* Vol.174, No.4, (February 2005), pp. 2242-2249, ISSN 0022-1767

Liu, Z. ; Liu, Q.; Pesce, J.; Anthony, R.M.; Lamb, E.; Whitmire, J.; Hamed, H.; Morimoto, M.; Urban, J.F.Jr. & Gause, W.C. (2004). Requirements for the development of IL-4-producing T cells during intestinal nematode infections: what it takes to make a Th2 cell *in vivo. Immunological Reviews,* Vol. 201, Issue 1, (October 2004), pp. 57–74, ISSN 0105-2896

Loke, P.; MacDonald, A.S. & Allen, J.E. (2000). Antigen-presenting cells recruited by *Brugia malayi* induce Th2 differentiation of naive CD4+ T cells. *European Journal of Immunology,* Vol.30, No.4, (April 2000), pp. 1127–1135, ISSN 0014-2980,

Loke, P.; MacDonald, A.S.; Roob, A.; Maizels, R.M. & Allen, J.E. (2000). Alternatively activated macrophages induced by nematode infection inhibit proliferation via cell-to-cell contact. *European Journal of Immunology,* Vol.30, No.9, (September 2000), pp. 2669-2678, ISSN 0014-2980

Löscher, T. & Saathoff, E. (2008). Eosinophilia during intestinal infection. *Best Practice & Research Clinical Gastroenterology,* Vol.22, Issue 3, (June 2008), pp. 511-536, ISSN 1521-6918

MacDonald, A.S. & Maizels, R.M. (2008). Alarming dendritic cells for Th2 induction. *The Journal of Experimental Medicine,* Vol.2005, No.1, (January 2008), pp. 13-17, ISSN 0022-1007

Maizels, R.M.; Balic, A.; Gomes-Escobar, N.; Nair, M.; Taylor, M.D. & Allen, J.E. (2004). Helminth regulation—masters of regulation. *Immunology Reviews,* Vol.201, Issue 1, (October 2004), pp. 89-116, ISSN 0105-2896

Maizels, R.M. & Yazdanbakhsh, M. (2003). Immune regulation by helminth parasites: cellular and molecular mechanisms. *Nature Reviews Immunology,* Vol.3, No.9, (September 2003), pp. 733-744, ISSN 1474-1733

Matzinger, P. (1994). Tolerance, danger, and the extended family. *Annual Review of Immunology,*Vol.12, (April 1994), pp. 991-1045, ISSN 0732-0582

May, R.M. &. Anderson, R.M. (1990). Parasite—host coevolution. *Parasitology,* Vol.100, supplement S1 S89-S101, ISSN 1469-8161

McKay, D.M. & Khan, W.I. (2003). STAT-6 is an absolute requirement for murine rejection of *Hymenolepis diminuta. Journal of Parasitology,* Vol.89, No.1, (February 2003), pp. 188-189, ISSN 0022-3395

Medzhitov, R. (2007). Recognition of microorganisms and activation of the immune response. *Nature,* Vol.449, No.7164, (October 2007), pp. 819-826, ISSN 0028-0836

Metwali, A.; Setiawan, T.; Blum, A.M.; Urban, J.; Elliott, D.E.; Hang, L. & Weinstock, J.V. (2006). Induction of CD8+ regulatory T cells in the intestine by *Heligmosomoides polygyrus* infection. *American Journal of Physiology Gastrointestinal and Liver Physiology,* Vol.291, No.2, (August 2006), pp. 253-259, ISSN 0193-1857

Mitchell, G.F. (1991). Co-evolution of parasites and adaptive immune responses. *Parasitology Today,* Vol.7, Issue 3, (March 1991), pp. 2-5, ISSN 0169-4758

Morar, R. & Feldman, C. (2003). Pulmonary echinococcosis. *European Respiratory Journal,* Vol.21, No.6, (June 2003), pp. 1069-1077, ISSN 0903-1936

Morimoto, M.; Morimoto, M.; Whitmire, J.; Xiao, S.; Anthony, R.M.; Mirakami, H.; Star, R.A.; Urban, J.F.Jr. & Gause, W.C. (2004). Peripheral CD4 T cells rapidly accumulate at the host: parasite interface during an inflammatory Th2 memory response. *The Journal of Immunology,* Vol.172, No.4, (February 2004), pp. 2424–2430, ISSN 0022-1767

Mouritsen, K.N. & Poulin, R. (2005). Parasites boosts biodiversity and changes animal community structure by trait-mediated indirect effects. *Oikos,* Vol.108, Issue 2, (February 2005), pp. 344-350, ISSN 0030-1299

Munder, M.; Eichmann, K. & Modolell, M. (1998). Alternative metabolic states in murine macrophages reflected by the nitric oxide synthase/arginase balance: competitive regulation by CD4+ T cells correlates with Th1/Th2 phenotype. *Journal of Immunology,* Vol.160, No. 11, (June 1998), pp. 5347-5354, ISSN 0022-1767

Mylonas, K.J.; Nair, M.G.; Prieto-Lafuente, L.; Paape, D. & Allen, J.E. (2009). Alternatively activated macrophages elicited by helminth infection can be reprogrammed to enable microbial killing. *Journal of Immunology,* Vol.182, No.5, (March 2009), pp. 3084-3094, ISSN 0022-1767

Neill, D.R.; Wong, S.H.; Bellosi, A.; Flynn, R.J.; Daly, M.; Langford, T.K.A.; Bucks, C.; Kane, C.M.; Fallon, P.G.; Pannell, R.; Jolin, H.E. & McKenzie, A.N. (2010). Nuocytes represent a new innate effector leukocyte that mediates type-2 immunity. *Nature,* Vol.464, Issue 7293, (April 2010), pp. 1367-1370, ISSN 0028-0836

Noverr, M.C.; Erb-Downward, J.R. & Huffnagle, G. B. (2003). Production of eicosanoids and other oxylipins by pathogenic eukaryotic microbes. *Clinical Microbiology Reviews,* Vol.16, No.3, (July 2003), pp. 517-533, ISSN 0893-8512

Ogilive, B.M. & Wilson, R.J.M. (1976). Evasion of the immune responsse by parasites. *British Medical Bulletin,* Vol.32, Issue 2, (May 1976), pp. 177-181, ISSN 0007-1420

Ozturk, G.; Aydinli, B.; Yildirgan, M.I.; Basoglu, M.; Atamanalp, S.S. & Polat, K.Y. (2007). Posttraumatic free intraperitoneal rupture of liver cystic echinococcosis: a case series and review of literature. *The American Journal of Surgery,* Vol.194, Issue 3, (September 2007), pp. 313-316, ISSN 0002-9610

Pacífico, L.G.G.; Marinho, F.A.V.; Fonseca, C.T.; Barsante, M.M.; Pinho, V.; Sales, P.A.Jr.; Cardoso, L.S.; Araujo, M.I.; Carvalho, E.M.; Cassali, G.D.; Teixeira, M. M. & Oliveira, S.C. (2009). *Schistosoma mansoni* antigens modulate experimental allergic asthma in a murine model: a major role for CD4+ CD25+ Foxp3+ T cells independent of Interleukin-10. *Infection and Immunity,* Vol.77, No.1, (January 2009), pp. 98-107, ISSN 0019-9567

Pedersen, S. & Saeed, I. (2002). Host age influence on the intensity of experimental *Trichuris suis* infection in pigs. *Parasite,* Vol.9, Issue 1, (March 2002), pp. 75-79, ISSN 1252-607X

Peng, Y.; Laouar ,Y.; Li, M.O.; Green, E.A. & Flavell, R.A. (2004). TGF-b regulates *in vivo* expansion of Foxp3-expressing CD4+CD25+ regulatory T cells responsible for protection against diabetes. *Proceedings of the National Academy of Sciences of the United States of America,* Vol.101, Issue 13, (March 2004), pp. 4572–4577, ISSN 0027-8424

Perrigoue, J.G.; Marshall, F.A. & Artis, D. (2008). On the hunt for helminths: innate immune cells in the recognition and response to helminth parasites. *Cellular Microbiology,* Vol.10, Issue 9, (September 2008), pp. 1757-1764, ISSN 1462-5814

Quinnell, R.J. (2003). Genetics of susceptibility to human helminth infections. *International Journal for Parasitology,*Vol.33, Issue 11, (September 2003), pp. 1219-1231, ISSN 0020-7519

Rajakumar, S.; Bleiss, W.; Hartmann, S.; Schierack, P.; Marko, A. & Lucius, R. (2006). Concomitant immunity in a rodent model of filariasis: The infection of *Meriones unguiculatus* with *Acanthocheilonema viteae. Journal of Parasitology,* Vol.92, No.1, (February 2006), pp. 41-45, ISSN 0022-3395

Read, A.F. & Sharping, A. (1995). The evolution of tissue migration by parasitic nematode. *Parasitology,* Vol.111, Issue 3, (September 1995), pp. 359-371, ISSN 1469-8161

Remoué, F.; Van, D.T.; Schacht, A.-M.; Picquet, M.; Garraud, O.; Vercruysse, J.; Ly, A.; Capron, A. & Riveau, G. (2001). Gender-dependent specific immune response during chronic human *Schistosomiasis haematobia. Clinical & Experimental Immunology,* Vol.124, Issue 1, (Aprill 2001), pp. 62-68, ISSN 0009-9104

Rimoldi, M.; Chieppa, M.; Salucci, V.; Avogadri, F.; Sonzogni, A.; Sampietro, G.M.; Nespoli, A.; Viale, G.; Allavena, P. & Rescigno, M. (2005). Intestinal immune homeostasis is regulated by the crosstalk between epithelial cells and dendritic cells. *Nature Immunology,* Vol.6, No.5, (May 2005), pp. 507-514, ISSN 1529-2908

Roberts, M.G. (1999). The immunoepidemiology of nematode parasites of farmed animals: a mathematical approachs. *Parasitology Today,* Vol.15, No.6, (June 1999), pp. 246-251, ISSN 0169-4758

Robinson, M.W.; Hutchinson, A.T.; Donnelly, S. & Dalton, J.P. (2010). Worm secretory molecules are causing alarm. *Trends in Parasitology,* Vol.26, No.8, (August 2010), pp. 371-372, ISSN 1471-4922

Rodríguez-Sosa, M.; Satoskar, A. R.; Calderon, R.; Gomez-Garcia, L.; Saavedra, R.; Bojalil, R. & Terrazas, L.I. (2002). Chronic helminth infection induces alternatively activated macrophages expressing high levels of CCR5 with low interleukin-12 production and Th2-biasing ability. *Infection and Immunity,* Vol.70, No.7, (July 2002), pp. 3656-3664, ISSN 0019-9567

Ruyssers, N.E.; De Winter, B.Y.; De Man, J.G.; Loukas, A.; Pearson, M.S.; Weinstock, J.V.; Van den Bossche, R.M.; Martinet, W.; Pelckmans, P.A. & Moreels, T.G. (2009).

Therapeutic potential of helminth soluble proteins in TNBS - induced colitis in mice. *Inflammatory Bowel Diseases*, Vol.15, Issue 4, (April 2009), pp. 491-500, ISSN 1078-0998

Rzepecka, J.; Lucius, R.; Doligalska, M.; Beck, S.; Rausch, S. & Hartmann, S. (2006). Screening for immunomodulatory proteins of the intestinal parasitic nematode *Heligmosomoides polygyrus*. *Parasite Immunology*, Vol.28, Issue 9, (September 2006), pp. 463-472, ISSN 0141-9838

Rzepecka J., Donskow-Schmelter K., Doligalska M. (2007). *Heligmosomoides polygyrus* infection down regulates eotaxin concentration and CCR3 expression on lung eosinophils in murine allergic pulmonary inflammation. *Parasite Immunology*,Vol. 29, Issue 8, (Jul 2007), pp. 405-413, ISSN 0141-9838

Schwartz, R.H. (2003). T cell anergy. *Annual Review of Immunology*, Vol.21, (April 2003), pp. 305-334, ISSN 0732-0582,

Semnani, R.T.; Venugopal, P.G.; Leifer, C.A.; Mostbock, S.; Sabzevari, H. & Nutman, T.B. (2008). Inhibition of TLR3 and TLR4 function and expression in human dendritic cells by helminth parasite. *Blood*, Vol.112, No.4, (August 2008), pp.1290-1298, ISSN 0006-4971

Setiawan, T.; Metwali, A.; Blum, A. M.; Ince, M. N.; Urban, J. F.; Elliott, D. E.; Weinstock, J. V. (2007). *Heligmosomoides polygyrus* promotes regulatory T cell cytokine production in normal distal murine intestine. *Infection and Immunity*, Vol.75, pp.4655-4663, ISSN 0019-9567

Silva, S.R.; Jacysyn, J.F.; Macedo M.S., & Faquim-Mauro, E.L. (2006). Immunosuppressive components of *Ascaris suum* down-regulate expression of costimulatory molecules and function of antigen-presenting cells via an IL-10-mediated mechanism. *European Journal of Immunology*, Vol.36, Issue 12, (December 2006), pp. 3227–3237, ISSN 0014-2980

Smith, P.; Mangan, N.E.; Walsh, C.M.; Fallon, R.E.; McKenzie, A.N. & van Rooijen N. (2007). Infection with a helminth parasite prevents experimental colitis via a macrophage-mediated mechanism. *The Journal of Immunology*, Vol.178, No.7, (April 2007), pp. 4557–466, ISSN 0022-1767

Soulsby, E.J.L. (1987). The evasion of the immune response and immunological unresponsiveness: Parasitic helminth infections. *Immunology Letters*, Vol.16, Issues 3-4, (December 1987), pp. 315-320, ISSN 0165-2478

Stadecker, M.J. (1992). The role of T cell anergy in the immunomodulation of schistosomiasis. *Parasitology Today*, Vol.8, Issue 6, (June 1002), pp. 199-204, ISSN 0169-4758

Stamler, J.S.; Singel, D.J. & Loscalzo, J. (1992). Biochemistry of nitric oxide and its redox-activated forms. *Science*, Vol. 258, No.5090, (December 1992), pp. 1898-1902, ISSN 0036-8075

Stear, M.J.; Bairden, K.; Duncan, J.L.; Holmes, P.H.; McKellar, Q.A.; Park, M.; Strain, S.; Murray, M.; Bishop, S.C. & Gettinby, G. (1997). How hosts control worms. *Nature*, Vol.389, Issue 6646, (September 1997), pp.27-27, ISSN 0028-0836

Stear, M.J. & Wakelin, D. (1998). Genetic resistance to parasitic infection. *Scientific and Technical Review-International Office of Epizootics*, Vol.17, Issue 1, (April 1998), pp. 143-153, ISSN 0253-1933

Steinman, R.M.; Turley, S.; Mellman, I. & Inaba, K. (2000). The induction of tolerance by dendritic cells that have captuted apoptotic cells. *The Journal of Experimental Medicine*, Vol.191, No.3, (February 2000), pp. 411-416, ISSN 0022-1007

Tan, T.H.P.; Edgerton, S.A.V.; Kumari, R.; McAlister, M.S.B.; Rowe, S.M.; Nagl, S.; Pearl, L.H.; Selkirk, M.E.; Bianco, A.E.; Totty, N.F.; Engwerda, C.; Gray, C.A. & Meyer, D.J. (2001). Macrophage migration inhibitory factor of the parasitic nematode *Trichinella spiralis. Biochemical Journal*, Vol.357, Issue 2, (July 2001), pp. 373-383, ISSN 0264-6021

Tawill, S.; Le Goff, L.; Ali, F.; Blaxter, M. & Allen, J.E. (2004). Both free living and parasitic nematodes induce a characteristic Th2 response is dependent on the presence of intact glycans. *Infection and Immunity*, Vol.72, No.1, (January 2004), pp. 398-407, ISSN 0019-9567

Taylor, J.J.; Krawczyk, C.M.; Mohrs, M. & Pearce, E.J. (2009). Th2 cell hyporesponsiveness during chronic murine schistosomiasis is cell intrinsic and linked to GRAIL expression. *The Journal of Clinical Investigation*, Vol.119, Issue 4, (April 2009), pp. 1019-1028, ISSN 0021-9738

Taylor, J.J.; Mohrs, M. & Pearce, F.J. (2006). Regulatory T cell responses develop in parallel to Th responses and control the magnitude and phenotype of the Th effector population. *The Journal of Immunology*, Vol.176, No.10, (May 2006), pp. 5839-5847, ISSN 0022-1767

Terhell, J.; Haarbrink, M.; Abadi, K.; Syafruddin; Maizels, R.M.; Yazdanbakhsh, M. & Sartono, E. (2001). Adults acquire filarial infection more rapidly than children: a study in Indonesian transmigrants. *Parasitology*, Vol.122, Issue 6, (Jun 2001), pp. 633-640, ISSN 1469-8161

Terrazas, L.I.; Walsh, K.L.; Piskorska, D.; McGuire, E. & Harn, D.A.,Jr. (2001). The schistosome oligosaccharide lacto-N-neotetraose expands Gr1+cells that secrete anti-inflammatory cytokines and inhibit proliferation of naïve CD4+ cells: a potential mechanism for immune polarization in helminths infections. *The Journal of Immunology*, Vol.167, No.9, (Nowember 2001), pp. 5294-5303, ISSN 0022-1767

Van der Boehmer, H. (1991). Positive and negative selection of the alpha beta T-cell repertoire in vivo. *Current Opinion in Immunology*, Vol.3, Issue 2, (April 1991), pp. 210-215, ISSN 0952-7915

Van der Kleij, D.; Latz, E.; Brouwers, J.F.H.M.; Kruize, Y.C.M.; Schmitz, M.; Kurt-Jones E.A.; Espevik, T.; de Jong, E.C.; Kapsenberg, M.L.; Golenbock, D.T.; Tielens, A.G.M. & Yazdanbakhsh, M. (2002). Novel host-parasite lipid cross-talk schistosomal lyso-phosphatidylserine activates tool-like receptor 2 and affects immune polarization. *Journal of Biological Chemistry*, Vol.277, (December 2002), pp. 48122-48129, ISSN 0021-9258

Van der Werf, M.J.; de Vlas, S.J.; Brooker, S.; Looman, C.A.N.; Nagelkerke, N.J.D.; Habbema, J.D.F. & Engels, D. (2003). Quantification of clinical morbidity associated with schistosome infection in sub-Saharan Africa. *Acta Tropica*, Vol.86, No.2-3, (May 2003), pp. 125-139, ISSN 0001-706X

Van Riet, E.; Hartagers, F.C. & Yazdanbakhsh, M. (2007). Chronic helminths infections induce immunomodulation: consequences and mechanisms. *Immunobiology*, Vol.212, Issue 6, (June 2007), pp. 475-490, ISSN 0171-2985

Velupillai, P. & Harn, D.A. (1994). Oligosacchride-specific induction of interleukin 10 production by B220+ cells from schistosome–infected mice: a mechanism for regulation of CD4+ T cell subsets. *Proceedings of the National Academy of Sciences of the United States of America,* Vol. 91, No.1, (January 1994), pp. 18-22, ISSN 0027-8424

Vermeire, J.J.; Cho, Y.; Lolis, E.; Bucala, R. & Cappello, M. (2008). Orthologs of macrophage migration inhibitory factor from parasitic nematodes. *Trends in Parasitology,* Vol.24, Issue 8, (August 2008), pp. 355-363, ISSN 1471-4922

Villanueva, P.O.F.; Harris, T.S.; Ricklan, D.E. & Stadecker, M.J. (1994). Macrophages from schistosomal egg granulomas induce unresponsiveness in specific cloned Th-1 lymphocytes in vitro and down-regulate schistosomal granulomatous disease in vivo. *Journal of Immunology,* Vol.152, No.4, (February 1994), pp. 1847-1855, ISSN 0022-1767

Wahid, F.N. & Behnke, J.M. (1992). Stimuli for acquired resistance to *Heligmosomoides polygyrus* from intestinal tissue resident L3 and L4 larvae. *International Journal for Parasitology,* Vol.22, Issue 6, (September 1992), pp. 699-710, ISSN 0020-7519

Wallet, M.A.; Sen, P. & Tisch, R. (2005). Immunoregulation of dendritic cells. *Clinical Medicine & Research,* Vol.3, No.3, (May 2005), pp. 166-175, ISSN 1554-6179

Wang, C-H. (1997). Study of biological properties of *Trichinella spiralis* newborn larvae and the antiparasitic mucosal immunity of the host. *Frontiers in Bioscience,* Vol.2, (July 1997), pp. d317-d330, ISSN 1093-4715

Warren, K.S. (1982). Schistosomiasis: host-pathogen biology. *Clinical Infection Diseases,* Vol.4, Issue 4, (July-August 1982), pp. 771-775, ISSN 1058-4838

WHO World Health Organization. Parasitic Diseases.: *http://www.who.int/vaccine_research/ diseases/soa_parasitic/en/index2.html.*

Wiegers, G.J. & Reul, J.M.H.M. (1998). Induction of cytokine receptors by glucocorticoids: functional and pathological significance. *Trends in Pharmacological Sciences,* Vol.19, Issue 8, (August 1998), pp. 317-321, ISSN 0165-6147

Wilkie, B.N.; Rupa, P. & Schmied, J. (2011). Practical immunoregulation: Neonatal immune response variation and prophylaxis of experimental food allergy in pigs. *Veterinary Immunology and Immunopathology,* (March 2011), doi:10.1016/j.vetimm.2011.03.010, ISSN 0165-2427

Wilson, M.S.; Taylor, M.D.; Balic, A.; Finney, C.A.; Lamb, J.R.; Maizels, R.M. (2005) Suppression of allergic airway inflammation by helminth-induced regulatory T cells. *The Journal of Experimental Medicine,* Vol.202, Issue 9, pp. 1199-212, ISSN 0022-1007

Wilson, M.S.; Taylor, M.D.; O'Gorman, M.T.; Balic, A.; Barr, T.A.; Filbey, K.; Anderton, S.M. & Maizels, R.M. (2010). Helminth-induced CD19+CD23hi B cells modulate experimental allergic and autoimmune inflammation. *European Journal of Immunology,* Vol.40, Issue 6, (June 2010), pp. 1682-1696, ISSN 0014-2980

Wohlleben, G.; Trujillo, C.; Müller, J.; Ritze, Y.; Grunewald, S.; Tatsch, U.; Erb, K.J. (2004). Helminth infection modulates the development of allergen-induced airway inflammation. *International immunology,* vol.16, pp. 585–596, ISSN 0953-8178

Yazdanbakhsh, M.; Van den Biggerlaar, A. & Maizels, R.M. (2001). Th2 responses without atopy: immunoregulation in chronic helminth infections and reduced allergic disease. *Trends in Immunology,* Vol.22, Issue 7, (July 2001), pp. 372-377, ISSN 1471-4906

11

Microbial Immunosuppression

Mohamed G. Elfaki[1], Abdullah A. Al-Hokail[2]
and Abdelmageed M. Kambal[3]
*[1]Infection and Immunity Department,
King Faisal Specialist Hospital and Research Centre, Riyadh,
[2]Department of Medicine, King Faisal Specialist Hospital and Research Centre, Riyadh,
[3]Department of Pathology, College of Medicine, King Saud University, Riyadh
Saudi Arabia*

1. Introduction

Immunosuppression is a condition characterized by immune dysfunction at either cellular or humoral levels [1]. Defective cellular levels include alterations in neutrophils, monocyte/macrophage, and natural killer (NK) cells for innate immunity or alterations in B or T lymphocytes for adaptive immunity [2, 3]. In contrast, immune dysfunction at the humoral level is largely due to alteration in soluble factors mediated by complement or chemokines for innate immunity [4] or due to alteration in antibodies or cytokines for adaptive immunity [5]. Most of these alterations are congenital in nature as evidenced in patients with primary immunodeficiency diseases. The defective compartment of the immune system determines the proclivity of the invading pathogens and the contracted infection is usually disseminating. Consequently, the inflicted immunosuppression is permanent unless reconstituted by immunoglobulin transfusions or bone marrow transplantation. On the other hand, secondary immunosuppression may be internal as a consequence of excessive adenosine release [6] into the extracellular space as evidenced in multiple organ failure (e.g. pancreas, kidney, liver) or it might be externally induced by a number of causal agents including infectious pathogens, immunosuppressive drugs, antimicrobial drugs, and anti-neoplastic drugs. The causal, pathophysiology, and methods used to evaluate immunosuppression due to pathogens are the focus of this chapter.

2. Immunosuppression induced by primary infections

Acquired immunosuppression due to pathogens is primarily caused by viruses that invade the cellular compartment of the immune system. The condition is seen in limited population of both humans and animals. In humans, it is caused by pathogens that selectively infect lymphocytes such as infection of T cells with human immunodeficiency virus (HIV) types I & II [7], or infection with human T-cell lymphotropic virus types I & II [8-10]. Human B lymphocytes, on the other hand, are prone to infection with Epstein-Barr virus (EBV) [11]. In animals, however, direct infection of immune cells that lead to immunosuppression is seen in cats infected with feline leukemia virus (FeLV) [12], cattle infected with bovine leukemia virus (BLV) [13] or in chickens infected with Marek's disease virus (MDV) [14] or infectious bursal disease (IBD) [15] virus. The striking feature in all of these infections is that immunosuppression is latently developed following viral replication that leads to lymphocytes depletion. Consequently the inflicted host develops immune anergy with increased susceptibility to opportunistic infections. Summary of the causal agents and the target cells involved in the induction of immunosuppression are presented in Table 1.

Causal agent	Host	Immune target cells	Disease	Immunologic sequelae
HIV-1&2	Humans	CD4+ T-cell	AIDS	- CD4 cells depletion; - Immune dysfunction; -IRIS after treatment with HAART
HTLV-1	Humans	CD4+ T-cell	ATL; HAM/TSP	↑ IFN-γ; ↑ TNF-α.
HTLV-2	Humans	CD8+ T-cell	Neuropathy	Immunosuppression
EBV	Humans	B cells	IMN; BL; HD; XLL; OHL	Immunosuppression
FeLV	Cats	CD4+ T-cell	Leukemia	Immunosuppression
BLV	Cattle	B cells	Leukemia; LS	Immunosuppression
MDV	Chickens	CD4+ T-cell	Marek's disease Marek's lymphoma	Immunosuppression
IBDV	Chickens	B cells	IBD	Immunosuppression

HIV= human immunodeficiency virus; AIDS = acquired immunodeficiency syndrome; IRIS= immune reconstitution inflammatory syndrome; HAART= highly active antiretroviral therapy; HTLV= human T-cell lymphotropic virus; ATL= adult T-cell leukemia; HAM/TSP=HTLV-1-associated myelopathy/ tropical spastic paraparesis; EBV= Epstein-Barr virus; IMN= infectious mononucleosis; BL= Burkitt's lymphoma; HD= Hodgkin's disease; XLL= X-linked lymphoproliferative syndrome; OHL= oral hairy leukoplakia; FeLV= feline leukemia virus; BLV= bovine leukemia virus; LS= Lymphosarcoma; MDV= Marek's disease virus; IBDV= infectious bursal disease virus; IBD= infectious bursal disease

Table 1. Common lymphotropic infections associated with immunosuppression

i. **HIV infection:** In HIV infection, immune dysfunction is likely due to combinatorial effects resulting from infection of immune cells (CD4+ T cells, macrophages, dendritic cells) with HIV, uncontrolled viral replication that impairs antigen presentation, increased mutations in *env* protein gp120 that leads to virus tropism and survival, increased activation of T helper cells by alloantigens, increased apoptosis by activated CD4+ T helper cells, down-regulation of CD4+ synthesis with functional impairment, and perturbation of cytokine pathways [7,16-19]. These immunologic defects can be partially restored in HIV patients treated with highly active antiretroviral therapy (HAART) [20]. Despite a reduced viral load and improved CD4+ T cells count, a paradoxical response known as immune reconstitution inflammatory syndrome (IRIS) has been evolved in HIV patients treated with HAART [21-23]. The induction of IRIS is worsened in HIV patients with preexisting opportunistic infections [24]. In essence, the severity of IRIS depends on CD4+ T cells count (≤ 100-200 cells/μl), degree of lymphocyte apoptosis or proliferation, and the degree of viral suppression and immune recovery after the initiation of treatment with HAART. All of these factors constitute a challenge to HIV vaccine development [25]. In animals, however, paradoxical immunosuppression associated with IRIS is rarely encountered due to the short life span of infected animals and variations in the care and management of sick animals compared to humans.

ii. **HTLV infection:** In HTLV infection, the virus preferentially infects CD4+ T cells and causes their transformation into malignant lymphoma *in vitro*. The majority of HTLV-infected patients are asymptomatic and few are carriers that may develop a chronic illness through time. The virus has 2 unique genes, *tax* and *rex*, in addition to the standard retroviral genes (*gag*, *pol*, and *env*) that play a central role in lymphocytes transformation. The HTLV-1 tax gene product is known to stimulate viral mRNA synthesis, interleukin (IL)-2 production, and IL-2 receptor (R) expression which are key elements for lymphocytes proliferation and transformation into malignant cells [9, 10]. The aberrant changes in T cells function during the transformation process may contribute to immunosuppression. However, in some patients, the humoral antibody response to HTLV antigens may be detected in sera of infected patients indicating that HTLV may not be the primary causes of all T cell lymphomas. In addition to T cell leukemia, some carriers of HTLV-1 may develop an inflammatory disease of the central nervous system called HTLV-1- associated myelopathy/tropical spastic paraparesis (HAM/TSP). Patients with HAM/TSP have increased HTLV-1 provirus load and increased numbers of HTLV-1-specific cytotoxic T lymphocytes (CTL, CD8+ T cells) that were restricted to the HTLV-1 tax protein. However, the HTLV-1-specific CTL of these patients have been demonstrated to produce IFN-γ and TNF-α that promote inflammation. Therefore, HTLV-1 tax-specific CTLs play a major role in the immunopathogenesis of HAM/TSP.

iii. **EBV infection:** Primary EBV infection causes infectious mononucleosis, a self limiting and silent disease in most inflicted patients. The virus exclusively infects B cells than any other cell type and persisted within the carrier's B cells to establish latent infection. *In vitro* EBV infection of human B lymphocytes has been demonstrated to induce B cell immortalization and proliferation [26]. The process carries the viral genome indefinitely and used for the generation of various lymphoblastoid cell lines. In addition to its B cells involvement, EBV infection has been demonstrated in epithelial cells of nasopharyngeal carcinoma as well as in the epithelial layer of oral hairy leukoplakia (OHL), a benign exclusive lesion in HIV individuals [11]. Despite its various clinical manifestations and lymphoid cells activation, EBV infection is common in immunocompromised patients. The control of EBV infection has been attributed to CTL (CD8+ T cells) [27] and the consequent immunosuppression is multifactorial effect.

iv. **FeLV infection:** Infection with FeLV is usually asymptomatic and is species-specific. Persistent infection emerges in carrier's cats and correlated well with persistent viremia that last for months [12]. The virus infects primarily T lymphocytes and spread to other lymphoid tissues including bone marrow and glandular epithelium. This broad infection lead to the development of leukemia, lymphoma, and non-regenerative anemia in persistently infected cats. Immunosuppression in pet cats showed suppressed antibody and T cell responses, prolonged allograft rejection times, thymic atrophy, and depletion of the paracortical zones in lymph nodes.

v. **BLV infection:** BLV infects primarily B cells and persisted to induce their transformation into cancerous cells after long latent periods [13]. In addition to B cells infection, BLV infect cells of the monocyte/macrophage lineage. Infection is usually silent but may progress to persistent lymphocytosis and tumor production. Immunosuppression due to BLV is largely contributed by altered gene expression for the cytokines IL-2, IL-6, IL-10, and IL-12, increased B cells apoptosis, down-regulation of TNF-α and its receptor, and alteration in cells signaling pathway.

vi. **MDV infection:** The pathogenesis of MDV that leads to lymphoma development with consequent immunosuppression [14] involves 4 stages: early cytolytic infection in which the virus spread from cell to cell and B cells were demonstrated as the primary targets for this stage; latent infection in which activated CD4+ T cells are the predominant targets in lymphoid organs as well as schwann cells of peripheral nerves and spinal ganglia; late cytolytic infection is characterized by permanent immunosuppression of T cells; and transformation stage in which T cells lymphoma develop with a dominant expression of Marek's disease tumor-associated surface antigen (MATSA). The resultant immunosuppression caused by MDV infection is largely attributed to loss of effector cells in major lymphoid organs, the bursa of Fabricius and the thymus as well as in bone marrow tissues. Consequently, this cytolytic infection leads to the development of atrophy at the bursa and thymus as well as aplasia in bone marrow cells. Studies by Calnek demonstrated that the degree of immunosuppression may be related to the pathotype of MDV isolates. However, the contribution of host factors in this immunosuppression needs to be elucidated.

vii. **IBDV infection:** Initial infection with IBDV involves lymphocytes and macrophages of gut- associated lymphoid tissues (GALT) followed by invasion of lymphoid follicles at the bursa of Fabricius, the primary source of B lymphocytes in avian species [15]. Since the bursa represents the primary target organ for viral replication, IgM positive B lymphocytes are the target cells for viral lysis. The consequent infection results in bursal atrophy and B cells depletion. Indeed, B cells depletion extends to other lymphoid tissues including the thymus, GALT, and the Harderian gland. Therefore, the production of antibodies will be impaired and the cellular immune response will be diminished in chickens infected with IBDV. The inflicted damage to the bursal tissue coupled with B cells depletion, and loss of T cells function contribute to the development of immunosuppression in chickens infected with IBDV. Restoration of immunity by adoptive transfer may be possible but no paradoxical inflammatory response has been demonstrated.

3. Immunosuppression induced by bacterial infections

It is well established that infection with some intracellular bacteria may have indirect effects on the immune system with consequent induction of immunosuppression. Among the leading causal agents, *Mycobacterium tuberculosis, Ehrlichia chaffeensis, Brucella melitensis, Coxiella burnetti, Bartonella* Sp. and *Nocardia farcinica*. However, in immunocompromised patients, infections with mycobacterial species or agents of bacterial pneumonia are commonly observed in clinical practice. In AIDS patients, disseminated infections with *Mycobacterium tuberculosis* or *Mycobacterium avium* complex are prominent [7, 28]. In contrast, deadly infection with *Nocardia farcinica* [29] has been reported in an immunocompromised patient with type II diabetes and end-stage renal failure. Thus, infection with opportunistic pathogens may be more deleterious to the host than infection caused by pathogens that primarily induce immunosuppression. In general, the underlying mechanism of immunosuppression due to bacteria varies according to the host-parasite cellular interactions, and the elicited host immune mediators that cause a shift in the balance between Th1 and Th2 responses. For instance, sustained production of transforming growth factor (TGF)-β has been associated with immunosuppression in patients with chronic brucellosis [30] or tuberculosis [31]. Further, other mechanisms exist for pathogens induced immunosuppression and they are largely attributed to a defective interaction between the microbe (bacteria, viruses, fungi, or protozoan parasites) and cells of the immune system (macrophages, dendritic cells, lymphocytes, natural killer). Support for this notion stems from the ability of certain intracellular pathogens to prevent phagolysosome biogenesis, inhibition of cellular autophagy, and inhibition of antigen presentation [28, 32-35]. The prototype models for these mechanisms have been established by several investigators who studied the interaction of *Mycobacterium tuberculosis* with the macrophage [36]. In essence, the induced immnuosuppression is the target of several microbial virulence factors in an effort to establish a disease process at their predilection sites. Major virulence factors associated with bacterial infection include toxin production, polysaccharide or polypeptide capsule formation, and secretion of degradative enzymes that promote tissue invasiveness, proteineous pili and mucosal adhesins. Individuals with prolonged immunosuppression offer a rich environment for microbial growth, replication, and pathogencicity conduction. Consequently, the resulting disease will be much exacerbated due to microbial abundance and invasiveness secondary to shift in balance between proinflammatory and anti-inflammatory factors of the host. Therefore, activation of the antimicrobial activity of leukocytes as well as induction of immune cytokines (interferon (IFN)-γ, interleukin (IL)-12, IL-2 and tumor necrosis factor (TNF)-α) are crucial elements in the restoration of cellular immunity [3] in patients with secondary immunosuppression due to bacteria.

In general, the extent of microbial immunosuppression is dependent on the balance of proinflammatory and anti-inflammatory mediators following injury and/or infection, disease duration (acute, chronic), immunocompetence of the inflicted host, dosage rate and treatment regimen of anti-microbial drugs used, and a synergy of these therapy, if exist. The balance between these factors had a major impact on the restoration of immunity and/or disease progression.

4. Immunosuppression induced by opportunistic viral infections

In clinical practice, the most common opportunistic viral infections that were encountered in immnuocompromised patients include, cytomegalovirus (CMV), Epstein-Barr virus (EBV), and human herpesvirus 8 (HHV8). In addition to their primary causes of disease in immunocompetent hosts, these viruses have been detected in blood and lesions of immnuocompromised patients with AIDS, renal and bone marrow transplants as well as in patients with neoplasms [24, 26, 37, 38]. Latency of infection is commonly encountered with these viruses while congenital infection is prominently seen in CMV. Therefore, newborns with immunological defects are at a highest risk of CMV disease. However, infection with HHV8 causes Kaposi's sarcoma, the most common cancer in patients with AIDS. The inflicted immunosuppression due to these viral infections is usually dual in nature and largely attributed to inhibition of T cell responses.

5. Immunosuppression induced by antimicrobial drugs

Although most antimicrobial drugs are safe and effective in patients with infectious diseases, some are toxic to the host cells causing alterations in immune cells function that may lead to immunosuppression [39]. Major immunotoxic effects attributed to antimicrobial drugs include neutropenia and agranulocytosis, autoimmune diseases development, or hypersensitivity reactions. These toxic effects had influenced the therapeutic choice of some antimicrobial drugs despite their clinical interventions. The mechanistic events involved in the alteration of immune cells with consequent immunosuppression are not well established. However, in clinical practice, the antiviral agents, Ganciclovir, Ribavirin, and Zidovudine as well as the antibacterial agents, Chloramphenicol, Rifampicin, Sulfa derivatives, Macrolides (Azithromycin, Clarithromycin, or Erythromycin) and β-lactam (Penicillins, Cephalosporins) antibiotics are leading causes of neutropenia, agranulocytosis, inhibition of phagocyte function, and immunotoxic effects on bone marrow precursor cells. The latter effect is dose dependent and usually diagnosed by adding the patient's serum and the antibiotic drug under investigation to an *in vitro* culture of bone marrow cells. However, in addition to toxic effects on immune cells, some antibacterial drugs or their metabolites have been implicated in allergic reactions as exemplified by the ß-lactam, Penicillin G. The sensitizing capacity of any antimicrobial drug depends solely on its ability to interact irreversibly with tissue proteins to form complexes that provoke immune effector cells. Consequently, an IgE-mediated allergic reaction would be induced and the competence of these patients to mount a specific immune response is paralyzed. Other immunologic caveats attributed to antibacterial drugs include production of immune complexes as shown in drug-induced systemic lupus erythematosus with Isoniazid, Sulfonamides, Streptomycins, and Penicillins or cell-mediated hypersensitivity reactions as shown in contact dermatitis with Penicillins, Neomycins, and Nitrofurantoin. Again, the immunocompetence of patients with drug-induced autoimmune disorders or hypersensitivity reactions would be jeopardized unless reconstituted. In any event, alterations in immune cells caused by these drugs are expected to affect the immune function with consequent immunosuppression. At this stage, the host is more prone to infection with several opportunistic pathogens.

In contrast, immunosuppression induced by immunosuppressant drugs had a profound effect on lymphocytes function [1]. Common drugs used for this purpose include Calcineurin inhibitors (Cyclosporine A or Tacrolimus), glucocorticoids, and Mycophenolate mofetil. The resultant immunosuppression induced by these drugs led the host to be more vulnerable to opportunistic infections as evidenced in most solid organ- transplants (e.g. kidneys, liver, and pancreas) or cancer patients [40]. In this population of immunocompromised patients, the predominately encountered opportunistic infections include *Mycobacterium tuberculosis*, *Mycobacterium* other than tuberculosis (MOTT), *Aspergillus* sp., *Crptococcus neoformans*, *cytomegalovirus*, and/or *pneumocystis jirovecii* pneumonia.

6. Immunological evaluation of immunosuppression

Despite the application of various treatment modalities for the control of infection in immunocompromised patients, a limited number of methods are available for the evaluation of immunosuppression. Most of the available methods rely on T or B cells function as exemplified by lymphocytes activation and proliferation, cytokines production, leukocytes count and expression, and specific antibody production. Although these methods are well established in several research studies, only ELISA for antibody and cytokine assays and flow cytometry for leukocyte counts and markers expression are commonly used in clinical referral laboratories. However, in routine diagnostic laboratories, none of these methods are approached properly. Therefore, there is an urgent need to scrutinize the fidelity of these methods in the evaluation of immunosuppression in most clinical laboratories. The rationale is to identify the immunocompetence of the host before the institution of any therapeutic intervention [41].

For routine isolation of lymphocytes and monocytes in anti-coagulant-treated blood, density gradient centrifugation [42] is used after lysis of red cells. For the isolation of neutrophils, dextran sedimentation is firstly used for the isolation of leukocytes-rich preparation followed by density gradient sedimentation in Percoll A. In both settings, the viability of leukocytes can be measured by trypan blue exclusion and phenotyping of leukocytes preparation can be established by flow cytometry using the commercially available monoclonal antibodies against leukocyte surface antigens (CD). HLA typing can be conducted similarly. For functional analysis of phagocytic cells (macrophages or neutrophils), limited methods are used including phagocytosis (ingestion), opsonisation (enhanced attachment), and chemotaxis (directed cell motility).

7. Conclusions

Immunosuppression is a sword of two edges; while it is beneficial when intentionally instituted to maintain the life in solid organ-transplants or cancer patients, it is perilous in patients with primary immunodeficiency diseases, patients with HIV infection, and/or patients with multiple organ failure. Therefore, the mediating factors must be scrutinized, the leukocyte counts and function must be stated and the pros and cons of an immunosuppressant medicine must be thoroughly evaluated before being prescribed.

8. Acknowledgements

The authors acknowledged the support of King Faisal Specialist Hospital and Research Centre, the King Saud University, and the King Abdulaziz City for Science and Technology for the financial support.

9. References

[1] Auphan, N., DiDonato, J.A., Rosette, C., Helmberg, A., and Karin, M., (1995). Immunosuppression by glucocorticoids: inhibition of NF-kβ activation through induction of I kappa biosynthesis, Science, 270: 286-290.

[2] Delves, P.J., and Roitt, I.M., (2000). The immune system. First of two parts, N. Engl. J. Med. 343: 37-49.

[3] Delves, P.J., and Roitt, I.M., (2000). The immune system. Second of two parts, N. Engl. J. Med. 343: 108-117.

[4] Figueroa, J.E., and Densen, P., (1991). Infectious diseases associated with complement deficiencies, Clin. Microbiol. Rev., 4: 359-395.

[5] Gaspar, H.B., Sharifi, R., Gilmour, K.C., and Thrasher, A.J., (2002). X-linked lymphoproliferative disease: clinical, diagnosis and molecular prospective, Br. J. Haematol. 119: 585-595.

[6] Haskó, G., Deitch, E.A., Szabó, C., Németh, Z.H., and Vizi, E.S., (2002). Adenosine: a potential mediator of immunosuppression in multiple organ failure, Curr. Opin. Pharmacol. 2: 440-444.

[7] Douek, D.C., Brenchley, J.M., Betts, M.R., Ambrozak, D.R., Hill, B.J., Okamoto, Y., Casazza, J.P., Kuruppu, J., Kuntsman, K., Wolinsky, K., Grossman, Z., Dybul, M., Oxenius, A., Price, D.A., Connors, M., and Koup, R.A., (2002). HIV preferentially infects HIV-specific CD4+ T cells, Nature, 417: 95-98.

[8] Uchiyama, T., (1997). Human T cell leukemia virus type 1(HTLV-1) and human diseases, Ann. Rev. Immunol. 15: 15-37.

[9] Yamano, Y., Cohen, C.J., Takenouchi, N., Yao, K., Tomaru, U., Li, H-C., Reiter, Y., and Jacobson, S., (2004). Increased expression of human T lymphocyte virus type 1 (HTLV-1) Tax11-19 peptide-human histocompatibility leukocyte antigen A*201 complexes on CD4+ CD25+ T cells detected by peptide-specific, major histocompatibility complex-restricted antibodies in patients with HTLV-1-associated neurologic disease, J. Exp. Med. 199: 1367-1377.

[10] Yamano, Y., Nagai, M., Brennan, M., Mora, C.A., Soldan, S.S., Tomaru, U., Takenouchi, N., Izumo, S., Osame, M., and Jacobson, S., (2002). Correlation of human T-cell lymphotropic virus type 1 (HTLV-1) mRNA with proviral DNA load, virus-specific CD8 (+) T cells, and disease severity in HTLV-1-associated myelopathy (HAM/TSP), Blood. 99: 88-94.

[11] Faulkner, G.C., Krajewski, A.S., and Crawford, D.H., (2000). The ins and outs of EBV infection, Trends Microbiol. 8:185-189.

[12] Neil, J.C., Fulton, R., Rigby, M., and Stewart, M., (1991). Feline leukemia virus: Generation of pathogenic and oncogenic variants, Curr. Top. Microbiol. Immunol. 171: 67-94.

[13] Gillet, N., Florins, A., Boxus, M., Burteau, C., Nigro, A., Vandermeers, F., Balon, H., Bouzar, A-B., Defoiche, J., Burny, A., Reichert, M., Kettmann, R., and Willems, L., (2007). Mechanisms of leukemogenesis induced by bovine leukemia virus: prospects for novel anti-retroviral therapies in human, Retrovirol. 4: 18.

[14] Calnek, B.W., (2001). Pathogenesis of Marex's disease virus infection, In: Kanji Hirai (Ed.), Marek's Disease, Springer-Verlag, Berlin Heidelberg, Germany, p. 25-49.

[15] Van den Berg, T.P., (2000). Acute infectious bursal disease in poultry: a review, Avian Pathol. 29: 175-194.

[16] Brenchley, J.M., Price, D.A., Schacker, T.W., Asher, T.E., Silvestri, G., Rao, S., Kazzaz, Z., Bornstein, E., Lambotte, O., Altman, D., Blazar, B.R., Rodriguez, B., Teixeira-Johnson, L., Landay, A., Martin, J.N., Hecht, F.M., Picker, L.J., Lederman, M.M., Deeks, S.G., and Douek, D.C., (2006). Microbial translocation is a cause of systemic immune activation in chronic HIV infection, Nat Med. 12: 1365-1371.

[17] Ho, D.D., Moudgil, T., and Alam, M., (1989). Quantitation of human immunodeficiency virus type 1 in the blood of infected persons, N. Engl. J. Med., 321: 1621-1625.

[18] Lyerly, H.K., Matthews, T.J., Langlois, A.J., Bolognesi, D.P., and Weinhold, K.J., (1987). Human T-cell lymphotropic virus III_B glycoprotein (gp120) bound to CD4 determinants on normal lymphocytes and expressed by infected cells serves as target for immune attack, Proc. Natl. Acad. Sci. USA, 84: 4601-4605.

[19] Trautmann, L., Janbazian, L., Chomont, N., Said, E., Gimmig, S., Bessette, B., Boulassel, M-R, Delwart, E., Sepulveda, H., Balderas, R.S., Routy, J-P., Haddad, E.K., and Sekaly, R-P., (2006). Upregulation of PD-1 expression on HIV-specific CD8+ T cells leads to reversible immune dysfunction, Nat. Med. 12: 1198- 1202.

[20] French, M.A., Price, P., and Stone, S.F., (2004). Immune restoration disease after antiretroviral therapy, AIDS.18:1615-1627.

[21] Cheng, V.C., Yuen, K.Y., Chan, W.M., Wong, S.S., Ma, E.S., and Chan, R.M., (2000). Immunerestitution disease involving the innate and adaptive response, Clin. Infect. Dis. 30: 882-892.

[22] Choi, Y., Townend, J., Vincent, T., Zaidi, I., Sarge-Njie, R., Jaye, A., and Clifford, D.B., (2011). Neurologic manifestations of human immunodeficiency virus-2: dementia, myelopathy, and neuropathy in West Africa, J. Neurovirol., 17: 166-175.

[23]Costello, D.J., Gonzalez, R.G., Frosch, M.P., (2011). Case 18-2011: A 35-year-old HIV-positive woman with headache and altered mental status, N. Engl. J. Med.364: 2343-2352.

[24] Guihot, A., Dupin, N., Marcelin, A.G., Gorin, I., Bedin, A-S., Bossi, P., Galicier, L., Oksenhendler, E., Autran, B., and Carcelain, C., (2006), Low T cell responses to human herpesvirus 8 in patients with AIDS-related and classic Kaposi sarcoma, J. Infect. Dis. 194: 1078-1088.

[25] Johnston, M.I., and Fauci, A.S., (2008). An HIV vaccine—Challenges and Prospects, N. Engl. J. Med. 359: 888-890.

[26] Calender, A., Billaud, M., Aubry, J-P., Banchereau, J., Vuillaume, M., and Lenoir, G., (1987). Epstein-Barr virus (EBV) induces expression of B-cell activation markers on *in vitro* infection of EBV-negative B-lymphoma cells, Proc. Natl. Acad. Sci. USA, 84: 8060-8064.

[27] Rickinson, A.B., and Moss, D.J., (1997). Human cytotoxic T lymphocyte responses to Epstein-Barr virus infection, Ann. Rev. Immunol. 15: 405-431.

[28] Deretic, V., Singh, S., Master, S., Harris, J., Roberts, E., Kyei, G., Davis, A., de Haro, S., Naylor, J., Lee, H-H., Vergne, I., (2006). *Mycobacterium tuberculosis* inhibition of phagolysosome biogenesis and autophagy as a host defence mechanism, Cellular Microbiol. 8: 719-727.

[29] Sonesson, A., Öqvist, B., Hagstam, P., Björkman-Burtscher, I.M., Miörner, H., and Petersson, A.C., (2004). An immunocompromised patient with systemic vasculitis suffering from cerebral abscesses due to *Nocardia farcinica* identified by 16S rRNA gene universal PCR, Nephrol. Dial. Transplant. 19: 2896-2900.

[30] Elfaki, M.G., and Al-Hokail, A.A., (2009). Transforming growth factor β production correlates with depressed lymphocytes function in humans with brucellosis. Microbes Infect, 11: 1089-1096.

[31] Toosi, Z., Gogate, P., Shiratsuchi, H., Young, T., and Ellner, J. J., (1995). Enhanced production of TGF-β by blood monocytes from patients with active tuberculosis and presence of TGF-β in tuberculous granulomatous lung lesions, J. Immunol. 154:465-473.

[32] Eisenstein, T.K., (2001). Implications of *Salmonella*-induced nitric oxide (NO) for host defense and vaccines: NO, an antimicrobial, antitumor, immunosuppressive and immunoregulatory molecule, Microbes Infect., 3: 1223-1231.

[33] Kurita-Ochiai, T., and Ochiai, K., (1996). Immunosuppressive factor from *Actinobacillus actinomycetemcomitans* down regulates cytokine production, Infect. Immun., 64: 50-54.

[34] Mariotti, S., Teloni, R., Iona, E., Fattorini, L., Romagnoli, G., Gagliardi, M.C., Orefici, G., and Nisini, R., (2004). *Mycobacterium tuberculosis* diverts alpha interferon-induced monocyte differentiation from dendritic cells into immunoprivileged macrophage-like host cells, Infect. Immun.72: 4385-4392.

[35] Vergne, I., Chua, J., Lee, H-H., Lucas, M., Belisle, J., and Deretic, V., (2005). Mechanism of phagolysosome biogenesis block by viable *Mycobacterium tuberculosis*, PNAS. 102: 4033-4038.

[36] Schlesinger, L.S., Azad, A.K., Torrelles, J.B., Roberts, E., Vergne, I., and Deretic, V., (2008). Determinants of phagocytosis, phagosome biogenesis and autophagy for *Mycobacterium tuberculosis*, In: Stefan H.E. Kaufmann, Warwick J. Britton (Eds), Handbook of Tuberculosis: Immunology and Cell Biology, Wiley-VCH Verlag GmbH & Co. KGaA, Weinheim, Germany, p. 1-22.

[37] Brander, C., Suscovich, T., Lee, Y., Nguyen, P.T., O'Conner, P., Seebach, J., Jones, N.G., van Gorder, M., Walker, B. D., and Scadden, D.T., (2000). Impaired CTL recognition of cells latently infected with Kaposi's sarcoma-associated herpes virus, J. Immunol. 165: 2077-2083.

[38] Wingard, J.R., Chen, D.Y., Burns, W.H., Fuller, D.J., Braine, H.G., Yeager, A.M., Kaiser, H., Burke, P.J., Graham, M.L., and Santos, G.W., (1988). Cytomegalovirus infection after autologous bone marrow transplantation with comparison to infection after allogeneic bone marrow transplantation, Blood 71: 1432-1437.

[39] Labro, M-T., (2005). Influence of antibacterial drugs on the immune system, In: Frans P. Nijkamp, Michael J. Parnham (Eds.), Principles of Immunopharmacology, 2nd edition, Birkhauser Verlag, Basel, Switzerland, p. 407-439.

[40] Wadhwa, P.D., and Morrison, V.A., (2006). Infectious complications of chronic lymphocytic leukemia, Semin. Oncol. 33: 240-249.

[41] Folds, J.D., and Schmitz, J.L., (2003). Clinical and laboratory assessment of immunity, J. Allergy Clin. Immunol. 111(suppl.2):S702-S711.

[42] Böyum, A., (1968). Isolation of mononuclear cells and granulocytes from human blood, Scand. J. Clin. Lab. Invest. Suppl. 97: 77-89.

12

Measles Virus Infection: Mechanisms of Immune Suppression

Xuelian Yu[1] and Reena Ghildyal[2]
[1]*Shanghai Municipal Centers of Disease Control and Prevention, Microbiology Laboratory, Shanghai,*
[2]*Respiratory Virology Group, Faculty of Applied Science, University of Canberra, Canberra*
[1]*PR China*
[2]*Australia*

1. Introduction

Measles virus (MV) is a highly contagious respiratory pathogen that causes systemic disease; most individuals recover with lifelong immunity to MV. Enormous progress toward measles elimination has been made worldwide, in large part due to the availability of a safe and effective vaccine (CDC, 2000; WHO, 2005; 2009; 2010). However, measles infections still cause 500,000 deaths annually, mostly due to subsequent opportunistic infections associated with MV induced immune-suppression (Wild, 1999). Prior to the introduction of vaccines and a global eradication programme coordinated by the World Health Organisation (WHO) (Wild, 1999), global death rates were as high as 7–8 million children annually. The introduction of a live measles vaccine has significantly reduced the incidence of acute measles in industrialized countries. In developing countries however, measles is still an important health problem and the major viral killer of children.

2. The disease

General symptoms of an acute MV infection consist of a maculopapular rash, dry cough, coryza, fever, conjunctivitis and photophobia, usually preceded by characteristic spots on the mucosal surface of the mouth, called Koplik spots. Complications consist of diarrroea, pneumonia, laryngotracheobronchitis, otitis media and stomatitis. In developing countries, increased case fatality is associated with age at infection and nutritional status. Around 0.1% of measles cases develop acute measles encephalitis during or shortly after acute measles with a mortality rate of 10-30%; maybe as a consequence of MV induced autoimmune reaction against brain antigens (Moench *et al.*, 1988). The most serious complications of MV infection occur within the central nervous system (CNS); three most common are acute disseminated encephalomyelitis (ADEM) (Liebert, 1997; Rima & Duprex, 2006), subacute sclerosing panencephalitis (SSPE) and, in immunocompromised individuals, measles inclusion body encephalitis (MIBE) (Chadwick *et al.*, 1982; Moench *et al.*, 1988).
ADEM occurs 5–6 days after the initial rash in about 1/1000 infected children (Leake *et al.*, 2004; Menge *et al.*, 2005). It is less common in vaccinees and children under 2 years of age

(Menge *et al.*, 2005; Nasr *et al.*, 2000; Rima & Duprex, 2006). Symptoms occur once the initial rash has disappeared and consist of a sudden recurrence of fever, decreased consciousness, seizures and multifocal neurological signs.
SSPE and MIBE are rare late complications of measles (Chadwick *et al.*, 1982; Moench *et al.*, 1988) and can occur months or even years after acute infection and are invariably fatal (Liebert, 1997; Rima & Duprex, 2006; Sips *et al.*, 2007). These fatal diseases exhibit virological and immunological features quite different from those seen in acute measles or measles encephalitis. Both diseases have their basis in a persistent MV infection in brain cells, where neurons, glial cells and endothelial cells can be infected. However, giant cell formation and budding virus particles as typically found in measles infection are virtually absent in SSPE and MIBE, indicating defective MV replication in CNS tissue. This is supported by the observation that MV cannot be isolated by standard procedures from diseased CNS tissue, and only occasionally by co-cultivation methods.

2.1 Clinical epidemiology

Immunization has altered the epidemiology of measles by reducing the susceptible individuals in the population, causing an increase in the average age at infection and resulting in a lengthening of the inter-epidemic period (Cutts & Markowitz, 1994). Very young infants are protected from measles by maternal antibody. In countries with poor immunization, the majority of measles patients are children because the older populations have gained immunity by natural infection. However, in countries with high rates of immunization, as elevated herd immunity reduces transmission and indirectly protects children from infection, the average age for measles patients has increased (Black, 1982). Therefore, when outbreaks occur in areas of sustained high vaccine coverage, an increasingly large portion of the cases may be in older individuals who are susceptible because of primary or secondary vaccine failure. For example in 1973, persons 20 years of age and older accounted for only 3% of cases. In 1994, adults accounted for 24%, and in 2001, for 48% of all reported cases.

2.1.1 Countries with no endemic measles virus

Measles is very rare in countries and regions of the world that are able to sustain high vaccination coverage. In North and South America, Finland, among others, endemic measles transmission has been interrupted through vaccination (see Figure 1A). In Europe, Australia, Mongolia, New Zealand, Philippines, the Pacific Island Nations and the Arab Gulf States, measles transmission has been interrupted or is at very low levels (WHO, 1995).
The importance of maintaining high vaccine coverage even after eradication has been achieved, is exemplified by the United States (USA) experience. During the 1980s, measles was very rare in USA, but from 1989 through 1991 a dramatic increase in cases occurred. A total of 27,786 cases were reported in 1990, of whom 64 died, the largest annual number of deaths from measles since 1971. The most important cause of the measles resurgence of 1989–1991 was low vaccine coverage (Lee *et al.*, 2004). After intensive efforts to vaccinate preschool-aged children, reported cases of measles declined rapidly. Since 1993, fewer than 500 cases have been reported annually, falling to <200 cases per year since 1997 (Papania *et al.*, 2004). A record low annual total of 37 cases were reported in 2004. There are still sporadic cases of measles in USA due to importation by visitors from other countries or US citizens travelling abroad becoming infected during travel and spreading the infection to unvaccinated or unprotected individuals (CDC, 2005).

2.1.2 Countries with endemic transmission of measles virus

Despite significant progress in Africa and Asia in reduction of measles-related mortality, countries like the Democratic Republic of Congo, Ethiopia, Niger, Nigeria (CDC, 2009), India and Pakistan (CDC, 2007) continue to sustain large numbers of measles-related deaths. In 2003 India reported more than 47,000 measles cases; the reported 115 measles-related deaths are likely to be an underestimate (Singh *et al.*, 1994; Sivasankaran *et al.*, 2006; WHO, 2008) (see Figure 1A). Reported vaccine coverage has been consistently high (>80%), but the estimated coverage is much lower (40–70%), and varies between states (WHO, 2008). Similarly Niger still reports large outbreaks (CDC, 2009); from November 2003 to June 2004,

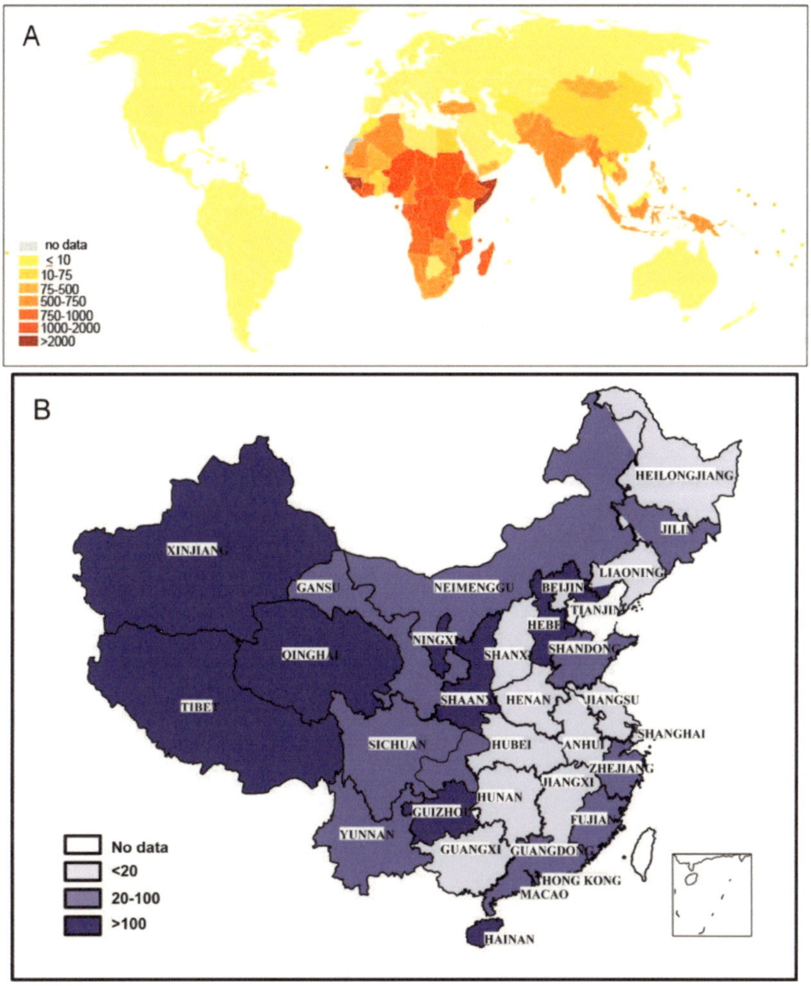

Fig. 1. Incidence of measles virus infection in the world and in China.
A. Regional map of the world, colour coded to show the incidence of measles per 100,000 population in any one year. Guide to the various colours used is shown on the left.
B. Average incidence of measles infection in China (2004-2007) Map of China showing various states, with colour coding to highlight areas of high (>100 cases per 100,000 population), mid (20-100) and low (<20) incidence. Guide to the colours used is shown on the left

11,073 cases were reported with 75% of cases and 86% of deaths being in children under five (WHO, 2008). Unacceptably high mortality related to measles epidemics in Niger, Nigeria, and Chad were reported during 2003-2005, with the overall case fatality ratios (CFRs) of 3.9%, 7.0% and 2.8%, respectively; CFR among under-fives were 4.6%, 10.8% and 4.0% (Grais *et al.*, 2007). The continuing high burden of preventable measles mortality during these epidemics results from poor access to appropriate treatment and the incomplete implementation of the WHO/UNICEF measles mortality-reduction strategy (Grais *et al.*, 2007).

3. Global vaccine initiative

In 2001, WHO and United Nations Children's Fund (UNICEF) developed a 5-year strategic plan to reduce global measles mortality by 50% in the year 2005, compared to 1999 levels (WHO/UNICEF, 2001). In regions with established measles elimination goals, the objective was to achieve and maintain interruption of indigenous measles transmission.
WHO estimates that measles is responsible for 4% of the 6 million annual deaths in children <5 years of age. Ninety-eight percent of these deaths occur in developing countries (Organization, 2005). In 2004, WHO reported an estimated 76% coverage of measles containing vaccines (MCV) world-wide (WHO, 2006). With 30 million estimated annual cases (WHO-UNICEF, 2001), most of them in unvaccinated individuals, MCV is still under-utilized. Of 23.3 million infants in 2007 who missed receiving their first dose of measles vaccine by the age of 12 months, 15.3 million (65%) reside in 8 highly populated countries (WHO, 2008).

3.1 Current status of measles eradication in the WHO Western Pacific region

In the WHO Western Pacific region (excluding China), reported confirmed measles cases decreased by 86% between 2000 and 2008 and measles mortality dropped by 92% (WHO/UNICEF, 2009). Progress has been made, and 24 of the 37 countries in this region have either achieved or nearly achieved elimination (WHO/UNICEF, 2009). However, China reported 109,023 measles cases in 2007 and 131,441 cases in 2008. A large measles outbreak in Japan resulted in >18,000 reported cases in 2007 and 11,015 cases in 2008. Intensified efforts to eliminate measles by Member States, particularly in China and Japan, are needed to achieve the WHO goal of measles elimination in the Western Pacific by 2012. China and Japan account for 82% of the region's population and >97% of its confirmed measles cases (WHO, 2009).

3.1.1 Current challenges in China

Prior to widespread use of measles vaccine, 2000 to 15000 cases per million population were reported each year in China (Wu, 2000). Monovalent measles vaccine was first used in China in 1965 and came into widespread use in 1978 when the China Expanded Program on Immunization (EPI) was established, covering all provinces in 1983 (Wang *et al.*, 2003; Ze, 2002). In 1986, the national 2-dose regimen was implemented (Wang *et al.*, 2003). To support continued progress in measles control, the Ministry of Health issued the *Plan for Acceleration of Measles Control in China* (CMOH, 1997b) and *National Strategic Plan for Measles Surveillance* in 1997 (CMOH, 1997a). These efforts enabled significant progress in measles control.

Measles prevalence varies significantly across the 31 provinces of China. The developed provinces of Eastern China have lower disease incidence with higher number of adult patients and more cases who have a history of immunisation but are susceptible because of primary or secondary vaccine failure. The resource-limited provinces located in Western China have a high measles prevalence with majority of patients being under 14 years of age with no measles vaccination history (CMOH, 1997a) (Figure 1B).

Although the developed Eastern provinces have moved ved from outbreak prevention to measles elimination, measles outbreaks still occur. A dramatic increase in measles cases in Zhejiang (see Figure 1B) was observed in 2005, with an incidence rate higher than 350 per million population (Zuo *et al.*, 2006). 51.4% of the total reported patients were migrant workers from other regions of China, of whom only 21.4% reported a vaccination history, in contrast to 33.5% of all patients who were permanent residents (Zuo *et al.*, 2006). In Shanghai, 2,838 measles cases were reported in 2005 (He *et al.*, 2006) compared with 415 in the previous year (Hu *et al.*, 2005). Migrant workers accounted for 68.1% of the total reported measles cases from 2000 to 2004 of whom, only 6.5% had a vaccination history (He *et al.*, 2006). Additional to the high measles incidence among hard to reach migrant workers, the Eastern provinces also face increased adult measles incidence. About 53.3% of measles patients were older than 20 years of age in Shanghai from 2000 to 2004 (He *et al.*, 2006), while 49.1% of the reported patients were older than 15 years in Zhejiang (Zuo *et al.*, 2006).

Different disease patterns were found in the less developed Western provinces including Qinghai, Tibet, Guizhou, and Xinjiang (Figure 1B). Measles epidemics occur every 3-4 years in these provinces. A dramatic increase in measles incidence was reported in 2004 in Xinjiang (301 cases per million population); 85% cases were younger than 14 years, and 32% of the patients had a vaccination history (Yu *et al.*, 2007b). Later in the same year, an effective measles mass vaccination campaign was implemented covering all children between 8 months and 14 years of age; only 259 measles cases (0.14 cases per million population) were reported in 2005 (Yu *et al.*, 2006). Similarly, in Guizhou, the measles incidence was 500 cases per million population in 2004; following a mass vaccination campaign, it decreased to 14.3 and 20.6 per million population respectively in 2005 and 2006 (Zhu *et al.*, 2008). In contrast to the Eastern provinces, the majority of the cases were children (Du *et al.*, 2010). Furthermore, in contrast to the developed provinces, fewer measles cases reported a vaccination history, e.g., only 18.1% and 32% of measles cases had measles vaccination history in Guizhou in 2008 (Du *et al.*, 2010) and in Xinjiang in 2004 (Yu *et al.*, 2007b), respectively. Clearly, region specific strategies are needed for control of measles in China.

In recent years, the percentage of pre-vaccination infants with measles has increased in all provinces (Zuo *et al.*, 2006). Multiple studies addressing this issue (Li, 2001; Lu *et al.*, 2008; Zhou *et al.*, 2003) suggest that the low antibody levels in child-bearing-women are insufficient to protect their babies from measles infection. Therefore, child-bearing-women should be included in the target population during measles mass vaccination campaigns.

Recent studies have found that liver dysfunction and pneumonia are very common in hospitalized adult measles patients as seen in outbreaks in Zhejiang and Shanghai (Jiang *et al.*, 2007; Kong & Zhang, 2009; Liang *et al.*, 2005; Ma & Song, 2009; Yu *et al.*, 2007a). Interestingly, the clinical manifestation of measles infection in hospitalized children is quite different, with almost no liver dysfunction being reported, while pneumonia is the most common complication (Kong & Zhang, 2009; Wang *et al.*, 2010; Yu *et al.*, 2009). The difference in the disease symptoms is not due to differing vaccination histories; most adult patients did not know their vaccination history (Liang *et al.*, 2005; Yu *et al.*, 2007a) and the majority of hospitalized children were infants <2 years of age without previous measles vaccination (Wang *et al.*, 2010; Yu *et al.*, 2009).

4. Infectious cycle of MV and clinical progression

MV has an incubation period of around 14 days and the infected person is contagious for around 2 to 4 days before the rash appears and then 2 to 5 days after the rash appears. So, in total the infected person can spread the disease to others for 4 to 9 days.

Initial infection is established in the respiratory tract with virus replication in tracheal and bronchial epithelial cells and pulmonary macrophages (Sakaguchi *et al.*, 1986). From the respiratory tract, spread extends to local lymphatic tissues. The MV infection runs its course for around 2 weeks usually without causing any complications (Griffin, 2006). Amplification of virus in regional lymph nodes results in viremia and spread of virus through the blood to infect a variety of organs including the skin, conjunctivae, kidney, lung, gastrointestinal tract, respiratory mucosa, genital mucosa, and liver (Esolen *et al.*, 1995; Esolen *et al.*, 1993; Forthal *et al.*, 1992; Peebles, 1967; Takahashi *et al.*, 1996). Viremia and systemic infection inevitably occur before host defence mechanisms control viral replication and clear infected cells (McChesney *et al.*, 1997). Lymphoid organs and tissues (e.g., thymus, spleen, lymph nodes, appendix, and tonsils) are prominent sites of virus replication (Sakaguchi *et al.*, 1986).

4.1 Clinical symptoms of measles

After an incubation period of 8-12 days, measles begins with increasing fever (to 39-40.5 °C) cough, coryza, and conjunctivitis (Robbins, 1962). Symptoms intensify over the next 2-4 days before the onset of rash and peak on the first day of rash. The rash is usually first noted on the face and neck, appearing as discrete erythematous lesions. The lesions increase in number for 2 or 3 days, especially on the trunk and the face, where they frequently become confluent. Discrete lesions are usually seen on the distal extremities, and with careful observation, small numbers of lesions can be found on the palms of 25%-50% of those infected (Robbins, 1962). The rash lasts for 3-7 days and then fades in the same manner as it appeared. An exaggerated desquamation is commonly seen in malnourished children (Morley, 1974; Robbins, 1962; Scheifele & Forbes, 1972). Fever usually persists for 2 or 3 days after the onset of the rash, and the cough may persist for as many as 10 days (Robbins, 1962).

Koplik's spots appearing as discrete, tiny, gray-white papules on a dull-red base on the buccal mucosa, usually appear 1 day before the onset of rash and persist for 2 or 3 days (Suringa *et al.*, 1970). Koplik's spots have been reported in 60%-70% of patients with measles but are probably present in most persons who develop measles (Babbott & Gordon, 1954). Photophobia from iridocyclitis, sore throat, headache, abdominal pain, and generalized mild lymphadenopathy are also common.

Milder forms of measles occur in children and adults with pre-existing partial immunity. Infants who have low levels of passively acquired maternal antibody and persons who receive blood products that contain antibody often have subclinical infections or minimal symptoms that may not be diagnosed as measles (Cherry *et al.*, 1972; Edmonson *et al.*, 1990). Vaccination protects 90% of recipients against disease, but after exposure to natural

measles, some vaccinees develop enhanced antibody response associated with mild symptoms and may have rash with little or no fever (Chen *et al.*, 1990; Smith *et al.*, 1982; Whittle *et al.*, 1999).
Atypical measles has been reported in children who received formalin inactivated (killed) measles vaccine that was in use in the USA from 1963 to 1968 (Fulginiti *et al.*, 1967). These children developed high fever, a rash that was most prominent on the extremities, often included petechiae and a high rate of pneumonitis (Fulginiti *et al.*, 1967; Rauh & Schmidt, 1965). Recent studies in monkeys indicate that this illness was caused by antigen-antibody immune complexes resulting from incomplete maturation of the antibody response to the vaccine (Polack *et al.*, 1999).

4.2 Disease progression

MV initially infects epithelial cells of the respiratory tract as well as pulmonary macrophages. MV subsequently infects regional lymph nodes, maybe disseminated via infected macrophages, and eventually establishes a systemic infection. The primary immune cell infected in blood is the monocyte, but T cells and B cells can be infected in vitro and probably *in vivo* as well (Grivel *et al.*, 2005; McChesney *et al.*, 1989). As MV infects immune cells, host innate immune response is inevitably activated to control viral replication and clear infected cells evidenced by up-regulated proinflammatory cytokines such as Interferon (IFN)-γ, Interleukin (IL)-2, etc. MV then spreads to the skin and conjunctivae leading to inflammation of the upper respiratory tract and conjunctivitis.
The lower respiratory tract and lungs are infected when MV spreads to lungs and leads to pneumonia. The infection of dermal endothelial cells can be accompanied by vascular dilatation, increased vascular permeability, mononuclear cell infiltration, and infection of surrounding tissue (Kimura *et al.*, 1975); infection of keratinocytes in the stratum granulosum of the overlying epidermis leads to focal keratosis and edema (Takahashi *et al.*, 1996) which displays as skin rash. Koplik's spots found on the oral mucosa are pathologically similar and involve the submucous glands. The rash and Koplik's spots occur about 2 weeks after infection marking the onset of a strong immune response which is effective in clearing virus and establishing long-term immunity (Roscic-Mrkic *et al.*, 2001). However, at this time numerous abnormalities of immune responses, such as MV-induced suppression of the immune system are also detected, which result in a greatly increased susceptibility to opportunistic bacterial infections that are largely responsible for the morbidity and mortality associated with measles (Borrow & Oldstone, 1995).

4.2.1 MV infection of CNS

Around 0.1% of measles cases develop acute measles encephalitis during or shortly after acute measles, with a mortality rate of 10-30%, maybe as a consequence of MV induced autoimmune reaction against brain antigens (Moench *et al.*, 1988).

4.2.1.1 Acute disseminated encephalomyelitis

ADEM occurs about 5–6 days after the initial rash in about 1/1000 infected children (Menge, et al., 2005; Leake et al., 2004; Nasr et al., 2000; Sips et al., 2007). Symptoms occur once the initial rash has disappeared and consist of a sudden recurrence of fever, decreased consciousness, seizures and multifocal neurological signs. The disease has an abrupt onset, often reaching its peak within the first 24 h with 20% mortality (Johnson, 1994). The cerebrospinal fluid usually shows a mild elevation of protein and mononuclear cells, but is normal in about one-third of patients (Menge, et al., 2005; Leake et al., 2004). The pathology of ADEM consists of a pattern of widespread perivascular demyelination and infiltration of mononuclear cells. Histologically, the pattern of demyelination resembles that observed in experimental allergic encephalomyelitis (EAE), an animal model of multiple sclerosis (Wegner, 2005). The exact pathological mechanism of this demyelination remains unclear. An autoimmune reaction has been suggested, but at present there is no consensus about the exact aetio-pathology of ADEM.

4.2.1.2 Measles inclusion body encephalitis

MIBE usually occurs between 2 and 6 months after MV infection in immunocompromised patients (Menge *et al.*, 2005; Nasr *et al.*, 2000; Rima & Duprex, 2006) and can follow both wild-type virus infection and vaccination (Aicardi *et al.*, 1977; Bitnun *et al.*, 1999; Mustafa *et al.*, 1993; Rima & Duprex, 2006; Valmari *et al.*, 1987). Prognosis is poor with a 76% mortality rate and all survivors retain a persistent neurological disorder (Mustafa *et al.*, 1993). Characteristic neuropathologic changes are glial cell proliferation and focal necrosis, with varying degrees of perivascular inflammation. Intranuclear and/or intracytoplasmic inclusion bodies are often present (Mustafa *et al.*, 1993). The diagnosis of MIBE can only be confirmed post mortem, by RT-PCR for MV RNA or by immunohistochemistry. A few cases have been described in which MIBE followed vaccination and here dysgammaglobulinaemia or a pre-existing undiagnosed immune abnormality was suggested to be a predisposing factor (Bitnun *et al.*, 1999; Valmari *et al.*, 1987). The mechanism of viral spread and persistence in the brain in MIBE patients is not well understood.

4.2.1.3 Subacute sclerosing panencephalitis

SSPE is thought to complicate about 1/1,000,000 cases of MV infection (Johnson, 1994; Rima & Duprex, 2006). SSPE occurs approximately 5 - 10 years after initial MV infection, with infection under the age of 2 being a risk factor (Jabbour *et al.*, 1972; Modlin *et al.*, 1979). In the early stage, children present with loss of attention span and neurological symptoms, typically stereotyped myoclonic jerks. As the disease progresses, they gradually slide into a vegetative state and eventually die from the infection (Ishikawa *et al.*, 1981). SSPE is an example of a chronic defective CNS infection (Connolly *et al.*, 1967). The factors that turn an acute MV infection into a chronic one are as yet unknown, although various mechanisms have been postulated over the years. Geographic clustering of SSPE occurs in several countries, and there is an increased incidence in children residing in rural areas (Halsey *et al.*, 1980). These data suggest that as-yet-undefined environmental factors, most likely another infectious agent, contribute to this disease.

4.2.2 Molecular basis of CNS disease

MV is an enveloped virus with a negative sense, single stranded RNA genome and belongs to the genus Paramyxovirus, within the *Paramyxoviridae* family, order *Mononegavirales.* Its genome is composed of six genes encoding the structural proteins, three of which form the viral envelope and three the ribonucleoprotein core (Figure 2A). The nucleoprotein (N) is the major component of the ribonucleoprotein core, the other two being the large (L) polymerase and the polymerase cofactor, phosphoprotein (P). The L polymerase catalyses the transcription and replication of the viral genome. The envelope is made up of the matrix protein (M), haemagglutinin protein (H), and fusion protein (F) (Griffin, 2006) (Figure 2A). The P gene also codes for two non-structural proteins, the C protein via an internal initiation site for translation and V via the insertion of a non-templated G nucleotide during transcription that results in a frameshift (see Figure 2B); C and V are implicated in inhibition of the host response.

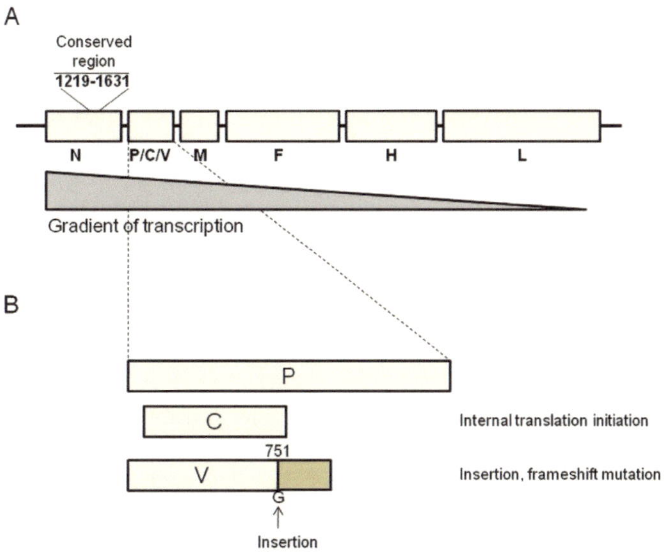

Fig. 2. Schematic diagram of the genome organisation of measles virus.
A. Schematic diagram showing the various genes. Gradient of transcription is indicated below the diagram. Conserved sequence within N gene that is used for molecular epidemiological studies to identify measles virus infection is shown.
B. The three gene products encoded by the P gene and the mechanism used to derive them. P protein is the full length gene product; C protein is translated from an internal open reading frame; V protein arises by the insertion of a non-templated G at position 751, resulting in a frameshift and a protein with a C-terminal high in cysteines

Early on it was recognised that the hyperimmune response in SSPE to MV antigens was directed against all MV proteins except the matrix (M) protein. The M gene of SSPE strains seems particularly vulnerable to mutations, affecting transcription, translation, stability, antigenicity, or function of M protein (Ayata *et al.*, 1989; Cattaneo *et al.*, 1988; Cattaneo *et al.*, 1986). cDNA cloning and sequencing of the entire M coding region established that one of the point mutations leads to a stop codon at triplet 12 of the M reading frame. It is unknown whether this defect, explaining by itself the lack of M protein, is related also to the block of M mRNA formation (Cattaneo *et al.*, 1986). Moreover, in a case of MIBE, 80% of the mutations affecting the viral M gene turned out to be uridine (U) to cytidine (C) transitions (Cattaneo *et al.*, 1988). The biased hypermutation is responsible for all but one of the missense mutations affecting the Biken M protein (a defective virus isolated from a patient with SSPE), which has a much shorter half-life *in vivo* than the M protein of the vaccine Edmonston strain. An extrinsic RNA mutational activity might alter MV RNA and gene expression in CNS infections (Wong *et al.*, 1989). The structural alterations and instability of the protein were attributed to multiple mutations in the amino and carboxyl regions. In primary neuron cultures, the mutated M protein prevents colocalization of the viral N with membrane glycoproteins, and is associated with accumulation of nucleocapsids in cell cytoplasm and nucleus. Defects in the levels of M protein are mediated by a number of mechanisms and mutations which affect the start codon making the protein unstable, enhance proteolytic degradation or lead to the generation of nonsense mutations (Cattaneo *et al.*, 1989; Hirano *et al.*, 1993). In some cases, translation of the M protein is complicated by a transcriptional defect that leads to an almost exclusive synthesis of dicistronic P-M mRNA (Ayata *et al.*, 1998; Cattaneo *et al.*, 1987; Cattaneo *et al.*, 1986; Seto *et al.*, 1999), due to a single mutation at the P gene end (Ayata *et al.*, 2002). Some SSPE strains have mutations in the F gene that variously result in an elongated or a shortened cytoplasmic domain (Billeter *et al.*, 1994; Ning *et al.*, 2002). A single amino acid substitution in the F protein transformed the non neuropathogenic wild-type MV IC323 strain into a lethal virus similar to the SSPE Osaka-2 strain in hamsters (Ayata *et al.*, 2010).

The demyelination observed in SSPE could be the result of several mechanisms. One possible mechanism involves CSF antibodies, which are produced in an unusually high level in SSPE and have been shown to be capable of lysing brain cells cultured from SSPE patients in vitro (Fujinami & Oldstone, 1980; Oldstone *et al.*, 1975). In addition, *in vivo* studies in rat models demonstrate that anti-measles antibodies not only promote viral persistence (Rammohan *et al.*, 1981) but possibly even decrease viral replication at the transcriptional level (Liebert *et al.*, 1990). Other theories propose that during latency, viral products accumulate in neurons and oligodendroglia and eventually lead to cell death and demyelination (Ikeda *et al.*, 1995). Furthermore, infiltration by CD4+ and CD8+ T cells and the release of inflammatory cytokines such as IFN-γ and TNF-α has been demonstrated, suggesting that cell-mediated damage to infected cells may also play a role (Hofman *et al.*, 1991).

5. Opportunistic infections

One major side-effect of MV induced immune-suppression (discussed below) is the plethora of opportunistic infections that follow. Multiple complications occur, such as diarrroea, pneumonia, laryngotracheobronchitis, otitis media, stomatitis and even encephalitis when measles virus spreads to the corresponding organ. More than half of measles cases in children aged under 5 years experienced acute respiratory infection and/or diarrhoea in the 30 days following rash onset in sub-Saharan Africa (Grais *et al.*, 2007). Measles related blindness is of multifactorial aetiology. While acute measles triggers corneal ulceration through viral proliferation in the cornea, nutritional keratomalacia is often the cause of blindness in the post-measles period. Although timely use of local antibiotic therapy to the eyes and administration of vitamin A supplements offer protection to the child who already has measles, vaccination is the best way to reduce the incidence of MV related eye disease. Live attenuated measles vaccine has been found to be safe and effective in malnourished children (Bhaskaram, 1995). The most common secondary infections following measles are caused by *Klebsiella pneumoniae, Streptococcus pneumoniae, Candida albicans, Haemophilus influenzae, Escherichia coli, Enterobacter cloacae,* and *Acinetobacter baumannii* (Yu *et al.*, 2009).

6. MV induced immune suppression

Measles is a major cause of childhood mortality in developing countries which is mainly attributed to the ability of MV to suppress general immune responses (Moss *et al.*, 2004). In most individuals, virus-specific immunity is efficiently induced and the immune response is successful, which eventually leads to clearance of MV from the host and confers long-lasting protection against re-infection. However, infection is also associated with persistence of viral RNA and development of immune-suppression, which can last up to 6 months after an acute infection (Kerdiles *et al.*, 2006b). Paradoxically, the induction of intense immune response in measles does occurs simultaneously with clinically relevant immune-suppression, a phenomenon that is not yet clearly understood. MV related immune-suppression includes loss of of delayed type hypersensitivity (DTH) responses (Garenne & Aaby, 1990; Katz, 1995) in immune individuals for several weeks following the rash, impaired proliferation of peripheral blood lymphocytes (Hirsch *et al.*, 1984) and allospecific cytotoxicity, which increases susceptibility to secondary infections while immune responses towards other pathogens are strongly impaired. This transient MV-induced immune-suppression is of important clinical significance, as it permits opportunistic infections to develop in infected children, leading to high infant morbidity and mortality (Kerdiles *et al.*, 2006b). The molecular basis for MV-induced immune-suppression is not completely understood. MV related severe immune-suppression includes both innate and adaptive immune responses and is probably caused via multiple mechanisms (Karp, 1999; Schneider-Schaulies *et al.*, 1995; Schneider-Schaulies & ter Meulen, 2002). Suppression of mitogen-induced lymphocyte proliferation can be induced by MV infection of lymphocytes or by lymphocyte exposure to a complex of the H and F surface glycoproteins without infection. Dendritic cells (DCs) are susceptible to MV infection and can transmit infection to lymphocytes. Apart from its direct effects on the immune system, MV also has indirect, longer-lasting effects on the immune system, in which the interaction between several viral proteins and the human host seems to play a role (Kerdiles *et al.*, 2006a; Kerdiles *et al.*, 2006b). MV-infected DCs are unable to stimulate a mixed lymphocyte reaction and can induce lymphocyte non-responsiveness through expression of MV glycoproteins.

Evidence of a role for many of these mechanisms was obtained *in vitro*, however, much has still to be learned about MV tissue tropism and its interactions with particular host cells such as DCs *in vivo* (Schneider-Schaulies *et al.*, 2001). Thus, multiple factors may contribute both to measles-induced immune-suppression and to the establishment of durable protective immunity. The mechanisms which contribute to the loss of the allostimulatory function of DCs include both virus release and active suppression mediated by MV-infected DCs, independent of virus production. Data from several studies suggest that carriage of MV by DCs may facilitate virus spreading to secondary lymphoid organs and that MV replication in DCs may play a central role in the general immune-suppression observed during measles. Therefore, contributions of measles virus to immune-suppression are likely multifactorial and include reduced DTH responses, T lymphocyte functional deficits, altered cytokine levels, inhibition of DC function, reduced immunoglobulin production, and inhibition of IFN-γ up-regulation of MHC-II molecules (Kerdiles *et al.*, 2006a).

Leopardi et al (Leopardi *et al.*, 1993) showed that in measles-infected monocytes, there was a 10-fold increase in the expression of MHC class II molecules. However, they showed that MV inhibited the IFN-γ-induced effect on HLA-DR expression in a human monocytic cell line. They also showed that MV affects presentation of exogenous antigen. Thus like HIV and influenza virus, MV interferes with class II processing by suppressing the production of class II molecules or impeding antigen trafficking (Peters & Sperber, 1999).

6.1 Lymphopenia

MV immune-suppression is associated with a pronounced lymphopenia as well as decreases in neutrophils and monocytes (Okada *et al.*, 2000). Measles is associated with suppression of mitogen-induced proliferative responses and lymphocyte response to monocyte signals is suboptimal (Griffin *et al.*, 1987) in measles infection in children (Esolen *et al.*, 1993; Griffin *et al.*, 1986), and in animal models (Hahm *et al.*, 2003; Niewiesk *et al.*, 2000). Monocytes persistently infected with MV exhibit suppression of NFκB activation, which represents a potential strategy of escape from the host immune system by MV via induced immunological silencing (Indoh *et al.*, 2007).

6.1.1 T lymphocytes

It is reported that MV infection results in remarkable lymphopenia in all measles cases with reduction in cell numbers of CD4+ T cells, CD8+ T cells, B cells, neutrophils, and monocytes in circulation, increased lymphocyte activation, and increased susceptibility to cell death of lymphocytes in children (Ryon *et al.*, 2002), in young adults (Okada *et al.*, 2000; Vinante *et al.*, 1999), in cultured peripheral blood mononuclear cells (PBMC) (Salonen *et al.*, 1989), and in animal models (Hahm *et al.*, 2003). Interestingly, in Chinese adult measles patients with no vaccination history, a general decrease in CD4+ and CD8+ T cells was not observed, although there was a trend toward lower levels compared with healthy donors (Yu *et al.*, 2008). An increase in the total CD3+T cells in PBMCs of Chinese adult measles patients was reported, possibly due to expansion of a CD3+CD4-CD8- T cell subset that defines a double negative Treg phenotype (Chen *et al.*, 2004), and can inhibit immune responses by directly killing effector T cells in an Ag-specific fashion, and produce IFN-γ and TNF-α in addition to other cytokines. The lymphopenia results primarily from depletion of infected and noninfected B and T lymphocytes. Profound lymphoid depletion may also occur in the thymus, lymph nodes, and spleen. With CD4+ T cell counts dropping, host defences may be bolstered by a compensatory increase in natural killer (NK) cell activity (Okada *et al.*, 2000). Similar to other immunosuppressive viruses, MV is lymphotropic and viral nucleic acid and proteins are detectable in PBMCs. It is considered central to MV-induced immune-suppression that PBMC isolated from patients largely fail to proliferate in response to antigen specific and polyclonal stimulation. The low abundance of MV-infected PBMC suggests that MV-induced immune-suppression is not directly caused by infection-mediated cell loss or fusion, but rather by indirect mechanisms such as deregulation of cytokines or surface contact-mediated signalling which may lead to apoptosis or impair the proliferative response of uninfected PBMC. In classical measles cases, infected lymphocytes detected as a minor population during the incubation period disappeared soon after onset of rash, whereas in the cases of serious illness, the infected cells persisted longer after the rash, correlating with reduction in cell numbers of CD4+ T cells, CD8+ T cells, B cells, neutrophils, and monocytes.

6.1.2 B lymphocytes

Mc-Chesney et al. found that MV infection of B cells leads to decreased antibody production when B cells are stimulated by mitogen (Casali *et al.*, 1984; McChesney *et al.*, 1986). More recently, Ravanel et al. have shown that the N protein of MV can bind to B cells through the Fcγ receptor and inhibit immunoglobulin (Ig) synthesis (Ravanel *et al.*, 1997). In contrast, MV-infected T cells still have the ability to produce cytokines required to help uninfected B cells differentiate into plasma cells and secrete Ig (McChesney *et al.*, 1987). Lack of HLA diversity may limit the range of peptides that can be presented to T helper or T cytotoxic lymphocytes, resulting in a decreased immune response to viral infections, as in children with a cumulative effect of increasing HLA homozygosity, in which homozygosity at increasing numbers of loci results in progressively lower measles-specific antibody levels (Jacobson *et al.*, 2003).

Significant lymphopenia due to apoptosis of uninfected cells is one of the principal causes for immune-suppression induced by MV infection, and is correlated with age-dependent severity of the disease (Okada *et al.*, 2000).

6.2 Modulation of T cell response

The initial T-cell response includes CD8+ and Th1 CD4+ T cells important for control of infectious virus. As viral RNA persists, there is a shift to a Th2 CD4+ T-cell response that likely promotes B-cell maturation and durable antibody responses but may suppress macrophage activation and Th1 responses to new infections. Type 2 polarisation of cytokine responses with an increase in the production of interleukin 4 (IL-4) and decrease in IL-2 and IFN-γ occurs during late stages of measles (Griffin & Ward, 1993). Production of the pro-inflammatory cytokine IL-12 is markedly suppressed in measles, providing a unifying mechanism for many of the immunological abnormalities associated with measles infection (Atabani *et al.*, 2001).

The principal players in the early nonspecific immune response are interferon α/β (IFN-α/β) induction, complement activation, natural killer cell (NK) and macrophage activation, and IFN-γ and interleukin-12 (IL-12) production. Although MV infection of cell lines *in vitro* has been shown to induce IFN (Volckaert-Vervliet & Billiau, 1977), the results with wild-type MV infection *in vivo* are conflicting and inconclusive. Active IFN-α/β has been documented *in vivo* after natural infection by MV in one study and shown to be absent in another (Crespi *et al.*, 1988; Shiozawa *et al.*, 1988; Tilles *et al.*, 1987). Levels of serum IFN and of the IFN-inducible oligoadenylate-synthetase (2-5OAS) gene transcript have been shown to rise after MV immunization with the live attenuated vaccine (Tilles *et al.*, 1987). With regard to other innate defence mechanisms, MV does not appear to hamper either complement activation *in vitro* or IFN-γ production *in vivo* (Patrick Sissons *et al.*, 1979). However, MV has been shown to depress IL-12 synthesis *in vitro* and to dampen NK cell activity *in vivo* (Griffin *et al.*, 1990b; Karp *et al.*, 1996). In addition to their antiviral function, IFN-α/β have potent effects in regulating specific immune response. They are thought to enhance differentiation of dendritic antigen-presenting cells and to contribute to prolonging T-lymphocyte lifespan (Luft *et al.*, 1998; Marrack *et al.*, 1999).

Viruses have evolved mechanisms to counter the antiviral effects of IFN or, in some cases, to suppress its production. Resistance to the antiviral effects of IFN is mediated by active inhibition of IFN-inducible gene function. IFN-resistant and -sensitive strains of MV can be isolated by cell culture, and it has been suggested that IFN-resistant strains of MV can contribute to the establishment of persistent infection of the CNS (Carrigan & Knox, 1990). This is relevant to the rare cases of persistent MV infection of the CNS giving rise to SSPE. It is not known which MV products contribute to IFN resistance, but studies in the closely related Sendai virus have shown that the nonstructural C protein counteracts the IFN-mediated antiviral state (Garcin *et al.*, 1999). MV infection *in vitro* has been shown to depress IL-12 production in both macrophages and DCs (Fugier-Vivier *et al.*, 1997). Macrophages, DCs, epithelial cells, and NK cells provide the initial sources of IFN-α/β, IL-12, and IFN-γ. MV may have established a redundancy of mechanisms to slow the innate immune response to allow early dissemination.

6.3 Cytokines in measles

Despite chemokines directing the migration of T cells to infected neurons, chemokine neutralization revealed that migration is not required for viral clearance, suggesting a cytokine-mediated antiviral mechanism. An increase in IFN-γ in MV-infected children compared with healthy controls has been observed in other studies and it may serve to inhibit viral growth and limit the spread of infection (Griffin *et al.*, 1990a). Children with measles display a transient increase in both IL-2 and IFN-γ, lasting for a few days following rash (Griffin & Ward, 1993; Ryon *et al.*, 2002), followed by sustained IL-4 production (Ryon *et al.*, 2002). A similar response was observed when a clinical isolate of MV was used to infect PBMCs (Dhiman *et al.*, 2005b). In contrast, adult patients demonstrate a sustained increase of IFN-γ and poor IL-4 secretion; an early IL-4 gene induction that was not reflected in protein secretion may be due to uptake of secreted IL-4 by cells, and does not necessarily reflect lack of protein production. Similar findings have been reported in a study where PBMCs from previously immunized adults were infected with MV. All subjects produced IFN-γ, and in subjects who produced both IFN-γ and IL-4, maximal IFN-γ production *in vitro* always greatly exceeded that of IL-4 (Dhiman *et al.*, 2005b). In Zambian children plasma IL-5 levels were lower in patients compared with controls (Ryon *et al.*, 2002). In contrast, a significant upregulation of IL-5 mRNA has been reported among seropositive adult donors after vaccination (Li *et al.*, 2001). The role of IL-5 in MV infection is not clear and data may be complicated by the underlying allergic status of the subjects.

Sustained high levels of IL-10 during convalescence suggest a role for this immunoregulatory cytokine in MV-induced immune-suppression. Plasma levels of IL-10 remain elevated for weeks in children with MV infection (Ryon *et al.*, 2002). The increased IL-10 levels may also be implicated in the decrease in IL-5 expression, because IL-10 is known to inhibit IL-5 production by T cells and in mouse models of allergic disease (Staples *et al.*, 2000). IL-10 has been shown to display a range of immune suppressive effects, including inhibition of APC function, induction of anergy, differentiation of Treg, and control of the expansion of other T cell populations (Kingsley *et al.*, 2002), and may be key to the observed decrease in monocyte/macrophages and innate immune responses observed in MV infection.

In brain tissue, IFN-γ is both necessary and sufficient to clear MV. Secretion of IFN-γ is stimulated by IL-12 in the brain, as neutralization of IL-12 results in loss of antiviral activity and stimulation of leukocytes with IL-12/IL-18 enhances their immune effector function of viral clearance. The IFN-γ signal is transduced within brain explants tissue by the Jak/STAT signalling pathway, as inhibition of Jak kinases results in a loss of antiviral activity driven by either brain-derived leukocytes or recombinant IFN-γ. These results reveal that primed T cells directly act to clear MV infection of the brain by using a noncytolytic IL-12- and IFN-γ-dependent mechanism in the CNS and that this mechanism relies upon Jak/STAT signalling.

6.4 Effects on DC function

As sensitisers of pathogen encounter and instructors of the adaptive immune response, DCs may play a decisive role in the induction and quality of the MV-specific immune activation. The ability of MV wild-type strains in particular, to infect DCs *in vitro* via the receptor binding H protein is clearly established. DC maturation is induced early after MV infection and is likely to be of crucial importance for the induction of MV-specific immunity. Several *in vitro* studies have demonstrated that MV infection of human DCs affects their phenotype and functions. Different types of DCs including Langerhans cells (Grosjean *et al.*, 1997), peripheral blood DCs (Schnorr *et al.*, 1997), CD34+-derived DCs (Grosjean *et al.*, 1997) and monocyte-derived DCs (Fugier-Vivier *et al.*, 1997) are permissive to MV infection. Viral infection induces formation of DC syncytia, followed by the loss of DC capacity to stimulate naive CD4+T cells (Fugier-Vivier *et al.*, 1997; Grosjean *et al.*, 1997) and acquisition of an active inhibitory function on CD4+ T cell proliferation in response to allogeneic noninfected DC (Grosjean *et al.*, 1997) or mitogens (Schnorr *et al.*, 1997). Inhibition of T-cell functions could be mediated through either transmission of infectious virus to T cells, leading to a block in the cell cycle (Naniche *et al.*, 1999) and/or delivery of inhibitory signals via infected DCs (Grosjean *et al.*, 1997). MV infection was shown to enhance apoptosis of DCs and to inhibit their CD40 ligand dependent terminal differentiation (Servet-Delprat *et al.*, 2000; 2000b). In addition, it induced cytotoxic activity by activation of the TNF-related apoptosis-inducing ligand (TRAIL) synthesis in DC and monocytes (Vidalain *et al.*, 2000). Although the infection of DCs is an attractive hypothesis to explain MV-induced immune-suppression, direct evidence for the presence of MV-infected DCs in children during measles remains to be demonstrated. Analysis of the presence of MV-infection in different cells of the immune system during measles suggests that the major mechanism for the induction of immune-suppression may not be a direct effect of virus replication in these cells. In fact, despite the small amount of virus-infected peripheral blood cells during measles (less than 1%), the severe suppression of the immune system can last for weeks (Borrow & Oldstone, 1995). Moreover, a number of immunological alterations during natural measles also occur to a lesser magnitude after vaccination with attenuated MV (Fireman *et al.*, 1969; Hussey *et al.*, 1996). Therefore, it is likely that MV-induced immune-suppression is induced not only by direct viral replication in haematopoietic cells, but also by indirect immunopathogenic mechanisms. Indeed, numerous recent studies indicate that MV proteins are sufficient to induce different aspects of MV-induced immune-suppression (Marie *et al.*, 2001; Ravanel *et al.*, 1997; Schlender *et al.*, 1996).

6.5 Type I interferons in measles

MV infection of cell lines *in vitro* has been shown to induce IFNα/β (Volckaert-Vervliet & Billiau, 1977), the results concerning wild-type MV infection *in vivo* are conflicting and inconclusive. Active IFNα/β have been documented *in vivo* after natural infection by MV in one study and shown to be absent in another (Crespi *et al.*, 1988; Shiozawa *et al.*, 1988; Tilles *et al.*, 1987). IFNα/β induction by MV is probably dependant on passage history of the virus and the cell type tested (Naniche *et al.*, 2000; Volckaert-Vervliet & Billiau, 1977; Volckaert-Vervliet *et al.*, 1978). Recent studies suggest that wild type MV isolates actively inhibit IFN synthesis and induce poor production of IFNα/β while the laboratory adapted and vaccine strains are potent stimulators (Yu, et al., 2008). Recombinant MV with defective V protein can grow in cell lines that do not produce IFN (Niewiesk *et al.*, 1997), *in vivo* studies demonstrate an important role of the V proteins as virulence factors (Patterson, 2000), and analysis of thymic xenografts revealed that V-deficient virus replication was delayed compared to that of wild-type or V-over-producing viruses (Valsamakis, 1998). MV V protein is capable of inducing cytokine inhibition by causing a defective IFN-induced STAT nuclear accumulation and nuclear redistribution, probably linking innate immune evasion to adaptive immune suppression by MV (Palosaari, 2003). MV C protein has also been shown to be a virulence factor (Escoffier *et al.*, 1999; Mrkic *et al.*, 2000; Patterson, 2000; Valsamakis, 1998) and to bind to the IFNα/β receptor (Yokota *et al.*, 2003); MV C protein inhibited the production of IFNα/β and IFNα/β signalling (Shaffer *et al.*, 2003). IFN-resistant and -sensitive strains of MV can be isolated by cell culture, and it has been suggested that IFN-resistant strains of MV may contribute to the establishment of persistent infection of the CNS (Carrigan & Knox, 1990). Systemic dissemination of C- and V-defective MVs is strongly impaired and upon intra- cerebral inoculation these viruses cause lethal disease less often than the parental strain. The attenuated candidate recombinant MV vaccine strains, which include C- and V-protein-defective viruses still replicate in animals at levels that are high enough to efficiently induce immunity and IFNα/β (Radecke and Billeter, 1996). Furthermore, robust production of IFNα in human myeloid DCs and epithelial cells was associated with increase in the level of virus-specific defective interfering RNA (DI RNA), subviral replicons originating from the viral genome associated with many RNA viruses (Lazzarini *et al.*, 1981). Wild type MV isolates contain undetectable levels of DI RNA and induce significantly lower production of IFN in mDCs.

6.6 Suppression of IL-12

IL-12 production by antigen-presenting cells is central to the orchestration of both innate and acquired cell-mediated immune responses to many pathogens. However, MV has been shown to depress IL-12 synthesis *in vitro* and to dampen NK cell activity *in vivo* (Griffin *et al.*, 1990b; Karp *et al.*, 1996). Production of IL-12 from DCs is also suppressed by MV (Karp *et al.*, 1998). The ability of MV to specifically ablate monocyte/macrophage and DC secretion of IL-12 provides a potentially unifying mechanism for many of the immunological abnormalities associated with MV infection. Specifically, (a) ablation of IL-12 activity, by antibodies or genetic deletion, compromises the ability to respond to a variety of infections; (b) DTH responses depend upon IL-12 production; (c) IL-12 stimulates NK activity; and (d) IL-12 is essential for the development as well as the expression of most Th1 responses. IL-12 failure may thus explain the propensity for developing superinfection, the absence of DTH reactivity, the meager NK cell activity, and the Th2 deviation in cytokine profiles seen in the aftermath of measles. IL-12 suppression would not explain lymphoproliferative defects, however. Although IL-12 is co-mitogenic for activated T and NK cells, it is not necessary for the proliferation of such cells. Interestingly, cytotoxic T cell and overall antibody responses develop normally in IL-12 knockout mice indicating that IL-12 suppression need not hinder the development of an effective anti-MV response.

Importantly, IL-12 production is significantly suppressed during natural infection of children with MV, with suppression lasting for weeks after acute presentation with measles (Karp & Wills-Karp, 2001).

The degree to which IFN-α/β induction and IL-12 synthesis are disrupted by MV may determine the virulence of a particular strain. Such virulent measles strains could thus replicate more efficiently and gain access more rapidly to the bone marrow and, on rare occasions, to the CNS. These hypotheses are based on *in vitro* studies and further studies in existing monkey models (Auwaerter *et al.*, 1999; McChesney *et al.*, 1997) are needed to determine if the pathogenesis of infection *in vivo* mirrors the *in vitro* observations presented.

7. Implications for treatment

Vitamin A treatment for children with measles in developing countries has been associated with a marked reduction in morbidity and mortality. The WHO recommends vitamin A administration to all children with measles in communities where vitamin A deficiency is a recognized problem and where the MV-related mortality rate exceeds 1%. Of note, low serum concentrations of vitamin A are found in children with severe measles in USA. Thus, supplemental vitamin A in patients aged 6 months to 2 years who are hospitalized with measles and its complications (e.g., croup, pneumonia, diarrhoea) should be considered (D'Souza & D'Souza, 2002a; b; Hussey & Klein, 1993; Markowitz *et al.*, 1989).

MV is susceptible to ribavirin *in vitro*. Although ribavirin (either intravenous (IV) or aerosolized) has been used to treat severely affected and immunocompromised adults with acute measles or SSPE (IV plus intrathecal high-dose IFNα) (Gururangan *et al.*, 1990), no controlled trials have been conducted; ribavirin is not approved by the US Food and Drug Administration (FDA) for this indication, and such use should be considered experimental.

For immunocompromised persons, immune globulins (IG) are indicated to prevent measles following exposure. If immediate protection against measles is required for immunocompromised persons with contraindications to measles vaccination, including exposed infants less than 1 year of age, passive immunization with IG, 0.5 mL/kg of body weight (maximum dose = 15 mL), should be administered intramuscularly as soon as possible after exposure. Exposed symptomatic HIV-infected and other severely immunocompromised persons should receive IG regardless of their previous vaccination status (recommended dose is 0.5 mL/kg of body weight if IG is administered intramuscularly; maximum dose = 15 mL), because measles vaccine may not be effective in such patients and the disease may be severe. Intramuscular IG may not be necessary if an HIV patient is receiving 100-400 mg/kg IGIV at regular intervals and the last dose was administered within 3 weeks of exposure to measles. Because the amounts of protein administered are similar, high-dose IGIV may be as effective as IG administered intramuscularly. However, no data are available concerning the effectiveness of IGIV in preventing measles. For immunocompromised persons receiving IG for measles prophylaxis, measles vaccination should be delayed for 6 months following IG administration. For persons receiving IG for replacement of humoral immune deficiencies (320 mg/kg intravenously), measles vaccination should be delayed until 8 months following IG administration (CDC, 1993).

8. Future perspectives

Huge strides have been made in reduction of measles incidence in most parts of the world following WHO global eradication programme, with several countries having interrupted the circulation of endemic virus. Unfortunately, the situation is different in the poorer developing and emerging nations, with high measles prevalence, low vaccine coverage and 500,000 childhood deaths annually. Within the Western Pacific region, of which China and Australia are a part, many countries have achieved success in controlling measles infections; but China and Japan still report localised outbreaks that seem to differ in frequency and in character between the developed and under-developed (poor) regions. A region specific vaccination programme is required to achieve control of the endemically circulating MV in China.

Measles infection very often induces characteristic immune-suppression that can extend for weeks following the acute disease, resulting in potentially fatal opportunistic infections. Despite intense research over the years, the mechanisms of MV induced immune-suppression are not completely defined; it is probably very complex with several mechanisms encompassing both the innate and adaptive responses being involved. The situation is further complicated by the fact that the mechanisms that are known are variably affected in different populations. The best characterised immunological change is the severe lymphopenia following MV infection. Immunosuppressive factors, e.g. IL-10 and suppressive cells, e.g. Treg have been shown to be elevated after acute MV infection in separate studies and may play major roles in causing immune-suppression. In various studies, a role for DCs, IL-12, and type I IFNs has been suggested. To date there is no unifying "model" of immune-suppression to connect all the findings. Additionally, as most studies have been performed in cell culture, it is not clear how many of the immunological findings can be directly co-related to natural infection. Success of the global measles vaccination programs has resulted in very rare occurrences of natural measles in developed nations. Clearly, investigations in the non-human primate model of measles are needed to better elucidate MV induced immune-suppression.

9. References

Aicardi, J., Goutieres, F., Arsenio-Nunes, M. L. & Lebon, P. (1977). Acute measles encephalitis in children with immunosuppression. *Pediatrics* 59, 232-239.

Atabani, S. F., Byrnes, A. A., Jaye, A., Kidd, I. M., Magnusen, A. F., Whittle, H. & Karp, C. L. (2001). Natural measles causes prolonged suppression of interleukin-12 production. *Journal of Infectious Diseases* 184, 1-9.

Auwaerter, P. G., Rota, P. A., Elkins, W. R., Adams, R. J., DeLozier, T., Shi, Y., Bellini, W. J., Murphy, B. R. & Griffin, D. E. (1999). Measles virus infection in rhesus macaques: altered immune responses and comparison of the virulence of six different virus strains. *Journal of Infectious Diseases* 180, 950-958.

Ayata, M., Hayashi, K., Seto, T., Murata, R. & Ogura, H. (1998). The matrix gene expression of subacute sclerosing panencephalitis (SSPE) virus (Osaka-1 strain): a comparison of two sibling viruses isolated from different lobes of an SSPE brain. *Microbiology Immunology* 42, 773-780.

Ayata, M., Hirano, A. & Wong, T. C. (1989). Structural defect linked to non-random mutations in the matrix gene of Biken strain subacute sclerosing panencephalitis virus defined by cDNA cloning and expression of chimeric genes. *Journal of Virology* 63, 1162-1173.

Ayata, M., Komase, K., Shingai, M., Matsunaga, I., Katayama, Y. & Ogura, H. (2002). Mutations affecting transcriptional termination in the P gene-end of subacute sclerosing panencephalitis viruses. *Journal of Virology* 76, 13062-13068.

Ayata, M., Takeuchi, K., Takeda, M., Ohgimoto, S., Kato, S., Sharma, L. B., Tanaka, M., Kuwamura, M., Ishida, H. & Ogura, H. (2010). The F Gene of the Osaka-2 Strain of Measles Virus Derived from a Case of Subacute Sclerosing Panencephalitis Is a Major Determinant of Neurovirulence. *Journal of Virology* 84, 11189-11199.

Babbott, F. L., Jr. & Gordon, J. E. (1954). Modern measles. *Am J Med Sci* 228, 334-361.

Bhaskaram, P. (1995). Micronutrient deficiencies in children--the problem and extent. *Indian Journal of Pediatrics* 62, 145-156.

Billeter, M. A., Cattaneo, R., Spielhofer, P., Kaelin, K., Huber, M., Schmid, A., Baczko, K. & ter Meulen, V. (1994). Generation and properties of measles virus mutations typically associated with subacute sclerosing panencephalitis. *Annals of the New York Academy of Sciences* 724, 367-377.

Bitnun, A., Shannon, P., Durward, A., Rota, P. A., Bellini, W. J., Graham, C., Wang, E., Ford-Jones, E. L., Cox, P., Becker, L., Fearon, M., Petric, M. & Tellier, R. (1999). Measles inclusion-body encephalitis caused by the vaccine strain of measles virus. *Clinical Infectious Diseaes* 29, 855-861.

Black, F. L. (1982). The role of herd immunity in control of measles. *Yale Journal of Biological Medicine* 55, 351-360.

Borrow, P. & Oldstone, M. B. (1995). Measles virus-mononuclear cell interactions. *Current Topics in Microbiology and Immunology* 191, 85-100.

Carrigan, D. R. & Knox, K. K. (1990). Identification of interferon-resistant subpopulations in several strains of measles virus: positive selection by growth of the virus in brain tissue. *Journal of Virology* 64, 1606-1615.

Casali, P., Rice, G. P. & Oldstone, M. B. (1984). Viruses disrupt functions of human lymphocytes. Effects of measles virus and influenza virus on lymphocyte-mediated killing and antibody production. *Journal of Experimental Medicine* 159, 1322-1337.

Cattaneo, R., Kaelin, K., Baczko, K. & Billeter, M. A. (1989). Measles virus editing provides an additional cysteine-rich protein. *Cell* 56, 759-764.

Cattaneo, R., Rebmann, G., Schmid, A., Baczko, K., ter Meulen, V. & Billeter, M. A. (1987). Altered transcription of a defective measles virus genome derived from a diseased human brain. *Embo Journal* 6, 681-688.

Cattaneo, R., Schmid, A., Eschle, D., Baczko, K., ter Meulen, V. & Billeter, M. A. (1988). Biased hypermutation and other genetic changes in defective measles viruses in human brain infections. *Cell* 55, 255-265.

Cattaneo, R., Schmid, A., Rebmann, G., Baczko, K., Ter Meulen, V., Bellini, W. J., Rozenblatt, S. & Billeter, M. A. (1986). Accumulated measles virus mutations in a case of subacute sclerosing panencephalitis: interrupted matrix protein reading frame and transcription alteration. *Virology* 154, 97-107.

CDC (1993). Use of Vaccines and Immune Globulins in Persons with Altered Immunocompetence. United States Centers for Disease Control and Prevention.

CDC (2000). Measles - United States. In *Morbidity and Mortallity Weekly*, pp. 557-560. Atlanta: Centers for Disease Control and Prevention.

CDC (2005). Global Measles and Rubella Laboratory Network, January 2004--June 2005. *MMR weekly of Center for Disease Prevention and Control* 54, 1100-1104.

CDC (2007). Progress in global measles control and mortality reduction, 2000-2006. *Morbidity and Mortality Weekly Report* 56, 1237-1241.

CDC (2009). Progress toward measles control - African region, 2001-2008. *Morbidity Mortality Weekly Report* 58, 1036-1041.

Chadwick, D. W., Martin, S., Buxton, P. H. & Tomlinson, A. H. (1982). Measles virus and subacute neurological disease: an unusual presentation of measles inclusion body encephalitis. *Journal of Neurological and Neurosurgical Psychiatry* 45, 680-684.

Chen, R. T., Markowitz, L. E., Albrecht, P., Stewart, J. A., Mofenson, L. M., Preblud, S. R. & Orenstein, W. A. (1990). Measles antibody: reevaluation of protective titers. *Journal of Infectious Diseases* 162, 1036-1042.

Chen, W., Ford, M. S., Young, K. J. & Zhang, L. (2004). The role and mechanisms of double negative regulatory T cells in the suppression of immune responses. *Cellular and Molecular Immunology* 1, 328-335.

Cherry, J. D., Feigin, R. D., Lobes, L. A., Jr., Hinthorn, D. R., Shackelford, P. G., Shirley, R. H., Lins, R. D. & Choi, S. C. (1972). Urban measles in the vaccine era: a clinical, epidemiologic, and serologic study. *Journal of Pediatrics* 81, 217-230.

CMOH (1997a). National Strategic Plan for Measles Surveillance. Edited by C. Ministry of Health. Beijing: Ministry of Health, China.

CMOH (1997b). Plan for accelerated measles control. Beijing: Ministry of Health, China.

Connolly, J. H., Allen, I. V., Hurwitz, L. J. & Millar, J. H. (1967). Measles-virus antibody and antigen in subacute sclerosing panencephalitis. *Lancet* 1, 542-544.

Crespi, M., Struthers, J. K., Smith, A. N. & Lyons, S. F. (1988). Interferon status after measles virus infection. *South African medical journal = Suid-Afrikaanse tydskrif vir geneeskunde* 73, 711-712.

Cutts, F. T. & Markowitz, L. E. (1994). Successes and failures in measles control. *Journal of Infectious Diseases* 170 Suppl 1, S32-41.

D'Souza, R. M. & D'Souza, R. (2002a). Vitamin A for preventing secondary infections in children with measles--a systematic review. *Journal of Tropical Pediatrics* 48, 72-77.

D'Souza, R. M. & D'Souza, R. (2002b). Vitamin A for the treatment of children with measles--a systematic review. *Journal of Tropical Pediatrics* 48, 323-327.

Dhiman, N., Ovsyannikova, I. G., Ryan, J. E., Jacobson, R. M., Vierkant, R. A., Pankratz, V. S., Jacobsen, S. J. & Poland, G. A. (2005b). Correlations among measles virus-specific antibody, lymphoproliferation and Th1/Th2 cytokine responses following measles–mumps–rubella-II (MMR-II) vaccination. *Clinical Experimental Immunology* 142, 498-504.

Du, W., Bian, Y. L., Xu, F., Wu, S. W., Dai, L. F. & Zhu, Q. (2010). An Analysis on Epidemiological Characteristics of Measles in Guizhou Province in 2008. *Journal of Guiyang medical College* 35, 493-495.

Edmonson, M. B., Addiss, D. G., McPherson, J. T., Berg, J. L., Circo, S. R. & Davis, J. P. (1990). Mild measles and secondary vaccine failure during a sustained outbreak in a highly vaccinated population. *Jama* 263, 2467-2471.

Escoffier, C., Manie, S., Vincent, S., Muller, C. P., Billeter, M. & Gerlier, D. (1999). Nonstructural C protein is required for efficient measles virus replication in human peripheral blood cells. *Journal of Virology* 73, 1695-1698.

Esolen, L. M., Takahashi, K., Johnson, R. T., Vaisberg, A., Moench, T. R., Wesselingh, S. L. & Griffin, D. E. (1995). Brain endothelial cell infection in children with acute fatal measles. *Journal of Clinical Investigation* 96, 2478-2481.

Esolen, L. M., Ward, B. J., Moench, T. R. & Griffin, D. E. (1993). Infection of monocytes during measles. *Journal of Infectious Diseases* 168, 47-52.

Fireman, P., Friday, G. & Kumate, J. (1969). Effect of measles vaccine on immunologic responsiveness. *Pediatrics* 43, 264-272.

Forthal, D. N., Aarnaes, S., Blanding, J., de la Maza, L. & Tilles, J. G. (1992). Degree and length of viremia in adults with measles. *Journal of Infectious Diseases* 166, 421-424.

Fugier-Vivier, I., Servet-Delprat, C., Rivailler, P., Rissoan, M. C., Liu, Y. J. & Rabourdin-Combe, C. (1997). Measles virus suppresses cell-mediated immunity by interfering with the survival and functions of dendritic and T cells. *Journal of Experimental Medicine* 186, 813-823.

Fujinami, R. S. & Oldstone, M. B. (1980). Alterations in expression of measles virus polypeptides by antibody: molecular events in antibody-induced antigenic modulation. *Journal of Immunology* 125, 78-85.

Fulginiti, V. A., Eller, J. J., Downie, A. W. & Kempe, C. H. (1967). Altered reactivity to measles virus. Atypical measles in children previously immunized with inactivated measles virus vaccines. *Jama* 202, 1075-1080.

Garcin, D., Latorre, P. & Kolakofsky, D. (1999). Sendai virus C proteins counteract the interferon-mediated induction of an antiviral state. *Journal of Virology* 73, 6559-6565.

Garenne, M. & Aaby, P. (1990). Pattern of exposure and measles mortality in Senegal. *Journal of Infectious Diseases* 161, 1088-1094.

Grais, R. F., Dubray, C., Gerstl, S., Guthmann, J. P., Djibo, A., Nargaye, K. D., Coker, J., Alberti, K. P., Cochet, A., Ihekweazu, C., Nathan, N., Payne, L., Porten, K., Sauvageot, D., Schimmer, B., Fermon, F., Burny, M. E., Hersh, B. S. & Guerin, P. J. (2007). Unacceptably high mortality related to measles epidemics in Niger, Nigeria, and Chad. *PLoS medicine* 4, e16.

Griffin, D. E. (2006). *Fields Virology, 5th Edition*: Lippincott, Williams & Wilkins.

Griffin, D. E., Johnson, R. T., Tamashiro, V. G., Moench, T. R., Jauregui, E., Lindo de Soriano, I. & Vaisberg, A. (1987). In vitro studies of the role of monocytes in the immunosuppression associated with natural measles virus infections. *Clinical Immunology and Immunopathology* 45, 375-383.

Griffin, D. E., Moench, T. R., Johnson, R. T., Lindo de Soriano, I. & Vaisberg, A. (1986). Peripheral blood mononuclear cells during natural measles virus infection: cell surface phenotypes and evidence for activation. *Clinical Immunology and Immunopathology* 40, 305-312.

Griffin, D. E. & Ward, B. J. (1993). Differential CD4 T cell activation in measles. *Journal of Infectious Diseases* 168, 275-281.

Griffin, D. E., Ward, B. J., Jauregui, E., Johnson, R. T. & Vaisberg, A. (1990a). Immune activation during measles: interferon-gamma and neopterin in plasma and cerebrospinal fluid in complicated and uncomplicated disease. *Journal of Infectious Diseases* 161, 449-453.

Griffin, D. E., Ward, B. J., Jauregui, E., Johnson, R. T. & Vaisberg, A. (1990b). Natural killer cell activity during measles. *Clinical Experimental Immunology* 81, 218-224.

Grivel, J. C., Garcia, M., Moss, W. J. & Margolis, L. B. (2005). Inhibition of HIV-1 replication in human lymphoid tissues ex vivo by measles virus. *Journal of Infectious Diseases* 192, 71-78.

Grosjean, I., Caux, C., Bella, C., Berger, I., Wild, F., Banchereau, J. & Kaiserlian, D. (1997). Measles Virus Infects Human Dendritic Cells and Blocks Their Allostimulatory Properties for CD4+ T Cells. *Journal of Exprimental Medicine* 186, 801-812.

Gururangan, S., Stevens, R. F. & Morris, D. J. (1990). Ribavirin response in measles pneumonia. *Journal of Infection* 20, 219-221.

Hahm, B., Arbour, N., Naniche, D., Homann, D., Manchester, M. & Oldstone, M. B. (2003). Measles virus infects and suppresses proliferation of T lymphocytes from transgenic mice bearing human signaling lymphocytic activation molecule. *Journal of Virology* 77, 3505-3515.

Halsey, N. A., Modlin, J. F., Jabbour, J. T., Dubey, L., Eddins, D. L. & Ludwig, D. D. (1980). Risk factors in subacute sclerosing panencephalitis: a case-control study. *American Journal of Epidemiology* 111, 415-424.

He, J. X., Yuan, J. L., Chen, Y. H., Xu, B. & Zhu, H. Y. (2006). Analysisi on Measles Surveillance Data of Luwan District of Shanghai. *Shanghai Journal of Preventive Medicine* 18, 177-.

Hirano, A., Ayata, M., Wang, A. H. & Wong, T. C. (1993). Functional analysis of matrix proteins expressed from cloned genes of measles virus variants that cause subacute sclerosing panencephalitis reveals a common defect in nucleocapsid binding. *Journal of Virology* 67, 1848-1853.

Hirsch, R. L., Griffin, D. E., Johnson, R. T., Cooper, S. J., Lindo de Soriano, I., Roedenbeck, S. & Vaisberg, A. (1984). Cellular immune responses during complicated and uncomplicated measles virus infections of man. *Clinical Immunology and Immunopathology* 31, 1-12.

Hofman, F. M., Hinton, D. R., Baemayr, J., Weil, M. & Merrill, J. E. (1991). Lymphokines and immunoregulatory molecules in subacute sclerosing panencephalitis. *Clinical Immunology and Immunopathology* 58, 331-342.

Hu, J. Y., Zhang, J. F., Tao, L. N. & Yuan, Z. A. (2005). Analysis on the Epidem iological Characteristics of M easles Outbreak in Shanghai from 2001 to 2004. *Chinese Journal of Expanded Programme on Immunizaiton* 11, 474-475.

Hussey, G. D., Goddard, E. A., Hughes, J., Ryon, J. J., Kerran, M., Carelse, E., Strebel, P. M., Markowitz, L. E., Moodie, J., Barron, P., Latief, Z., Sayed, R., Beatty, D. & Griffin, D. E. (1996). The effect of Edmonston-Zagreb and Schwarz measles vaccines on immune response in infants. *Journal of Infectious Diseases* 173, 1320-1326.

Hussey, G. D. & Klein, M. (1993). Routine high-dose vitamin A therapy for children hospitalized with measles. *Journal of Tropical Pediatrics* 39, 342-345.

Ikeda, K., Akiyama, H., Kondo, H., Arai, T., Arai, N. & Yagishita, S. (1995). Numerous glial fibrillary tangles in oligodendroglia in cases of subacute sclerosing panencephalitis with neurofibrillary tangles. *Neuroscience Letters* 194, 133-135.

Indoh, T., Yokota, S., Okabayashi, T., Yokosawa, N. & Fujii, N. (2007). Suppression of NF-kappaB and AP-1 activation in monocytic cells persistently infected with measles virus. *Virology* 361, 294-303.

Ishikawa, A., Murayama, T., Sakuma, N. & Saito, Y. (1981). Subacute sclerosing panencephalitis: atypical absence attacks as first symptom. *Neurology* 31, 311-315.

Jabbour, J. T., Duenas, D. A., Sever, J. L., Krebs, H. M. & Horta-Barbosa, L. (1972). Epidemiology of subacute sclerosing panencephalitis (SSPE). A report of the SSPE registry. *Jama* 220, 959-962.

Jacobson, R. M., Poland, G. A., Vierkant, R. A., Pankratz, V. S., Schaid, D. J., Jacobsen, S. J., Sauver, J. S. & Moore, S. B. (2003). The association of class I HLA alleles and antibody levels after a single dose of measles vaccine. *Human Immunology* 64, 103-109.

Jiang, T. J., Zhao, M., Zhou, Z. N., Yan, H. M., Xie, Y. X., Zhao, P. & Shi, L. (2007). Reserch on the Correlated Factors of Liver Dysfunction in Measles Patients. *Chinese Hepatology* 12, 287-288.

Johnson, R. T. (1994). The virology of demyelinating diseases. *Ann Neurol* 36 Suppl, S54-60.

Karp, C. L. (1999). Measles: immunosuppression, interleukin-12, and complement receptors. *Immunological Reviews* 168, 91-101.

Karp, C. L. & Wills-Karp, M. (2001). Complement and IL-12: yin and yang. *Microbes and Infection* 3, 109-119.

Karp, C. L., Wysocka, M., Ma, X., Marovich, M., Factor, R. E., Nutman, T., Armant, M., Wahl, L., Cuomo, P. & Trinchieri, G. (1998). Potent suppression of IL-12 production from monocytes and dendritic cells during endotoxin tolerance. *European Journal of Immunolopgy* 28, 3128-3136.

Karp, C. L., Wysocka, M., Wahl, L. M., Ahearn, J. M., Cuomo, P. J., Sherry, B., Trinchieri, G. & Griffin, D. E. (1996). Mechanism of suppression of cell-mediated immunity by measles virus. *Science* 273, 228-231.

Katz, M. (1995). Clinical spectrum of measles. *Current Topics in Microbiology and Immunology* 191, 1-12.

Kerdiles, Y. M., Cherif, B., Marie, J. C., Tremillon, N., Blanquier, B., Libeau, G., Diallo, A., Wild, T. F., Villiers, M. B. & Horvat, B. (2006a). Immunomodulatory properties of morbillivirus nucleoproteins. *Viral Immunology* 19, 324-334.

Kerdiles, Y. M., Sellin, C. I., Druelle, J. & Horvat, B. (2006b). Immunosuppression caused by measles virus: role of viral proteins. *Reviews in Medical Virology* 16, 49-63.

Kimura, A., Tosaka, K. & Nakao, T. (1975). Measles rash. I. Light and electron microscopic study of skin eruptions. *Archives of Virology* 47, 295-307.

Kingsley, C. I., Karim, M., Bushell, A. R. & Wood, K. J. (2002). CD25+CD4+ regulatory T cells prevent graft rejection: CTLA-4- and IL-10-dependent immunoregulation of alloresponses. *Journal of Immunology* 168, 1080-1086.

Kong, H. L. & Zhang, J. X. (2009). Analysis on Epidemiological and Clinical Characteristics from 120 Mealses Patients. *Clinical Medicine Research* 4, 63.

Lazzarini, R. A., Keene, J. D. & Schubert, M. (1981). The origins of defective interfering particles of the negative-strand RNA viruses. *Cell* 26, 145-154.

Leake, J. A., Albani, S., Kao, A. S., Senac, M. O., Billman, G. F., Nespeca, M. P., Paulino, A. D., Quintela, E. R., Sawyer, M. H. & Bradley, J. S. (2004). Acute disseminated encephalomyelitis in childhood: epidemiologic, clinical and laboratory features. *Pediatric Infectious Disease Journal* 23, 756-764.

Lee, B., Ying, M., Papania, M. J., Stevenson, J., Seward, J. F. & Hutchins, S. S. (2004). Measles Hospitalizations, United States, 1985-2002. *Journal of Infectious Diseases* 189, S210-215.

Leopardi, R., Ilonen, J., Mattila, L. & Salmi, A. A. (1993). Effect of measles virus infection on MHC class II expression and antigen presentation in human monocytes. *Cellular Immunology* 147, 388-396.

Li, H., Hickman, C. J., Helfand, R. F., Keyserling, H., Anderson, L. J. & Bellini, W. J. (2001). Induction of cytokine mRNA in peripheral blood mononuclear cells of infants after the first dose of measles vaccine. *Vaccine* 19, 4896-4900.

Li, Y. B. (2001). Observation on association of measels antibody levels between mothers and their infants. *Infectious Disease Information* 14, 186-188.

Liang, X. Y., Xiang, H. & Zhou, J. X. (2005). Analysis on clinical symtoms of 224 adult measles patients. *Chinese Journal for Experiment Clinical Virology* 19, 99.

Liebert, U. G. (1997). Measles virus infections of the central nervous system. *Intervirology* 40, 176-184.

Liebert, U. G., Schneider-Schaulies, S., Baczko, K. & ter Meulen, V. (1990). Antibody-induced restriction of viral gene expression in measles encephalitis in rats. *Journal of Virology* 64, 706-713.

Lu, L., Zhang, M. J., Li, M. H., Liu, Y., Xu, B., Chen, Y. H., Zhu, H. Y., Ju, L. W., Zhang, Z. X., Qiu, X. F., Zhu, L. L. & Jiang, Q. W. (2008). Study on measle immunization level of pregnant women and newborn babies. *Chinese Journal of Disease Control and Prevention* 12, 287-288.

Luft, T., Pang, K. C., Thomas, E., Hertzog, P., Hart, D. N., Trapani, J. & Cebon, J. (1998). Type I Interferons enhance the terminal differentiation of dendritic cells. *Journal of Immunology* 161, 1947-1953.

Ma, X. L. & Song, X. A. (2009). The Clinical Observation of Liver Dysfunction in Measles Patients *Chinese Journal for Clinical Medicine* 18, 77.

Marie, J. C., Kehren, J., Trescol-Biemont, M. C., Evlashev, A., Valentin, H., Walzer, T., Tedone, R., Loveland, B., Nicolas, J. F., Rabourdin-Combe, C. & Horvat, B. (2001). Mechanism of measles virus-induced suppression of inflammatory immune responses. *Immunity* 14, 69-79.

Markowitz, L. E., Nzilambi, N., Driskell, W. J., Sension, M. G., Rovira, E. Z., Nieburg, P. & Ryder, R. W. (1989). Vitamin A levels and mortality among hospitalized measles patients, Kinshasa, Zaire. *Journal of Tropical Pediatrics* 35, 109-112.

Marrack, P., Kappler, J. & Mitchell, T. (1999). Type I interferons keep activated T cells alive. *Journal of Experimental Medicine* 189, 521-530.

McChesney, M. B., Fujinami, R. S., Lampert, P. W. & Oldstone, M. B. (1986). Viruses disrupt functions of human lymphocytes. II. Measles virus suppresses antibody production by acting on B lymphocytes. *Journal of Experimental Medicine* 163, 1331-1336.

McChesney, M. B., Fujinami, R. S., Lerche, N. W., Marx, P. A. & Oldstone, M. B. (1989). Virus-induced immunosuppression: infection of peripheral blood mononuclear cells and suppression of immunoglobulin synthesis during natural measles virus infection of rhesus monkeys. *Journal of Infectious Diseases* 159, 757-760.

McChesney, M. B., Kehrl, J. H., Valsamakis, A., Fauci, A. S. & Oldstone, M. B. (1987). Measles virus infection of B lymphocytes permits cellular activation but blocks progression through the cell cycle. *Journal of Virology* 61, 3441-3447.

McChesney, M. B., Miller, C. J., Rota, P. A., Zhu, Y. D., Antipa, L., Lerche, N. W., Ahmed, R. & Bellini, W. J. (1997). Experimental measles I: Pathogenesis in the normal and the immunized host. *Virology* 233, 74-84.

Menge, T., Hemmer, B., Nessler, S., Wiendl, H., Neuhaus, O., Hartung, H. P., Kieseier, B. C. & Stuve, O. (2005). Acute disseminated encephalomyelitis: an update. *Archives of Neurology* 62, 1673-1680.

Modlin, J. F., Halsey, N. A., Eddins, D. L., Conrad, J. L., Jabbour, J. T., Chien, L. & Robinson, H. (1979). Epidemiology of subacute sclerosing panencephalitis. *Journal of Pediatrics* 94, 231-236.

Moench, T. R., Griffin, D. E., Obriecht, C. R., Vaisberg, A. J. & Johnson, R. T. (1988). Acute measles in patients with and without neurological involvement: distribution of measles virus antigen and RNA. *Journal of Infectious Diseases* 158, 433-442.

Morley, D. C. (1974). Measles in the developing world. *Proceedings of the Royal Society of Medicine* 67, 1112-1115.

Moss, W. J., Ota, M. O. & Griffin, D. E. (2004). Measles: immune suppression and immune responses. *International Journal of Biochemistry and Cell Biology* 36, 1380-1385.

Mrkic, B., Odermatt, B., Klein, M. A., Billeter, M. A., Pavlovic, J. & Cattaneo, R. (2000). Lymphatic dissemination and comparative pathology of recombinant measles viruses in genetically modified mice. *Journal of Virology* 74, 1364-1372.

Mustafa, M. M., Weitman, S. D., Winick, N. J., Bellini, W. J., Timmons, C. F. & Siegel, J. D. (1993). Subacute measles encephalitis in the young immunocompromised host: report of two cases diagnosed by polymerase chain reaction and treated with ribavirin and review of the literature. *Clinical Infectious Diseases* 16, 654-660.

Naniche, D., Reed, S. I. & Oldstone, M. B. (1999). Cell cycle arrest during measles virus infection: a G0-like block leads to suppression of retinoblastoma protein expression. *Journal of Virology* 73, 1894-1901.

Naniche, D., Yeh, A., Eto, D., Manchester, M., Friedman, R. M. & Oldstone, M. B. (2000). Evasion of host defenses by measles virus: wild-type measles virus infection interferes with induction of Alpha/Beta interferon production. *Journal of Virology* 74, 7478-7484.

Nasr, J. T., Andriola, M. R. & Coyle, P. K. (2000). ADEM: literature review and case report of acute psychosis presentation. *Pediatric Neurology* 22, 8-18.

Niewiesk, S., Eisenhuth, I., Fooks, A., Clegg, J. C., Schnorr, J. J., Schneider-Schaulies, S. & ter Meulen, V. (1997). Measles virus-induced immune suppression in the cotton rat (Sigmodon hispidus) model depends on viral glycoproteins. *Journal of Virology* 71, 7214-7219.

Niewiesk, S., Gotzelmann, M. & ter Meulen, V. (2000). Selective in vivo suppression of T lymphocyte responses in experimental measles virus infection. *Proceedings of the National Academy of Sciences U S A* 97, 4251-4255.

Ning, X., Ayata, M., Kimura, M., Komase, K., Furukawa, K., Seto, T., Ito, N., Shingai, M., Matsunaga, I., Yamano, T. & Ogura, H. (2002). Alterations and diversity in the cytoplasmic tail of the fusion protein of subacute sclerosing panencephalitis virus strains isolated in Osaka, Japan. *Virus Research* 86, 123-131.

Okada, H., Kobune, F., Sato, T. A., Kohama, T., Takeuchi, Y., Abe, T., Takayama, N., Tsuchiya T & Tashiro, M. (2000). Extensive lymphopenia due to apoptosis of uninfected lymphocytes in acute measles patients. *Archives of Virology* 145, 905-920.

Oldstone, M. B., Bokisch, V. A., Dixon, F. J., Barbosa, L. H., Fuccillo, D. & Sever, J. L. (1975). Subacute sclerosing panencephalitis: destruction of human brain cells by antibody and complement in an autologous system. *Clinical Immunology and Immunopathology* 4, 52.

Organization, W. H. (2005). .The world health report 2005. In *make every mother and child count*. Edited by WHO. Geneva: WHO.

Palosaari, H., Parisien, J., Rodriguez, J., Ulane, C., Horvath, C., . , . Takeuchi, K., Kadota, S., Takeda, M., Miyajima, N., Nagata, K., . (2003). STAT protein interference and suppression of cytokine signal transduction by measles virus V protein. *Journal of Virology* 77, 7635-7644.

Papania, M. J., Seward, J. F., Redd, S. B., Lievano, F., Harpaz, R. & Wharton, M. E. (2004). Epidemiology of Measles in the United States,1997-2001. *Journal of Infectious Diseases* 189, S61-68.

Patrick Sissons, J. G., Schreiber, R. D., Perrin, L. H., Cooper, N. R., Muller-Eberhard, H. J. & Oldstone, M. B. (1979). Lysis of measles virus-infected cells by the purified cytolytic alternative complement pathway and antibody. *Journal of Experimental Medicine* 150, 445-454.

Patterson, J. B., Thomas, D., Lewicki, H., Billeter, M. A. & Oldstone,M. B. A. (2000). V and C proteins of measles virus function as virulence factors in vivo. *Virology* 267, 80-89.

Peebles, T. C. (1967). Distribution of virus in blood components during the viremia of measles. *Arch Gesamte Virusforsch* 22, 43-47.

Peters, V. B. & Sperber, K. E. (1999). The effect of viruses on the ability to present antigens via the major histocompatibility complex. *Microbes and Infection* 1, 335-345.

Polack, F. P., Auwaerter, P. G., Lee, S. H., Nousari, H. C., Valsamakis, A., Leiferman, K. M., Diwan, A., Adams, R. J. & Griffin, D. E. (1999). Production of atypical measles in rhesus macaques: evidence for disease mediated by immune complex formation and eosinophils in the presence of fusion-inhibiting antibody. *Nature Medicine* 5, 629-634.

Rammohan, K. W., McFarland, H. F. & McFarlin, D. E. (1981). Induction of subacute murine measles encephalitis by monoclonal antibody to virus haemagglutinin. *Nature* 290, 588-589.

Rauh, L. W. & Schmidt, R. (1965). Measles Immunization with Killed Virus Vaccine. Serum Antibody Titers and Experience with Exposure to Measles Epidemic. *American Journal of Diseases of Children* 109, 232-237.

Ravanel, K., Castelle, C., Defrance, T., Wild, T. F., Charron, D., Lotteau, V. & Rabourdin-Combe, C. (1997). Measles virus nucleocapsid protein binds to FcgammaRII and inhibits human B cell antibody production. *Journal of Experimental Medicine* 186, 269-278.

Rima, B. K. & Duprex, W. P. (2006). Morbilliviruses and human disease. *J Pathol* 208, 199-214.

Robbins, F. C. (1962). Measles: clinical features. Pathogenesis, pathology and complications. *American Journal of Diseases of Children* 103, 266-273.

Roscic-Mrkic, B., Schwendener, R. A., Odermatt, B., Zuniga, A., Pavlovic, J., Billeter, M. A. & Cattaneo, R. (2001). Roles of macrophages in measles virus infection of genetically modified mice. *Journal of Virology* 75, 3343-3351.

Ryon, J. J., Moss, W. J., Monze, M. & Griffin, D. E. (2002). Functional and phenotypic changes in circulating lymphocytes from hospitalized zambian children with measles. *Clinical Diagnosis Laboratory Immunology* 9, 994-1003.

Sakaguchi, M., Yoshikawa, Y., Yamanouchi, K., Sata, T., Nagashima, K. & Takeda, K. (1986). Growth of measles virus in epithelial and lymphoid tissues of cynomolgus monkeys. *Microbiology and Immunology* 30, 1067-1073.

Salonen, R., Ilonen, J. & Salmi, A. A. (1989). Measles virus inhibits lymphocyte proliferation in vitro by two different mechanisms. *Clinical Experimental Immunology* 75, 376-380.

Scheifele, D. W. & Forbes, C. E. (1972). Prolonged giant cell excretion in severe African measles. *Pediatrics* 50, 867-873.

Schlender, J., Schnorr, J. J., Spielhoffer, P., Cathomen, T., Cattaneo, R., Billeter, M. A., ter Meulen, V. & Schneider-Schaulies, S. (1996). Interaction of measles virus glycoproteins with the surface of uninfected peripheral blood lymphocytes induces immunosuppression in vitro. *Proceedings of the National Academy of Sciences U S A* 93, 13194-13199.

Schneider-Schaulies, J., Dunster, L. M., Schneider-Schaulies, S. & ter Meulen, V. (1995). Pathogenetic aspects of measles virus infections. *Veterinary Microbiology* 44, 113-125.

Schneider-Schaulies, S., Niewiesk, S., Schneider-Schaulies, J. & ter Meulen, V. (2001). Measles virus induced immunosuppression: targets and effector mechanisms. *Current molecular medicine* 1, 163-181.

Schneider-Schaulies, S. & ter Meulen, V. (2002). Measles virus and immunomodulation: molecular bases and perspectives. *Expert Reviews in Molecular Medicine* 4, 1-18.

Schnorr, J. J., Xanthakos, S., Keikavoussi, P., Kampgen, E., ter Meulen, V. & Schneider-Schaulies, S. (1997). Induction of maturation of human blood dendritic cell precursors by measles virus is associated with immunosuppression. *Proceedings of the National Academy of Sciences, USA* 94, 5326-5331.

Servet-Delprat, C., Vidalain, P. O., Bausinger, H., Manie, S., Le Deist, F., Azocar, O., Hanau, D., Fischer, A. & Rabourdin-Combe, C. (2000). Measles virus induces abnormal differentiation of CD40 ligand-activated human dendritic cells. *Journal of Immunology* 164, 1753-1760.

Servet-Delprat, C., Vidalain, P. O., Bausinger, H., Manie, S., Le Deist, F., Azocar, O., Hanau, D., Fischer, A. & Rabourdin-Combe, C. (2000b). Measles virus induces abnormal differentiation of CD40 ligand-activated human dendritic cells. *Journal of Immunology* 164, 1753-1760.

Seto, T., Ayata, M., Hayashi, K., Furukawa, K., Murata, R. & Ogura, H. (1999). Different transcriptional expression of the matrix gene of the two sibling viruses of the subacute sclerosing panencephalitis virus (Osaka-2 strain) isolated from a biopsy specimen of patient brain. *Journal of Neurovirology* 5, 151-160.

Shaffer, J. A., Bellini, W. J. & Rota, P. A. (2003). The C protein of measles virus inhibits the type I interferon response. *Virology* 315, 389-397.

Shiozawa, S., Yoshikawa, N., Iijima, K. & Negishi, K. (1988). A sensitive radioimmunoassay for circulating alpha-interferon in the plasma of healthy children and patients with measles virus infection. *Clinical Experimental Immunology* 73, 366-369.

Singh, J., Sharma, R. S. & Verghese, T. (1994). Measles mortality in India: a review of community based studies. *Journal of Communicable Diseases* 26, 203-214.

Sips, G. J., Chesik, D., Glazenburg, L., Wilschut, J., De Keyser, J. & Wilczak, N. (2007). Involvement of morbilliviruses in the pathogenesis of demyelinating disease. *Reviews in Medical Virology* 17, 223-244.

Sivasankaran, S., Manickam, P., Ramakrishnan, R., Hutin, Y. & Gupte, M. D. (2006). Estimation of Measles Vaccination Coverage Using the Lot Quality Assurance Sampling Method Tamilnadu, India, 2002--2003. *Morbidity and Mortality Weekly* 55, 16-19.

Smith, F. R., Curran, A. S., Raciti, K. A. & Black, F. L. (1982). Reported measles in persons immunologically primed by prior vaccination. *Journal of Pediatrics* 101, 391-393.

Staples, K. J., Bergmann, M., Barnes, P. J. & Newton, R. (2000). Stimulus-specific inhibition of IL-5 by cAMP-elevating agents and IL-10 reveals differential mechanisms of action. *Biochemical Biophysical Research Communications* 273, 811-815.

Suringa, D. W., Bank, L. J. & Ackerman, A. B. (1970). Role of Measles Virus in Skin Lesions and Koplik's Spots. *New England Journal of Medicine*, 1139-1142.

Takahashi, H., Umino, Y., Sato, T. A., Kohama, T., Ikeda, Y., Iijima, M. & Fujisawa, R. (1996). Detection and comparison of viral antigens in measles and rubella rashes. *Clinical Infectious Diseases* 22, 36-39.

Tilles, J. G., Balkwill, F. & Davilla, J. (1987). 2',5'-Oligoadenylate synthetase and interferon in peripheral blood after rubella, measles, or mumps live virus vaccine. *Proceedings of the Society for Experimental Biology and Medicine Society for Experimental Biology and Medicine (New York, NY)* 186, 70-74.

Valmari, P., Lanning, M., Tuokko, H. & Kouvalainen, K. (1987). Measles virus in the cerebrospinal fluid in postvaccination immunosuppressive measles encephalopathy. *Pediatric Infectious Disease Journal* 6, 59-63.

Valsamakis, A., Schneider, H., Auwaerter, P. G., Kaneshima, H.,Billeter, M. A. & Griffin, D. E. (1998). Recombinant measles viruses with mutations in the C, V, or F gene have altered growth phenotypes in vivo. *Journal of Virology* 72, 7754-7761.

Vidalain, P. O., Azocar, O., Lamouille, B., Astier, A., Rabourdin-Combe, C. & Servet-Delprat, C. (2000). Measles virus induces functional TRAIL production by human dendritic cells. *Journal of Virology* 74, 556-559.

Vinante, F., Krampera, M., Morosato, L., Rigo, A., Romagnani, S. & Pizzolo, G. (1999). Peripheral T lymphocyte cytokine profile (IFNgamma, IL-2, IL-4) and CD30 expression/release during measles infection. *Haematologica* 84, 683-689.

Volckaert-Vervliet, G. & Billiau, A. (1977). Induction of interferon in human lymphoblastoid cells by Sendai and measles viruses. *Journal of General Virology* 37, 199-203.

Volckaert-Vervliet, G., Heremans, H., De Ley, M. & Billiau, A. (1978). Interferon induction and action in human lymphoblastoid cells infected with measles virus. *Jouranl of General Virology* 41, 459-466.

Wang, L. X., Zeng, G., Lisa, A. L., Yang, Z. W., Yu, J. J., Zhou, J., Liang, X. F., Xu, C. & Bai, H. Q. (2003). Progress in accelerated measles control in the People's Republic of China, 1991-2000. *Journal of Infectious Diseases* 187 Suppl 1, S252-257.

Wang, P., Zha, C. M. & Liu, X. J. (2010). Observation on 382 Infant Measles Patients with Complicaitons. *Nurse Journal of China PLA* 27, 777-778.

Wegner, C. (2005). Pathological differences in acute inflammatory demyelinating diseases of the central nervous system. *International MS Journal* 12, 13-19, 12.

Whittle, H. C., Aaby, P., Samb, B., Jensen, H., Bennett, J. & Simondon, F. (1999). Effect of subclinical infection on maintaining immunity against measles in vaccinated children in West Africa. *Lancet* 353, 98-102.

WHO-UNICEF (2001). Joint Statement on Strategies to Reduce Measles Mortality Worldwide. Geneva: World Health Organization

WHO (1995). Measles. Progress towards global control and regional elimination, 1998--1999. *Weekly Epicemiological Record* 74, 429?424.

WHO (2005). Global Measles and Rubella Laboratory Network, January 2004-June 2005. *MMWR Morbidity Mortality Weekly Report* 54, 1100-1104.

WHO (2006). Progress in reducing global measles deaths: 1999–2004. *Weekly Epidemiological Record* 10, 89-96.

WHO (2008). Progress in global measles control and mortality reduction, 2000–2007. *Weekly Epidemiological Record* No. 49, 441-448.

WHO (2009). Progress towards the 2012 measles elimination goal in WHO's Western Pacifi c Region, 1990–2008. *Weekly Epidemiological Record* 27, 271-279

WHO (2010). Measles reported cases In *Vaccine-preventable Diseases Vaccine Monitoring System 2010 Global Summary Reference Time Series*. Edited by V. a. B. Immunization. Geneva: World Health Organization.

WHO/UNICEF (2001). Measles: mortality reduction and regional elimination.Strategic plan 2001–2005. In *WHO/V&B/0113 Rev 1*. Edited by W. H. Organization. Geneva: World Health Organization.

WHO/UNICEF (2009). Strengthening Immunization Services through Measles Control, Joint Annual Measles Report 2009, p. 10: WHO/UNICEF.

Wild, T. F. (1999). Measles vaccines, new developments and immunization strategies. *Vaccine* 17, 1726-1729.

Wong, T. C., Ayata, M., Hirano, A., Yoshikawa, Y., Tsuruoka, H. & Yamanouchi, K. (1989). Generalized and localized biased hypermutation affecting the matrix gene of a measles virus strain that causes subacute sclerosing panencephalitis. *Journal of Virology* 63, 5464-5468.

Wu, T. (2000). The History and Current Status for Measles Control and Prevention in China. *Chinese Journal of Epidemiology* 21, 143－146.

Yokota, S., Saito, H., Kubota, T., Yokosawa, N., Amano, K. & Fujii, N. (2003). Measles virus suppresses interferon-alpha signaling pathway: suppression of Jak1 phosphorylation and association of viral accessory proteins, C and V, with interferon-alpha receptor complex. *Virology* 306, 135-146.

Yu, G., Chen, Q. F., Liu, J. R., Lin, X. L., Zhang, H. L., Chen, Y. P. & Li, C. C. (2009). Analysis on 429 Pneumonia in Children Measles Patients. *Zhejiang Preventive Medicine* 21, 29-30.

Yu, X., Qian, F., Sheng, Y., Xie, D., Li, D., Huang, Q., Zhang, Y., Yuan, Z. & Ghildyal, R. (2007a). Clinical and genetic characterization of measles viruses isolated from adult patients in Shanghai in 2006. *Journal of Clinical Virology* 40, 146-151.

Yu, X., Wang, S., Guan, J., Mahemuti, Purhati, Gou, A., Liu, Q., Jin, X. & Ghildyal, R. (2007b). Analysis of the cause of increased measles incidence in Xinjiang, China in 2004. *Pediatric Infectious Disease Journal* 26, 513-518.

Yu, X. L., Cheng, Y. M., Shi, B. S., Qian, F. X., Wang, F. B., Liu, X. N., Yang, H. Y., Xu, Q. N., Qi, T. K., Zha, L. J., Yuan, Z. H. & Ghildyal, R. (2008). Measles virus infection in adults induces production of IL-10 and is associated with increased CD4+ CD25+ regulatory T cells. *Journal of Immunol* 181, 7356-7366.

Yu, X. L., Liu, Q. M., Guan, J., Mahemuti, K., Reyihan, G., Xu, X., Cui, H. & Gou, A. L. (2006). Evaluation Measles Mass Campaign of Xinjiang Uygur Autonomous Region in 2004. *Chinese Journal of Expanded Programme on Immunizaiton* 12, 373-375.

Ze, W. Y. (2002). *Expanded Programme on Immunization*. Shanghai: Shanghai Publishing House of Scientific and Technological Literature.

Zhou, H., Zhao, W. Y., Luo, X. M., Lv, H., Y. & Gao, S. Z. (2003). Surveillance on measles antibody level of pregnant women and the immune efficiency in their babies. *Chinese Journal of Disease Surveillance* 18, 380-381.

Zhu, Q., Tong, Y. B., Zhang, D. Y., Du, W., Wu, S. W. & Xu, F. (2008). Measles Mass Campaign Experience and Effect Evaluation on Measles Vaccine in Guizhou Province. *Chinese Journal of Vaccines and Immunization* 14, 23-26.

Zuo, S. Y., Xu, X. Q., Xia, W., Liang, X. F., Xu, W. B., Zhang, Y., An, Z. J., Cheng, H. M., Wang, X. J. & Yu, J. J. (2006). Epidemiology Investigation and Analysis on Measles Prevalence in Zhejiang Province in 2005. *Chinese Journal of Expanded Programme on Immunizaiton* 12, 342-349.

13

Immunoregulation: A Proposal for an Experimental Model

Marcela Šperanda[1] and Ivica Valpotić[2]
[1]*University of J. J. Strossmajer, Faculty of Agriculture in Osijek,*
[2]*University of Zagreb, Faculty of Veterinary Medicine, Zagreb*
Croatia

1. Introduction

The scope of the chapter is to describe principles and mechanisms of activation and regulation of porcine intestinal immune system, especially during postnatal development. The pig is an essential source of food Worldwide, and thus, immunological research in swine husbandry and nutrition is performed to develop a safe and sustainable meat production. The study of the swine mucosal immune system is important because induction and maintenance of protective immune mechanisms will be at the cost of energy which will be lost for productive purpose. Also, certain degree of mucosal immune response is necessary to protect against chronic and acute infectious diseases that can cause losses in production, but on the other side, overacting immune responses can be detrimental for the host. Further, the pig is important biomedical model for applied experimental studies in different areas of physiology or clinical medicine. In particular, the pig is important for transplantation research, both for the development of surgical techniques and as xenotransplant donor. Thus, it is of importance to understand porcine immunology and to obtain insight into the structure and functional characteristics of their humoral and cellular immune system, both systemic and local. Herein, we propose the pig as a model for immunoregulation at the mucosal surfaces of the gut. The gut and gut associated lymphoid tissue (GALT) has dual roles in mammals organism: digestion and apsorption of nutrients as well as protecting the body from harmful pathogens and inducing tolerogenic responses to self-antigens, food particles and commensals. The unique architecture of the GI tract facilitates both of these functions.The purpose of this chapter is to review the existing literature on developmental aspects of antigen handling and processing by intestinal mucosal immune system of developing pigs.

The immune defence system of the gut consists of lymphoid tissues and cells distributed along the gastrointestinal tract. Important features that characterize the mucosal immune system are:

- Mucosa-associated lymphoid tissue (MALT or GALT-gut associated lymphoid tissue) with local and regional lymph nodes (LNs) where the induction of immune responses is established (Payer's patches and the mesenterial lymph nodes)
- Certain subpopulation of lymphoid cells at the mucosal surfaces
- Mucosal homing, that means specific recirculation of mucosal lymphocytes towards mucosae
- Predominant mucosal immunoglobulin is IgA secreted at the mucosal surface.

2. Intestinal mucosal immune system (IMIS): Paradoxycal role to protect and/or tolerate

The concept of mucosal immunity includes response to harmful antigens and also control of harmless antigens to prevent inflammation, well known as mucosal or oral tolerance. Therefore the mucosal immune system has to retain the ability to respond actively to pathogens, while avoiding active potentially inflammatory responses to pathogens. For that reason, the organisms have decision-making pathways embedded with the immunological architecture of the mucosal immune system. If a little dietary antigen access to the general circulation a systemic immune response may be prevented by the activities of regulatory T cells. Oral tolerance develops to the antigen. It involves either cellular suppression or clonal anergy and it is directed against Th1 cells (Gad, 2005). Which mechanism would be involved depends on several things. The feeding of novel protein antigens is associated with the presence of mucosal IgA responses despite the appearance of systemic oral tolerance. There is a strong genetic influence on the extent of systemic tolerance induced by feeding. Dose of orally administered antigen is important. Low doses invoke priming; high doses provoke clonal anergy (oral tolerance). Several studies, including humans, swine and mice, demonstrated that small quantities of food proteins absorb intact across the intestinal epithelium in adults and neonates (Bailey et al, 1994; Telemo et al, 1991). Recent studies of the phenomenon of oral tolerance suggest that it is variable and age-dependent (Bailey & Haverson, 2006) as well as the present of commensal microbial flora in the intestine.

2.1 Structure of the intestinal mucosal immune system (IMIS)

The mucosal immune system is described as the subset of immunological components, which appear in or associated with mucosal tissues. In mammals, there is clear distinction between primary lymphoid tissue, such as the bone marrow and the thymus, and secondary lymphoid tissue such as the spleen and organised lymph nodes and Payer's patches. Since mucosal tissues are exposed to the harmless and harmful antigens, mechanisms must activate appropriate, but different responses to different types of antigens. Therefore we use classic differentiation mucosal immune system on the organised and the diffuse lymphoid tissues.

The organised lymphoid tissues include the Payer's patches and the mesenteric lymph nodes. There's role is recognition of luminally presented antigens through different pathways:

1. Some antigens cross the epithelium membrane of the villi owing the dendritic lineage which are underneath the intestinal epithelium. Dendritic cells with dendrites uptake antigen through the epithelium by manipulation tight-cell junction (Rescigno et al., 2001, MacPherson & Uhr, 2004). Dendritic cells may also phagocytose epithelial cells together with environmental antigens (Huang et al., 2000) or ensure crossing the epithelium intact, transcellularly or paracellularly (Jang et al., 2004). Mucosal dendritic cells migrate through afferent lymphatics to the mesenteric lymph nodes, where they can present antigen in T-cell areas. So, the mesenteric lymph nodes are important for initiation or expansion of mucosal immune responses (Mowat, 2003).
2. Antigen may be taken up directly to the Payer's patches mediated by specialised M-cells or paracellularly by dendritic cells. Migration of this cells to the T-cell zones results in T-cell activation, migration and induction of responses in the follicle of the Payer's patch. Primed T- and B-cells emigrate from the patches in efferent lymphatics (Brandtzaeg & Pabst, 2004).

3. Intact antigen absorbed across the mucosal epithelium may reach the lymphatics directly and be transported to the lymph nodes and into blood, where it can interact with components of the systemic immune system (Telemo el al., 1991).
4. Antigens may cross the enterocytes epithelial membrane in the form of exosomes. Pig enterocytes do not express MHC II proteins on their surfaces, but capillary lymphoid tissue epithelium in the pig's intestine expresses high levels of MHC II molecules, so it could be possible that these cells release exosomes directly into blood (Wilson et al., 1996).

The diffuse lymphoid tissues

Different cells and molecules are present into mucus membrane of the pigs' gastrointestinal tract.

1. Intestinal epithelium contains some amount of leucocytes. The predominant lymphocyte population express the CD8 coreceptors, unconventional subset of T-cells expressing a CD8αα homodimer and the TCR chains (Hayday et al., 2001). The majority of lymphocytes in the intestinal epithelium express CD2. A high proportion of lymphocytes express $CD8^{+}$ in adults which do not appear in piglets until 7 weeks onwards (Whary et al., 1995). In young pigs, intestinal epithelium lymphocytes are mostly $CD2^{-}CD4^{-}CD8^{-}$, and during the first few weeks of life $CD2^{+}CD4^{-}CD8^{-}$ appear.
2. Lamina propria underneath the epithelium is well supplied with leukocytes and in pigs shows a high level of organisation (Wilson et al., 1996). Theirs' APCs expressing MHC II protein class. Immature dendritic cells are present in large numbers within the villi and co-localise with T-cells expressing the CD4 coreceptor in the pig, but expressing the low affinity FcγRIII (Bailey & Haverson, 2006). The point is that diffuse mucosal tissue has the first role in immune regulation, rather than active defensive responses. At the same time, these plastic cells may easiliy be switched from regulatory to active responses (Mellman & Steinman, 2001).
3. The endothelium of the capillary plexus beneath the epithelial basement membrane expresses MHC II molecules as good as dendritic cells. There are also dendritic cells within the villi and help to promote CD4 co-receptor with T-cells.
4. Lamina propria around intestinal crypts consists of cells staning for immunoglobulin (IgA, presumably plasma cells) and myeloid lineage cells have more characteristic of macrophages and granulocytes (Vega-Lopez et al., 1993). Plasma cells are predominantly IgA^{+}, IgM^{+} and some IgG^{+}cells are present.

2.2 The role of antigen presenting dendritic cells

The role of population of dendritic cells (DCs) in the intestine and associated lymphoid tissues is of great interest because theirs influence in maintenance of tolerance towards the commensal microflora and in protection against pathogens. There are unique functional properties of populations of intestinal DC, as well as the type of signals that are necessary for them to mediate these functions. The intestine and GALT have network of cells with antigen-presenting function, including macrophages, DCs (CD11c) and plasmacytoid DCs (Smith et al., 2005; Iwasaki A, 2007). Various subpopulations of DCs are present in the organized lymphoid tissue of the intestine, Payer's patches and mesenteric lymph nodes, through the small intestine and lamina propria (Johansson & Kelsall, 2005). Dendritic cells have a central role in the activation of resting T cells and the initiation of primary responses. DCs acquire antigen (Ag) in peripheral tissues and transport it to lymph nodes (LNs) for presentation to lymphocytes (Banchereau & Steinman, 1998). DCs migrate constitutively from peripheral tissue when they have acquired foreign Ag, but also in the absence of any antigenic or inflammatory stimuli (Huang et al., 2000). However, DCs continually migrate from the intestine to mesenteric LNs in the absence of overt antigenic stimulation (Liu et al., 1998). Plasmacytoid dendritic cells (pDC) recognize pathogen molecules, particularly viral, and play crucial roles in the inate defense and regulation of adaptive immune responses (Colonna et al., 2004). pDCs function primarily via TLRs and ligation of these receptors stimulates the secretion of large amounts of cytokines, particularly IFN (Asselin-Paturel & Trinchieri, 2005).

Theirs functional properties vary according to their anatomical location. Activated DC from the Payer's patches produce higher levels of interleukin 10 (IL-10), than splenic DC (Iwasaki & Kelsall, 1999). Naive CD4 T-cells activated by DC from the Payer's patches produce higher levels of IL-4 and IL-10, indicative of a T helper (T_H2) type phenotype, than those activated by splenic DC. Surface phenotypic analysis of CD11c1 DC populations revealed that Payer's patches DCs expressed higher levels of major histocompatibility complex class II molecules, but similar levels of costimulatory molecules and adhesion molecules compared with splenic DCs. But, the level of IFN-g produced by T cells primed with spleen DCs was significantly higher than that produced by T cells primed with PP DCs. While presentation of antigen by DCs *in vitro* leads to T cell activation, the same may not apply *in vivo*, and there is circumstantial evidence that DCs may be able to present Ag in a tolerogenic manner (Finkelman et al., 1996, Viney et al., 1998).

Activated pDCs secrete proinflammatory cytokines, change their morphology from a round cell to dendritic cell-like, up-regulate MHC and costimulatory molecules and become effective APCs. Human pDCs activated by CD40L or influenza virus can induce proliferation and polarization of T cells. Mature pDCs efficiently stimulate T cells and drive a potent TH1 polarization in vitro, which is mediated by the synergistic effect of interleukin 12 and type I interferon. In vivo, mature pDCs are found in secondary lymphoid organs, where they represent the principal source of type I interferon during inflammation (Cella et al., 2000). Mice pDCs activated with virus have shown to activate naive CD8+ T cells and to promote and polarization of Ag-experienced unpolarized CD4+ T cells (Krug et al., 2003). pDCs have a role in tolerogenic responses, as they can induce development of anergic T cells or T cells with regulatory function in vitro (Moseman et al., 2004). It is known now that depletion of pDCs can lead to airway hyperactivity to normally inert inhaled Ags, and that adoptive transfer of Ag-loaded pDCs before sensitization could prevent the induced asthma (De Heer et al., 2004). In this case Ag bearing pDCs was isolated from lung and the draining LN which suggested that similarly to classical DC, pDCs may acquire Ag at mucosal sites and transport it to the induce tolerogenic responses. There was no evidence for migration pDC in afferent lymph under steady state condition. However, Yrlid et al., (2006) showed that pDCs are not present in afferent lymph draining another mucosal tissue, especially the intestine. It is possible that the absence of pDCs in intestinal lymph is only in steady-state condition. These experiments suggest that pDCs present in mucosal tissues and liver do not induce tolerogenic or immunogenic Ag-specific T cell responses by acquiring Ag in the periphery and transporting it via afferent lymph to the draining lymph node. The mechanisms of acquiring Ag from periphery is unknown, potential mechanisms include delivery by classical DCs or exosomes or release of DC fragments (Villadangos & Heath, 2005).

Dendritic cells in human are classified according to their cell-surface receptor expression into several subsets. In the Payer's patches, conventional DCs are $CD11c^{hi}CD11b^{+}CD8\alpha^{-}$, $CD11c^{hi}CD11b^{-}CD8\alpha^{-}$ and $CD11c^{hi}CD11b^{-}CD8\alpha^{+}$ subtypes, with unique anatomical localisation and functional properties. These DC can also be described in terms of their expression of the chemokine receptors CX_3C chemokine receptor 1 (CX_3CR1) and CC chemokine receptor 6 (CCR6, Salazar-Gonzalez et al., 2006). CX_3CR1^{+} DCs were found to be associated with the follicle-associated epithelium in the steady state, whereas $CCR6^{+}$ was recruited from the subepithelial dome to the follicle-associated epithelium during infection (Salazar-Gonzalez et al., 2006). An additional population of CD11cmid plasmacytoid DCs are present in the Payer's patches and MLN, but they do not migrate from the intestine to the MLN (Yrlid et al., 2006). Similar subset composition we can find in the small intestinal lamina propria DCs. DCs in the small-intestinal lamina propria were found to express CX_3CR1 (Niess et al., 2005). In the colon, DCs appear to be concentrated within isolated lymphoid follicles, with very few present in the lamina propria under steady-state conditions. MLNs contain population of DCs written before, but they are both migratory DCs arriving from the intestinal lamina propria in the steady-state and resident DCs that have developed from blood-home precursors. Functional differences depend on developmental origins, local environmental conditions and maturation states (Coombes & Powrie, 2008). $CD11b^{+}$ DCs can be found in the subepithelial dome of the Payer's patches, whereas $CD8\alpha^{+}$ is present in the inter-follicular region. While $0CD11b^{+}$ DCs from the Payer's patches produce IL-10 and prime Th2 cells, $CD8\alpha^{+}$ and $CD11b^{-}CD8\alpha^{-}$ were shown to produce IL-12 and interferon-γ (IFN-γ) by T-cells. Jejunal lamina propria in pigs contains large number of MHC class II cells, which could be divided into at least three subsets based upon expression of other markers. The majority of MHC class II co-expressed on $CD45^{+}$ cells, and second population of cells expressing CD16, SwC3 and CD45. Actually, there are $CD45^{+}$ and $CD45^{-}$ cells which very differ morphologically. The $CD45^{+}$ cells are large, strongly adherent and had bilobed nuclei. The CD^{-} is smaller and elongated with dense oval nuclei (Stokes & Bailey, 2000). Haverson & Riffault (2006) found that $CD45^{+}$ population was potent stimulators of primary responses, but $CD45^{-}$ stromal population were unable to generate any proliferative response. Further, there are identified some unusual APC DC such as expressing both CD11c and MHC II at low intensity. These DC produced immune-regulatory cytokines such as IL-10 and type I IFN, suggesting a role in immunoregulation and tolerance induction. These intestinal DCs are capable of presenting antigen and induce tolerance, but also can response to inflammatory stimuli to allow T cell priming and protective immunity (Mowat, 2005).

DCs are separate lineage that is present in the steady state, but they have ability to run pro-inflammatory responses. Alternatively, these cells may represent population of DCs in steady state but becomes more dominant during inflammation (Coombes & Powrie, 2008). Intestinal macrophages display some characteristics compared with splenic macrophages or those that derive from blood monocytes (Smythies et al., 2005). Human intestinal macrophages retain phagocytic and bactericidal activity, but they lack CD14 expression, which is obligatory for the Toll-like receptor 4 (TLR4)-mediated recognition of ligands. These cells showed an impaired ability to produce proinflammatory cytokines. These modifications might contribute to intestinal immune homeostasis by ensuring the contact of intestinal APCs with microbial products do not result in the generation of potentially destructive inflammatory responses.

2.3 Intraepithelial and lamina propria lymphocytes (IEL, LPL)

Different antigens enter the body from the intestine: food proteins, commensal gut flora, invading pathogens, toxins. The digestive tube is lined by a continuous monolayer of epithelial cells. That intestinal epithelial cells (IEC) act as a physical barrier, separating the contents of a luminal environment from the layers of tissue comprising the interior milieu (Gewirtz et al., 2002). IEC also participate in the innate immune response of the intestine like a physical barrier, mucus secretion, antibacterial peptide synthesis and participation in the cytokine/chemokine network (Oswald, 2006).

2.3.1 Intraepithelial Lymphocytes (IEL)

At the basolateral surfaces of intestinal epithelial cells there are intestinal intraepithelial lymphocytes (IEL) which play important roles in the homeostasis of intestinal microenvironment. Intraepithelial lymphocytes (IEL) are predominantly T lymphocytes, a major subpopulation of γδ i-IEL is produced from uncommitted precursors at extrathymic sites (Bandeira et al., 1991; Poussier & Julius, 1994). T cells appear to have both proinflammatory and regulatory functions: they can act as a bridge between innate and adaptive immunity early in responses and can down-modulate inflammatory responses (Newton et al., 2006).

In samples of proximal and distal small intestine of five 6-month-old pigs (Vega-Lopez et al., 1995) were studied CD2, CD4 (helper/inducer T-cells), CD8 (suppressor/cytotoxic T cells), accessory cell marker (monocyte/granulocyte) and MHC Class II (DRw) receptor. $CD2^+$ cells were found in high numbers in both the epithelium and the lamina propria. Two subpopulations of intraepithelial lymphocytes were identified: apically in the epithelium there were $CD2^+CD4^-CD8^-$(double negative) cells, whereas cells expressing CD8 marker were concentrated around the basement membrane. $CD4^+$cells were localized in the lamina propria towards the villus core. Accessory cells were distributed in crypts and the villus base and more cells were found in ileum than in duodenum. In contrast, MHC Class II^+ cells were located predominantly in villi, just underneath the basement membrane, forming a sheath of cells between the $CD8^+$ and the $CD4^+$ cells. Pig IEL express CD2 and have an increased proportion of CD8+ cells (Stokes et al., 2001; Davis et al., 2004). However, neonatal pigs are mostly $CD2^-CD4^-CD8^-$, and $CD8^+$ IEL cannot be recognized until the animal matures. Bailey et al. (2001) confirmed the infiltration of $CD8^+$ T cells within the intestinal lamina propria of the villi from 4 week of age onward. It has also been demonstrated that phenotypic changes in porcine IEL are influenced by exposure to environmental antigens (Pabst & Rothkotter, 1999, Bailey et al., 2005). McCracken et al. (1999) reported that the number of $CD8^+$ T lymphocytes per 100 m of villus isolated from the intestinal jejunum was increased post weaning.

According to morphology, size, and sedimentation density of lymphocytes, Hayday et al., (2001) have proposed that IEL be classified into 2 subgroups: Type a and Type b. As Type a IEL would be included intraepithelial lymphocytes that are thymus-dependent, activated within the peripheral circulation, that express the αβ T-cell receptor, and that recognize antigen in the context of major histocompatibility complex I or II. Type b IEL are thymus-independent cells that express T-cell receptors that are $\gamma\delta^+$, $\gamma\delta^+CD8\alpha\alpha^+$, or $\alpha\beta^+CD8\alpha\alpha^+$. Both types of IEL are cytolytic effectors that secrete cytokine and chemokine mediators. Havran et al. (2005) supported the idea that intraepithelial $\gamma\delta^+$ T cells are involved in tissue repair, lysis of damaged epithelial cells, and inflammatory cell recruitment (qualified like innate immune response), while type a IEL are more indicative of an adaptive response. Egan et al

(2011) showed that αβ and not γδ T-cell IELs mediate intestinal damage in mice after parasite infection. In that case IELs did not function alone to cause inflammatory lesions, but acted with $CD4^+$ T lymphocytes from the lamina propria (LP). IEL has ability to bind to E cadherin on IEC, which is facilitated by the expression of αEβ7 integrin (Cepek et al., 1994). Zuckermann and Gaskins (1996) reported that mucosa-associated lymphoid tissues had significantly smaller proportions of $CD4^+$ and/or $CD8^+$ T cells than lymph nodes and CD4/CD8 double positive cells accounted for a larger proportion of the total $CD4^+$ lymphocytes than in lymph nodes. The mid-section of the continuous Peyer's patch in the ileum contained 7% CD4 single positive, 8% CD8 single positive and 4% CD4/CD8 double positive lymphocytes.

2.3.2 Lamina Propria Lymphocytes (LPL)

The gastrointestinal lamina propria is composed of smooth muscle cells, fibroblasts, blood vessels and lymphatics that make up a highly vascular layer of loose connective tissue underlying and supporting the mucosal epithelium. There are macrophages, dendritic cells, neutrophils, mast cells, and lymphocytes that participate in lamina propria effector functions (Hunyady et al., 2000). The population of lymphocytes that resides in the lamina propria has been classified as heterogeneous, and the organization of these cells is classified as random (Bailey et al., 2005). These characteristics are consistent with the effector function of lamina propria lymphocytes, which enables these cells to participate in immunosurveillance and to respond actively to potential pathogens (Burkey et al., 2009). Mixed population of T lymphocytes include helper $CD4^+$ in adult swine settled in lamina propria of the villi and suppressor/cytotoxic $CD8^+$ lymphocytes closer to epithelial cells (Vega-Lopez et al., 1993). The same author found that lamina propria comprise the unique population of $CD2^+CD4^+CD8^+$ lymphocytes (about 30%), as well as $CD2^+$ and $SWC3^+$ (swine workshop cluster) monocyte-granulocyte cells. Important differences in lamina propria lymphocytes exist between humans and swine that may relate to the function of these compartmentalized cells. In the small intestine of pigs, lymphocytes have been categorized as diffuse or organized (Pabst & Rothkotter, 1999). For the most species, intraepithelial lymphocytes and lymphocytes contained in the lamina propria are considered diffuse lymphocytes. In contrast, the gut mucosa of the pig has a greater degree of organization compared with the gut mucosa of rodents and humans (Bailey et al., 2001). For example, Vega-Lopez et al. (1993) observed that plasma cells are preferentially localized to the intestinal crypts and T cells to the intestinal villi. The same authors also observed a spatial separation between $CD4^+$ and $CD8^+$ T cells within the lamina propria of intestinal villi. In addition, researchers have observed differences in cytokines secreted by activated porcine and murine lamina propria T lymphocytes compared with human lamina propria T lymphocytes (Harriman et al., 1992; Bailey et al., 1994). The significance of the differences that exist in pigs has not been fully elucidated. It has been suggested that lamina propria lymphocytes, in addition to their effector function, also have a role in immunoregulation (Bailey et al., 2001). Lamina propria T cells differ from peripheral T cells in that they have a greater threshold of activation, produce increased concentrations of cytokines on stimulation, and have a phenotype associated with immunologic memory (Wittig & Zeitz, 2003).

2.4 Gut cytokines

Cytokines are small peptide molecules derived either from traditionally immune cells (lymphocytes, macrophages) or produced by epithelial cells, endothelial cells and fibroblasts

(Pie et al., 2003). They are powerful mediators that regulate the appropriate host defence against enteric pathogens and other luminal events, and participate in the maintenance of tissue integrity. Cytokines receptors are located on both immune and non-immune cells, and every change in the number, location and distribution of these receptors exert a significant impact on the function of the gut. Syntesis of proinflammatory cytokines can have a strong influence on gut integrity and epithelial functions, permeability to macromolecules and transport of nutrients and ions (McKay & Baird, 1999).

The usefulness of gut immunity depends on tissue integrity, cell function, clinical states, the site of primed immune or others cells. Production of cytokines depends also on mucosal micropopulation. Daudelin et al. (2011) found that expression of IL-8 in the ileum was significantly greater in the pigs challenged with ETEC F4 than in the nonchallenged animals, but IL-8 gene expression was significantly increased with probiotic addition (*P. acidilactici* + *S. cerevisiae boulardii*), compared to the control group. Other *in vitro* studies indicate an increase in IL-8 production following the stimulation of porcine intestinal epithelial cells, Caco-2 cells or a porcine macrophage cell line (3D4/31) with ETEC F4 (Roselli et al, 2006; Pavlova et al., 2008). Probiotic bacteria such as *Bifidobacterium lactis* BB12 stimulated IL-6 production in primary murine intestinal epithelial cells (Ruiz et al., 2005). In addition, this cytokine plays an important role in the regulation of immune intestinal response, barrier fortification, activation of neutrophils and B cell IgA isotype switching (Haller et al., 2000). Similarly, ileal TNF-a gene expression tended to be upregulated in the *P. acidilactici* + *S. cerevisiae boulardii* group in comparison with the control group, which means that the administration of probiotics induced a stronger inflammatory reaction than the feeding of an antibiotic enriched diet (Daudelin et al., 2011). The pattern of cytokine secretion by pig intestinal epithelium depend on the strain of bacteria used (Bailey, 2009). In study by Roselli et al., (2007), *Lactobacillus sobrius* reduced the amount of IL-8 secreted by IPEC-1 in response to ETEC, by stimulation of IL-10 secretion.

There are many reported studies in which feed supplements enhance a component of the immune system. Rodrigues et al., (2007) reported that viable probiotics are more efficient than inactivated probiotics to induce immunostimulation and intestinal modifications in piglets, thus improving their health and development. More IgA expressing cells were found in the mesenteric lymph nodes with the probiotic with viable cells than observed in the inactivated cells treatment. It should be very careful in comparisons and judgments in regard of specific probiotic/prebiotic strains, environment conditions, animal's age and feed composition. Nutrition can also modulate the intestinal cytokine level. Wu et al., (1999) found marked decrease in the levels of IL-10 and IL-4 in mice avoiding enteral feeding.

The roles of gut epithelium are regulation of tissue permeability, absorption of nutrients and ions, secretion and contraction of smooth muscle necessary for mixing contents. Following antigen stimulation, naive $CD4^+$ T cells proliferate and differentiate into various T cell subsets including T helper (Th)1, Th2 and Th17 effectors cells, and T regulatory cells-Treg (Vignali et al., 2008). The development of Th1 cells is the typical response to intracellular pathogens, such as bacteria or viruses. Th1 cells mediate through their secreted cytokines: interferon gamma (IFN-γ), tumor necrosis factor alpha (TNF-α), IL-1β, IL-2, IL-12. Th2 cells are initiated by IL-4 and develop in response to allergens or parasite infection. Cytokines that induce Th2 cells are IL-4, IL-5, IL-13. The third T-effector cell lineage is Th17 subset, which also participate in antimicrobial immunity and inflammatory pathology (Bailey, 2009). Commensal microbial flora drives accumulation of Th17 T cells in healthy, SPF compared to germ-free mice, but numbers and activation state further increase in colitis

(Niess et al., 2008). The differentiation of $CD4^+$ T cells into Trag plays a critical role in maintaining immunological tolerance to self antigen or suppressing excessive immune responses (Vignali et al., 2008). Mucosally activated T cells may differ from systemic T cells better towards interleukin-4 (IL-4) than IL-2, by polyclonal lines from murine lamina propria cells (Bailey et al., 1994). Some cytokines expressed by the intestinal epithelium and have great influence on the epithelial cells growth and homeostasis are TGF-β, IL-1α, IL-6. IL-8, IL-1β and TNF-α upregulated in response to microbial infection. After an ischemic or ischemia/reperfusion type injuries the levels of TNF-α and IL-6 released from the rats' gut (Grotz et al, 1999). The recent study suggests that gut microflora may have adverse effects by modulating gut cytokines, which would alter other components of gut function, and may make the host susceptible to other infectious and metabolic processes. The portal and systemic TNF and IL-6 levels were higher in those rats whose GI tracts were colonized with **E. coli** (bacterial overgrowth) than in rats with either normal intestinal microflora or whose intestinal flora had been decontaminated with oral antibiotics. The disruption of the normal intestinal microflora may result in bacterial overgrowth with enteric bacilli that can subsequently translocate to distant organs and the systemic circulation.

3. Natural products and biological substances as immune response modifiers

Since 2006 the European-wide directives are restricting the non-clinical use of antibiotic growth promoters (AGPs) in food animal production. To accommodate the withdrawal of AGPs it now becomes urgent to provide relevant health criteria and scientifically founded recommendations for alternatives to in-feed antibiotics. Since the 1980's intriguing reports have appeared suggesting that vast variety of substances of natural origin can restore, stimulate or suppress nonspecific and specific immunity in domestic food animals and, hence improve their growth and performance, acting as immune response modifiers (IRMs). The scope of this chapter is to compile recent knowledge on the exogenous immunomodulation of the immune responses in the pig as an important biomedical model. With the growing knowledge of porcine immune system and its endogenous modulation, it has been clarified that exogenous immunomodulation represents an important prophylactic/therapeutic approach aiming at stimulating natural host defenses through the use of a broad spectrum of immunomodulating/growth-promoting agents of a natural origin generally termed IRMs. With combined efforts of basic and clinical veterinary immunologists, animal producers and feed manufacturers, immunomodulation will bring into veterinary medicine, particularly in swine production, the same type of curative revolution as antibiotics have in the combat against infectious diseases. However, it is essential to select fully evaluated IRMs which may act either as nonspecific immunostimulators or synergistically as adjuvants with vaccines. Although, numerous of these substances have been successfully used in *in vivo* nutritional investigations in pig, substantiation of their efficacy is still lacking. Herein we will comparatively analyze immunomodulating properties of some IRMs such as prebiotics, probiotics and immunomodulators (including microbiotics, fungibiotics, phytobiotics and zoobiotics) from several sources applied *in vivo* in different concentrations using domestic swine as a model organism in relation to immunostimulatory effects of some exogenous IRMs of microbial or animal origin tested *in vitro* and *in vivo* on suckling and weaned pigs in our laboratory.

3.1 Early days of IRMs

Since the mid 1980's intriguing reports have appeared suggesting that vast variety of substances of natural or synthetic origin act as IRMs and can restore, stimulate or suppress the innate and adaptive immunity in domestic food animals and, hence improve their growth and performance (Blecha and Charley, 1990). The enormous number of empirical studies of exogenous effects of manipulation of the immune system of the pig by IRMs and feed additives have been carried out (reviewed by Valpotić, 2000; Gallois et al., 2009; Bailey, 2009).

The naturally occurring substances with a long history as immunomodulators are the herb extracts described by Chinese traditional medicine originated from plants *Angelica sinensis* and *Cynachus auriculatus,* which are well known today as IRMs (Weng et al., 1987) or antimicrobials (Kawakita et al., 1987). Today is possible to extract, characterize and classify the substances with putative immunomodulatory properties from different natural sources. Based on their biological or chemical origin bioactive substances with properties of IRMs have been classified by Poli (1984). Further, Reizenstein & Mathe (1984) divided IRMs on the basis of their origin to biological and synthetic substances. Moreover, a number of chemotherapeutics exhibited immunomodulatory activities (Sedlacek et al., 1986). The IRMs of importance for veterinary medicine were further classified into three categories as: physiological products, microbial products and synthetic compounds (Mulcahy & Quinn, 1986). Generally, the IRMs may be divided into substances of endogenous origin, normally produced by the genome of the host and those of exogenous origin which are not products of mammalian genome, but may stimulate production of endogenous IRMs and modulate the immune response of the host (Roth, 1988). The capacity of tested endogenous (neuropeptides, hormones, cytokines, immunoglobulins, peptides) and exogenous IRMs (plant and microbial extracts, synthetic compounds, feed additives, drugs) to improve immune status of laboratory and domestic animal species has been thoroughly reviewed (Wybran, 1988; Georgiev, 1991, 1993; Valpotić, 2000). The synthesis of all these classifications, supplemented with newly emerged bioactive organisms/substances is given in the Table 1.

Origin of IRMs	Type of immunomodulation	Group/source of IRMs	Bioactive molecules/organisms
ENDOGENOUS	Physiological	- hormones - cytokines - acute phase proteins - enzymes - nucleic acids	thymic hormones, lymphokins, monokins, inteferons, TNFα/β, CSF, CRP, haptoglobin, neopterins, NOS, immunogenic RNA/DNA
	Neuroendocrine	- hormones - neuropeptides	ACTH, glucocorticoids, somatostatin, prolactin, TSH, opioids (enkephalin, endorfin, dinorfin, neurotensin)
	Behavioral	- brain-immune system - interactions	neurotrasmitters (VIP, SP), cytokines (IL-1, TNFα, IL6, IL-8), hormones (ACTH, β–endorfin, thyreotropin, cortisol)

Origin of IRMs	Type of immunomodulation	Group/source of IRMs	Bioactive molecules/organisms
EXOGENOUS	Biological	- microbiotics - fungibiotics - phytobiotics - zoobiotics and their products/by-products/derivatives	viruses (Duphamun® – inactivated avipox virus, Baypamun®-inactivated *Parapoxvirus ovis*), bacteria (*P. acnes, E. coli, M. bovis, S. pyogenes, L. casei, S. olivoreticuli, K. pneumoniae), yeasts (S. cerevisiae)* and their derivatives (mannan, glucan), fungi (*T. inflatum, L. edodes, C. albicans, A. bisporus*) and their derivatives (mannan, glucan, lentinan) , plant and algal extracts (carotenoids, flavonoids, polyphenols, saponin, fucan, carvacol, thymol, curcumin, laminarin, phycarin, fucoidan), animal products (bee venom, royal gelly, propolis, fish oil) and animal by-products (colostrum, lactoferrin, spray-dried plasma, purified IgG or total Igs)
	Chemical	- natural compounds - synthetic compounds - metals/microelements	lipopolysaccharide, peptidoglycan, muramil dipeptide, levamisole, POE-POP copolymer, isoprinisine, indometacine, ascorbic acid derivatives, ciprofloxacin, ^{132}Ge organic compounds, organic acids (acetic, benzoic, citric, formic, fumaric, lactic, phosphoric, propionic, sorbic, tartaric), acetic salts (K/Na-benzoate, Na-butyrate/citrate, K-formate/sorbate, Ca-lactate/propionate), Zn, Fe, Cu, Se.
	Nutritive	- nutrients - nutraceuticals	nucleotides, aminoacids (arginine, cysteine, glutamine),carotenoids, flavonoids, n-3 , polyunsaturated fatty acids, vitamins (A and E), minerals (Zn, zeolites)

Table 1. Classification of IRMs based on genetic origin, group/source and type of immunomodulation

TNF = tumor necrosis factor; CSF = colony-stimulating factor; CRP = C-reactive protein; NOS = nitricoxide synthase; ACTH = adrenocorticotropic hormone; TSH = thyroid stimulating hormone; VIP = vasoactive intestinal peptide; SP = substance P; IgG = immunoglobulin G; POE-POP = polyoxiethylene polyoxipropylene

The most common protocol for studies of IRMs effectiveness involves feeding (or application via other routes) the test bioactive substance or compound to young animals, recording feed intake and growth rate as a measures of the efficiency of the animal overall, and recording immunological parameters as direct measures of contribution of the IRMs effect on immunological function. The results from such studies generally fall into two categories. In the first, application of IRMs resulted in an increase in a specific parameter of the immune system. Recently reported studies in which feed supplements enhance a component of porcine immune system have generally focused on increases in IgA, cytokines or serum/intestinal leukocyte subsets. In the second, feed supplementation had no effect or decreased measures of the mucosal immune system. A modification of this protocol is to challenge test and control pigs with a specific pathogen or antigen (including vaccines), where outcomes have been similarly variable (reviewed by Blecha & Charley, 1990; Valpotić, 2000, Gallois et al., 2009; Bailey, 2009).

It should be apparent from the previous discussion regarding modulation of growth and immune functions that the observation of increased, decreased or unchanged measures of these parameters by themselves cannot be interpreted as beneficial or harmful. Each of the studies reports important finding, but an understanding of the mechanisms and, perhaps more importantly, the ability to predict which IRM or feed additive may be beneficial under particular environmental conditions, is going to require many more studies and an overall meta-analysis of the data. The advantage of working with the pig for these studies is that large field trials can be carried out under a range of environmental challenges (intensive, extensive rearing systems) in association with detailed study protocols comprising defined and well characterized IRMs.

Following a brief description of historical aspects on IRMs, we will focus on a group of exogenous bioactive organisms/substances that have been suggested to show immunomodulatory properties, particularly in the pig model systems.

3.2 Nonspecific immunomodulation in swine: A state of art

Unlike specific immunmodulation or vaccination, nonspecific immunmodulation is a complex concept in scientific terms because there is the necessity to balance immunostimulation against excessive activation of the immune system which is usually damaging and growth-inhibiting. Also, certain IRMs when used as immunostimulants are likely to exhibit immunosuppressive effect at increased doses. Clearly a more robust, rapid and sustained immune response would be desirable. Pigs selected for high humoral and cellular immune responses had better growth rates than pigs with low immune responses (Wilkie & Mallard, 1999). In pig production, this is of particular importance during the weaning transition when pigs are subjected to major stressful events, making them highly susceptible to digestive disorders. At that time, the development of both innate and adaptive systemic and local intestinal immunity is critical in preventing the potential harmful effects of pathogenic agents. Strategies aiming at stimulating natural defenses of swine through the use of IRMs able to modulate immune functions have gained increased interest in animal research, and different bioactive components sharing properties of IRMs have been the subject of *in vivo* and/or *in vitro* investigations in pigs (Blecha & Charley, 1990; Valpotić, 2000, Gallois & Oswald, 2008; Gallois et al., 2009).

Nonspecific immunostimulation primarily implies stimulation of the innate or nonspecific immunity which comprises monocytes/macrophages, neutrophils, NK cells, intraepithelial lymphocytes, complement, CRP, haptoglobin and cytokines, such as IFNs, but also certain T- and B-lymphocyte subsets of adaptive or specific immunity. The aim of immunomodulating substances is to help pigs develop "appropriate/optimal" active responses from both innate and adaptive immunity. However, these substances generally termed IRMs have to fulfill a variety of properties from technical and regulatory viewpoints, but also should share a positive image towards the public (Gallois et al., 2009). Thus, products/derivatives from natural sources will probably be easily accepted by the public and legislation.

3.2.1 The effects of IRMs as natural alternatives to AGP in pig production

Until recently, problems of enteric infections in food animal production have been overcome by adding sub-therapeutic doses of AGPs in-feed to enhance production efficiency in swine industry (Cromwell, 2002). Concerns about potential risks for human health due to use and misuse of AGPs in animal feeds (Dewey et al., 1997) have led to their ban throughout EU (Regulation EC no. 1831/2003). These criteria which are commonly accepted within EU must be usable for objective assessment of alternatives to in-feed AGPs (Gallois et al., 2009) and must be acceptable for swine producers, feed manufacturers and consumers. To accommodate to withdrawal of AGPs it now becomes urgent to provide relevant gut health criteria for a large-scale production of pigs and scientifically founded recommendations for alternatives to in-feed AGPs. More recently focus has shifted from specific immunization to another non-antibiotic approach offered by the use of IRMs, and prebiotics/probiotics in non-specific immune/nutritive stimulation of resistance to enteric infections. Such strategies aiming at stimulating natural host defence through the use of substances of natural or synthetic origin able to modulate immune functions have gained increasing interest in food animal research (Mulcahy & Quinn, 1986; Blecha & Charley, 1990; Valpotić, 2000; Gallois & Oswald, 2008; Gallois et al., 2009). This chapter will focus on groups of in-feed alternatives to AGPs originated from fungi and their derivatives, termed fungibiotics (Table 2), plants and their extracts, termed phytobiotics (Table 3) and animal products and by-products, termed zoobiotics (Table 4) that have been suggested to exhibit immunomodulatory properties and that have been tested in *in vivo* studies in pigs.

A variety of polysaccharides from different natural sources, particularly yeast derivatives β-D-glucans and α-D-mannans (Brown & Gordon, 2003) have been recognized to be responsible for modulating the immune responses in farm animals, including pigs (Table 2) through specific interactions with different immune cells (Kogan & Kocher, 2007). Numerous preparations derived from yeast cell walls, fungi (Table 2), marine algae or plants (Table 3), particularly rich in glucans and mannans, have been investigated in pigs. The BGC extracted from the cell wall of baker's yeast *Saccharomyces cerevisiae* is the most common source used for pig in-feed complements. It is a β-1,3-glucan with long β-1,6-glucan branches, whose structure is different from the β-glucans extracted from bacteria (linear β-1,3-glucans), fungi (short β-1,6-glucans branched β-1,3-glucans) and cereals (β-1,3/1,4-glucans), and thus, their different chemical structures would be expected to be reflected in their different bioactivities (Tzianabos, 2000). Much interest has been paid to the effects of BGC and MOS on porcine systemic immune responses, particularly innate immunity, whereas literature dealing with their effects on local intestinal immunity is very scarce (Table 2). Generally, the effects of BGC on porcine immunity are not predictable and their ability to act as growth-promoters is also not reliable. Their beneficial effects on health were difficult to detect since many of the studies have been performed in "clean" environments where morbidity/mortality rates are low. As for BGC, the influence of MOS on porcine immunity is not always reliable, as well as their effects on pigs performances and health, particularly following challenge infections with enteric pathogens (Table 2).

Literature dealing with β-glucans as potential alternatives to in-feed AGPs and their impact on pig immunity has been reviewed recently (Špoljarić et al., 2011).

Stressor/challenge or vaccinal organism	IRM applied in-feed or *per os*	Effects on immune and production parameters	Reference
Weaning	β-glucan polysaccharide (BGC; single oral dose of 100μg or 1mg/pig)	NT; Increased average body weight	Schoenherr et al. (1994)
Weaning	BGC (0.1%)	None on blood neutrophil function; Lower average daily feed intake; None on average body weight.	Dritz et al. (1995)
Weaning /*Streptoccocus suis* -immunization	BGC (0.025-0.05%)	None on phagocytic function of macrphages/neutrophils; Decreased level of haptoglobin in plasma; Increase of average body weight; Higher average daily feed intake. None on feed conversion.	
E.coli vaccine/Partus	BGC (0.05%)	Increased levels of specific colostral/milk antibodies; None on no. of liveborn/stillborn pigs; Decreased average body weight; Slower recovery from neonatal diarrheal disease.	Decuypere et al. (1998)
Weaning	BGC (0.05%)	Decreased serum level of antibody to F6 antigen or without influence on antibodies to F4, F5 and LT antigens; Increased average body weight; Without influence on incidence of diarrhea.	
Weaning	BGC (0.4%)	Increased proportion of $CD8^+$ and decreased proportion of $CD4^+$ T cells; Decreased no. of granulocytes/monocytes; None on average body weight and average daily feed intake; Decreased incidence of diarrhea.	Kim et al. (2000)
Weaning	α-mannan oligosaccharide (MOS; 0.1%)	None on blood proportions of $CD4^+$ or $CD8^+$ cells.	
Weaning	MOS (0.2%)	Without influence on proliferative response of PBL.	Davis et al. (2002)
Weaning/$F4^+$ *E. coli* challenge	MOS (3%) from brewer's yeast)	None on serum levels of IgA, IgM and IgG following challenge or without challenge.	White et al. (2002)

Stressor/challenge or vaccinal organism	**IRM applied in-feed or *per os***	**Effects on immune and production parameters**	**Reference**
Weaning/ *Salmonella enterica* - challenge	MOS (0.15%)	Increased serum concentration of haptoglobin; None on serum level of Il-6; Without influence on hyperthermia after challenge infection; None on growt performance.	Burkey et al. (2004)
Weaning	MOS (0.3%)	Without influence on no. of intestinal macrophages; Increased phagocytosis of macrophages from JLP. Lowered ratio of $CD3^+ CD4^+/CD3^+ CD8^+$ blood T cells due to a higher proportion of $CD8^+$ T cells. Decreased no. of blood neutrophils.	Davis et al. (2004a)
Weaning	MOS (0.2- 0.3%)	Decreased proliferative responses of PBL to PWM or PHA;	Davis et al. (2004b)
Weaning/PRRS virus - vaccination	BGC (0.015-0.03%)	Tendency of serum haptoglobin increase; None of lymphocyte proliferation; Without influence on increase in level of specific antibody to PRRS virus; None on average body weight and feed conversion; Increased average daily feed intake.	Hiss and Sauerwein, (2003)
Weaning/ Ovoalbumin - or LPS - immunization + LPS *in vitro*	BGC (0.005%)	Short-term increase of humoral immunity to ovoalbumin; Increased release of IL-10, and decreased IL-6 and TNFα production after *in vitro* or *in vivo* stimulation of PBL with LPS; NT.	Li et al. (2005)
Weaning/LPS - immunization	BGC (0.005%)	Increased plasma levels of IL-6, TNFα and IL-10; Without influence on somatotropin level.	Li et al. (2006)
Weaning	BGC (0.005%)	Decreased reactivity of PBL to PHA or ConA mitogens; Increased average daily feed intake and body weight: None on feed conversion.	
Weaning/Atrophici rhinitis – vaccination + in-feed antibiotics	BGC (0.02-0.04%)	Slightly changed level of antibody specific for *Pasteurella multocida* sv. A and D; Increased proportion of $CD4^+$ and tendency of increased proportion of $CD8^+$ PBL; Increased average body weight; Better feed digestibility.	Hahn et al. (2006)

Stressor/challenge or vaccinal organism	IRM applied in-feed or *per os*	Effects on immune and production parameters	Reference
Weaning/LPS - immunization	BGC (2.5%)	Increased intestinal TNFα and IL-1β, but also Il-1 receptor antagonist mRNA; None in blood TNFα level and leukocyte count.	Eicher et al. (2006)
Weaning	MOS (0.1%)	Reduced recruitment of lymphocytes into intestinal lamina propria; Profiles of intestinal and PBL subsets influenced.	Lizardo et al. (2008)
Weaning/F4+ ETEC - immunization	BGC (0.05%); from fungus *Sclerotium rolfsii*)	Decreased serum level of antibody to F4 antigen; Increased numbers of IgM^+ and IgA^+ plasma cells in JPP/IPP, and decreased in MLN; Lower susceptibility for $F4^+$ ETEC infection; Lower incidence of fecal isolates of $F4^+$ ETEC bacteria; Milder or totally reduced diarrhea.	Stuyven et al. (2009)
Weaning/ *S. enterica* sv. Typhimurium - immunization	BGC (0.2%)	NT; None on average body weight; Lower incidence of *S.enterica* sv. Typhimurium in feces:	Price et al. (2010)
Weaning/$F4^+$ ETEC - immunization	Yeast fermentation product (0.2% XPC®) from *S. cerevisiae*)	Increased PCV of blood leukocytes; Increased average daily feed intake, Smaller no. of adherent ETEC to ileal mucosa; Decreased no. of *Eneterobacteria* in ileal content; Improved growth and gut health status.	Kiarie et al. (2011)

Table 2. *In vivo* immunomodulatory effects of dietary supplementation of fungibiotics on porcine immune and production parameters

Weaning = from 2-4 weeks; BGC = β glucans given either in diets or orally originated from bakers yeast *S. cerevisiae* ,except where sources were given in parenthesis; LT = thermo labile toxin, PRRS = porcine reproductive and respiratory syndrome; PWM = pokeweed mitogen; PHA = phytohaemagglutinin, ConA = concanavalin A; NT = not tested

Stressor/challenge or vaccinal organism	IRM applied in-feed or *per os*	Effects on immune and production parameters	Reference
Weaning*/ *S. enterica* sv. Typhimurium - immunization	Fucan polysaccharide (0.5-2.0%) from seaweed *Ascophillum nodosum*)	Increased feed intake, but decreased feed efficiency; Without influence on immune responses; Challenge infection had only moderate effects on pigs; Increased activation of alveolar macrophages to secrete prostaglandin E2 (PGE2); None on secretion of IL-10 by splenocytes.	Turner et al. (2002a)
Weaning/ *S. enterica* sv. Typhimurium - immunization	Saponin (0.0125-0.05%) from *Quillaja saponaria*)	Without influence on feed intake and growth rate followinh challenge infection with *S. enterica;* None o serum levels of haptoglobin, α-1-acid glycoprotein and IgM postinfection; Slightly weaker phagocytic function of blood leukocytes with higher dose of saponin.	Turner et al. (2002b)
Weaning	Saponin/Curcumin (0.02-0.03%) from *Q. saponaria/Curcuma longa*)	Without influence on immune response (curcumin); Increased concentrations of IgA, IgG and CRP (saponin); Decreased feed : weight gain ratio and, thus, feed utilization; Improved health status of pigs.	Ilsley et al. (2005)
Weaning	Carvacol, thymol (0.3%) from *Cinnamomum spp., Capsicum annum* and Oregano feed additive™)	Increased proportions of $CD4^{+}$, $CD8^{+}$ and $CD4^{+}$/ $CD8^{+}$ T cells in peripheral blood and MLN Protection of low-weight pigs from disease.	Walter and Bilkei (2004)
Weaning	Sugar cane extract - polysaccharides ?) (0.5-2.0g/kg of BW) from *Saccharum officinarum*	Increased NK cell cytotoxicity and phagocytosis of monocytes/neutrophils; Low morbidity and mortality rates.	Lo et al. (2005)
Weaning	Chicory acid, alkamids (1.8 cobs for 6 weeks) from *Echinacea purpurea*)	None on growth performance; Slightly increased feed efficiency; Nonaffected blood parameters – cell count and proliferation of PBL; Improved health status of pigs;	Maass et al. (2005)

Stressor/challenge or vaccinal organism	IRM applied in-feed or *per os*	Effects on immune and production parameters	Reference
Weaning/ *Erysipelothrix rhusiopathiae* - vaccination	Chicory acid, alkamids (1.5 cobs and 4-6 ml juice/day for 9 weeks) from *E. purpurea*	Enhanced response to vaccine against *Erysipelothrix rhusiopathiae;* Increased serum level of specific antibody.	
Weaning/LPS - immunization	BGC (0.05-0.1%) from Chinese herb *Astragalus membranaceus*)	Increased plasma levels of IL-1β, PGE2 and cortisol; Enhanced reactivity of PBL to ConA; Increased production of IL-2 following the immunization;. None on average body weight and feed conversion; Decreased average body weight after immunization with LPS; Increased average daily feed intake; Higher plasma level of glucose. Increaed plasma levels of IL-1β and PGE2 after LPS immunization.	Mao et al. (2005)
Weaning/Ovoalbumin - immunization	BGC (0.01-0.1%) from *A. membranaceus)*	Incresed blood leukocyte count; Increased proportion of $CD4^+$ T cells; Increased blood concentrations of IL-2 and IFNγ following the immunization; Non-affected levels of IL-4 and IL-10; None on specific antibody titers following immunization with ovoalbumin.	Yuan et al. (2006)
Weaning	Carvacol, cinnamaldehyde, capsicum oleoresin (0.03%) from *Origanum spp.*)	None on subsets of mononuclear cells from IPP; Decreased percentage of B cells in ileal/colonic lymph nodes.	Nofrarias et al. (2006)
Weaning	Carvacol, thymol (0.05-0.15%) from Phytogenic™ additive)	Without influence on plasma levels of CRP and haptoglobin.	Muhl & Liebert (2007)

Stressor/challenge or vaccinal organism	IRM applied in-feed or *per os*	Effects on immune and production parameters	Reference
Weaning/LPS or Ovoalbumin-immunization	Flavonoids, polyphenols (1%) from Bahzen™ Chinese herbal medicine)	Increased blood leukocyte count; Enhanced release of serum IL-6 and TNFα following LPS immunization; Increased levels of blood IgG and activity of neutrophils; Without influence on specific antibody responses to SRBC or ovoalbumin; Improved growth rate.	Lien et al. (2007)
Weaning	BGC (0.15%) from brown algae *L. digitata* and/or *L. hyperborean)*	Increased expression of mRNA for IL-8; Increased no. of monocytes; Decreased no. of enterobacteria, bifidobacteria and lactobacilli in colon/cecum; Lowered height of intestinal vili in duodenum/jejunum.	Reilly et al. (2008)
Level of gases in fattening unit	BGC (?) from barley and oats – diets (13.5MJ/kg) with either or with their combination	NT; Lower digestibility of feed; Increased no. of *Bifidobacterium spp*. and *Lactobaillus spp*. in colon; Decreased concentration of ammonia.	O'Shea et al. (2010)
Weaning/LPS-immunization	Laminarin (300 or 600 parts/million ppm) from *L. digitata*)	Increased IL-6 and IL-8 gene expression in colon following LPS immunization; Reduced population of *Enterobacteria* in colon; Increased expression of mucin genes in ileum/colon	Smith et al. (2011)

Table 3. *In vivo* immunomodulatory effects of dietary supplementation of phytobiotics on porcine immune and production parameters

* At 2-4 weeks of age; BW = body weight; NK = natural killer; SRBC = sheep red blood cells. BGC= β glucans

Seaweed extracts are known to have immunomodulatory properties on the immune parameters in mice (Vetvicka & Ivyn, 2004) and pigs (Reilly et al., 2008; Leonard et al., 2010). Empirical evidences suggest that plant extracts may also offer benefits in stimulating the immune system, and thus, preventing disease in monogastric food animals (Wenk, 2003). A variety of plant-derived products have gained increasing interest as potential feed additives for poultry and swine (Windisch et al., 2008). Plants, and their bioactive components, are very diverse and their potential to enhance pig immunity and health has only been scarcely tested *in vivo* (Table 3).

The most of these studies have used a mixture of compounds (Kommera et al., 2006; Manzanilla et al., 2006), which does not allow the investigation of the immunomodulating properties of a specific bioactive component. However, Chinese pharmacopoeia describes the use of numerous herbal formulations to cure wide variety of diseases. Among those, Bahzen is a medicine composed of eight different plants (*Atractylodes ovata, Codonopsis pilosula, Poria cocos, Glycyrrhiza uralensis, Angelica sinensis, Ligusticum chuanxiong, Paeonia albiflora and Rehmannia glutinosa*) whose extracts have been tested *in vivo* in pigs (Lien et al., 2007). In spite positive image of medical plants in the public opinion a lack of data on the bioactive components of particular plants and the large diversity of their species, it has proved difficult to prepare extracts of equivalent potency, and thus the results of investigations on their influence on pig immunity remains inconclusive.

The most promising results among IRMs tested have been obtained with animal by-products of commercial slaughtering facilities such as purified porcine Igs or IgG (Valpotić et al., 1989a, b) and spay-dried porcine/bovine plasma (Coffey & Cromwell, 2001), whose positive effects would be provided by specific allogenic/xenogenic antibodies as well as by non-specific competition of glycan moieties of plasma glycoproteins with bacteria for intestinal receptors (Table 4). Namely, plasma from both porcine and bovine origins are characterized by a rich protein content, whose Igs can represent 24% to 25% (Niewold et al., 2007), and the IgG fraction would appear to be the main component responsible for the growth-promoting properties (Pierce et al., 2005). The major positive effect of animal product such as bee glue or propolis given in-feed (0.2%) is in reducing numbers of air-born bacteria in pig facilities (Bevilacqua et al., 1997) and the colonization of intestinal mucosa of weaned pigs by potentially harmful bacteria (Špoljarić, personal communication). The effects of spray-died porcine plasma (SDPP) on local intestinal immune responses have been widely studied in pigs (Table 4) and are concordant that SDPP prevents infiltration of GALT by immune cells and decreases jejunal proinflammatory cytokines, reflecting a lower antigenic challenge and suggesting that SDPP would be efficient in helping pigs fight against enteric infections (Jiang et al., 2000; Bosi et al., 2004; Nofrarias et al., 2006, 2007). Concerning systemic immune responses, a supplementation of the diet with SDPP did not modulate blood immune cells (Jiang et al., 2000; Nofrarias et al., 2006, 2007) or cytokines under basal conditions (Touchette et al, 2002), but when immunized with LPS, SDPP-fed pigs showed increased serum levels of proinfammatory cytokines associated with severe intestinal damage, suggesting that these pigs would be more susceptible to certain immunological challenges (Touchette et al., 2002). The growth-promoting properties of plasmas are more commonly observed with SDPP than from with that from bovine origin (vanDijk et al., 2001). The health-promoting properties of SDPP in pigs perorally challenged with an ETEC strain are usually reported as reduction in incidence/severity of postweaning diarrhea and growth promotion (Bosi et al., 2004; Niewold et al., 2007). Bovine colostrum has been shown to enhance intestinal mucosa restoration by stimulating migration of enterocytes and by decreasing apoptosis of apical epithelial cells in weaned pigs (Huguet et al., 2007). The use of lactoferrin is promising, as it seems to be efficient in preventing postweaning diarrhea in pigs (Wang et al., 2007).

Stressor/challenge or vaccinal organism	**IRM applied in-feed or *per os***	**Effects on immune and production parameters**	**Reference**
Partus/weaning*	Porcine plasma Igs (single peroral dose of 10 mg/pig or pretreatment of PBL with a same dose)	Increased reactivity of PBL from suckling pigs to PHA a T- cell mitogen; Decreased reactivity of PBL from suckling pigs to PWM a B.cell mitogen; Non-affected reactivity of PBl from weaned pigs to PHA, ConA or PWM; Better survival of during preweaning period.	Valpotić et al. (1989a)
Microbial load/ population density of pigs	Propolis (vaporized in farm facility)	Reduced no. of CFU in the air; Improved health of weaners.	Bevilacqua et al. (1997)
Weaning	Spray-dried porcine plasma (SDPP; 10%)	Decreased infiltration of GALT by macrophages and lymphocytes, None on blood leukocyte count; Promotion of growth.	Jiang et al. (2000)
Weaning/LPS-immunization	SDPP (7%)	None on serum IFNγ or TNFα levels; Increased serum IFNγ or TNFα levels following immunization with LPS; Severe damage of intestinal mucosa.	Touchette et al. (2002)
Weaning(LPS-immunization	SDPP (7%)	Increased serum Il-6 and Il-1β following immunization with LPS; Without influence on mRNA cytokine levels in liver, thymus or spleen; Decreased serum CRP, but not haptoglobin level.	Frank et al. (2003)
Weaning/F4+ ETEC-challenge	SDPP (6%)	Decreased expression of proinfammatory cytokines IL-8 and TNFα; Lower serum IgA level; Lower histopathologic score due to a better defense against ETEC infection. Increased average body weight.	Bosi et al. (2004)
Weaning/F4+ ETEC-challenge	SDPP (7%)	None on serum IL-6 level; Prevention of growth retardation and clinical signs of diarrheal disease.	Yi et al. (2005)

Stressor/challenge or vaccinal organism	**IRM applied in-feed or *per os***	**Effects on immune and production parameters**	**Reference**
Weaning	SDPP (6%)	Decreased infiltration of GALT by immune cells; None on no. of blood leukocytes; Promotion of growth.	Nofrarias et al. (2006)
Weaning	SDPP (6%)	Decreased infiltration of GALT by immune cells; None on no. of blood leukocytes; Increased average body weight..	Nofrarias et al. (2007)
Weaning/Rotavirus + $F4^+$ ETEC- challenges	SDPP (8%)	Reduced postweaning diarrhea and increased growth; Increased specific antibody against LT of ETEC; Decreased ETEC excretion. Competition of glycan moieties of glycoproteins from SDPP with intestinal receptors for F4 fimbrial antigens.	Niewold et al. (2007)
Weaning	Bovine colostrum (1g or 5g/day/pig for 3 weeks)	Increased profiles of IL-2, IFNγ and IL-12 (Th1) or IL-4 and IL-10 cytokines (Th2) in IPP (more Th2 than Th1); More pronounced Th1 profile of cytokines in JLP; Decreased total no. of mononuclear cells in IPP, but their proliferative responses were increased; Decreased $CD21^+$ cell count and increased $CD3^+$ $CD4^+$ cell subset 3 weeks postweaning; Systemic immune responses non-affected.	Boudry et al. (2007)
Weaning	Lactoferrin (0.1%)	Increased blood level of IL-2 and C4 component of complement; None on IL-1α or C3 blood concentrations; Enhanced proliferation of PBL and splenocytes stimulated with PHA or ConA; Increased serum levels of IgG, IgA and IgM, Prevention of diarrhea.	Shan et al. (2007)
Weaning	SDPP (2.5 or 5.0%)	Decreased level of TNFα in colon, but not in ileum; Decreased level of IFNγ in ileum and colon; Reduced diarrheal disease.	Peace et al. (2011)

Table 4. In vivo immunomodulatory effects of dietary supplementation of zoobiotics on porcine immune and production parameters

* At 2-4 weeks of age; SDPP= spray dried porcine plasma; CFU = colony forming units; IFN = interferon; IL = interleukin

3.2.2 Croatian experiences with IRMs in veterinary medicine

In the following, the capacity of selected natural substances of microbial, fungal and animal origin to improve performances and the immune status of swine is reviewed based on *in vivo* or *in vitro* investigations performed in Croatian scientific community (Table 5). In our opinion, two main reasons are responsible for this research interest of a group of veterinary immunologists in Croatia: (i) at that time (the end of 1980') literature dealing with IRMs as natural alternatives to in-feed AGPs and their impact on porcine immunity was scarce, and (ii) more recently (since 2006 in the EU) the total ban of in-feed AGPs and trends in research work on that topic may arise in the following years.

Indeed, to accommodate to withdrawal of AGPs it now becomes urgent for Croatia as a member candidate and for Croatian scientific community to follow-up forthcoming EU regulations and keep-up with scientific trends in veterinary immunology in order to provide relevant health criteria and scientifically founded recommendations for alternatives to in-feed AGPs.

For each type of substance, only major elements concerning experimental designs, such as the immune/performance parameters which have been studied by differentiating the systemic and local intestinal immune responses were given. In spite of the fact that in most of the experiments *in vivo* application of IRMs has been performed parenterally, the gut mucosal immune cells have been prevalently studied. Thus, immune reactions after such applications of natural IRMs cannot directly be linked to a defined site of origin. So far, it is often difficult to explain whether their reaction pattern depends on intestinal mucosal or systemic immune responses. However, intestinal mucosal immune responses can occur independently of systemic immunity (Hannant, 2002).

Considering experimental designs in the context of testing IRMs (Table 5) it is necessary to mention that in the most cases stressful events such as birth and weaning (accompanied with ETEC challenge and non-ETEC vaccination) have been used as a model systems. To help pigs to cope with postweaning transition, various nutritional approaches have been proposed, including supplementation the diet with substances that increase appetence or have anti-microbial and/or immunostimulating properties (Lalles et al., 2007). Amongst the alternatives to in-feed AGPs, the IRMs, including preparation of inactivated *Parapoxvirus ovis* (Valpotić et al., 1993; Grgić et al., 1995; Šver et al., 1996a; Krsnik et al., 1999, Šperanda et al., 2008) and yeast derivatives such as Progut® (mixture of α-mannans, β-glucans, nucleotides and peptides) and BioMOS® (α-mannan oligosaccharide) are attracting greater attention (Šperanda et al., 2008, Valpotić, 2009; Špoljarić et al., 2011). Indeed, the correct functional development of the gut and GALT is of crucial importance in controlling potential pathogens during neonatal and postweaning period. Weaning affects the ontogeny of immune functions, largely as a consequence of the withdrawal of milk and catabolism of colostral antibodies, which have important implications for passively modulating immune responses through both suppressive and enhancing pathways. In accordance with this phenomenon, plasma-derived porcine IgG acted *in vitro* as an IRM on PBL reactivity to T- or B-cell mitogens from weaned pigs (Valpotić et al., 1989).

Finally, to assess the impact of in-feed IRMs simultaneously on immunity and on performances and health, the pigs used in these experiments (Table 5) were kept under commercial farm conditions implying that they were exposed to immune/infectious challenges. Thus, the studies performed may reflect immune functions and dysfunctions occurring following exogenous immunomodulation.

Stressor/ challenge or vaccinal strain	IRM applied		Effects on immune and production parameters	Reference
	in vivo	*in vitro*		
Partus	-	PGM	Increased no. of macrophages and decreased proliferation of PBL; Better survival of neonates	Valpotić et al. (1987)
Partus/weaning*	-	Porcine IgG**	Increased T and decreased B cell proliferation.	Valpotić et al. (1989b)
Weaning	-	PGP	Increased no. of leukocytes/lymphocytes.	Vijtiuk et al. (1992)
Weaning	-	PGP or PGM	Increased proliferation of PBL/splenocytes.	Vijtiuk et al. (1993)
Partus	BPM	-	Enhanced lacteal/colostral immunity in primiparous sows/neonatal pigs; Decreased mortality of pigs from litters of gilts	Valpotić et al. (1993)
Weaning/F4ac+ ETEC or non-ETEC strains	BPM	-	Increased proliferative responses of lymphocytes from IPP and MLN	Grgić et al. (1995)
Weaning/F4ac+ ETEC strain	BPM	-	Increased proliferative responses of lymphocytes from JLP, IPP and MLN; Increased no. of $CD2a^+$ and $CD8a^+$ T cells in JLP	Šver et al. (1996a)
	-	LPS	Increased proliferative responses of lymphocytes from GALT	
Weaning/ F4ac+ non-ETEC strain 2407	BPM		Higher level of total protein and IgG Incresed no. of leucocytes and share of neutrophils/lymphocytes	Šperanda et al. (2008)
Weaning/F4ac+ F6+ ETEC strain	-	MDP	Increased no. of $CD21^+$ B cells in MLN.	Šver et al. (1996b)
Regrouping***	BPM	-	Decreased no. of stillborn pigs	Krsnik et al. (1999)
Weaning	PGT	-	Increased growth rate; Non-affected no. of blood neutrophils; Increased proportions of $CD4^+$ and $CD8^+$ T cells; Increased no. of PBL.	Šperanda et al. (2008)
Weaning	MOS	-	Increased proportion of $CD45^+$, $CD4^+$, $CD8^+$ and $CD21^+$ PBL; Increased no. of $CD45RA^+$ lymphoid cells in IFA and IPP; Enhanced phagocytosis of granulocytes	Valpotić (2009)

Table 5. Immune and production parameters in conventionally reared pigs following in vivo or in vitro treatment with exogenous IRMs of either microbial origin or fungibiotics/zoobiotics
*At 4-weeks of age, **Purified from swine plasma, ***Primiparous/multiparous sows; PGM/PGP = peptidoglycan monomer/polymer from cell wall of *Brevibacterium divaricatum*; PBL = peripheral blood lymphocytes; BPM = Baypamun® (inactivated *Parapoxvirus ovis*); IPP = ileal Peyer's patches; MLN = mesenteric lymph node; ETEC = enterotoxigenic *E. coli* strain; JLP = jejunal lamina propria; LPS = lipopolysaccharide from cell wall of *Escherichia coli*; GALT = gut-associated lymphoid tissues; MDP = muramyl dipeptide synthetic analogue of molecule from Wax D component of plasmatic membrane of mycobacteria; MOS = mannan oligosaccharide from cell wall of *Saccharomyces cerevisiae* ; IFA = interfollicular areas

4. Conclusions: Potentials and limitations

Considerable efforts have been focused to understanding of enteric infectious diseases, their diagnosis, including biology of pathogens, host resistance and therapy in intensive large-scale production of food animals, particularly pigs. Conversely, little is known on prevention of such diseases through immunomodulatory and dietary strategies because these problems have been overcome thus far by adding sub-therapeutic doses of AGPs in-feed in swine industry to enhance production efficiency. The AGPs were used not only to improve growth but also to control enteric infections during critical periods such as birth and weaning. Numerous reports have suggesting that vast variety of substances of natural origin termed IRMs, including bioactive components of feed, *i. e.* nutraceuticals (prebiotics, probiotics, minerals) and of organisms, including their products or derivatives, *i. e.* immunomodulators (microbiotics, fungibiotics, phytobioticy, zoobiotics) can modulate (stimulate, suppress or restore) nonspecific and specific immunity in young pigs. Such strategy underlying pharmacological manipulation of the immune system, *i. e.* immunomodulation is to identify parameters of the host response that will indicate enhancement/suppression or restoration to a level of an "optimal immune response", to allow the host better combat against invading microbes during the course of infection. With growing knowledge of porcine immune system and its endogenous modulation, it has been stated in the literature that exogenous modulation using broad spectrum of IRMs represents an important prophylactic/therapeutic approach in prevention/treatment of both stress- and microbial-induced disorders accompanied birth or weaning, particularly enteric infections. Such substances should be effective in protection of gut health, and at same time harmless for animal and environment, and should be capable of stimulating/restoring of gut physiological and immune functions, and thus, could be particularly important during development and maturation of intestinal mucosal immune system. However, it is essential to select fully evaluated agent which may act either as an IRM or synergistically as an adjuvant with vaccines.

As highlighted in this chapter, substances whose immunomodulatory properties often issue from *in vitro* studies are not exhibiting putative potentials when tested *in vivo*, particularly as feed additives. Namely, studies where variety of IRMs (such as yeast derivatives or plant extracts) have been fed to pigs have shown inconsistent results, suggesting that their ability to target particular immune cells through the oral route is questionable. The main causes are: the influence of environment, feed content, present commensals, possible inflammation or ischemia type injuries, which may shift the mucosal immune response as well as the whole gut functions. Consequently, influence of IRMs on pig immunity remains inconclusive. The most promising results to date have been obtained with animal by-products and precuts, such as spray-dried plasma or propolis, respectively. The heterogeneity of these experiments can partly explain the discrepancies on their efficacy due to: (i) variable composition of feed additives, (ii) different time of supplementation, (iii) diversity of experimental designs or measured parameters, and (iv) the level of additive in the final diet often remains unknown as well as (v) the composition of additive itself is not revealed/defined. Moreover, while the effects of in-feed IRMs on systemic immunity are quite well documented, the local intestinal immune responses have only receive little attention despite the fact that the study of systemic immune responses may not reflect immune functions following dietary treatments with IRMs occurring in the GALT. In spite of all these experiments in the context of testing immunomodulatory compounds of various origin, one main problem is to define what "optimal" immune functions should be targeted. For instance, if there is evidence that immunosuppressive effect is expected to prevent potentially damaging immune-mediated reactions, such as chronic inflammation, stimulation of the active immunity is not required for development and education of the immune system. This is particularly true for GALT where a homeostatic balance has to be reached to both tolerate harmless antigens from commensal bacteria or diet, and eliminate harmful antigens from pathogenic microbes. The definition of an "optimal" immune function is thus highly complex, and in the context of food animal production, it could be defined as the one that offers both the best growth and health status to animal. This, however, implies that pigs are exposed to normal commercial rearing conditions in which they are submitted to immune/infectious challenges in order to objectively assess the impact of in-feed IRMs simultaneously on immunity and on performances and health.

In the future, the effects of in-feed/oral additives on the development of immune responses in the GALT should be more largely documented, as their effects are mainly expected in this compartment. Thus, such studies should include:

- well characterized relevant model systems of young pigs on multidisciplinary basis, and usable for an uniform evaluation of their performances, gut health criteria and optimal functioning of the GALT;
- fully defined IRMs, particularly their bioactive substance(s);
- pharmacokinetic studies intended to know the fate of these substances in the organism, in order to precise their site of action and physiological/immunological effects;
- scientifically founded statement regarding relationship between immunomodulatory effects induced by dietary IRMs and health status of pigs, as the final goal of using such substances in pig nutrition is to promote their performance, health and welfare.

5. References

Asselin-Paturel, C. & Trinchieri, G. (2005). Production of type I interferons: plasmacytoid dendritic cells and beyond. *J. Exp. Med.* 202, pp. 461-465

Bailey, M. & Haverson, K. (2006). The postnatal development of the mucosal immune system and mucosal tolerance in domestic animals. *Vet. Res.* 37, pp. 443-453

Bailey, M. (2009). The mucosal immune system: Recent developments and future directions in the pig. *Develop. Comp. Immunol.* 33, pp. 375-383

Bailey, M. &Haverson, K., Inman, C., Harris, C., Jones, P., Corfield, G., Miller, B. & Stokes C. (2005). The influence of environment on development of the mucosal immune system. *Vet. Immunol. Immunopathol.* 108, pp. 189–198

Bailey, M., Hall, L., Bland, P. W. & Stokes C. R. (1994). Production of cytokines by lymphocytes from spleen, mesenteric lymph node and intestinal lamina propria of pigs. *Immunology* 82, pp. 577–583

Bailey, M., Plunkett, F. J., Rothkotter, H. J., Vega-Lopez, M. A., Haverson, K. & Stokes C. R. (2001). Regulation of mucosal immune responses in effector sites. *Proc. Nutr. Soc.* 60, pp. 427–435

Banchereau, J. & Steinmann, R. M. (1998). Dendritic cells and the control of immunity. *Nature,* 392, pp. 245-252

Bandeira A., Itohara, S., Bonneville M., Burlen-Defranoux 0., Mota-Santos T., Coutinho A. & Tonegava S. (1991). Extrathymic origin of intestinal intraepithelial lymphocytes bearingT-cell antigen receptor γδ. *Proc. Nati. Acad. Sci.* 88, pp. 43-47

Bevilacqua, M, Bevilacqua, M., Serra, E., Vianello, A., Garrou, E., Sparagna, B., Barale, U. & Zaccagna, C. A. (1997). Natural resin association such as incense and propolis in zootechnology.*Agriculture Ecosystems Environment*. 62, pp. 247-252

Blecha F. & Charley B. (1990). Rationale for using immunoptentiators in domstic food animals. In: Immunomodulation in domestic food animals. F. Blecha i B. Charley pp. 3-19. Academic Press, San Diego, CA, USA.

Bosi, P., Casini, L., Finamore, A., Cremokolini, C., Merialdi, G., Trevisf. Nobili, P. & Mangheri E. (2004). Spray-dried plasma improves growth performance and reduces inflammatory status of weaned pigs challenged with enterotoxigenic Escherichia coli K88. *J. Anim. Sci.* 82, pp. 1764-1772

Boudry, C., Buldgen, A., Portetelle, D., Collard, A., Thewis, A. & Dehoux, J. P. (2007). Effects of oral supplementation with bovine colostrum on the immune system of weaned piglets. *Res. Vet. Sci.* 83, pp. 91-101

Brandtzaeg, P. & Pabst, R. (2004). Let's go mucosal: communication on slippery ground. *Trends in Immunology* 25, pp. 570-577

Brown, G.D. & Gordon, S. (2003). Fungal β-glucans and mammalian immunity. *Immunity* 19, pp. 311- 315

Burkey, T. E., Dritz, S. S., Nietfeld, J. C., Johnson, B. J. & Minton, J. E. (2004). Effect of dietary mannanoligosaccharide and sodium chlorate on the growth performance, acute-phase response, and bacterial shedding of weqaned pigs challenged with Salmonella enterica serotype Typhimurium, *J. Anim. Sci.* 82, 397-404

Burkey, T. E., Skjolaas K. A. & Minton J. E. (2009). Porcine mucosal immunity of the gastrointestinal tract. *J. Anim. Sci.* 87, pp. 1493-1501

Cella, M., Facchetti, F., Lanzavecchia, A. & Colonna M. (2000). Plasmacytoid dendritic cells activated by influenza virus and CD40L drive a potent TH1 polarization. *Nature Immunology* 1, pp. 305–310

Cepek, K. L., Shaw, S. K., Parker, C. M., Russel G. J., Morrow J. S., Rimm, D. L. & Brenner M. B. (1994). Adhesion between epithelial cells and T lymphocytes mediated by E-cadherin and the alpha E beta 7 integrin. *Nature* 372, pp. 190–193

Coffey, R. D. & Cromwell, G. L. (2001). Use of spray-dried animal plasma in diets for weaning pigs. Pig News Information 22, pp. 39N-48N

Colonna, M., Trinchieri, G. & Liu Y. J. (2004). Plasmacytoid dendritic cells in immunity. *Nat Immun*, 5, pp. 1219-1226

Coombes Janine L. & Powrie F. (2008). Dendritic cells in intestinal immune regulation. *Nature* 8, pp. 435-446

Cromwell, G. L. (2002). Why and how antibiotics are used in swine production. *Animal Biotechnol.* 13, 7-27

Daudelin, J. F., Lessard, M., Beaudoin, F., Nadeau E., Bissonnette N., Boutin, Y., Brousseau, J. P., Lauzon, K. & Fairbrother, J. M. (2011). Administration of probiotics influences F4 (K88)-positive enterotoxigenic Escherichia coli attachment and intestinal cytokine expression in weaned pigs. *Vet Res* pp. 42, 69

Davis, M. E., Maxwell, C. V., Brown, D. C., Derodas, B. Z., Johnson, Z. B., Kegles, E. B., Hellwig, D. H. & Dvorak, R. A. (2002). Effect of dietary mannan oligosaccharide and (or) pharmacological additions of copper sulfate on growth performance and immunocompetence of weanling and growing/finishing pigs. *J. Anim.Sci.* 80, pp. 2887-2894.

Davis, M. E., Maxwell, C. V., Erf, G. F., Brown,D. C. & Wistuba, T. J. (2004a). Dietary supplementation with phosphorylated mannans improves growth response and modulates immune function of weanling pigs. *J. Anim.Sci.* 82, pp. 1882-1891

Davis, M. E., Brown, D. C., Maxwell, C. V., Johnson, Z. B., Kegley, E. B., & Dvorak, R. A. (2004b). Effect of phosphorylated mannans and pharmacological additions of zinc oxide on growth and immunocompetence of weanling pigs. *J. Anim.Sci.* 82, pp. 581-587

De Heer, H. J., Hammad, H., Soullié, T., Hijdra, D., Vos, N., Willart, M. A. M., Hoogsteden, H. C. &. Lambrecht, B. N. (2004). Essential Role of Lung Plasmacytoid Dendritic Cells in Preventing Asthmatic Reactions to Harmless Inhaled Antigen. *J. Exp. Med.* 200(1), pp. 89–98

Decuypere, J., Dierick, N. & Boddez, S. (1998). The potentials for immunostimulatory substances (β-1,3/1,6 glucans) in pig nutrition. *J. Animal Feed Sci.* 7, pp. 259-265

Dewey, C. E., Cox, B. D., Straw, B. E., Bush, E. J. & Hurd, H. S. (1997). Associations between off-label feed additives and farm size, veterinary consultant use, and animal age. *Prev. Vet. Med.* 31, pp. 133-146

Dritz, S. S., Kielian, T. L., Goodland, R. D., Nelssen, J. L., Tokach, M. D., Chengappa, M. M., Smith, J. E. & Blecha, F. (1995). Influence of dietary beta-glucan on growth performance, nonspecific immunity, and resistance to Streptoccocus suis infection in weanling pigs. *J. Animal Sci.* 73, pp. 3341-3350

Egan, C. E., Maurer, K. J., Cohen, S. B., Mack, M., Simpson K. W. & Denkers E. Y. (2011). Synergy between intraepithelial lymphocytes and lamina propria T cells drives intestinal inflammation during infection. *Mucosal Immunology advance* online publication 27 July 2011. doi:10.1038/mi.2011.31 /

Eicher, S. D., Mckee, C. A., Carroll, J. A. & Pajor, E. A. (2006). Supplemental vitamin C and yeast cell wall β-glucan as growth enhancers in newborn pigs and as immunomodulators after an endotoxin challenge after weaning. *J. Anim. Sci.* 84, pp. 2352-2360

Finkelman, F. D., Lees, A., Birnbaum, R., Gause, W. C. & Morris S. C. (1996). Dendritic cells can present antigen in vivo in a tolerogenic or immunogenic fashion. *J. Immunol.* 157, pp. 1406-1414

Frank, J. W., Carroll, J. A., Allee, G. L. & Zannelli, M. E. (2003). The effects of thermal environment and spray-dried plasma on the acute-phase responseof pigs challenged with lipopolysaccharide. *J. Anim. Sci* 81, pp. 1166-1176

Gad M. (2005). Regulatory T cells in experimental colitis. *Curr. Top. Mocrobiol. Immunol.* 293, pp. 179-208

Gallois, M., Rothkötter, H. J., Bailey, M., Stokes, C. R. & Oswald, I. P. (2009). Natural alternatives to in-feed antibiotics in pig production: can immunomodulators play a role? *Animal* 3, pp. 1644-1661

Gallois, M. & Oswald, I. P. (2008). Immunomodulators as efficient alternatives to in-feed antimicrobials in pig production? Arch. Zootechn. 11, pp. 15-32.

Georgiev, V. S. T. (1991). Immunomodulating peptides:of natural and synthetic origin. *Med. Res. Rev.* 11, pp. 81-119

Gergiev, V. S. T. (1993). Immunomodulating drugs: major advances in research and development. *Ann. N. Y. Acad. Sci.* 685, pp. 1-10

Gewirtz, A. T., Liu, Y., Sitaraman, S. V. & Madara, J. L. (2002). Intestinal epithelial pathobiology: past, present and future. *Best Pract. Res. Clin. Gastroenterol.* 16, pp. 851-867

Grgić A., Vijtiuk N., Radeljević D., Šver L. & Valpotić I. (1995). In vitro effect of Baypamun® (BPM) on porcine gut lymphoid cell function after experimental infection with F4ac+ enterotoxigenic Escherichia coli (ETEC) or non–ETEC strains. *Veterinar* 38, pp. 12–15

Grotz, M. R. W., Deitch, E. A., Ding, J., Xu, D., Huang Q. & Regel, G. (1999). Intestinal cytokine response after gut ischemia. Role of gut barrier failure. *Ann of Surgery*. 229 (4), pp. 478-486.

Hahn, T. W., Lohakare, J. D., Lee, S. L., Moon, W. K. & Chae, B. J. (2006). Effects of supplementation of beta-glucans on growth performance, nutrient digestibility, and immunity in weaned pigs. *J. Anim. Sci.* 84, pp. 1422-1428.

Haller, D., Bode, C., Hammes, W. P., Pfeifer, A. M. A., Schiffrin, E. J., & Blum, S. (2000). Nonpathogenic bacteria elicit a differential cytokine response by intestinal epithelial cell/leucocyte co-cultures. *Gut*, 47(1), pp. 79-87

Hannant, D. (2002). Mucosal immunology: overview and potential in veterinary species. *Vet. Immunol. Immunopathol.* 87, pp. 265-267

Harriman, G. R., Hornqvist E. & Lycke N. Y. (1992). Antigenspecific and polyclonal CD4+ lamina propria T-cell lines: Phenotypic and functional characterization. *Immunology* 75. pp. 66–73

Haverson, K. & Riffault, S. (2006). Antigen presenting cells in mucosal sites of veterinary species. *Vet. Res.* 37, pp. 339-358

Havran, W. L., Jameson, J. M. & Witherden, D. A. (2005). Epithelial cells and their neighbours. III. Interactions between intraepithelial lymphocytes and neighbouring epithelial cells. *Am. J. Physiol. Gastrointest. Liver Physiol.* 289, pp. G627–G630

Hayday, A., Theodoridis, E., Ramsburg E. & Shires J. (2001). Intraepithelial lymphocytes: Exploring the third way in immunology. *Nat. Immunol.* 2, pp. 997–1003

Hiss, S. & Sauerwein, H. (2003).Influence of dietary β-glucan on growth performance, lymphocyte proliferation, specific immune response and haptoglobin plasma concentrations in pigs. *J. Anim. Physiol. Nutrit.* (Berlin) 87, pp. 2-11.

Huang, F.P., Platt, N., Wykes, M., Major, J. R., Powell, T. J., Jenkins, C. D. & MacPherson, G. G. (2000). A discrete subpopulation of dendritic cells transports apoptotic intestinal epithelial cells to T cell areas of mesenteric lymph nodes. *J Exp Med.* 191, pp. 435-443

Huguet, A., Le Normand, L., Fauquant, J., Kaeffer, B. & Le Huerou-Luron, I. (2007). Influence of bovine colostrum on restoration of intestinal mucosa in weaned piglets. *Livestock Sci.* 108, pp. 20-22

Hunyady, B., Mezey, E. & Palkovits M. (2000). Gastrointestinal immunology: Cell types in the lamina propria—A morphological review. *Acta Physiol. Hung.* 87, pp. 305–328

Ilsley, S. E., Miller, H. M. & Kamel, C. (2005). Effects of dietary quillaja saponin and curcumin on the performance and immune status of weaned piglets. *J. Anim. Sci.* 83, pp. 82-88

Iwasaki, A. & Kelsal, B. L. (1999). Freshly isolated Peyer's patch, but not spleen, dendritic cells produce interleukin 10 and induce the differentiation of T helper Type 2 cells. *Jou. Exper. Med.* 190, (2), pp. 229–239

Iwasaki, A. (2007). Mucosal dendritic cells. Annu. Rev. Immunol. 25, pp. 381-418

Jang, M. H., Kweon, M.N., Iwatani, K., Yamamoto, M., Terahara, K., Sasakawa, C., Suzuki, T., Nochi, T., Yokota, Y., Rennert, P. D., Hiroi, T., Tamagawa, H., Iijima, H., Kunisawa, J., Yuki, Y. & Kiyono, H. (2004). Intestinal villous M cells: an antigen entry site in the mucosal epithelium. *Proc. Natl. Acad. Sci. USA.* 101, pp. 6110-6115

Jiang, R., Chang, X., Stoll, B., Fan, M. Z., Arthington, J., Weaver, E., Campbell, E. & Burrin, D. G. (2000). Dietrary plasma protein reduces small intestinal growth and lamina propria cell densityin early weaned pigs. *J. Nutrition* 130, pp. 21-26

Johansson, C. & Kelsall B. L. (2005). Phenotype and function of intestinal dendritic cells. *Semin. Immunol.* 17, pp. 284-294

Kawakita, T., Yamada, A., Mitsuyama, M., Kumazawa, Y. & Nomoto, K. (1987). Protective effect of a traditional Chinese medicine, Xiao Chai-Hu-Tang (Japanese name: Shosaiko-To), on Pseudomonas aeruginosa infection in mice. *Immunopharmacol. Immunotoxicol.* 9, pp. 523-540

Kiarie, E., Bhandari, S., Scott, M., Krause, D. O. & Nyachoti, M. (2011). Growth performance and gastrointestinal microbial ecology responses of piglets received Saccharomyces cerevisiae fermentation products after an oral challenge with Escherichia coli (K88). *J. Anim. Sci.* 89, pp. 1062-1078

Kim, J.D., Hyun, Y., Sohn, K. S., Woo, H. J., Kim, T. J. & Han, I. K. (2000). Effects of immunostimulators on growth performance and immune response in pigs weaned at 21 days of age. *J. Anim. Feed Sci.* 9, pp. 333-346

Kogan, G. & Kocher, A. (2007). Role of yeast cell wall polysaccharides in pig nutrition and health protection. *Livestock Sci.* 109, pp. 161-165

Kommera, S. K., Mateo, R. D., Neher, F. J. & Kim, S. W. (2006). Phytobiotics and organic acids as potential alternatives to the use of antibiotic in nursery pig diets. *Asian-Australasian J. Anim. Sci.* 19, pp. 1784-1789

Krsnik B., Yammine R., Pavičić Ž., Balenović T., Njari B., Vrbanac I. &Valpotić I. (1999). Experimental model of enterotoxigenic Escherichia coli infection in pigs: potential for an early recognition of colibacillosis by monitoring of behavior. *Comp Immunol Microbiol Infect Dis* 22, pp. 261–273

Krug, A., Veeraswamy, R., Perkosz, A., Kanagawa, O., Unuane, E. R., Colonna, M. & Cella, M. (2003). Interferon-producing cells fail to induce proliferation of naive T cells but can promote expansion and T helper 1 differentiation of antigen-experienced unpolarized T cells. *J. Exp. Med.* 197, pp. 899-906

Lalles, J. P., Bosi, P., Smidt, H. & Stokes, C. R. (2007). Weaning-A challenge to gut physiology. *Livestock Sci.* 108, pp. 82-93

Leonard, S., Sweeney, G., T., Bahar, B., Lynch, B. P. & O'doherty, J. V. (2010). Effect of maternal fish oil and seaweed extract supplementation on colostrum and milk composition, humoral immune response, and performance of suckled pigs. *J. Anim. Sci.* 88, pp. 2988-2997

Li J., Li, D. F., Zing, J. J., Cheng, Z. B. & Lai, C. H. (2006). Effects of β-glucan extracted from Saccharomyces cerevisiae on growth performance, and immunological and somatotropic responses of pigs challenged with Escherichia coli lipopolysaccharide. *J. Anim. Sci.* 84, pp. 2374-2381

Li, J., Zing, J.J., Li, D. F., Wang, X., Zhao, L., Lv, S. & Huang, D. (2005). Effects of β-glucan extracted from Saccharomyces cerevisiae on humoral and cellular immunity in weaned pigs. *Arch. Anim. Nutr.* 59, pp. 303-312

Lien, T. F., Horng, Y. M. & Wu, C. P. (2007). Feasibility of replacing antibiotic feed promoters with the Chinese traditional herbal medicine Bazhen in weaned piglets. *Livestock Sci.* 107, pp. 97-102

Liu, L. M., Zhang, M., Jenkins, C. & MacPherson (1998). Dendritic cell heterogeneity in vivo: two functionally different dendritic cell population in rat intestinal lymph can be distinguished by CD4 expression. *J. Immunol.* 161, pp. 1146-1155

Lizardo, R. , Nofrarias, M., Guinvarch, J., Justin, A. L., Auclair, E. & Brufau, J. (2008). Influence de l'incorporation de levures Saccharomyces cerevisiae ou de leurs parois dans l'aliment sur la digestion et les performances zootechniques des porcelets an post-sevrage. In: *40emes Journees de la Recherche Porcine*, Paris, France, pp. 183-190

Lo, D. Y., Chen, T. H., Chien, M. S., Koge, K., Hosono, A., Kaminogawa, S. & Lee, W. C. (2005). Effects of sugar cane extract on the modulation of immunity in pigs. *J. Vet. Med. Sci.* 67, pp. 591-597

Maass, N., J. Bauer, B. R. Paulicks, B. M. Bohmer & Roth-Maier, D. A. (2005). Efficiency of Echinacea purpurea on performance and immune status in pigs. *J. Anim Physiol. Anim. Nutr.* (Berlin) 89, pp. 244-252

MacPherson, A.J. & Uhr, T. (2004). Induction of protective IgA by intestinal dendritic cells carrying commensal bacteria. Science 303, pp. 1662-1665Moseman, E.A., Liang, X., Dawson, A.J., Panoskaltsis-Mortari, A., Krieg, A.M., Liu, Y.J., Blazar, B.R. & Chen, W. (2004). Human plasmacytoid dendritic cells activated by CpG oligodeoxynucleotides induce the generation of CD4+CD25+ regulatory T cells. *J. Immunol.* 173, pp. 4433–4442

Manzanilla, E. G., Nofrarias, M., Anguita, M., Castillo, M., Perez, J. F., Martin-Orue, S. M., Kamel, C. & Gasa, J. (2006). Effects of butyrate, avilamycin, and plant extract combination on the intestinal equilibrium of early-weaned pigs. *J. Anim. Sci.* 84, pp. 2743-2751

Mao X. F., Piao, X. S., Lai, C. H., Li, D. F., Xing, J. J. & Shi, B. L. (2005). Effects of beta-glucan obtained from the Chinese herb Astragalus membranaceus and lipopolysaccharide challenge on performance, immunological, adrenal, and somatotropic responses of weanling pigs *J. Anim. Sci.* 83, pp. 2775-2782

McCracken B.A., Spurlock M.E., Roos M.A., Zuckermann F.A. & Gaskins H.R. (1999). Weaning anorexia may contribute to local inflammation in the piglet small intestine, *J. Nutr.* 129, pp. 613–619

McKay, D. M. & Baird, A. W. (1999). Cytokine regulation of epithelial permeability and ion transport. *Gut*, 44, pp. 283-289

Mellman, I. & Steinman, R. M. (2001). Dendritic cells: specialized and regulated antigen processing machines. *Cell* 106, pp. 255-258

Mowat, A. M. (2003). Anatomical basis of tolerance and immunity to intestinal antigens. *Nat. Rev. Immunol.* 3, pp. 331-341

Mowat, A. M. (2005). Dendritic cells and immune responses to orally administrated antigens. *Vaccine* 23, pp. 1797-1799

Muhl, A. & Liebert, F. (2007). No impact of a phytogenic feed additive on digestion and unspecific immune reaction in piglets. *J. Anim. Physiol. Anim. Nutr.* (Berlin) 91, pp. 426-431

Mulcahy, G. & Quinn, P. J. (1986). A review of immunomodulators and their application in veterinary medicine. *J. Vet. Pharmacol. Therap.* 9, pp. 119-139.

Newton D. J., Andrew, E. M., Dalton, J., Mears, E. R. & Carding S. R. (2006). Identification of novel γδ T-Cell subsets following bacterial infection in the absence of Vγ1+ T cells: Homeostatic Control of γδ T-Cell Responses to pathogen infection by Vγ1+ T Cells, *Infection and immunity*, 74 (2), pp. 1097–1105

Niess, J. H., Brand, S., Gu, X., Landsman, L., Jung, S., McCormick, B. A., Vyas, J. M., Boes, M., Ploegh, H. L., Fox, J. G., Littman, D. R. & Reinecker H. C. (2005). CX3CR1-mediated dendritic cell access to the intestinal lumen and bacterial clearance. *Science* 14, pp. 254-258

Niess, J. H., Leithauser, F., Adler, G., & Reinmann, J. (2008). Commensal gut flora drives the expansion of proinflammatory CD4 T cells in the colonic lamina propria under normal and inflammatory conditions. *J of Immunol* 180, pp. 559-568

Niewold, T. A., Van Dijk, A. J., Greenen, P. L., Roodink, H., Margry, R. & Van Der Meulen, J. (2007). Dietary specific antibodies in spray-dried immune plasma prevent enterotoxigenic Escherichia coli F4 (ETEC) post weaning diarrhoea in piglets. *Vet. Microbiol.* 124, pp. 362-369

Nofrarias, M., Manzanilla, E. G., Pujols, J., Gibert, X., Majo, N., Segales, J. & Gasa, J. (2006). Effects of spray-dried porcine plasma and plant extracts on intestinal morphology and on leukocyte cell subsets of weaned pigs. *J. Anim. Sci.* 84, pp. 2735-2742

Nofrarias, M., Manzanilla, E. G., Pujols, J., Gibert, X., Majo, N., Segales, J. & Gasa, J. (2007). Spray-dried porcine plasma affects intestinal morphology and immune cell subsets of weaned pigs. *Livestock Sci.* 108, pp. 299-302

O'shea, C. J., Sweeney, T., Lynch, M. B., Gohan, D. A., Callan, J. J. & O'doherty, J. V. (2010). Effect of β-glucans contained in barley- and oats-based diets and exogenous enzyme supplementation on gastrointestinal fermentation of finisher pigs and subsequent manure odor and ammonia emission. *J. Anim. Sci.* 88, pp. 1411-1420

Oswald, I. P. (2006). Role of intestinal epithelial cells in the innate immune defence of the pig intestine. *Vet. Res.* 37, pp. 359-368

Pabst, R., & Rothkotter H. J. (1999). Postnatal development of lymphocyte subsets in different compartments of the small intestine of piglets. Vet. *Immunol. Immunopathol.* 72, pp. 167–173

Pavlova, B., Volf, J., Alexa, P., Rychlik, I., Matiasovic, J. & Faldyna M. (2008). Cytokine mRNA expression in porcine cell lines stimulated by enterotoxigenic Escherichia coli. *Vet Microbiol* 2008, 132(1-2), pp. 105-110

Peace, R. M., Campbell, J., Polo, J., Crenshaw, J., Russell, L. & Moeser, A. (2011). Spray-Dried Porcine Plasma Influences Intestinal Barrier Function, Inflammation, and Diarrhea in Weaned Pigs. *J. Nutr.* 141, pp. 1312-1317.

Pie, S., Lalles, J. P., Blazy, F., Laffitte, J., Seve, B. & Oswald, I. P. (2003). Weaning is associated with an upregulation of expression of inflammatory cytokine in the intestine of piglets. *J. Nutr.* 134, pp. 641-647

Pierce, J. L., Cromwell, G. L., Lindemann, M. D., Russell, L. E. & Weaver, E. M. (2005). Effects of spray-dried animal plasma and immunoglobulins on performance of early weaned pigs. *J. Anim. Sci.* 83, pp. 2876-2885

Poli, G. (1984). Immunomodulators. In: *Adjuvants, interferon and non-specific immunity.* Cancellotti, F. M., D. Galassi, eds. pp. 111-126. Luxembourg, EEC.

Poussier, P & Julius, M. (1994). Thymus independent T-cell development and selection in the intestinal epithelium. Ann. Rev. Immunol. 12, pp. 521-553.

Price, K.L., Totty, H. R., Lee, H. B., Utt, M. D., Fritzner, G. E., Yoon, I., Ponder, M. A. & Escobar, J. (2010). Use of Saccharomyes cerevisiae fermentation product on growht performance and microbiota of weaned pigs during Salmonella infection. *J. Anim. Sci.* 88, pp. 3896-3908

Reilly, P., O'doherty, J. V., Pierce, K. M., Callan, J. J., O'sullivan, J. T. & Sweeney, T. (2008). The effects of seaweed extract inclusion on gut morphology, selected intestinal microbiota, nutrient digestibility, volatile fatty acid concentrations and the immune status of the weaned pig. *Animal* 2, pp. 1465-1473

Reizenstein, P. & Mathe, G. (1984). Immunomodulating agents. In: *Immune modulation agents and their mechanisms*. Fenichel, R. L., M. A. Chirigos, eds. pp. 347-361. New York, Dekker.

Rescigno, M., Urbano, M., Valzasina, B., Francolini, M., Rotta, G., Bonasio, R., Granucci, F., Krachenbuhl, J. P. & Ricciardi-Castagnoli (2001). Dendritic cells express tight junction proteins and penetrate gut epithelial monolayers to sample bacteria. *Nat. Immunol.* 2, pp. 361-367

Rodrigues, M. M. A., Silva D. D. A., Taketomi E. A. & Hernandez-Blazquez F. J. (2007). IgA production, coliforms analysis and intestinal mucosa morphology of piglets that received probiotics with viable or inactivated cells. *Pesq. Vet. Bras.* 27(6), pp. 241-245

Roselli, M., Finamore, A., Britti, M. S. & Mengheri, E. (2006). Probiotic bacteria Bifidobacterium animalis MB5 and Lactobacillus rhamnosus GG protect intestinal Caco-2 cells from the inflammation-associated response induced by enterotoxigenic Escherichia coli K88. Br *J Nutr* 95(6), pp. 1177-1184.

Roselli, M., Finamore, A., Britti, M. S., Konstantinov, S. R., Smidt, H. & de Vos W. M. (2007). The novel porcine Lactobacillus sobrius strain protects intestinal cells from enterotoxigenic Escerichia coli K88 infection and prevents membrane barrier damage. *J of Nutr*, 137, pp. 2709-2816

Roth, J. A. (1988). Enhancement of nonspecific resistence to bacterial infection by biologic response modifiers. In: *Virulence mechanisms of bacterial pathogens*. Roth, J. A. , ed. pp. 329-342. Washington, D. C., American Soc. Microbiol.

Ruiz, P. A., Hoffmann, M., Szcesny, S., Blaut, M. & Haller D. (2005). Innate mechanisms for Bifidobacterium lactis to activate transient pro-inflammatory host responses in intestinal epithelial cells after the colonization of germ-free rats. *Immunology*, 115(4), pp. 441-450

Salazar-Gonzalez, R. M. Niess, J. H., Zammit, D. J., Ravindran, R., Srinivasan, A., Maxwell, J. R., Stoklasek, T., Yadav, R., Williams, I. R., Gu, X., McCormick, B. A., Pazos, M. A., Vella, A. T., Lefrancois, L., Reinecker, H. C. & McSorley S. J. (2006). CCR6-mediated dendritic cell activation of pathogen-specific T cells in Peyer's patches. *Immunity*, 24, pp. 623-632

Sauerwein, H., Schmitz, S. & Hiss, S. (2007). Effects of a dietary application of a yeast cell wall extract on innate and acquired immunity, on oxidative status and growth performance in weanling piglets and on the ileal epithelium in fattened pigs. *J. Anim. Physiol. Nutr.* 91, pp. 369–380

Schoenherr, W. D., Pollmann, D. S. & Coalson, J. A. (1994). Titration of MacroGard™ - S on growth performance of nursery pigs. *J. Anim. Sci.* 72 (Suppl. 2), p. 57

Sedlacek, H. H., Dickneite, G. & Schorlemmer, H. U. (1986). Chemotherapeutics. A questionable or promising project. Comp. *Immunol. Microbiol. Infect. Dis.* 9, pp. 99-119

Shan, T., Wang, Y., Liu, J. & Xu, Z. (2007). Effect of dietary lactoferrin on the immune functions and serum iron level of weanling piglets. *J. Anim. Sci.* 85, pp. 2140-2146

Smith, A. G., O'doherty, J. V., Reilly, P., Ryan, M. T., Bahar, B. & Sweeney, T. (2011). The effects of laminarin derived from Laminaria digitata on measurements of gut health: selected bacterial populations, intestinal fermentation, mucin gene expression and cytokine gene expression in pig. *Br. J. Nutr.* 105, pp. 669-677

Smith, P. D., Ochsenbauer-Jambor, C. & Smythies, L. E. (2005). Intestinal macrophages: unique effector cells of the innate immune system. *Immunol. Rev.* 206, pp. 49-159

Smythies, L. E., Sellers, M., Clements, R. H., Barnum, M. M., Meng, G., Benjamin, W. H., Orenstein, J. M., & Smith, P. D. (2005). Human intestinal macrophages display profound inflammatory anergy despite avid phagocytic and bacteriocidal activity. *J Clin Invest.* 3; 115(1), pp. 66–75

Šperanda, M., Điđara, M., Šperanda, T., Domaćinović, M., Valpotić, H., Kovačević, J., Antunović, Z. & Novoselec, J. (2008). Hydrolyzed brewery yeast product like immunomodulator in weaned piglets. *Archiva Zootechnica.* 11, pp. 52-60

Šperanda, M.; Šperanda, T., Šerić, V., Liker, B. Balenović, T., Gros, M., Antunović, Z., Popović, I., Popović, M. Valpotić, I. (2008). Auswirkungen von der unspezifischen und spezifischen Immunmodulation auf immunhämathologische Parameter bei entwöhnten Ferkel. *Tierärztliche Umschau.* 63 (10), 557-562

Špoljarić, D., Fumić, T., Kezić, D., Valpotić, H., Fabijanić, V., Popović, M., Sladoljev, S., Mršić, G. & Valpotić, I. (2011). β-glucans natural immune response modifiers insufficiently known in veterinary medicine. *Vet. stanica* 42, pp. 361-376

Stokes, C. R., & Bailey M. (2000). The porcine gastrointestinal lamina propria: an appropriate target for mucosal immunisation? *Journal of Biotechnology* 83, pp. 51-55

Stokes, C. R., Bailey M. & Haverson K. (2001). Development and function of the pig Gastrointestinal Immune System. In: *Digestive Physiology of Pigs.* J. E. Lindberg & Ogle, B. pp. 59–66 ed. CAB Int., New York, NY

Stuyven, E., Cox, E., Vancaeneghem, S., Arnouts, S., Deprez, P. & Goddeeris, B. M. (2009). Effect of beta-glucan on an ETEC infection in piglets. *Vet. Immunol. Immunopathol.* 128, pp. 60-66

Šver L., Njari B., Gerenčer M., Radeljević D., Bilić V. & Valpotić I. (1996a) Parapoxvirus-induced modulation of porcine gut immune cells primed with Escherichia coli antigens. *Vet arhiv* 66, pp. 1–12

Šver L., Trutin-Ostović K., Žubčić D., Casey T. A., Dean-Nystrom E. A. & Valpotić I. (1996b). Porcine gut T, B and null/□□ TCR+ cell quantification in the protective immunity to fimbrial/toxin antigens of Escherichia coli. *Period biol* 98, pp. 473–478

Telemo, E.; Bailey, M., Miller, B. G., Stokes, C. R. & Bourne, F. J. (1991). Dietary antigen handling by mother and offsprting. *Scand. J. Immunol.* 34, pp. 689-696

Touchette, K. J., Carroll, J. A., Allee, G. L., Matteri, R. L., Dyer, C. J., Beausang, L. A. & Zannelli, M. E. (2002). Effect of spray-dried plasma and lipopolysaccharide exposure on weaned pigs: I. Effects on the immune axis of weaned pigs. *J. Anim. Sci.* 80, pp. 494-501

Turner, J. L., Dritz, S. S., Higgins, J. J. & Minton, J. E. (2002a). Effects of Ascophillum nodosum extract on growth performance and immune function of young pigs challenged with Salmonella typhimurium. *J. Anim. Sci.* 80, pp. 1947-1953

Turner, J. L., Dritz, S. S., Higgins, J. J., Herkelman, J. E. & Minton, K. L. (2002b). Effects of a Quillaja saponaria extract on growth performance and immune function of young pigs challenged with Salmonella typhimurium. *J. Anim. Sci.* 80, pp. 1939-1946

Tzianabos, A.O. (2000). Review - polysaccharide immunomodulators as therapeutic agents: structural aspects and biologic function. *Clin. Microbiol. Rev.* 13, pp. 523–533

Valpotić I., Gerenčer M., Žuvanić J., Modrić Z. & Bašić I. (1989a) Modulating effect of allogeneic immunoglobulins on the reactivity of lymphocytes in suckling and weaned piglets. *Period biol* 91, pp. 39–40

Valpotić I., Gerenčer, M. & Bašić, I. (1989b). In vitro modulating effects of porcine immunoglobulin G on mitogens-induced lymphocyte responce in precolostral, suckling and weaned piglets. *Vet Immunol Immunopathol* 22, pp. 113-122

Valpotić I., Vijtiuk N., Radeljević D., Bilić V., Krsnik B., Vrbanac I. & Laušin M. (1993). Nonspecific immunization of primiparous sows with Baypamun® enhances lacteal immunity in their offspring. *Vet arhiv* 63, pp. 161–172

Valpotić, H. (2009). Effects of nutraceuticals and immunmodulators on productivity, immunity and health status of weaned pigs. Dissertation. Veterinary Faculty, University of Zagreb, Croatia, pp. 73-92

Valpotić, I. (2000). Immunomodulation in domestic animals. *Hrv. vet. vjesnik* 23, pp. 4-10

Valpotić, I., Lučinger, S., Gerenčer, M., Ćurić, S., Radeljević, D., Vrbanac, I. & Bašić, I. (1987). Enhancement of resistance in suckling pigs by immunomodulators. *Proc. 9th Symposium of Yugoslavian Swinebreeders, Osijek*, pp. 395-400

van Dijk, A. J., Everts, H., Nabuurs, M. J. A., Margry, R. J. C. F. & Beynen, A. C. (2001). Growth performance of weanling pigs fed spray-dried animal plasma: a review. *Livestock Prod. Sci.* 68, pp. 263-274

Vega-López M. A., Telemo E., Bailey M., Stevens K. & Stokes C. R. (1993). Immune cell distribution in the small intestine of the pig: immunohistological evidence for an organized compartmentalization in the lamina propria. *Veterinary Immunology and Immunopathology* 37 (1), pp. 49-60

Vega-López, M. A., Bailey, M., Telemo, E. & Stokes, C. R. (1995). Effect of early weaning on the development of immune cells in the pig small intestine. *Vet Immunol Immunopathol.* 44(3-4), pp. 319-27

Vetvicka, V. & Yvin, J. C. (2004). Effects of marine β-1,3-glucan on immune reactions. Int. *Immunopharmacology* 4, pp. 721-730

Vignali, D. A. A., Collison, L. W. & Workman C. J. (2008). How regulatory T cells work. *Nat Rew Immun* 8, pp. 523-532

Vijtiuk N., Košuta D., Bašić I. & Valpotić I. (1993). In vivo modulating effects of bacterial peptidoglycans on PHA-induced responses of porcine PBL and splenocytes. *Immunobiology* 188, pp. 274–280

Vijtiuk N., Košuta D., Valpotić I., Krsnik B. & Bašić I. (1992). Effect of peptidoglycan polymer isolated from Brevibacterium divaricatum on porcine immunohematological parameters. *Vet arhiv* 62, pp. 203–211

Villadangos, J.A. & Heath, W.R. (2005). Life cycle, migration and antigen presenting functions of spleen and lymph node dendritic cells: Limitations of the Langerhans cells paradigm. *Semin. Immunol.* 17, pp. 262–272

Viney, J. L., Mowat, A. M., Omalley, J. M., Williamson, E. & Fanger, N. A. (1998). Expanding dendritic cells in vivo enhances the induction of oral tolerance. J. Immunol. 160, pp. 5815-5825

Walter, B. M. & Bilkei, G. (2004). Immunomodulatory effect of dietary oregano etheric oils on lymphocytes from growth-retarded, low-weight growing-finishing pigs and productivity. *Tijdschrift Diergeneeskunde* 129, pp. 178-181

Wang, Y. Z., Shan, T. Z., Xu, Z. R., Feng, J. & Wang, Z. Q. (2007). Effects of the lactoferrin (LF) on the growth performance, intestinal microflora and morphology of weanling pigs. *Animal Feed Sci. Technol.* 135, pp. 263-272

Weng, X. C., Zang, P., Gong, S. S., & Xiai, S. W. (1987). Effect of immunomodulating agents on murine IL-2 production. *Immunol. Invest.* 16, pp. 79-86

Wenk, C. (2003). Herbs and botanicals as feed additives in monogastric animals. Asian-Autralasian J. *Anim. Sci.* 16, pp. 282-289.

Whary, M.T., Zarkower, A., Confer, F. & Ferguson, F. (1995). Age-related differences in subset composition and activation responses of intestinal intraepithelial and mesenteric lymph node lymphocytes from neonatal swine. *Cell. Immunol.* 163, pp. 215-221

White, L. A., Newman, M. C., Cromwell, G. L. & Lindemann, M. D. (2002). Brewers dried yeast as a source of mannan oligosaccharides for weanling pigs. *J. Anim. Sci.* 80, pp. 2619-2628

Wilkie, B. & Mallard, B. (1999). Selection for high immune response: an alternative approach to animal health maintenance? *Vet. Immunol. Immunopathol.* 72, pp. 231-235

Wilson, A. D., Haverson, K., Southgate, K., Bland, P. W., Stokes, C. R. & Bailey, M. (1996). Expression of major histocompatibility complex class-II antigens on normal porcine intestinal endothelium. *Immunology* 88, pp. 98-103.

Windisch, W.M., Schedle, K., Plitzner, C. & Kroismayr, A. (2008). Use of phytogenic products as feed additives for swine and poultry. *J. Anim. Sci.* 86, pp. E140-E148

Wittig, B. M. & Zeitz M. (2003). The gut as an organ of immunology. *Int. J. Colorectal Dis.* 18, pp. 181–187.

Wu, Y., Kudsk, K. A. DeWitt, R. C., Tolley, E. A. & Li, J. (1999). Route and type of nutrition influence IgA-mediating intestinal cytokines. *Ann. Surg.* 229, pp. 662-667

Wybran, J. (1988). Immunoregulatory agents: synthetic compounds, microbial extracts, Chinese herbs, neuropeptides and intravenous immunoglobulins. *Curr. Opin. Immunol.* 1, pp. 275-281

Yi, G. F., Carroll, J. A., Allee, G. L., Gaines, A. M., Kendall, D. C., Usry, J. L., Toride, Y. & Izuru, S. (2005). Effect of glutamine and spray-dried plasma on growth performance, small intestinal morphology, and immune responses of Escherichia coli K88+ challenged weaned pigs. *J. Anim. Sci.* 83, pp. 634-643

Yrlid, U., Cerovic, V., Milling, S., Jenkins, C. D , Zhang, J. Crocker, P. R., Klavinskis, Linda S. & MacPherson G. G. (2006). Plasmacytoid Dendritic Cells Do Not Migrate in Intestinal or Hepatic Lymph. *The Journal of Immunology*, 177, pp. 6115-6121

Yuan, S. L., Piao, X. S., Li, D. F., Kim, S. W., Lee, H. S. & Guo, P. F. (2006). Effects of dietary Astragalus polysaccharide on growth performance and immune function in weaned pigs. *Animal Sci* 62, pp. 501-507

Zuckermann, F. A. & Gaskins H. R. (1996). Distribution of porcine CD4/CD8 double-positive T lymphocytes in mucosa-associated lymphoid tissues. *Immunology*, 87 (3), pp. 493–499

Part 2

Transplantation and Novel Therapies

14

Cellular Therapies for Immunosuppression

Nathalie Cools, Viggo F. I. Van Tendeloo and Zwi N. Berneman
Laboratory of Experimental Hematology, Vaccine & Infectious Disease Institute,
University of Antwerp
Belgium

1. Introduction

Almost all current therapeutic approaches to inhibit destructive immune responses in autoimmunity are based on antigen non-specific agents, such as cyclosporine A, which systemically suppress the function of virtually all immune effector cells. This indiscriminate immunosuppression, however, often causes serious and sometimes life-threatening side-effects. Indeed, long-term use of immunosuppressive drugs leads to nephrotoxicity and metabolic disorders, as well as manifestations of hyperimmunosuppression such as opportunistic infections and cancer. It is evident, that treatment would be greatly improved by targeting the fundamental cause of pathogenic immune responses in autoimmunity, i.e. loss of tolerance to self-antigens. For this, manipulation of the immune system in autoimmune diseases should ideally arise in specific tolerance for the self-antigens that stimulate chronic activation of the immune system resulting in long term remissions.

New – more antigen-specific and targeted - therapies are intensively being investigated for the treatment of human diseases (Sabatos-Peyton et al., 2010; Dazzi et al., 2007; Miller et al., 2007). In this context, a variety of cellular therapies have been designed to elicit or amplify immune responses. These cell-based activation immunotherapies have proven to be effective for cancer and infectious diseases. Although still in its infancy, the use of well specified and functionally characterized cellular products as treatment modality for autoimmune disorders and in transplantation tolerance is gaining interest. Indeed, experiences with hematopoietic stem cells and cell types with regulatory properties support the concept of resetting immune tolerance and have made cell-based therapies for autoimmune diseases a realistic alternative. At this point however, it is not yet clear which cell type among a broad arsenal of different tolerogenic entities is best with regard to safety, efficacy and related costs.

This review will explore the molecular and cellular mechanisms underlying T cell tolerance and will focus on emerging cell-based therapies pertaining to reduce, suppress or redirect existing immune responses to self-antigens in human diseases.

2. Control and regulation of immune responses

2.1 Tolerance induction

Immune tolerance is the process by which the body naturally does not launch an immune system attack against its own tissues. A variety of tolerance mechanisms have been described to exist naturally and to be responsible for protection of the body's own tissue from immune injuries, while effectively fighting pathogens. Central tolerance to self-antigens results primarily from apoptotic deletion of autoreactive T cells during intrathymic T cell development (Burnet, 1959a; Burnet, 1959b). However, some limitations of this process have been observed resulting in escape of potentially autoreactive T cells (Steinman & Nussenzweig, 2002). Therefore additional mechanisms to induce tolerance occur in the periphery. These include (i) T cell anergy (i.e. the induction of functional hyporesponsiveness to antigens) (Schwartz, 2003), (ii) T cell deletion (i.e. the elimination of autoreactive T cells by apoptosis) (Kurts et al., 1998) and (iii) active suppression of the immune response by regulatory T cells (Cools et al., 2007a). Collectively these mechanisms are known as peripheral tolerance. Despite these mechanisms, some autoreactive T cells may escape and be present in the periphery. Their activation may lead to autoimmune disease. These diseases result in cell and tissue destruction by autoreactive T cells or autoantibodies and the accompanying inflammatory processes. Common autoimmune diseases include rheumatoid arthritis (RA), systemic lupus erythematosis (SLE), type 1 diabetes, multiple sclerosis (MS), Sjogren's syndrome, and inflammatory bowel disease (IBD).

2.2 T cell activation

The current paradigm is that the outcome of the immune response is determined by the relative balance between cells that are capable of causing tissue damage, such as T helper type 1 (Th1), type 2 (Th2) and type 17 (Th17) cells versus cells that are designed to suppress immune responses and limit damage, such as regulatory T cells (Treg). It is generally accepted that antigen-presenting cells (APC), particularly dendritic cells (DC), play a central role in the control and maintenance of this delicate balance depending on the level of inflammation in the microenvironment in which T cell activation takes place (Cools et al., 2007b).

(Auto)immune reactions are set in motion with the uptake, processing and presentation of self-antigens through APC. Nevertheless, it is commonly believed now that generation of T cell-mediated (auto)immunity requires a 3-signal T cell activation process (Curtsinger et al., 1999; Curtsinger et al., 2003) (Figure 1). The first signal is provided by the presentation of (self-)antigens by major histocompatibility complex (MHC) molecules on the APC to the T cell receptor (TCR) on the T cell. At this site, antigen recognition will take place which will create an immune synapse determining subsequent T cell fate. Next, interaction of costimulatory molecules on APC and T cells ensures appropriate activation of naïve T cells (Greenfield et al., 1998). For instance, the costimulatory factors CD80 and CD86 bind to CD28 on naïve T cells resulting in activation and proliferation of T cells. Absence of the second signal results in T cell anergy. Besides effector T cell activation, costimulation is also required for the activation and expansion of different regulatory T cell subsets (Salomon et al., 2000). Currently, it is generally accepted that (an) additional signal(s) (i.e. "signal 3"), such as CD40 ligation and/or the production of pro- or anti-inflammatory cytokines are involved in APC-driven polarization of naïve T cells into effector T cell populations. Indeed depending on the cytokines present upon T cell activation, naïve CD4+ T helper cells can acquire a variety of immune effector phenotypes (Strom & Koulmanda, 2009; Zhou et al., 2009). In brief, when CD4+ T cells are activated in the presence of interleukin (IL)-12, they become IFN-γ-producing Th1 cells; while CD4+ T cells that are activated in the presence of

IL-4 will differentiate into Th2 cells producing IL-4, IL-5 and IL-13. Expression of the transcription factor FOXP3 and subsequent generation of Treg is induced by transforming growth factor (TGF)-β, in the absence of additional pro-inflammatory cytokines. In contrast, expression of TGF-β in concert with IL-6 and IL-21 induces IL-17-producing T cells (Th17) (Bettelli et al., 2007; Weaver & Hatton, 2009; Jäger & Kuchroo, 2010).

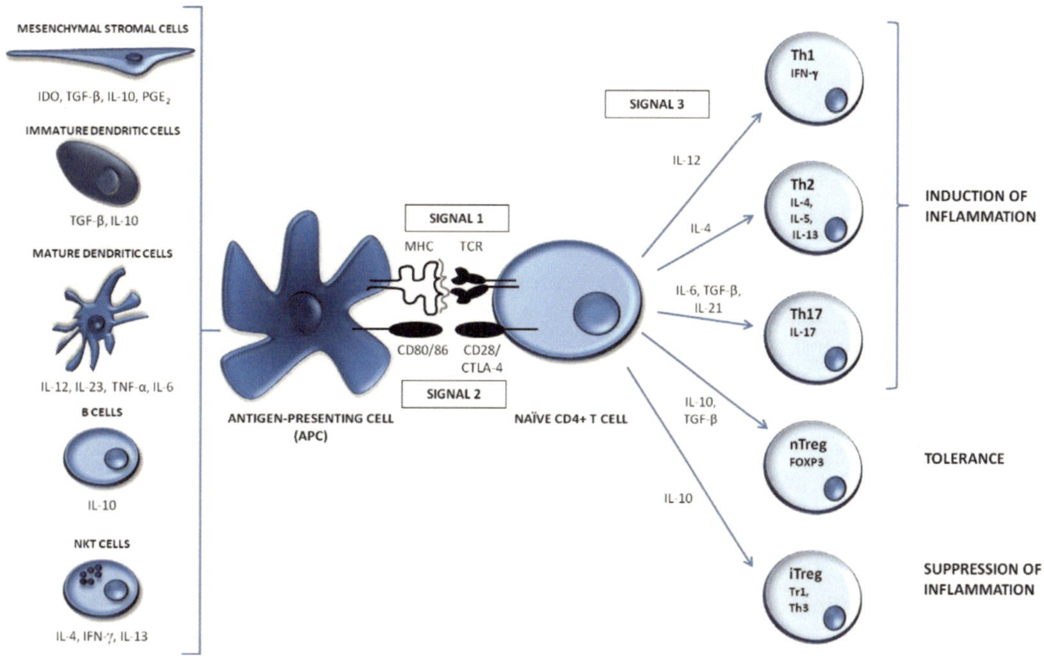

Fig. 1. Molecular mechanisms of T cell activation. Currently, it is accepted that generation of T cell-mediated immunity requires at least 3 signals. In brief, antigen presentation (= "signal 1"), costimulation (= "signal 2"), and the production of immunoregulatory cytokines (= "signal 3") are required for the activation and expansion of different effector and regulatory T cell subsets

It might be evident that the immunological basis of the therapeutic effect of a variety of biological agents used for the induction of immunosuppression lies in the interaction with one, or more, of the above molecular signals. Therefore, immunosuppressants developed for their ability to alter T cell function can generally be divided into 3 categories: (i) TCR-directed agents, (ii) costimulatory antagonists, and (iii) antagonists of cytokines and cytokine receptors. First, Fc receptor (FcR)-non-binding CD3-specific antibodies carrying mutations of the IgG1 Fc chain with elimination of glycosylation sites, are minimally depleting and result in T cell apoptosis and anergy by altering the TCR-CD3 complex and/or induction of Treg. The early results from clinical trials using anti-CD3 antibodies, i.e. Otelixizumab (ChAgly CD3), Tepilizumab [hOKT3γ1(Ala-Ala)], and Visilizumab, in a variety of autoimmune disorders are encouraging (Keymeulen et al., 2005; Bisikirsha et al., 2005; Plevy et al., 2007). Second, agents that block T cell costimulation are currently being tested as maintenance drug in transplant patients. In this context, Abatacept (CTLA4-Ig) blocks the interaction between CD28 expressed on the surface of T cells and CD80/CD86 on the surface of APC. Additionally, Alefacept interferes with the activation of T cells by preventing the interaction between CD2 on T cells and LFA-3 on APC (Vincenti & Luggen, 2007). Furthermore, cytokine- and/or cytokine receptor-directed therapies are also in development in order to promote immunosuppression. Indeed, TNF-α blockers have been extensively used and validated as an efficacious treatment for RA, Crohn's disease and psoriasis (Feldman et al., 1998; Victor et al., 2003). This approach clearly represents one of the greatest successes in biological response-modifying therapies. In addition, the therapeutic efficacy of an anti-IL-12/IL-23 (p40) monoclonal antibody (i.e. Ustekinumab) has been demonstrated in patients with active Crohn's disease (Mannon et al., 2004) and psoriasis (Krueger et al., 2007; Leonardi et al., 2008), but not in MS patients (Segal et al., 2008). For completeness, also biologicals that interfere with lymphocyte trafficking have been approved for the treatment of autoimmune disease. Thus far, the most successfull drug in this class is Natalizumab, a monoclonal antibody to α4-integrin (Yednock et al., 1992; Stüve et al., 2006) blocking the entry of leukocytes into the central nervous system. In addition, Fingolimod (FTY-720) holds promise as a new treatment for MS by promoting tissue retention (O'Connor et al., 2009). In fact, lymphocytes are trapped in the lymph nodes, which reduces peripheral lymphocyte counts and the recirculation of lymphocytes to the inflamed tissues (Mandala et al., 2002; Mehling et al., 2008).

Unlike conventional immunosuppressants for the treatment of patients with autoimmune diseases, biologicals only bind to immune cells or to products secreted by immune cells, thereby reducing or preventing toxicity to non-immune system tissues.

3. Cell therapy approaches aiming at minimizing T cell activation

At present, existing immunomodulatory drugs do not specifically target pathogenic autoreactive T lymphocytes. It is therefore evident, that the "holy grail" for the treatment of autoimmune disease is the development of treatment strategies in which only the pathogenic autoreactive T cells are safely inactivated in an antigen-specific manner, while leaving the remainder of the immune system undisturbed. Therefore, strong efforts are currently undertaken to circumvent various systemic side effects that may occur after overall modulation of protective immunity by harnessing peripheral regulatory mechanisms. Indeed, the anticipated induction of antigen-specific immunosuppression may operate via a number of cell-intrinsic (e.g. anergy) and/or cell-extrinsic (e.g. Treg) mechanisms. Potential candidate cell populations that bear immunomodulating and regulatory properties comprise stem cells of various origins, as well as immune cells such as Treg, DC, NKT and B cells.

3.1 Stem cells

3.1.1 Hematopoietic stem cells (HSC)

Hematopoietic stem cells (HSC) are cells capable of self-renewal and reconstitute all types of blood cells. For this, research on HSC is now providing new approaches to remove autoreactive immune cells and to subsequently generate a new, properly functioning immune system. Although the approach to use high dose myeloablative therapy combined with subsequent hematopoietic stem cell transplantation (HSCT) was first described more than 50 years ago for the treatment of malignant conditions, this principle was adopted in recent years for treatment of various autoimmune diseases. It is evident that complete

immunoablation is a drastic way to achieve maximal treatment efficiency in autoimmune diseases (Teng et al., 2005), with potentially lethal complications such as cardiotoxicity or overt opportunistic infections. For this, HSCT is only considered in patients suffering from severe and progressive autoimmune disease and refractory to conventional immunosuppressants. In contrast to complete ablation of autoreactive T cells, recent immune reconstituting data suggest that non-myeloablative or reduced intensity conditioning protocols could also allow the normal immune-regulatory mechanisms to recontrol the system (Muraro et al., 2005).
To obtain cells for autologous HSCT, stem cells are mobilized from the bone marrow to the peripheral blood, before patient conditioning, using various protocols [e.g. granulocyte colony-stimulating factor (G-CSF)]. Subsequently, the autologous HSC are collected through leukapheresis. After this, the patient is prepared for the transplant by potent immunosuppressive treatment, usually by chemotherapy and/or radiotherapy, in order to eliminate autoreactive T cells. Thereafter, peripheral blood cells or bone marrow cells enriched for HSC or previously purified CD34+ HSC are re-injected and newly developing B and T cells are introduced to self-antigens and controlled by the natural tolerance mechanisms. In most trials, the patient's own stem cells have been used (i.e. autologous HSCT), however small series and case reports of allogeneic HSCT have been reported (Oyama et al., 2001; Burt et al., 2004). Although the advantage of allogeneic HSCT is clear, namely introducing a "healthy" immune system, limited experience is available with regard to this approach for treatment of autoimmune disease. Indeed, the increased toxicity and potential risk of graft-versus-host disease (GVHD) is associated with significant morbidity and mortality of allogeneic HSCT (Griffith et al., 2006).
Several mechanisms may apply for correction of autoimmunity by HSCT. As mentioned above, potent immunosuppressive treatment attributes to the elimination of autoreactive T and B cells. However, incomplete immunoablation may account for the suboptimal responses and high risk rates of early relapse seen in some clinical trials of autologous HSCT. Although HSCT targets a wide array of immune effector cells non-specifically, it has become evident that the therapeutic efficacy of HSCT cannot merely be the consequence of the profound immunosuppression. In contrast, resetting of the abnormal immune regulation underlying the autoimmune conditions most likely attributes to the success of this therapeutic approach. This was well illustrated by Traynor and colleagues who found that following HSCT the deregulated T cell receptor repertoires were restored to those of healthy individuals (Traynor et al., 2000). From this, it can be postulated that re-establishing tolerance in T cells contributes to the beneficial effect of HSCT and thereby decreases the likelihood of disease re-occurrence. Besides the risk associated with allogeneic HSCT, this approach is associated with durable and complete remission in a small number of patients. It is postulated that elimination of autoreactive host lymphocytes by allogeneic donor T cells contributes to this beneficial effect, known as graft–versus–autoimmunity (GVA) effect. However, as stated above, this benefit comes with the associated risk of GVHD. Furthermore tolerance to self-antigens, after allogeneic HSCT, may also be achieved by mixed hematopoietic chimerism, i.e. a state in which HSC of the recipient and donor co-exist and thus also multi-lineage hematopoietic populations. When both donor and host cells contribute to hematopoiesis, the new T cell repertoire in the recipient thymus is rendered tolerant to antigens expressed by hematopoietic cells of both origins.

According to the EBMT/EULAR database (Daikeler et al., 2011), MS is the most frequent diagnosis for which HSCT is being used. Other indications are scleroderma, RA, juvenile idiopathic arthritis (JIA), SLE, Crohn's disease, ulcerative colitis, and vasculitis (Burt et al., 2003; Popat & Krance, 2004; Hough et al., 2005; Tyndall & Saccardi, 2005). Today, HSCT can induce long-term remission lasting for more than six years without any treatment and with a significant decrease in the risks of HSCT, in particular for patients with severe autoimmune disease refractory to conventional treatment. Nonetheless, the major limitation of HSCT in autoimmune patients remains that a considerable amount of treatment-related complications have been reported (e.g. infections, graft failure and malignant relapses), which accounted for the majority of the transplant-related mortality. Currently, several phase III clinical trials are ongoing to evaluate the prospects of autologous HSCT as a cellular treatment strategy for severe autoimmune disease.

3.1.2 Mesenchymal stromal cells (MSC)

Recently another cell, the mesenchymal stromal cell (MSC), has generated great interest for its ability to induce immunosuppression. In pioneering studies, Friedenstein et al. reported more than 30 years ago fibroblast-like cells that could be isolated from bone marrow via their inherent adherence to plastic in culture (Friedenstein et al., 1974). MSC are now known as cells of stromal origin that have the ability of self-renewal and multipotency, which allows their differentiation into various tissues of mesodermal origin (osteocytes, chondrocytes and adipocytes) and other embryonic lineages, and may be isolated from bone marrow, skeletal muscle, adipose tissue, synovial membranes and other connective tissues, and blood. Although still subject of debate, MSC are defined by using a combination of phenotypic markers and functional properties. A generally accepted phenotypic profile of human MSC includes the expression of CD73, CD105 and CD90 as well as the absence of expression of hematopoietic (CD45) and vascular (CD31) markers (Pittenger et al., 1999; Dominici et al., 2006).

MSC are relatively non-immunogenic, i.e. they do not normally express MHC or costimulatory molecules such as CD80 and CD86. Moreover, MSC exert a profound immunosuppressive and anti-inflammatory effect *in vitro* and *in vivo*, which has made these cells of particular interest for therapeutic application (Marigo & Dazzi, 2011). The mechanisms underlying the immunosuppressive effect of MSC remain to be clarified. However, it has been demonstrated that preliminary "licensing" of MSC by inflammatory environmental conditions, such as IFN-γ, is needed to acquire their immunosuppressive properties (Jones et al., 2007). In turn, MSC skew the inflammatory environment into an anti-inflammatory environment both directly, through mechanisms mediated by soluble factors [TGF-β (Di Nicola et al., 2002), indoleamine 2,3-dioxygenase (IDO) (Meisel et al., 2004), hepatocyte growth factor (HGF) (Di Nicola et al., 2002), nitric oxide (Sato et al., 2007), IL-10 (Batten et al., 2006) and prostaglandin E2 (Aggarwal & Pittenger, 2005)] and cell contact [e.g. via the inhibitory molecule programmed death 1 (PD-1) (Augello et al., 2005)], and indirectly via the recruitment of other regulatory networks that involve APC (Beyth et al., 2005) and Treg (Prevosto et al., 2007). Although MSC-induced unresponsiveness lacks any selectivity, its effect is directed mainly at the level of T cell proliferation, as evidenced by cell cycle arrest of MSC-induced anergic T cells. Additionally, recent studies suggest that MSC may induce a cytokine profile shift in the Th1/Th2 balance towards the anti-inflammatory Th2 phenotype (Haniffa et al., 2007; Zhou et al., 2008). Indeed, MSC have been shown to decrease the production of IFN-γ, IL-2 and TNF-α, whilst they increase IL-4 secretion (Aggarwal & Pittenger, 2005). Furthermore, MSC suppress the cytolytic effects of cytotoxic T cells (Rasmusson et al., 2003). However, the effects of MSC on immune responses are not confined to T cells. Indeed, it has been demonstrated that MSC are also capable of inhibiting proliferation of IL-2- and IL-15-stimulated natural killer (NK) cells (Sotiropoulou et al., 2006; Spaggiari et al., 2006), as well as alter the function of B cells and APC. Indeed, MSC affect terminal differentiation of B cells demonstrated by an altered release of humoral factors. Moreover, they increase B cell viability, while inhibiting B cell proliferation through cell cycle arrest of B lymphocytes in the G0/G1 phase (Tabera et al., 2008; Asari et al., 2009). In addition, MSC-derived prostaglandin E2 was shown to act on macrophages by stimulating the production of IL-10 (Németh et al., 2009) and on monocytes by blocking their differentiation towards DC as well as on dendritic cell maturation and function, as demonstrated by a decreased cell-surface expression of MHC class II and costimulatory molecules, and a decreased production of IL-12 and TNF-α (Spaggiari et al., 2009; Jiang et al., 2005; Nauta et al., 2006). Finally, MSC have been reported to promote both *in vitro* and *in vivo*, the formation of potent CD4+CD25+ as well as CD8+ Treg (Prevosto et al., 2007; Maccario et al., 2005), although the precise mode of action is still subject of active research.

Although better understanding of the underlying mechanisms is still required, accumulating evidence with regard to their immunomodulatory properties suggests that MSC have great potential to suppress immune responses in various clinical settings. While MSC represent only a rare fraction in bone marrow and other tissues (i.e. 0.001-0.01% of the total nucleated cells), they can be expanded *ex vivo*, under clinical-grade conditions, to significant numbers from a small bone marrow aspirate in 8 to 10 weeks (DiGirolamo et al., 1999; Sekiya et al., 2002). Treatment of several auto-immune diseases, such as type 1 diabetes, RA, MS (Zappia et al., 2005), and GVHD (Le Blanc et al., 2004; Le Blanc et al., 2008; Lazarus et al., 2005) was performed with administration of MSC derived from allogeneic donors. Several phase I and II clinical trials have been conducted, and encouraging results have been generated from these studies. For example, it has recently been demonstrated that MSC may promote reconstitution of the bone marrow stroma after chemotherapy and enhance HSC engraftment. Indeed, sustained hematopoietic engraftment in pediatric patients was shown after co-transplantation of donor MSC with allogeneic HSC (Ball et al., 2007). In addition, MSC infusion has resulted in striking improvement of therapy-resistant, acute GVHD, as demonstrated by a complete response of 30 out of 55 patients in a multi-center phase II clinical trial (LeBlanc et al., 2008). Although clinical results obtained so far confirm feasibility and safety of the *in vivo* application of MSC without major adverse events, another report has shown an increased risk of relapse in leukemia patients who were co-transplanted with MSC in order to prevent acute GVHD after allogeneic HSCT (Ning et al., 2008), as compared with patients receiving standard HSCT.

3.2 Dendritic cells

A major therapeutic goal in autoimmune diseases is to provide inhibitory mechanisms with the capacity to suppress inappropriate immune activation in an antigen-specific manner with minimal risk and damage to the host. In this perspective, we discuss the role of dendritic cells (DC) and regulatory T cells (Treg) in the design of new cell-based and antigen-specific therapeutic strategies to suppress autoreactive immune responses.

DC are a highly specialized population of white blood cells that are capable of orchestrating the adaptive immune responses (Cools et al., 2007b). In their immature state, DC reside in the peripheral tissues (skin, airways and intestine) where they function as the "sentinels" of the immune system, i.e. they patrol the body to capture antigens, including self-antigens, invading pathogens and certain malignant cells. In the classical view, antigen-loaded DC migrate to the secondary lymphoid organs and the internalized antigen is processed and presented to T cells in a MHC-dependent manner (Trombetta et al., 2005). Depending on the context in which the antigen was captured, DC induce tolerance or immunity. Indeed, in a steady-state condition DC remain immature, expressing only small amounts of MHC and costimulatory molecules, and are believed to induce T cell anergy or regulatory T cells (Lutz & Schuler, 2002). Upon encounter of so-called danger signals, DC undergo a complex maturation process from antigen-capturing cells into antigen-presenting cells, essential for triggering T cell proliferation and differentiation into helper and effector T cells with unique functions and cytokine profiles.

DC are heterogeneous and can be divided into two major subsets: plasmacytoid DC and conventional or myeloid DC, which show several distinct phenotypic and biological features (O'Doherty et al., 1994). Plasmacytoid DC (pDC) originate from a lymphoid progenitor cell in lymphoid organs and are characterized by the production of high amounts of type I interferon in response to viral stimuli (Cella et al., 1999). For this, pDC are believed to be primarily involved in innate immunity (Swiecki & Colonna, 2010; Reizis et al., 2011). On the other hand, a myeloid progenitor cell differentiates towards different DC populations in the bone marrow (Liu, 2001). Subsequently, DC subsets circulate throughout the body: Langerhans cells migrate towards the skin epidermis and interstitial DC migrate towards the skin dermis and various other tissues (airways, liver and intestine). Circulating or migrating DC are found in the blood and in the afferent lymphatics, respectively. In human blood, differences in DC subsets can be identified based on a different expression of Toll-like Receptors (TLR) (Kadowaki et al., 2001), cytokine receptors and cytokines (Kohrgruber et al., 1999), as well as a difference in migratory potential (Penna et al., 2001), indicating a different function in induction and regulation of the immune response by various subtypes [for review on DC subsets see (Ju et al., 2010)].

DC appear to be essential for both central tolerance in the thymus and peripheral tolerance (Liu et al., 2007). Indeed, mature thymic DC present self-antigens to developing T and B cells and subsequently delete lymphocytes with autoreactivity above a certain threshold (Steinman et al., 2003). In addition, DC induce peripheral tolerance through induction of T cell anergy and T cell deletion and through activation of Treg. Antigen presentation in the absence of costimulation can lead to impaired clonal expansion and T cell anergy (Schwartz, 2003). Furthermore, there is increasing evidence that under steady-state conditions antigen presentation by immature DC leads to T cell deletion and peripheral tolerance. In this context, a discrete subset of human DC expressing indoleamine 2,3-dioxygenase (IDO) have been identified (Munn et al., 2002; Mellor & Munn, 2004). IDO is a catabolic enzyme responsible for the degradation of tryptophan, an amino acid essential for T cell proliferation. Additionally, signalling through CD95 (Fas ligation) by DC may be involved in tolerance induction (Süss & Shortman, 1996). Finally, it has also been documented that DC are able to prime Treg in order to maintain tolerance to self-antigens, foreign peptides and allo-antigens (Banerjee et al., 2006; Fehérvári & Sakaguchi, 2004; Kretschmer et al., 2005).

While the pivotal role of DC in immunity is clearly established and results of early studies using DC-based therapeutic vaccines in cancer patients (Van Tendeloo et al., 2011) and HIV-infected individuals (Connolly et al., 2008) are encouraging, the fact that DC are also involved in tolerance induction has provided the prospect for the use of DC to suppress noxious immune responses in allergy, autoimmunity and transplantation (Hilkens et al., 2010). Dendritic cell-based immunotherapeutic strategies for autoimmune and allergic diseases can be developed either by targeting antigen to DC *in vivo* or by culturing the cells *in vitro*, pulsing with antigen and injecting them back into patients. On the one hand, antigens coupled to antibodies specific for DC markers, such as 33D1 or DEC-205, have already been used to deliver antigens to DC *in vivo*, resulting in antigen-specific tolerance which in contrast could not be attained by injection of the same peptide in the Freund's adjuvant (Hawiger et al., 2001; Bonifaz et al., 2002). On the other hand, administration of immature DC has already been shown to induce antigen-specific T cell tolerance. Indeed, when iDC pulsed with influenza matrix protein (IMP) and keyhole limpet hemocyanin (KLH), a general stimulator of CD4+ T cells, were injected, a decline in influenza-specific CD8+ IFN-γ-secreting T cells was observed, while peptide-specific IL-10-secreting T cells appeared (Dhodapkar et al., 2001; Dhodapkar & Steinman, 2002). Aforementioned results suggest that DC can induce antigen-specific T cell tolerance *in vitro* as well as *in vivo*, and have prompted a number of groups to translate these findings into clinical applications. A phase I clinical trial using vitamin D3-treated tolerogenic DC will be started in RA patients at Newcastle University (Harry et al., 2010; Hilkens et al., 2010) (http://clinicaltrials.gov/ct2/show/study/NCT012352858). Furthermore, genetic manipulation of DC by overexpressing immune–regulatory molecules or inhibiting or silencing immune–stimulatory molecules promotes tolerogenic function. In line with this, a first safety study using tolerogenic DC treated with antisense oligonucleotides targeting the primary transcripts of the CD40, CD80, and CD86 costimulatory molecules has recently started at the University of Pittsburg (http://clinicaltrials.gov/ct2/show/study/NCT00445913).

3.3. Regulatory T cells

Different T cell subsets have been identified with the ability to suppress immune responses and are currently subdivided based on expression of cell surface markers, production of cytokines and mechanisms of action. Two broad categories of Treg have been described. The first are naturally-occurring thymic-derived regulatory T cells (nTreg) which constitutively express the IL-2 receptor α chain (CD25), and comprise 1-10% of the CD4+ T cell population in healthy adults. These cells also express the intracellular transcription factor forkhead box P3 (FOXP3) (Ziegler, 2006), which has demonstrated to be critical for the generation of Treg (Gavin et al., 2007; Bacchetta et al., 2006), and its genetic deficiency results in autoimmune and inflammatory diseases (Wildin & Freitas, 2005). Recently, a unique CpG-rich island within an evolutionary conserved region upstream of exon 1, named TSDR (Treg-specific demethylation region), was demonstrated to be unmethylated in nTreg (Lal & Bromberg, 2009a; Lal et al., 2009b). Demethylation of this region resulted in strong and stable induction of FOXP3. In contrast, conventional CD4+ T cells display methylation of the FOXP3 locus. This finding has led to new methods of analysing Treg based on quantitative analysis of methylation patterns of the key transcription factor FOXP3, which may be valuable for quality assessment of *ex vivo* expanded Treg (Wieczorek et al., 2009). There is accumulating evidence that 2 subsets of nTreg exist: a first population that is derived directly from the thymus; the second derives from CD4+CD25- T cell precursors in the periphery. In addition, several other studies have reported the existence of various subsets of (antigen-)induced or adaptive Treg. There are at least two populations of induced Treg (iTreg), subdivided according to different expression of immunosuppressive cytokines: CD4+ regulatory T cells type 1 (Tr1) express high levels of interleukin (IL)-10 (Roncarolo et al., 2006; Battaglia et al., 2004), while T helper 3 (Th3) regulatory T cells secrete large amounts of TGF-β (Faria & Weiner, 2006; Carrier et al., 2007). In addition, we have shown the presence of IL-10/TGF-β double-positive Tr1 cells at the single cell level (Cools et al., 2008). Ultimately, only the demonstration of actual suppressive function confirms the presence of Treg.

Numerous immunosuppressive mechanisms described thus far suggest that multiple, redundant mechanisms are required for optimal Treg function *in vivo*. Indeed Treg mediate suppressive effects by several mechanisms including cell contact-mediated suppression, competition for growth factors and secretion of soluble suppressive factors. Several *in vitro* studies have demonstrated that Treg suppress proliferation and IFN-γ production by effector T cells through a direct cell contact-dependent mechanism between suppressor and effector cells, possibly mediated by the expression of cell surface markers, such as glucocorticoid-induced tumor necrosis factor (TNF) receptor-related protein (GITR), cytotoxic T lymphocyte-associated antigen (CTLA-4) and galectin-1 (Shevach, 2009; Garín et al., 2007). Also, cell surface-bound TGF-β has been reported to mediate cell contact-dependent immunosuppression by Treg (Nakamura et al, 2001). Another mechanism for Treg to affect effector T cell activation can be established by modulating DC function. For example, ligation of CD80/CD86 on DC by CTLA-4 on Treg results in expression and activation of IDO (Fallarino et al., 2003), a catabolic enzyme involved in tryptophan degradation. Furthermore, soluble factors such as the immunosuppressive cytokines IL-10, IL-35 (Collison et al., 2007) and TGF-β have been implicated in the suppressive function of Treg. The roles of these cytokines in immunosuppression include cell cycle arrest and inhibition of proliferation, induction of apoptosis, and suppression of DC maturation and function (Li & Flavell, 2008). Moreover, Treg can express cytotoxic molecules, such as granzyme A, granzyme B and perforin, inducing apoptosis of target cells (Grossman et al., 2004; Gondek et al., 2005). Finally, Treg may also attenuate immune responses by competing with effector cells for essential growth factors, such as IL-2 which has been demonstrated to be essential for both Treg and effector cell function (Busse et al., 2010). It is evident from the studies delineated above that the precise mechanisms of suppression by Treg has yet to be fully elucidated.

Various studies have confirmed the importance and therapeutic potential of Treg. A number of commonly used non-specific therapies have been documented to induce immunomodulatory cytokines and to alter Treg function. For instance, rapamycine (sirolimus), an oral inhibitor of the mammalian target of rapamycin (mTor) pathway, promotes the *de novo* generation and enhances the suppressive capacity of Treg (Gao et al., 2007; Monti et al., 2008). This is in contrast to calcineurin inhibitors which inhibit Treg induction. While the action of these drugs is non-specific, strategies to specifically induce Treg are currently the subject of active investigation. These approaches are based on the fact that exposure to antigen increases Treg frequency and/or potency by either expanding nTreg or inducing the generation of induced Treg from cells that do not originally possess regulatory activity (Long & Wood, 2009). They include adoptive transfer of *ex vivo* generated and/or expanded CD4+CD25+ Treg, and the induction of appropriate Treg populations in patients *in vivo*. Since Treg comprise only a small proportion of peripheral blood CD4+ T cells in human, *ex vivo* expansion of these cells prior to administration to the patient is required. The most commonly used expansion protocol at present is based on stimulation by anti-CD3/anti-CD28 beads in the presence of high doses of recombinant IL-2, supplemented in some protocols with rapamycin (Trzonkowski et al., 2009). This approach is advantageous since the expanded cells can be phenotypically and functionally characterized prior to infusion. Currently, several clinical trials using adoptively transferred Treg are ongoing (Riley et al., 2009). In a phase I/II clinical trial in 28 patients receiving HSCT together with conventional T cells as well as Treg, long-term protection from GVHD and robust immune reconstitution was demonstrated (Di Ianni et al., 2011). In addition, Trzonkowski et al. did not report unexpected adverse effects using *ex vivo* expanded Treg in humans for the treatment of GVHD following HSCT (Trzonkowski et al., 2009). To date, further clinical studies are being planned to test the therapeutic potential of Treg in view of immunosuppression in autoimmunity and in solid organ transplantation.

3.4 Other immune effector cells

3.4.1 B cells

B cells can play a variety of pathogenic roles in human autoimmune diseases. On the one hand, they may serve as potent self-antigen-presenting cells and on the other hand after differentiation into plasma cells they can secrete auto-antibodies that through complexing antigen can promote local inflammatory reactions. Indeed, two major B cell subsets have been demonstrated: (i) early lineage CD20+CD79+CD27+ B cells function primarily as APC expressing MHC and costimulatory antigens that sustain T cell-mediated cellular responses, and (ii) late lineage CD138+ mature plasma cells and CD38+ plasma blasts that relate to the humoral response (Zarkhin et al., 2008; Zarkhin et al., 2010). From these results it is evident that B cells contribute to immunity through production of antibodies, antigen presentation to T cells and secretion of cytokines. The role of B cells as an essential component of the autoimmune reaction that sustains the chronic inflammation has been underlined by successful therapeutic B cell depletion with anti-CD20 monoclonal antibodies. Indeed, rituximab - a chimeric anti-CD20 monoclonal antibody - has been proven to be highly beneficial for patients with certain autoimmune diseases, including RA, MS and type 1 diabetes. However, this treatment also resulted in aggravation of symptoms in a few patients, suggesting that B cells can also protect from autoimmune pathology. In this context, IL-10-producing regulatory CD1d+CD5+ B cells are able to downregulate autoimmune disease initiation, onset, or severity in experimental autoimmune encephalomyelitis (EAE), collagen-induced arthritis, contact hypersensitivity, and inflammatory bowel disease, indicating that B cells can also be essential for immunosuppression of autoreactive T cell responses (Iwata et al., 2011; DiLillo et al., 2010). Therefore, B cell-mediated regulation of the immune system may be of great interest for the development of new cell-based therapies for immunosuppression. Indeed, adoptive transfer of *in vitro* activated B cells isolated from successfully treated mice limited disease severity, suggesting a possible role for regulatory B cells (Yanaba et al., 2008).

3.4.2 Natural killer T cells

A T cell subset with regulatory properties that additionally exhibit natural killer cell characteristics has been identified in mice and humans [extensively reviewed elsewhere (Hegde et al., 2010; Pratschke et al., 2009; Wu & Van Kaer, 2009)]. These natural killer T (NKT) cells are a subset of innate lymphocytes that recognize endogenous or exogenous glycolipids in the context of CD1d molecules expressed by APC, such as monocytes, DC and myeloid suppressor cells. Upon antigenic stimulation NKT cells produce a variety of immunomodulatory cytokines, which endow these cells with potent immunoregulatory properties. Therefore, NKT cells have been tested in animal models of various autoimmune diseases, such as type 1 diabetes, experimental autoimmune encephalomyelitis, arthritis and SLE, but so far only with moderate success.

3.4.3 Peripheral blood mononuclear cells (PBMC)

An alternative approach for effective immunosuppression for treatment of autoimmune disease involves the coupling of self-antigen-derived peptides to cellular vehicles using chemical fixatives (Miller et al., 2007). The induction of immunosuppression by this method is indirect and implies that the fixed cells rapidly undergo apoptotic cell death following fixation and subsequently carry over intact peptides to tolerogenic APC for processing and presentation (Smith & Miller, 2006; Turley & Miller, 2007).

To date, the group of Roland Martin from the University of Hamburg (Germany) has started a phase I/IIa study to evaluate the therapeutic use of autologous peripheral blood mononuclear cells (PBMC) in MRI-proven relapsing-remitting MS patients. These PBMC are coupled with a cocktail of 7 myelin peptides associated with MS pathogenesis against which demonstrable responses can be detected in patient subsets (Lutterotti et al., 2008). This first-in-man exploratory study will provide proof-of-concept of the potential for this cell-based immune-therapeutic approach.

4. Conclusion

Cell-based immunotherapy presents an appealing venue as a substantial component of future individualized treatment modalities for a broad scope of medical fields, including cancer immunotherapies, autoimmune diseases and transplantation tolerance.

Increasing knowledge with regard to the biology, function and mode of immunosuppression of immunoregulatory cell populations opens up new possibilities for antigen-specific manipulation of autoimmunity. Ultimately, this will lead to their clinical application. Nonetheless, the complexity and heterogeneity of autoimmunity, in which multiple dysregulated cell types on various genetic backgrounds are involved, may require integration of several tolerance induction mechanisms to restore tolerance. Therefore, the opportunity to intervene before the appearance of epitope spreading (Miller et al., 2007) using tolerogenic strategies in combination with broader immunosuppressive agents, should be further explored. For instance, induction of immunosuppression may be preceded by treatment with biologicals which can function to reduce the self-antigen-specific T cell frequency to a level that can be effectively and permanently suppressed. Strategies that have shown immunosuppressive effects in animal models include the combination of costimulatory blockade reagents and T cell depletion, as well as adoptively transferred Treg (Chen et al., 2005; Bresson & von Herrath, 2008).

Additionally, also the therapeutic benefit of autologous HSCT could be boosted by the addition of regulatory cell populations, such as tolerogenic DC, Treg, or MSC, which have potent immunosuppressive properties.

Numerous questions still remain in view of the translation of bench findings to the bedside. One challenge for immune tolerance induction is the identification of disease subsets to be considered in evaluating treatment response as well as careful and proper choice of patients to be included for clinical trials evaluating the effects of cellular therapies for immunosuppression. Another quest is how to qualitatively and quantitatively measure immunosuppression in patients. In this context, immunological assays may be used as measures of the effect of immune therapies, although their relationship to the disease process remains speculative. As an example, cellular proliferation assays to islet-specific proteins have distinguished responses in diabetic patients from healthy control subjects (Herold et al., 2009). Ideally, therapies for immunosuppression must also be durable. This means that the ability to regulate the autoimmune response has to be permanent or at least for many years following intervention, for instance via the generation of self-antigen-specific Treg. Nevertheless, major concerns to administer a specified cell product as a tolerizing regimen relates to the risk of *in vivo* re-activation, particularly in response to any underlying inflammatory microenvironment. By means of example, it has indeed been shown that a minority of adoptively transferred Treg lose their FOXP3 expression and can even differentiate into effector T cells (Komatsu et al., 2009). Moreover, a number of groups have identified the ability of Treg to differentiate into proinflammatory Th17 cells (Koenen et al., 2008; Voo et al., 2009). Therefore, such side effects need to be blocked and – in the case of DC - several reports demonstrate that exposure to anti-inflammatory cytokines and immunosuppressive agents can condition DC to a tolerogenic state (Steinman & Banchereau, 2007). Recently, we have shown that *in vitro* exposure of *ex vivo* generated DC from MS patients to IL-10 results in IL-10-, but not IL-12-, secreting DC with low expression levels of CD80/86 and an effective capacity to suppress myelin-specific T cell responses *in vitro* (Cools et al., manuscript submitted for publication). Importantly, further *in vitro* treatment of DC with maturation stimuli did not induce phenotypic changes or modifications in the cytokine secretion profile. Other related safety issues include immunogenicity, carcinogenicity, sensitization to donor HLA, lack of clear mechanistic understanding and cost-benefit relations. In particular the absence of transformation potential of *ex vivo* cultured cells needs to be documented before infusion into (immune-compromised) patients, since failure of immune surveillance mechanisms may favour the development of tumors *in vivo*.

In conclusion, improved understanding of the disease pathogenesis of autoimmunity, the genetic defects underlying different forms of autoimmune diseases, and the mechanisms by which regulatory cell populations suppress autoreactive T and B cells will better define the ultimate role of cellular therapies in the treatment of autoimmune disease.

5. Acknowledgement

This work was supported by grant no. G.0168.09 of the Fund for Scientific Research – Flanders, Belgium (FWO-Vlaanderen), by the grants of the University of Antwerp through the Special Research Fund (BOF), Medical Legacy Fund, and the Methusalem funding program, by a grant of the Hercules Foundation - Belgium, by grants of the Charcot

Foundation - Belgium and of the "Belgische Stichting Roeping" - Belgium. NC is a postdoctoral fellow of the Fund for Scientific Research (FWO)-Flanders.

6. References

Aggarwal S, Pittenger MF. (2005). Human mesenchymal stem cells modulate allogeneic immune cell responses. Blood, 105(4):1815-22.

Asari S, Itakura S, Ferreri K, Liu CP, Kuroda Y, Kandeel F, Mullen Y. (2009). Mesenchymal stem cells suppress B-cell terminal differentiation. Exp Hematol, 37(5):604-15.

Augello A, Tasso R, Negrini SM, Amateis A, Indiveri F, Cancedda R, Pennesi G. (2005). Bone marrow mesenchymal progenitor cells inhibit lymphocyte proliferation by activation of the programmed death 1 pathway. Eur J Immunol, 35(5):1482-90.

Bacchetta R, Passerini L, Gambineri E, Dai M, Allan SE, Perroni L, Dagna-Bricarelli F, Sartirana C, Matthes-Martin S, Lawitschka A, Azzari C, Ziegler SF, Levings MK, Roncarolo MG. (2006). Defective regulatory and effector T cell functions in patients with FOXP3 mutations. J Clin Invest, 116(6):1713-22.

Ball LM, Bernardo ME, Roelofs H, Lankester A, Cometa A, Egeler RM, Locatelli F, Fibbe WE. (2007). Cotransplantation of ex vivo expanded mesenchymal stem cells accelerates lymphocyte recovery and may reduce the risk of graft failure in haploidentical hematopoietic stem-cell transplantation. Blood, 110(7):2764-7.

Banerjee DK, Dhodapkar MV, Matayeva E, Steinman RM, Dhodapkar KM. (2006). Expansion of FOXP3high regulatory T cells by human dendritic cells (DCs) in vitro and after injection of cytokine-matured DCs in myeloma patients. Blood, 108(8):2655-61.

Battaglia M, Gianfrani C, Gregori S, Roncarolo MG. (2004). IL-10-producing T regulatory type 1 cells and oral tolerance. Ann N Y Acad Sci, 1029:142-53.

Batten P, Sarathchandra P, Antoniw JW, Tay SS, Lowdell MW, Taylor PM, Yacoub MH. (2006). Human mesenchymal stem cells induce T cell anergy and downregulate T cell allo-responses via the TH2 pathway: relevance to tissue engineering human heart valves. Tissue Eng, 12(8):2263-73.

Bettelli E, Korn T, Kuchroo VK. (2007). Th17: the third member of the effector T cell trilogy. Curr Opin Immunol, 19(6):652-7.

Beyth S, Borovsky Z, Mevorach D, Liebergall M, Gazit Z, Aslan H, Galun E, Rachmilewitz J. (2005). Human mesenchymal stem cells alter antigen-presenting cell maturation and induce T-cell unresponsiveness. Blood, 105(5):2214-9.

Bisikirska B, Colgan J, Luban J, Bluestone JA, Herold KC. (2005). TCR stimulation with modified anti-CD3 mAb expands CD8+ T cell population and induces CD8+CD25+ Tregs. J Clin Invest. 115(10):2904-13.

Bonifaz L, Bonnyay D, Mahnke K, Rivera M, Nussenzweig MC, Steinman RM. (2002). Efficient targeting of protein antigen to the dendritic cell receptor DEC-205 in the steady state leads to antigen presentation on major histocompatibility complex class I products and peripheral CD8+ T cell tolerance. J Exp Med, 196(12):1627-38.

Bresson D, von Herrath M. (2008). Resuscitating adaptive Tregs with combination therapies? Novartis Found Symp, 292:50-60; discussion 60-7, 122-9, 202-3.

Burnet M. (1959a). Auto-immune disease. I. Modern immunological concepts. Br Med J, 2(5153):645-650.

Burnet M. (1959b). Auto-immune disease. II. Pathology of the immune response. Br Med J, 2(5154):720-725.

Burt RK, Marmont A, Arnold R, Heipe F, Firestein GS, Carrier E, Hahn B, Barr W, Oyama Y, Snowden J, Kalunian K, Traynor A. (2003). Development of a phase III trial of hematopoietic stem cell transplantation for systemic lupus erythematosus. Bone Marrow Transplant, 32 Suppl 1:S49-51.

Burt RK, Oyama Y, Verda L, Quigley K, Brush M, Yaung K, Statkute L, Traynor A, Barr WG. (2004). Induction of remission of severe and refractory rheumatoid arthritis by allogeneic mixed chimerism. Arthritis Rheum, 50(8):2466-70.

Busse D, de la Rosa M, Hobiger K, Thurley K, Flossdorf M, Scheffold A, Höfer T. (2010). Competing feedback loops shape IL-2 signaling between helper and regulatory T lymphocytes in cellular microenvironments. Proc Natl Acad Sci U S A, 107(7):3058-63.

Carrier Y, Yuan J, Kuchroo VK, Weiner HL. (2007). Th3 cells in peripheral tolerance. I. Induction of Foxp3-positive regulatory T cells by Th3 cells derived from TGF-beta T cell-transgenic mice. J Immunol, 178(1):179-85.

Cella M, Jarrossay D, Facchetti F, Alebardi O, Nakajima H, Lanzavecchia A, Colonna M. (1999). Plasmacytoid monocytes migrate to inflamed lymph nodes and produce large amounts of type I interferon. Nat Med, 5(8):919-23.

Chen Z, Benoist C, Mathis D. (2005). How defects in central tolerance impinge on a deficiency in regulatory T cells. Proc Natl Acad Sci U S A, 102(41):14735-40.

Collison LW, Workman CJ, Kuo TT, Boyd K, Wang Y, Vignali KM, Cross R, Sehy D, Blumberg RS, Vignali DA. (2007). The inhibitory cytokine IL-35 contributes to regulatory T-cell function. Nature, 450(7169):566-9.

Connolly NC, Whiteside TL, Wilson C, Kondragunta V, Rinaldo CR, Riddler SA. (2008). Therapeutic immunization with human immunodeficiency virus type 1 (HIV-1) peptide-loaded dendritic cells is safe and induces immunogenicity in HIV-1-infected individuals. Clin Vaccine Immunol, 15(2):284-92.

Cools N, Ponsaerts P, Van Tendeloo VF, Berneman ZN. (2007a). Regulatory T cells and human disease. Clin Dev Immunol, 2007:89195.

Cools N, Ponsaerts P, Van Tendeloo VF, Berneman ZN. (2007b). Balancing between immunity and tolerance: an interplay between dendritic cells, regulatory T cells, and effector T cells. J Leukoc Biol, 82(6):1365-74.

Cools N, Van Tendeloo VF, Smits EL, Lenjou M, Nijs G, Van Bockstaele DR, Berneman ZN, Ponsaerts P. (2008). Immunosuppression induced by immature dendritic cells is mediated by TGF-beta/IL-10 double-positive CD4+ regulatory T cells. J Cell Mol Med, 12(2):690-700.

Curtsinger JM, Lins DC, Mescher MF. (2003). Signal 3 determines tolerance versus full activation of naive CD8 T cells: dissociating proliferation and development of effector function. J Exp Med, 197(9):1141-1151.

Curtsinger JM, Schmidt CS, Mondino A, Lins DC, Kedl RM, Jenkins MK, Mescher MF. (1999). Inflammatory cytokines provide a third signal for activation of naive CD4+ and CD8+ T cells. J Immunol, 162(6):3256-3262.

Daikeler T, Labopin M, Di Gioia M, Abinun M, Alexander T, Miniati I, Gualandi F, Fassas A, Martin T, Schwarze CP, Wulffraat N, Buch M, Sampol A, Carreras E, Dubois B, Gruhn B, Güngör T, Pohlreich D, Schuerwegh A, Snarski E, Snowden J, Veys P,

Fasth A, Lenhoff S, Messina C, Voswinkel J, Badoglio M, Henes J, Launay D, Tyndall A, Gluckman E, Farge D. (2011). Secondary autoimmune diseases occurring after HSCT for an autoimmune disease: a retrospective study of the EBMT Autoimmune Disease Working Party. Blood, Epub ahead of print.

Dazzi F, van Laar JM, Cope A, Tyndall A. (2007). Cell therapy for autoimmune diseases. Arthritis Res Ther, 9(2):206.

Dhodapkar MV, Steinman RM, Krasovsky J, Munz C, Bhardwaj N. (2001). Antigen-specific inhibition of effector T cell function in humans after injection of immature dendritic cells. J Exp Med, 193(2):233-8.

Dhodapkar MV, Steinman RM. (2002). Antigen-bearing immature dendritic cells induce peptide-specific CD8(+) regulatory T cells in vivo in humans. Blood, 100(1):174-7.

Di Ianni M, Falzetti F, Carotti A, Terenzi A, Castellino F, Bonifacio E, Del Papa B, Zei T, Ostini RI, Cecchini D, Aloisi T, Perruccio K, Ruggeri L, Balucani C, Pierini A, Sportoletti P, Aristei C, Falini B, Reisner Y, Velardi A, Aversa F, Martelli MF. (2011). Tregs prevent GVHD and promote immune reconstitution in HLA-haploidentical transplantation. Blood, 117(14):3921-8.

Di Nicola M, Carlo-Stella C, Magni M, Milanesi M, Longoni PD, Matteucci P, Grisanti S, Gianni AM. (2002). Human bone marrow stromal cells suppress T-lymphocyte proliferation induced by cellular or nonspecific mitogenic stimuli. Blood, 99(10):3838-43.

Digirolamo CM, Stokes D, Colter D, Phinney DG, Class R, Prockop DJ. (1999). Propagation and senescence of human marrow stromal cells in culture: a simple colony-forming assay identifies samples with the greatest potential to propagate and differentiate. Br J Haematol, 107(2):275-81.

DiLillo DJ, Matsushita T, Tedder TF. (2010). B10 cells and regulatory B cells balance immune responses during inflammation, autoimmunity, and cancer. Ann N Y Acad Sci, 1183:38-57.

Dominici M, Le Blanc K, Mueller I, Slaper-Cortenbach I, Marini F, Krause D, Deans R, Keating A, Prockop Dj, Horwitz E. (2006). Minimal criteria for defining multipotent mesenchymal stromal cells. The International Society for Cellular Therapy position statement. Cytotherapy, 8(4):315-7.

Fallarino F, Grohmann U, Hwang KW, Orabona C, Vacca C, Bianchi R, Belladonna ML, Fioretti MC, Alegre ML, Puccetti P. (2003). Modulation of tryptophan catabolism by regulatory T cells. Nat Immunol, 4(12):1206-12.

Faria AM, Weiner HL. (2006). Oral tolerance and TGF-beta-producing cells. Inflamm Allergy Drug Targets, 5(3):179-90.

Fehérvári Z, Sakaguchi S. (2004). Control of Foxp3+ CD25+CD4+ regulatory cell activation and function by dendritic cells. Int Immunol, 16(12):1769-80.

Feldman M, Taylor P, Paleolog E, Brennan FM, Maini RN. (1998). Anti-TNF alpha therapy is useful in rheumatoid arthritis and Crohn's disease: analysis of the mechanism of action predicts utility in other diseases. Transplant Proc, 30(8):4126-7.

Friedenstein AJ, Chailakhyan RK, Latsinik NV, Panasyuk AF, Keiliss-Borok IV. (1974). Stromal cells responsible for transferring the microenvironment of the hemopoietic tissues. Cloning in vitro and retransplantation in vivo. Transplantation, 17(4):331-40.

Gao W, Lu Y, El Essawy B, Oukka M, Kuchroo VK, Strom TB. (2007). Contrasting effects of cyclosporine and rapamycin in de novo generation of alloantigen-specific regulatory T cells. Am J Transplant, 7(7):1722-32.

Garín MI, Chu CC, Golshayan D, Cernuda-Morollón E, Wait R, Lechler RI. (2007). Galectin-1: a key effector of regulation mediated by CD4+CD25+ T cells. Blood, 109(5):2058-65.

Gavin MA, Rasmussen JP, Fontenot JD, Vasta V, Manganiello VC, Beavo JA, Rudensky AY. (2007). Foxp3-dependent programme of regulatory T-cell differentiation. Nature, 445(7129):771-5.

Gondek DC, Lu LF, Quezada SA, Sakaguchi S, Noelle RJ. (2005). Cutting edge: contact-mediated suppression by CD4+CD25+ regulatory cells involves a granzyme B-dependent, perforin-independent mechanism. J Immunol, 174(4):1783-6.

Greenfield EA, Nguyen KA, Kuchroo VK. (1998). CD28/B7 costimulation: a review. Crit Rev Immunol, 18(5):389-418.

Griffith LM, Pavletic SZ, Tyndall A, Gratwohl A, Furst DE, Forman SJ, Nash RA. (2006). Target populations in allogeneic hematopoietic cell transplantation for autoimmune diseases--a workshop accompanying: cellular therapy for treatment of autoimmune diseases, basic science and clinical studies, including new developments in hematopoietic and mesenchymal stem cell therapy. Biol Blood Marrow Transplant, 12(6):688-90.

Grossman WJ, Verbsky JW, Barchet W, Colonna M, Atkinson JP, Ley TJ. (2004). Human T regulatory cells can use the perforin pathway to cause autologous target cell death. Immunity, 21(4):589-601.

Haniffa MA, Wang XN, Holtick U, Rae M, Isaacs JD, Dickinson AM, Hilkens CM, Collin MP. (2007). Adult human fibroblasts are potent immunoregulatory cells and functionally equivalent to mesenchymal stem cells. J Immunol, 179(3):1595-604.

Harry RA, Anderson AE, Isaacs JD, Hilkens CM. (2010). Generation and characterisation of therapeutic tolerogenic dendritic cells for rheumatoid arthritis. Ann Rheum Dis, 69(11):2042-50.

Hawiger D, Inaba K, Dorsett Y, Guo M, Mahnke K, Rivera M, Ravetch JV, Steinman RM, Nussenzweig MC. (2001). Dendritic cells induce peripheral T cell unresponsiveness under steady state conditions in vivo. J Exp Med, 194(6):769-79.

Hegde S, Fox L, Wang X, Gumperz JE. (2010). Autoreactive natural killer T cells: promoting immune protection and immune tolerance through varied interactions with myeloid antigen-presenting cells. Immunology, 130(4):471-83.

Herold KC, Brooks-Worrell B, Palmer J, Dosch HM, Peakman M, Gottlieb P, Reijonen H, Arif S, Spain LM, Thompson C, Lachin JM; Type 1 Diabetes TrialNet Research Group. (2009). Validity and reproducibility of measurement of islet autoreactivity by T-cell assays in subjects with early type 1 diabetes. Diabetes, 58(11):2588-95.

Hilkens CM, Isaacs JD, Thomson AW. (2010). Development of dendritic cell-based immunotherapy for autoimmunity. Int Rev Immunol, 29(2):156-83.

Hough RE, Snowden JA, Wulffraat NM. (2005). Haemopoietic stem cell transplantation in autoimmune diseases: a European perspective. Br J Haematol, 128(4):432-59.

Iwata Y, Matsushita T, Horikawa M, Dilillo DJ, Yanaba K, Venturi GM, Szabolcs PM, Bernstein SH, Magro CM, Williams AD, Hall RP, St Clair EW, Tedder TF. (2011).

Characterization of a rare IL-10-competent B-cell subset in humans that parallels mouse regulatory B10 cells. Blood, 117(2):530-41.
Jäger A, Kuchroo VK. (2010). Effector and regulatory T-cell subsets in autoimmunity and tissue inflammation. Scand J Immunol, 72(3):173-84.
Jiang XX, Zhang Y, Liu B, Zhang SX, Wu Y, Yu XD, Mao N. (2005). Human mesenchymal stem cells inhibit differentiation and function of monocyte-derived dendritic cells. Blood, 105(10):4120-6.
Jones S, Horwood N, Cope A, Dazzi F. (2007). The antiproliferative effect of mesenchymal stem cells is a fundamental property shared by all stromal cells. J Immunol, 179(5):2824-31.
Ju X, Clark G, Hart DN. (2010). Review of human DC subtypes. Methods Mol Biol, 595:3-20.
Kadowaki N, Ho S, Antonenko S, Malefyt RW, Kastelein RA, Bazan F, Liu YJ. (2001). Subsets of human dendritic cell precursors express different toll-like receptors and respond to different microbial antigens. J Exp Med, 194(6):863-9.
Keymeulen B, Vandemeulebroucke E, Ziegler AG, Mathieu C, Kaufman L, Hale G, Gorus F, Goldman M, Walter M, Candon S, Schandene L, Crenier L, De Block C, Seigneurin JM, De Pauw P, Pierard D, Weets I, Rebello P, Bird P, Berrie E, Frewin M, Waldmann H, Bach JF, Pipeleers D, Chatenoud L. (2005). Insulin needs after CD3-antibody therapy in new-onset type 1 diabetes. N Engl J Med, 352(25):2598-608.
Koenen HJ, Smeets RL, Vink PM, van Rijssen E, Boots AM, Joosten I. (2008). Human CD25highFoxp3pos regulatory T cells differentiate into IL-17-producing cells. Blood, 112(6):2340-52.
Kohrgruber N, Halanek N, Gröger M, Winter D, Rappersberger K, Schmitt-Egenolf M, Stingl G, Maurer D. (1999). Survival, maturation, and function of CD11c- and CD11c+ peripheral blood dendritic cells are differentially regulated by cytokines. J Immunol, 163(6):3250-9.
Komatsu N, Mariotti-Ferrandiz ME, Wang Y, Malissen B, Waldmann H, Hori S. (2009). Heterogeneity of natural Foxp3+ T cells: a committed regulatory T-cell lineage and an uncommitted minor population retaining plasticity. Proc Natl Acad Sci U S A, 106(6):1903-8.
Kretschmer K, Apostolou I, Hawiger D, Khazaie K, Nussenzweig MC, von Boehmer H. (2005). Inducing and expanding regulatory T cell populations by foreign antigen. Nat Immunol, 6(12):1219-27.
Krueger GG, Langley RG, Leonardi C, Yeilding N, Guzzo C, Wang Y, Dooley LT, Lebwohl M; CNTO 1275 Psoriasis Study Group. (2007). A human interleukin-12/23 monoclonal antibody for the treatment of psoriasis. N Engl J Med, 356(6):580-92.
Kurts C, Heath WR, Kosaka H, Miller JF, Carbone FR. (1998). The peripheral deletion of autoreactive CD8+ T cells induced by cross-presentation of self-antigens involves signaling through CD95 (Fas, Apo-1). J Exp Med, 188(2):415-420.
Lal G, Bromberg JS. (2009a). Epigenetic mechanisms of regulation of Foxp3 expression. Blood, 114(18):3727-35.
Lal G, Zhang N, van der Touw W, Ding Y, Ju W, Bottinger EP, Reid SP, Levy DE, Bromberg JS. (2009b). Epigenetic regulation of Foxp3 expression in regulatory T cells by DNA methylation. J Immunol, 182(1):259-73.
Lazarus HM, Koc ON, Devine SM, Curtin P, Maziarz RT, Holland HK, Shpall EJ, McCarthy P, Atkinson K, Cooper BW, Gerson SL, Laughlin MJ, Loberiza FR Jr, Moseley AB,

Bacigalupo A. (2005). Cotransplantation of HLA-identical sibling culture-expanded mesenchymal stem cells and hematopoietic stem cells in hematologic malignancy patients. Biol Blood Marrow Transplant, 11(5):389-98. PubMed PMID: 15846293.

Le Blanc K, Frassoni F, Ball L, Locatelli F, Roelofs H, Lewis I, Lanino E, Sundberg B, Bernardo ME, Remberger M, Dini G, Egeler RM, Bacigalupo A, Fibbe W, Ringdén O; Developmental Committee of the European Group for Blood and Marrow Transplantation. (2008). Mesenchymal stem cells for treatment of steroid-resistant, severe, acute graft-versus-host disease: a phase II study. Lancet, 371(9624):1579-86.

Le Blanc K, Rasmusson I, Sundberg B, Götherström C, Hassan M, Uzunel M, Ringdén O. (2004). Treatment of severe acute graft-versus-host disease with third party haploidentical mesenchymal stem cells. Lancet, 363(9419):1439-41.

Leonardi CL, Kimball AB, Papp KA, Yeilding N, Guzzo C, Wang Y, Li S, Dooley LT, Gordon KB; PHOENIX 1 study investigators. (2008). Efficacy and safety of ustekinumab, a human interleukin-12/23 monoclonal antibody, in patients with psoriasis: 76-week results from a randomised, double-blind, placebo-controlled trial (PHOENIX 1). Lancet, 371(9625):1665-74.

Li MO, Flavell RA. (2008). Contextual regulation of inflammation: a duet by transforming growth factor-beta and interleukin-10. Immunity, 28(4):468-76.

Liu YJ, Soumelis V, Watanabe N, Ito T, Wang YH, Malefyt Rde W, Omori M, Zhou B, Ziegler SF. (2007). TSLP: an epithelial cell cytokine that regulates T cell differentiation by conditioning dendritic cell maturation. Annu Rev Immunol, 25:193-219.

Liu YJ. (2001). Dendritic cell subsets and lineages, and their functions in innate and adaptive immunity. Cell, 106(3):259-62.

Long E, Wood KJ. (2009). Regulatory T cells in transplantation: transferring mouse studies to the clinic. Transplantation, 88(9):1050-6.

Lutterotti A, Sospedra M, Martin R. (2008). Antigen-specific therapies in MS - Current concepts and novel approaches. J Neurol Sci, 274(1-2):18-22.

Lutz MB, Schuler G. (2002). Immature, semi-mature and fully mature dendritic cells: which signals induce tolerance or immunity? Trends Immunol, 23(9):445-9.

Maccario R, Podestà M, Moretta A, Cometa A, Comoli P, Montagna D, Daudt L, Ibatici A, Piaggio G, Pozzi S, Frassoni F, Locatelli F. (2005). Interaction of human mesenchymal stem cells with cells involved in alloantigen-specific immune response favors the differentiation of CD4+ T-cell subsets expressing a regulatory/suppressive phenotype. Haematologica, 90(4):516-25.

Mandala S, Hajdu R, Bergstrom J, Quackenbush E, Xie J, Milligan J, Thornton R, Shei GJ, Card D, Keohane C, Rosenbach M, Hale J, Lynch CL, Rupprecht K, Parsons W, Rosen H. (2002). Alteration of lymphocyte trafficking by sphingosine-1-phosphate receptor agonists. Science, 296(5566):346-9.

Mannon PJ, Fuss IJ, Mayer L, Elson CO, Sandborn WJ, Present D, Dolin B, Goodman N, Groden C, Hornung RL, Quezado M, Yang Z, Neurath MF, Salfeld J, Veldman GM, Schwertschlag U, Strober W; Anti-IL-12 Crohn's Disease Study Group. (2004). Anti-interleukin-12 antibody for active Crohn's disease. N Engl J Med, 351(20):2069-79.

Marigo I, Dazzi F. (2011). The immunomodulatory properties of mesenchymal stem cells. Semin Immunopathol, Epub ahead of print.

Mehling M, Brinkmann V, Antel J, Bar-Or A, Goebels N, Vedrine C, Kristofic C, Kuhle J, Lindberg RL, Kappos L. (2008). FTY720 therapy exerts differential effects on T cell subsets in multiple sclerosis. Neurology, 71(16):1261-7.

Meisel R, Zibert A, Laryea M, Göbel U, Däubener W, Dilloo D. (2004). Human bone marrow stromal cells inhibit allogeneic T-cell responses by indoleamine 2,3-dioxygenase-mediated tryptophan degradation. Blood, 103(12):4619-21.

Mellor AL, Munn DH. (2004). IDO expression by dendritic cells: tolerance and tryptophan catabolism. Nat Rev Immunol, 4(10):762-74.

Miller SD, Turley DM, Podojil JR. (2007). Antigen-specific tolerance strategies for the prevention and treatment of autoimmune disease. Nat Rev Immunol, 7(9):665-77.

Monti P, Scirpoli M, Maffi P, Piemonti L, Secchi A, Bonifacio E, Roncarolo MG, Battaglia M. (2008). Rapamycin monotherapy in patients with type 1 diabetes modifies CD4+CD25+FOXP3+ regulatory T-cells. Diabetes, 57(9):2341-7.

Munn DH, Sharma MD, Lee JR, Jhaver KG, Johnson TS, Keskin DB, Marshall B, Chandler P, Antonia SJ, Burgess R, Slingluff CL Jr, Mellor AL. (2002). Potential regulatory function of human dendritic cells expressing indoleamine 2,3-dioxygenase. Science, 297(5588):1867-70.

Muraro PA, Douek DC, Packer A, Chung K, Guenaga FJ, Cassiani-Ingoni R, Campbell C, Memon S, Nagle JW, Hakim FT, Gress RE, McFarland HF, Burt RK, Martin R. (2005). Thymic output generates a new and diverse TCR repertoire after autologous stem cell transplantation in multiple sclerosis patients. J Exp Med, 201(5):805-16.

Nakamura K, Kitani A, Strober W. (2001). Cell contact-dependent immunosuppression by CD4(+)CD25(+) regulatory T cells is mediated by cell surface-bound transforming growth factor beta. J Exp Med, 194(5):629-44.

Nauta AJ, Kruisselbrink AB, Lurvink E, Willemze R, Fibbe WE. (2006). Mesenchymal stem cells inhibit generation and function of both CD34+-derived and monocyte-derived dendritic cells. J Immunol, 177(4):2080-7.

Németh K, Leelahavanichkul A, Yuen PS, Mayer B, Parmelee A, Doi K, Robey PG, Leelahavanichkul K, Koller BH, Brown JM, Hu X, Jelinek I, Star RA, Mezey E. (2009). Bone marrow stromal cells attenuate sepsis via prostaglandin E(2)-dependent reprogramming of host macrophages to increase their interleukin-10 production. Nat Med, 15(1):42-9.

Ning H, Yang F, Jiang M, Hu L, Feng K, Zhang J, Yu Z, Li B, Xu C, Li Y, Wang J, Hu J, Lou X, Chen H. (2008). The correlation between cotransplantation of mesenchymal stem cells and higher recurrence rate in hematologic malignancy patients: outcome of a pilot clinical study. Leukemia, 22(3):593-9.

O'Connor P, Comi G, Montalban X, Antel J, Radue EW, de Vera A, Pohlmann H, Kappos L; FTY720 D2201 Study Group. (2009). Oral fingolimod (FTY720) in multiple sclerosis: two-year results of a phase II extension study. Neurology, 72(1):73-9.

O'Doherty U, Peng M, Gezelter S, Swiggard WJ, Betjes M, Bhardwaj N, Steinman RM. (1994). Human blood contains two subsets of dendritic cells, one immunologically mature and the other immature. Immunology, 82(3):487-93.

Oyama Y, Papadopoulos EB, Miranda M, Traynor AE, Burt RK. (2001). Allogeneic stem cell transplantation for Evans syndrome. Bone Marrow Transplant, 28(9):903-5.

Penna G, Sozzani S, Adorini L. (2001). Cutting edge: selective usage of chemokine receptors by plasmacytoid dendritic cells. J Immunol, 167(4):1862-6.

Pittenger MF, Mackay AM, Beck SC, Jaiswal RK, Douglas R, Mosca JD, Moorman MA, Simonetti DW, Craig S, Marshak DR. (1999). Multilineage potential of adult human mesenchymal stem cells. Science, 284(5411):143-7.

Plevy S, Salzberg B, Van Assche G, Regueiro M, Hommes D, Sandborn W, Hanauer S, Targan S, Mayer L, Mahadevan U, Frankel M, Lowder J. (2007). A phase I study of visilizumab, a humanized anti-CD3 monoclonal antibody, in severe steroid-refractory ulcerative colitis. Gastroenterology, 133(5):1414-22.

Popat U, Krance R. (2004). Haematopoietic stem cell transplantation for autoimmune disorders: the American perspective. Br J Haematol, 126(5):637-49.

Pratschke J, Stauch D, Kotsch K. (2009). Role of NK and NKT cells in solid organ transplantation. Transpl Int, 22(9):859-68.

Prevosto C, Zancolli M, Canevali P, Zocchi MR, Poggi A. (2007). Generation of CD4+ or CD8+ regulatory T cells upon mesenchymal stem cell-lymphocyte interaction. Haematologica, 92(7):881-8.

Rasmusson I, Uhlin M, Le Blanc K, Levitsky V. (2007). Mesenchymal stem cells fail to trigger effector functions of cytotoxic T lymphocytes. J Leukoc Biol, 82(4):887-93.

Reizis B, Bunin A, Ghosh HS, Lewis KL, Sisirak V. (2011). Plasmacytoid dendritic cells: recent progress and open questions. Annu Rev Immunol, 29:163-83.

Riley JL, June CH, Blazar BR. (2009). Human T regulatory cell therapy: take a billion or so and call me in the morning. Immunity, 30(5):656-65.

Roncarolo MG, Gregori S, Battaglia M, Bacchetta R, Fleischhauer K, Levings MK. (2006). Interleukin-10-secreting type 1 regulatory T cells in rodents and humans. Immunol Rev, 212:28-50.

Sabatos-Peyton CA, Verhagen J, Wraith DC. (2010). Antigen-specific immunotherapy of autoimmune and allergic diseases. Curr Opin Immunol, 22(5):609-15.

Salomon B, Lenschow DJ, Rhee L, Ashourian N, Singh B, Sharpe A, Bluestone JA. (2000). B7/CD28 costimulation is essential for the homeostasis of the CD4+CD25+ immunoregulatory T cells that control autoimmune diabetes. Immunity, 12(4):431-440.

Sato K, Ozaki K, Oh I, Meguro A, Hatanaka K, Nagai T, Muroi K, Ozawa K. (2007). Nitric oxide plays a critical role in suppression of T-cell proliferation by mesenchymal stem cells. Blood, 109(1):228-34.

Schwartz RH. (2003). T cell anergy. Annu Rev Immunol, 21:305-34.

Segal BM, Constantinescu CS, Raychaudhuri A, Kim L, Fidelus-Gort R, Kasper LH; Ustekinumab MS Investigators. (2008). Repeated subcutaneous injections of IL12/23 p40 neutralising antibody, ustekinumab, in patients with relapsing-remitting multiple sclerosis: a phase II, double-blind, placebo-controlled, randomised, dose-ranging study. Lancet Neurol, 7(9):796-804.

Sekiya I, Larson BL, Smith JR, Pochampally R, Cui JG, Prockop DJ. (2002). Expansion of human adult stem cells from bone marrow stroma: conditions that maximize the yields of early progenitors and evaluate their quality. Stem Cells 20(6):530-41.

Shevach EM. (2009). Mechanisms of foxp3+ T regulatory cell-mediated suppression. Immunity, 30(5):636-45.

Smith CE, Miller SD. (2006). Multi-peptide coupled-cell tolerance ameliorates ongoing relapsing EAE associated with multiple pathogenic autoreactivities. J Autoimmun, 27(4):218-31.

Sotiropoulou PA, Perez SA, Gritzapis AD, Baxevanis CN, Papamichail M. (2006). Interactions between human mesenchymal stem cells and natural killer cells. Stem Cells, 24(1):74-85.

Spaggiari GM, Abdelrazik H, Becchetti F, Moretta L. (2009). MSCs inhibit monocyte-derived DC maturation and function by selectively interfering with the generation of immature DCs: central role of MSC-derived prostaglandin E2. Blood, 113(26):6576-83.

Spaggiari GM, Capobianco A, Becchetti S, Mingari MC, Moretta L. (2006). Mesenchymal stem cell-natural killer cell interactions: evidence that activated NK cells are capable of killing MSCs, whereas MSCs can inhibit IL-2-induced NK-cell proliferation. Blood, 107(4):1484-90.

Steinman RM, Banchereau J. (2007). Taking dendritic cells into medicine. Nature, 449(7161):419-26.

Steinman RM, Hawiger D, Nussenzweig MC. (2003). Tolerogenic dendritic cells. Annu Rev Immunol, 21:685-711.

Steinman RM, Nussenzweig MC. (2002). Avoiding horror autotoxicus: the importance of dendritic cells in peripheral T cell tolerance. Proc Natl Acad Sci U S A, 99(1):351-358.

Strom TB, Koulmanda M. (2009). Recently discovered T cell subsets cannot keep their commitments. J Am Soc Nephrol, 20(8):1677-80.

Stüve O, Marra CM, Jerome KR, Cook L, Cravens PD, Cepok S, Frohman EM, Phillips JT, Arendt G, Hemmer B, Monson NL, Racke MK. (2006). Immune surveillance in multiple sclerosis patients treated with natalizumab. Ann Neurol, 59(5):743-7.

Süss G, Shortman K. (1996). A subclass of dendritic cells kills CD4 T cells via Fas/Fas-ligand-induced apoptosis. J Exp Med, 183(4):1789-96.

Swiecki M, Colonna M. (2010). Unraveling the functions of plasmacytoid dendritic cells during viral infections, autoimmunity, and tolerance. Immunol Rev, 234(1):142-62.

Tabera S, Pérez-Simón JA, Díez-Campelo M, Sánchez-Abarca LI, Blanco B, López A, Benito A, Ocio E, Sánchez-Guijo FM, Cañizo C, San Miguel JF. (2008). The effect of mesenchymal stem cells on the viability, proliferation and differentiation of B-lymphocytes. Haematologica, 93(9):1301-9.

Teng YK, Verburg RJ, Sont JK, van den Hout WB, Breedveld FC, van Laar JM. (2005). Long-term followup of health status in patients with severe rheumatoid arthritis after high-dose chemotherapy followed by autologous hematopoietic stem cell transplantation. Arthritis Rheum, 52(8):2272-6.

Traynor AE, Schroeder J, Rosa RM, Cheng D, Stefka J, Mujais S, Baker S, Burt RK. (2000). Treatment of severe systemic lupus erythematosus with high-dose chemotherapy and haemopoietic stem-cell transplantation: a phase I study. Lancet, 356(9231):701-7.

Trombetta ES, Mellman I. (2005). Cell biology of antigen processing in vitro and in vivo. Annu Rev Immunol, 23:975-1028.

Trzonkowski P, Bieniaszewska M, Juścińska J, Dobyszuk A, Krzystyniak A, Marek N, Myśliwska J, Hellmann A. (2009). First-in-man clinical results of the treatment of patients with graft versus host disease with human ex vivo expanded CD4+CD25+CD127- T regulatory cells. Clin Immunol, 133(1):22-6.

Turley DM, Miller SD. (2007). Peripheral tolerance induction using ethylenecarbodiimide-fixed APCs uses both direct and indirect mechanisms of antigen presentation for prevention of experimental autoimmune encephalomyelitis. J Immunol, 178(4):2212-20.

Tyndall A, Saccardi R. (2005). Haematopoietic stem cell transplantation in the treatment of severe autoimmune disease: results from phase I/II studies, prospective randomized trials and future directions. Clin Exp Immunol, 141(1):1-9.

Van Tendeloo VF, Van de Velde A, Van Driessche A, Cools N, Anguille S, Ladell K, Gostick E, Vermeulen K, Pieters K, Nijs G, Stein B, Smits EL, Schroyens WA, Gadisseur AP, Vrelust I, Jorens PG, Goossens H, de Vries IJ, Price DA, Oji Y, Oka Y, Sugiyama H, Berneman ZN. (2010). Induction of complete and molecular remissions in acute myeloid leukemia by Wilms' tumor 1 antigen-targeted dendritic cell vaccination. Proc Natl Acad Sci U S A, 107(31):13824-9.

Victor FC, Gottlieb AB, Menter A. (2003). Changing paradigms in dermatology: tumor necrosis factor alpha (TNF-alpha) blockade in psoriasis and psoriatic arthritis. Clin Dermatol, 21(5):392-7.

Vincenti F, Luggen M. (2007). T cell costimulation: a rational target in the therapeutic armamentarium for autoimmune diseases and transplantation. Annu Rev Med, 58:347-58.

Voo KS, Wang YH, Santori FR, Boggiano C, Wang YH, Arima K, Bover L, Hanabuchi S, Khalili J, Marinova E, Zheng B, Littman DR, Liu YJ. (2009). Identification of IL-17-producing FOXP3+ regulatory T cells in humans. Proc Natl Acad Sci U S A, 106(12):4793-8.

Weaver CT, Hatton RD. (2009). Interplay between the TH17 and TReg cell lineages: a (co-)evolutionary perspective. Nat Rev Immunol, 9(12):883-9.

Wieczorek G, Asemissen A, Model F, Turbachova I, Floess S, Liebenberg V, Baron U, Stauch D, Kotsch K, Pratschke J, Hamann A, Loddenkemper C, Stein H, Volk HD, Hoffmüller U, Grützkau A, Mustea A, Huehn J, Scheibenbogen C, Olek S. (2009). Quantitative DNA methylation analysis of FOXP3 as a new method for counting regulatory T cells in peripheral blood and solid tissue. Cancer Res, 69(2):599-608.

Wildin RS, Freitas A. (2005). IPEX and FOXP3: clinical and research perspectives. J Autoimmun, 25 Suppl:56-62.

Wu L, Van Kaer L. (2009). Natural killer T cells and autoimmune disease. Curr Mol Med, 9(1):4-14.

Yanaba K, Bouaziz JD, Haas KM, Poe JC, Fujimoto M, Tedder TF. (2008). A regulatory B cell subset with a unique CD1dhiCD5+ phenotype controls T cell-dependent inflammatory responses. Immunity, 28(5):639-50.

Yednock TA, Cannon C, Fritz LC, Sanchez-Madrid F, Steinman L, Karin N. (1992). Prevention of experimental autoimmune encephalomyelitis by antibodies against alpha 4 beta 1 integrin. Nature, 356(6364):63-6.

Zappia E, Casazza S, Pedemonte E, Benvenuto F, Bonanni I, Gerdoni E, Giunti D, Ceravolo A, Cazzanti F, Frassoni F, Mancardi G, Uccelli A. (2005). Mesenchymal stem cells ameliorate experimental autoimmune encephalomyelitis inducing T-cell anergy. Blood, 106(5):1755-61.

Zarkhin V, Chalasani G, Sarwal MM. (2010). The yin and yang of B cells in graft rejection and tolerance. Transplant Rev (Orlando), 24(2):67-78.

Zarkhin V, Kambham N, Li L, Kwok S, Hsieh SC, Salvatierra O, Sarwal MM. (2008). Characterization of intra-graft B cells during renal allograft rejection. Kidney Int, 74(5):664-73.

Zhou H, Jin Z, Liu J, Yu S, Cui Q, Yi D. (2008). Mesenchymal stem cells might be used to induce tolerance in heart transplantation. Med Hypotheses, 70(4):785-7.

Zhou L, Chong MM, Littman DR. (2009). Plasticity of CD4+ T cell lineage differentiation. Immunity, 30(5):646-55.

Ziegler SF. (2006). FOXP3: of mice and men. Annu Rev Immunol, 24:209-26.

15

Low Immunogenic Potential of Human Neural Stem Cells

L. De Filippis[1], L. Rota Nodari[1] and Maurizio Gelati[2]
[1]*Department of Biotechnologies and Biosciences, Università Milano Bicocca, Milan,*
[2]*Laboratorio Cellule Staminali, Cell Factory e Biobanca,*
Azienda Ospedaliera "Santa Maria", Terni
Italy

1. Introduction

Grafting of neural stem cells into the mammalian central nervous system (CNS) has been performed for some decades now, both in basic research and clinical applications for neurological disorders such as Parkinson's and Huntington's disease, stroke, and spinal cord injuries. Albeit the "proof of principle" status that neural grafts can reinstate functional deficits and rebuild damaged neuronal circuitries, many critical roadblocks have still to be overcome to reach clinical applications. Among these are the manifold immunological aspects that are encountered during the graft–host interaction in vivo. In this chapter we will elucidate different aspects of cellular therapy, particularly using CNS derived stem cells and their ability to modulate immune system in order to avoid rejection and/or affect inflammatory reactions related to neurodegenerative diseases.

2. Neural transplantation for the therapy of neurodegenerative diseases

2.1 NSCs: Use into humans and animal models

Grafting of neural stem cells (NSCs) into the mammalian central nervous system in association with their ability to induce active neurogenesis in the adult CNS has fostered a flurry of studies to investigate the exploitation of NSC for the therapy of neurodegenerative disorders including both genetic diseases like Metachromatic Leukodystrophy (MLD), Huntington's Disease (HD), Alzheimer's Disease (AD) (sporadic) and idiopathic diseases like Parkinson's Disease (PD), AD, Multiple Sclerosis (MS), Amyotrophyc Lateral Sclerosis (ALS), stroke.

Regenerative medicine strongly relies on the capacity of intrinsic subsets of cells to replenish the damaged ones. Although for a long time the CNS was thought to be a "perennial", i.e. post-mitotic tissue, the discovery of active neurogenesis in the adult mammalian brain has debunked this dogma and spurred ongoing research efforts to focus on stem/ precursor cell therapy to treat neurodegeneration and neurotrauma.

Given the intrinsic resilience of NSC to fast proliferation and prompt expansion in vivo, the spontaneous recovery of most CNS injuries remains limited and a feasible strategy to support the endogenous NSC-mediated therapy would be the autologous transplantation of adult stem cells from various tissue compartments than the CNS. Different sources of stem cells have been proposed, but they mostly generate a restricted range of cell phenotypes.

Induced pluripotent stem cells (iPS) have been recently proposed for autologous transplantation, but a major drawback of these genetically manipulated cells is the high risk of cancer formation, mainly due to the uncontrolled integration of retroviral vectors and recombination events.
Therefore, the most feasible candidates to clinical neurological applications are currently the embryonic stem cells (ESCs) and adult somatic stem cells, particularly NSCs.
ESCs are the most primitive type of stem cells properly belonging to the human body and are pluripotent, meaning that they are able to generate all the types of cells present in the human body. As such and thanks to their easy handling and proliferation ex vivo, they would represent ideal candidates to provide a wide array of cell types for the therapy of different disorders. Alas, the limited availability of primary tissue due to ethical concerns and their remarkable teratogenic potential in vivo has strongly discouraged their application in clinical trials. On the contrary, NSC are mostly considered as the optimal cell type for cell-mediated therapy of neural disorders because they share the same tissue origin of the damaged cells they are meant to replenish and are amenable to local environmental cues able to commit their differentiation choice (Cao et al. 2001;Shihabuddin et al. 2000;Suhonen et al. 1996). Accordingly, NSC have been shown to exert multiple therapeutic effects, such as secretion of neurotrophic factors and cytokines, scavenging of toxic molecules, immunomodulation of inflammatory milieu, where neural cell replacement plays only a minor role in the recovery of CNS damage (Bacigaluppi et al. 2009;Behrstock et al. 2006;Ebert et al. 2008;Lindvall and Kokaia 2010). The major roadblock to their procurement from an autologous tissue source can be currently circumvented by their derivation from the fetal human brain, while the requirement for immunosuppression to prevent transplant rejection remains object of conflicting debates.
Above all the disavantages of using immunosuppressive treatment during stem cells therapies include an increased risk for opportunistic infections (Garrido et al. 2006), toxic side effects (Rezzani 2006) and potential negative effects on donor cells as recently described (Guo et al. 2007) for cyclosporin treatment able to reduce cell proliferation and affect differentiation of rat NSCs in vitro.
In this manuscript we will discuss about NSC immunogenic potential and the exploitation of -mild- and/or transient immune suppressive protocols after NSC transplantation.

3. Neural stem cells

Somatic adult NSCs are undifferentiated cells that reside in specialized regions, namely the niche, of the fetal and adult CNS; they possess life-long self-renewal ability and a multipotent differentiation potential, given their ability to generate neurons, astrocytes and oligodendrocytes. Reynolds and Weiss (Reynolds and Weiss 1992) have first demonstrated a stem cell niche in the CNS. In particular, the finding of adult neurogenesis in the SVZ, which leads to the generation of neural progenitors migrating to the olfactory bulbs and to the cortex, has favoured the idea that newborn neurons might subserve cognitive functions and contribute to the homeostasis of the telencephalic-diencephalic area.
Therefore, NSCs maintain the functional and structural integrity of the brain in physiological conditions, thus contributing to tissue homeostasis and repair throughout adulthood (Gage et al. 1998;Reynolds and Weiss 1992;Temple and Alvarez-Buylla 1999). Alas, given the inherent resilience of NSC to rapidly expand into the adult CNS, there is limited spontaneous recovery after brain damage (Popa-Wagner et al. 2009;Romanko et al.

2004), so the integration of new functional neurons following injury can be achieved by transplanting exogenous cells. In vitro, NSCs can be propagated as free-floating aggregates called neurospheres or as a cell monolayer (on adhesion) and demonstrate the same characteristics of self-renewal and potential to differentiate into functionally mature neural cells. The establishment of protocols to isolate and culture NSC as stable cell lines able to maintain unaltered their functional properties over passaging ex vivo, has allowed to set up important model systems for studying neurogenic processes during development and neurobiological mechanisms for maintaining cellular complexity and plasticity. Moreover, compelling evidence from transplantation experiments in animal models suggested the potential use of NSC lines in novel cell-based therapies for brain injury and neurodegenerative disease. Interesting, functional recovery by NSC transplantation was mostly reached through alternative mechanisms rather than cell replacement (Pluchino et al. 2005). These mechanisms include neuroprotection and reduction of host cell death (Chu et al. 2004), enhancement of endogenous angiogenesis after stroke (Jiang et al. 2005), immunomodulatory effects on inflammatory damage (Pluchino, et al. 2005;Rota Nodari et al. 2010;Ziv et al. 2006a) and scavenging of neurotoxic molecules (Emsley et al. 2004).

Thus far, cells with stem-like properties have been identified in the mammalian CNS, including that of humans, throughout development and adulthood (Alvarez-Buylla et al. 2001;Gage 2000;Temple 2001). In particular, NSCs have been derived from germinative zones of the brain such as the hippocampal dentate gyrus, olfactory bulb, subventricular zone, subcallosal zone and spinal cord of embryonic, neonatal, and adult rodents (Gritti et al. 1996;Reynolds and Weiss 1992;Weiss et al. 1996). The SVZ has the greatest potential for neurogenesis and is one of the best characterized niches in the adult brain (Doetsch 2003). It consists of a cell layer adjacent to the ependymal layer which lines the lateral ventricles and contains three major cell types. The stem-like cells (type B cells) have an astroglial phenotype express the glial-fibrillary acidic protein (GFAP), are slow-proliferating but endowed of long-term self-renewal ability (Alvarez-Buylla and Garcia-Verdugo 2002). They give rise to transiently amplifying progenitor cells (type C cells) which are typically GFAP- and express at meaning levels distal-less homeobox 2 (Dlx2) and Epidermal Growth Factor Receptor (EGFR) genes (Pastrana et al. 2009). These type C cells can, in turn, originate migrating neuroblasts (type A cells) which acquire the expression of polisyalylated form of neural cell adhesion molecule (PSA-NCAM) and of doublecortin (Dcx) and migrate to the olfactory bulbs through the a physiological pathway named -rostral migratory stream- (RMS). Altogether these cell characteristics suggest that NSCs are the best candidate in advanced therapies on neurodegenerative/inflammatory diseases. Indeed in the last decade NSC were used to putative treatment in a number of different diseases.

4. Therapeutic potential of NSC

4.1 NSCs: Therapy, proof of concept

Experimentation with intracerebral transplantation of NSCs into animal models has helped to individuate strategies to develop pharmacological and cell replacement therapies for different neurodegenerative pathologies (Anderson et al. 2001), including both genetic diseases like metachromatic leukodystrophy, Huntington's disease and sporadic Alzheimer's disease (AD), and idiopathic diseases like Parkinson's disease (PD), multiple sclerosis (MS), amyotrophic lateral sclerosis (ALS), and stroke (Kim and de Vellis 2009).

In particular, Pluchino et al. recently showed that following intravenous or intracerebral injection in mice affected by an experimental form of MS (EAE), fetal hNSCs can selectively reach brain and spinal cord areas affected by the demyelinating-inflammatory process and contribute to myelin restoration and reduction of astrogliosis in those damaged areas (Pluchino et al. 2009;Pluchino et al. 2003). However, a crucial step toward successful clinical application of NSC-mediated therapy is to unravel how immunocompetent *in vitro* expanded hNSCs are, whether they are amenable to host rejection following transplantation, and whether they present immunomodulatory besides neuroprotective effects after nervous system lesions. The major disadvantage of immune suppression is to excessively undermine the immunity of the patient and the ensuing enhancement of sensitiveness to multiple infections. For a long time a widely held view was that whatever immune activity in the brain was detrimental to the neuronal tissue. However recent studies have elucidated a neuroprotectant role of immune response on neural repair, which basically relies on the mutual interaction between infiltrating blood-immune cells, microglia and neuronal cells, namely a cross-play of regenerative signals generated by the "neurovascular niche" (Madri 2009). Indeed it has been recently shown that both traumatic injury and chronic neurodegeneration induce the activation of resident microglia and infiltration of T-cells and macrophages from the blood vessels, which can exert evident beneficial besides detrimental effects on the surrounding neural tissue (Beers et al. 2006;Glezer et al. 2007;Neumann et al. 2006;Schwartz and Moalem 2001;Ziv, et al. 2006a;Ziv et al. 2006b). These results in combination with unsuccessful clinical studies (in some cases leading to an exacerbation of the disease) radically revised the theory of immune suppression as a therapeutic approach for neurodegenerative disorders. Moreover, the use of immune suppression in order to prevent the rejection of donor NSC transplants can block the immune mediated guidance cues required for the "homing" of NSC to the lesion sites (Ben-Hur 2008). In particular, Fibroblast Growth Factor 2 (FGF2) (Craig et al. 1996;Kuhn et al. 1997), tumor necrosis factor-a (TNF-α) and Interferon-γ (IFN-γ) have been shown to induce cell mobilization (Ben-Hur et al. 2003), while other cytokines drive NSC migration to the lesion through specific physiological pathways, such as the monocyte chemoattractant protein-1 (MCP-1) (Belmadani et al. 2006), hepatocyte growth factor (HGF) (Lalive et al. 2005), Epidermal Growth Factor (EGF), platelet Growth Factor (PDGF) (Armstrong et al. 1990), and stromal derived growth factor (SDF-1 or CXCL12) (Imitola et al. 2004b).

Interestingly, the majority of hNSC lines expanded *in vitro* display low dissimilitaries in the major histocompatibility complex (MHC) expression pattern, most likely owing to different culture conditions and to the origin of the primary tissue.

The presence of MHC class I and II molecules on human NSC isolated by our group (Figure 1), or described by Akesson and colleagues (Akesson et al. 2009) would presumably predict a risk for rejection after transplantation. However, Akesson demonstrated that neither NSCs nor differentiated cells were recognized by alloreactive lymphocytes.. Indeed, human NSCs and newly formed astrocytes, but not neurons, suppressed lymphocyte stimulation to alloantigens, suggesting low risk for alloreaction and a role as immunomodulators. Despite these results, in accordance with providing evidence of NSCs low immunogenicity (Odeberg et al. 2005) and ability to produce TGF-β cytokine with a potent bystander effect on limpho/monocytes (Ubiali et al. 2007), the presence of MHC class I and II molecules on hNSCs implies a risk for recognition by alloreactive T cells after transplantation, thus indicating a potential risk for immunological rejection due to MHC incompatibility and subsequent requirement of immunosuppressive treatment to avoid rejection.

The disadvantages of using immunosuppressive treatment include an increased risk for opportunistic infections, toxic side effects and potential negative effects on donor cells.

Notwithstanding several clinical trials harnessing various sources of neural stem cells such as ESC-derived progenitors, spinal cord NSC and fetal NSC are currently ongoing (www.clinicaltrials.org).

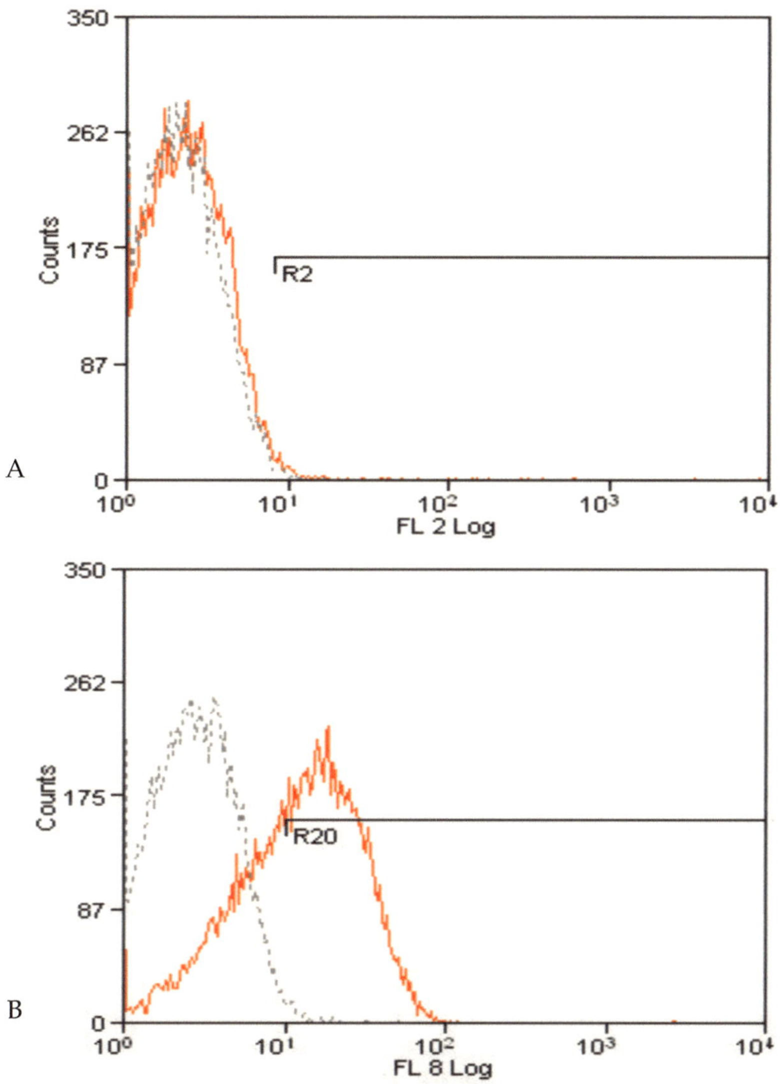

Fig. 1. Cytofluorimetric analysis of HLA class I and II on cultured human neural stem cells (hNSC). A) absence of HLA DR (Class II) on hNSC cell surface. B) Expression of HLA ABC (Class I) on hNSC cell surface

5. Establishment of human NSC lines for clinical application

5.1 NSCs: Cells "clinical grade" produced under GMPs guidelines

Our hNSCs have now been serially expanded under chemically defined conditions and are being cryopreserved, establishing a Good Manufacturing Practice (GMP)-grade, hNSCs bank. In order to certify these cells by the GMP standard, a panel of cellular, functional and biochemical criteria must be met prior to cell release, which include, but are not limited to, karyotype analysis, stable differentiation and growth capacity, and lack of biological contamination by adventitious agents.

In our GMP facility designed to produce human neural stem cells for advanced therapies, quality control is only part of overall quality assurance for cell lines which includes: evaluation and quality control measures for cells and critical reagents coming into the laboratory, control of the laboratory environment, equipment and procedures, control of data arising from cell culture, control of the delivery of research materials, including cells, to other laboratories and traceability of raw material, especially tissue from donors.

Four critical characteristics of cell cultures are fundamental to assure the quality of cell culture work:

1. Identity, i.e., the cells need to possess a specific behaviour:
   i. Self Renewal: growth kinetic stable for a elevated number of passages in vitro
   ii. Multipotency: NSCs are able to differentiate into 3 neural lineages (Astrocytes, Neuron and oligodendrocytes) after growth factors (EGF and bFGF) removal
2. Purity, i.e., freedom from microbiological contamination (all the assays need to be performed according to official Europeian Pharmacopeia, current edition)
   i. Sterility (Bacteria and fungi)
   ii. Mycoplasma
   iii. Bacterial Endotoxins
   iv. Viral contamination
   v. BSE (at least a risk analysis)
3. Maintenance of stable functional properties over passaging *in vitro*
   i. Growth curve: constant positive slope over passages
   ii. Constant ratio neurons/astrocytes/oligodendrocytes upon differentiation assay
   iii. Karyology (healthy karyotype asset and deeper analysis like SKY or comparative genomic hybridisation)
4. Tumorigenicity, i.e., Cell lines not toxic or tumorigenic
   i. Growth factor dependence: the cells died into a few passages after EGF and bFGF removal from culture medium.
   ii. No tumor signs after transplantation into the brain of Nude mice (Figure 2). The cells are able to migrate, differentiate and integrate into host tissue.

Because all of the characteristics above mentioned, raw material (media, cell culture plastic disposable, etc.) were obtained from GMP certified suppliers. Human Neural Stem Cells were produced into controlled environment (class A surrounded by Class B) according to Annex I Vol.4 European GMP Guidelines. Tissue samples were obtained from screened donors according to European Guidelines on "Certain technical requirements for the donation, procurement and testing of human tissues and cell" (Implementing Directive 2004/23/EC of the European Parliament and of the Council).

6. Current immunosuppression in transplant

6.1 Immunosuppressive drugs in cells transplant

Immunosuppression after transplantations is complex and improved therapeutic strategies have contributed to ameliorate the quality of the patient's life and to enhance the survival of the graft; however, the adverse effects associated with immunosuppressive compounds and

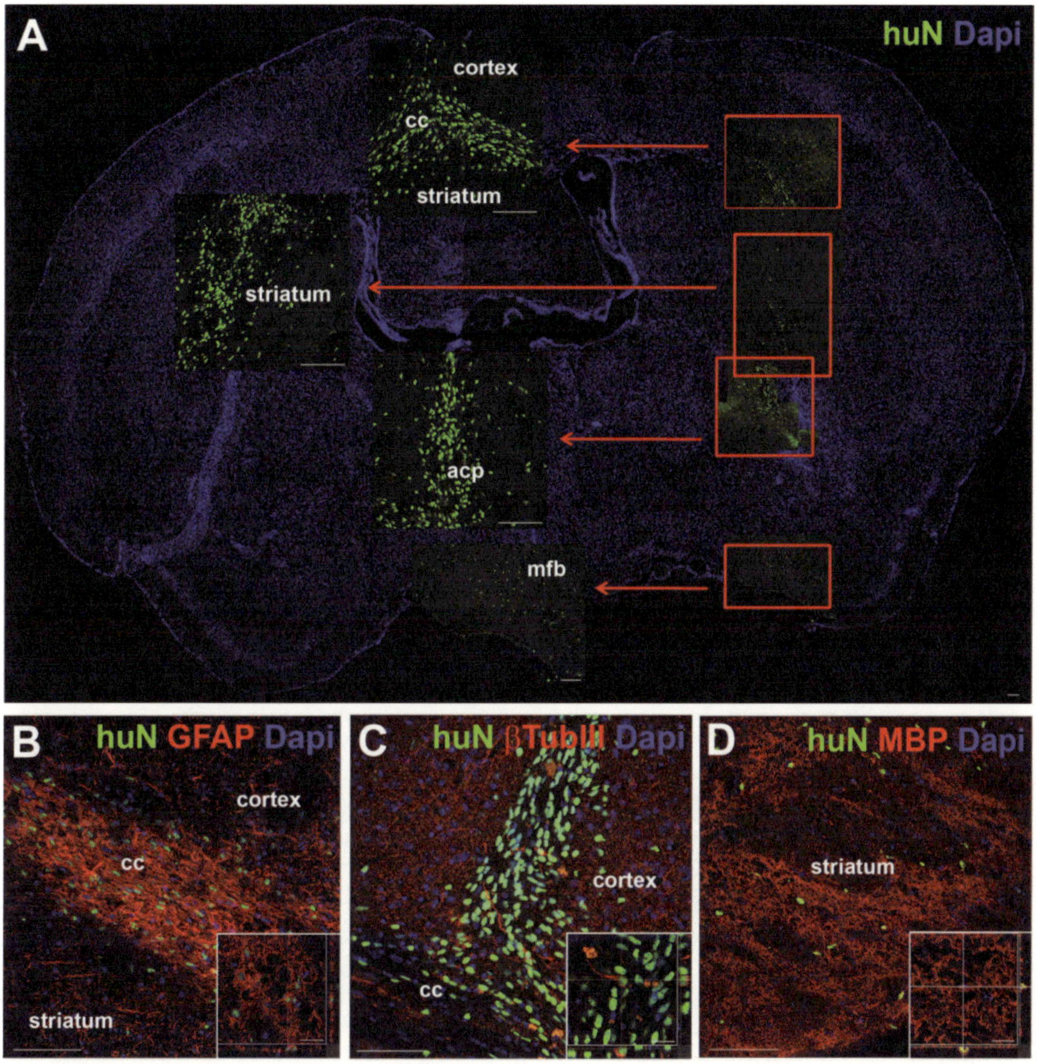

Fig. 2. Panel A-D) Nude mice were injected in striatum with hNSCs. Six months after transplantation mice with hNSCs were sacrificed and immunohistochemistry analysis showed that hNSCs engraft efficiently and migrate throughout the injected hemisphere. (A) Brain map showing the localization of huN+ cells the cells colonized cortex, cc, striatum, acp and mfb. B-D Confocal microscopy analysis showing integration and differentiation of hNSC at 6 months from transplantation into the striatum of nude mice. A) migration of gfp-Transduced hNSC along the corpus callosum and to the striatum of the ipsilateral emisphere. B-D) expression of differentiation and proliferation markers by hNSC identified as human-Nuclei (huN)-immunoreactive cells. Immunostaining with the astroglial marker Glial Fibrillary Acidic Protein (GFAP, B), the neuronal protein β-TubulinIII (C) and the late oligodendroglial marker Myelin Basic Protein (MBP, D). Insets show huN+/MBP colocalization. Nuclei are shown by dapi staining (blue). Scale bars: in A=100μm; in B-D=75μm inset scale bar: B-D=12-17μm. apc: posterior part of anterior commissure; cc: corpus callosum; mfb = medial forebrain bundle

DRUG		MECHANISM OF ACTION	EFFECTS	ADVERSE EFFECTS
Cyclosporine	Calcineurin inhibitor	Binding to the cytosolic protein cyclophilin of immunocompetent lymphocytes and preventing the production of IL-2.	Induction and mainteinance of immunosuppression	Nephrotoxicity, hypertension, hyperkalemia, hypomagnesemia, nausea, intestinal diseases, hypertrichosis, gingival hyperplasia, hyperlipidemia, infection, malignancy
Tacrolimus (FK-506)	Macrolide antibiotic (calcineurin inhibitor)	Reducing peptidyl-prolyl isomerase activity by binding to the immunophilin FKBP12 and creating a new complex FKBP12-FK506 which inhibits both T-lymphocyte signal transduction and IL-2 transcription.	Maintenance immunosuppression and for rescue therapy in patients with refractory rejection under cyclosporine based therapy	Infection, cardiac damage, hypertension, liver and kidney problems, hyperkalemia, hypomagnesemia, hyperglycemia, diabetes mellitus, itching, lung damage, neurological problems,
Sirolimus (Rapamycin)	Macrolide	Binding the cytosolic protein FK-binding protein 12 and inhibiting the response to IL-2 and the activation of T and B-cells.	Maintenance immunosuppression and protection from chronic rejection	Hyperkalemia, hypomagnesemia, hyperlipidemia, leukopenia, anemia, healing and joint pain
Mycophenolate mofetil (MMF)	Prodrug of Mycophenolic Acid	Inhibiting inosine monophoshate dehydrogenase impairing B and T-cells proliferation.	Maintenance immunosuppression and protection from chronic rejection	Nausea, vomiting, diarrhea, leukopenia, anemia and thrombocytopenia
Azathiopine	Purine analogue	Decreasing DNA and RNA synthesis and inhibiting the proliferation of fast-growing lymphocytes (T and B-cells particulary)	Maintenance immunosuppression	Leukopenia, thrombocytopenia, hepatitis, cholestasis, alopecia
Corticosteroids	Steroids hormones	Preventing interleukin IL-1 and IL-6 production by macrophages and inhibiting all stages of T-cells activation	Induction, maintenance immunosuppression and protection from acute rejections	Cushing diseases, bone disease, glucose intolerance, infections
Muromonab-CD3 (OKT-3)	Monoclonal Antibody of IgG_{2A} clones to the CD3 portion of the T-cell recepto	Blocking T-cell function	Induction of immunosuppression and protection from acute rejection (primary treatment or steroid-resistant)	Cytokine release syndrome (fever, dyspnea, wheezes, headache, hypotension) and pulmonary edema.

Table 1. Immunosuppression regimens used for clinical applications on human patients

the risks of inducing a long-term immunosuppression represent a challenging issue for researches and clinicians. Total body radiation after organs' transplantation was among the first protocols of immunosuppression, but it resulted as extremely severe and led inexorably to the death of all the patients. Therefore, steroid alone were used without success. With the development of 6-mercaptopurine (Purinethol), followed by azathioprine (Imuran) in the 1960s, pharmacological immunosuppression became the standard protocol after both organs and cells transplantation until 1980s, when cyclosporine (Sandimmune and Neoral) was introduced as the first calcineurin inhibitor. Calcineurin is a protein phosphatase also known as protein phosphatase 3, PPP3CA, which activates the T cells of the immune system and can be blocked by drugs. Cyclosporine was initially used in combination with azathioprine and steroids and was credited with a dramatic improvement of graft survival. Cyclosporin is thought to bind to the cytosolic protein cyclophilin (an immunophilin) of immunocompetent lymphocytes, especially T-lymphocytes. This complex of ciclosporin and cyclophilin inhibits the phosphatase calcineurin, which under baseline conditions induces the transcription of interleukin-2. The drugs also inhibits lymphokine production and interleukin release, leading to a reduced function of effector T-cells. In 1994 another calcineurin inhibitor, the macrolide antibiotic Tacrolimus (or FK-506), active against helper T cells, became available and gradually supplanted cyclosporine in many clinical Institutes. It has been largely used for maintenance of the immunosuppression and for rescue therapy in patients with refractory rejection under cyclosporine-based therapy. However, the risk of both acute and chronic nephrotoxicity attributed to calcineurin inhibitors has strongly suggested the development of protocols free of these agents as most desirable.

At the present, numerous immunosuppressive drugs and protocols have been designed for transplantation (Table 1), but a protocol which is highly effective with minimal side effects has still to be identified. In this view, although the brain is commonly considered partially "immunoprivileged", a specific immunosuppression regimen has to provide the best conditions allowing graft survival, preventing the patient from the additional burden of an immune reaction against the graft (Barker and Widner 2004).

Actually, the precise sequelae of events leading from antigen recognition to lymphocyte activation and proliferation has still to be elucidated. However, recent findings, concerning the molecular actions of cyclosporine A (CsA) and the new immunosuppressive drugs, Tacrolimus and Rapamycin, have provided important novel breakthroughs in the biochemical processes involved. Interestingly, none of the T-cell directed immunosuppressants is, by itself, anti-lymphocyitic. Conversely, these molecules act as "molecular adaptors" which mediate the interaction between specific intracellular drug-binding proteins and target molecules. Several additional drugs are currently used as immunomodulatory agents, eventually in combination with Calcinneurin inhibitors. Most of these, like steroids, azathioprine, MMF, sirolimus, are routinely used in peripheral organ allograft programs with a unique and different mode of action to that of tacrolimus and cyclosporin A (Table1). The use of adjuvants agents allows clinicians to achieve adequate immunosuppression while decreasing the dose and the toxicity of individual agents.

In neural transplantation, immunomodulators have been used experimentally, in particular with xenografts. Antibodies against T-cell receptor anti-TCR and T cells have been used to enhance the survival of intracerebral neural xenografts in rats (Okura et al. 1997;Wood et al. 1996). Also the use of blockers of T-cells costimulatory molecules have been explored as alternative route to tolerance, therefore highlighting the value of targeting this arm of the immune response for xenograft survival (Larsson et al. 2003;Larsson et al. 2002).

7. Low immunogenic potential of NSC

We already obtained some evidence of hNSCs efficacy and immunogenic tolerance upon transplantation into animal models of neurological disorders (Rota Nodari, et al. 2010) such as transient global ischemia, which is a model of vascular dementia and resembles several pathological features of AD. At 3 days from global ischemic injury, hNSC were unilaterally implantated into the corpus callosum or the hippocampal fissure of adult rat brains. After 1 month, hNSCs were detected to migrate through the corpus callosum (Fig.3), into the cortex or throughout the dentate gyrus of the hippocampus and by the fourth month, to reach the ipsilateral subventricular zone, the CA1-3 hippocampal layers and the controlateral hemisphere, showing to be non-tumorigenic and to undergo a proper regional differentiation into GABAergic and GLUTAmatergic neurons (Rota Nodari, et al. 2010). Notably, these results could be accomplished using transient immunosuppression, i.e administering cyclosporine for 15 days following the ischemic event. A wide array of studies have shown that NSCs are not susceptible to immunological rejection (Bjorklund et al. 2003;Mendez et al. 2008;Olstorn et al. 2007;Wennersten et al. 2006) even when transplanted in animal models like EAE, characterized by a constitutively activated immunological response(Pluchino, et al. 2003;Pluchino, et al. 2005). Similar results were also obtained in a different context: after transplantation into the adult rat brain lesioned by focal demyelination (Ferrari et al., submitted), hNSCs demonstrated to integrate into the NSC host niche and to migrate toward the lesioned corpus callosum, where they properly differentiated into myelinating oligodendrocytes. No sign of tumorigenicity was ever

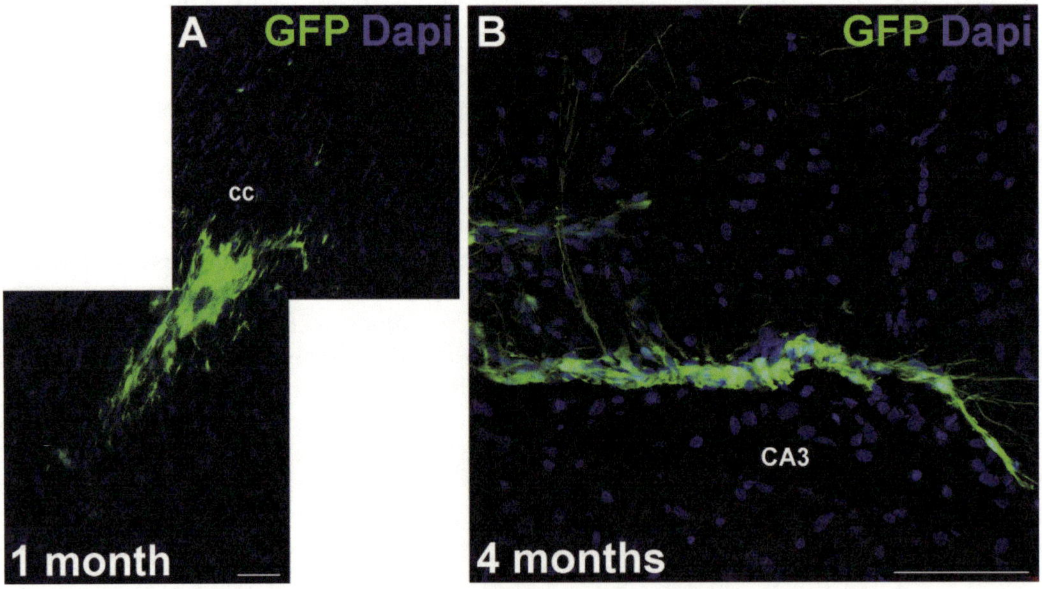

Fig. 3. hNSC transduced with a lentiviral vector carrying the reporter gene gfp were transplanted into the brain of adult rats after 3 days from lesioning by transient global ischemia. Confocal microscopy analysis showing hNSC-GFP integration into the corpus callosum (A) (1 month from transplantation) and in the hippocampal CA3 layer (B) (4 months from transplantation) under transient immunosuppression. Total nuclei are shown by dapi staining (blue). Scale Bar: 50μm. cc: corpus callosum; CA3: hippocampal layer

detected upon transplantation of hNSCs (unpublished observation) nor of hNSC immortalized with proliferating genes as c-myc, c-myc T58A and v-myc (De Filippis et al. 2008; De Filippis et al. 2007). These results have confirmed that hNSC are scarcely immunogenic. Consistently, parallel analysis of hNSC in vitro by cytofluorimetric assays showed that hNSC display only a very faint expression of HLA DR compared to a normal expression of HLA A, B and C (see Figure 1). Moreover, recent studies have shown that hNSCs may also exert their therapeutic potential through an immunomodulatory action (Bacigaluppi, et al. 2009; Pluchino, et al. 2009; Pluchino, et al. 2005).

8. NSC-mediated immunomodulation of the inflammatory component in neurodegenerative disorders

Besides neurodegeneration *per se*, one of the hallmarks characterizing most neurodegenerative disorders like stroke, AD, PD, ALS, MLD, is the development of an inflammatory environment, which can contribute to tissue damage (Glass et al. 2010). Although for a long time the NSC-mediated therapy was basically aimed at replacing damaged neural cells (Lindvall et al. 2004; Pluchino, et al. 2003), the local immune response has been shown to play a key role in recruitment of neural precursors to the lesion site. When neuroinflammation is prevailing over neurodegeneration, NSC have been shown to promote long-lasting neuroprotection and to exert unexpected immune-like functions (Pluchino, et al. 2005). Pluchino et al. (Pluchino, et al. 2005) showed that after systemic injection into a mouse model of multiple sclerosis, transplanted NSC are recruited into perivascular niche areas, where they retain undifferentiated features, proliferate and promote CNS repair through a cross-talk with inflammatory CNS-infiltrating T cells. A dual role in the regulation of both neurogenesis and oligodendrogenesis of adult neural progenitor cells is played by microglia (Streit 2002), so that the two physiological processes can be blocked by inflammation-associated microglia or induced by IL-4/IFN-γ associated to T-helper cells (Butovsky et al. 2006). Several studies have demonstrated that T cells able to recognize CNS antigens can foster spontaneous recovery from CNS injuries through an active cross-talk with local microglia (Hauben et al. 2000;Hofstetter et al. 2003;Moalem et al. 1999;Yoles et al. 2001). Consistently, T cell-based vaccination of mice with a myelin-derived peptide appeared to synergistically promote functional recovery after spinal cord injury when combined with transplantation of neural precursors into the cerebro-spinal fluid (Ziv, et al. 2006a). It's important to consider that immune cells are involved in the control of neurogenesis even under physiological conditions (Ziv, et al. 2006b). However, under pathological environment, the outcome of the interplay between inflammation, synaptic transmission and neurodegeneration is strongly conditioned by the short- or long-term persistence of inflammation (Centonze et al. 2010;Pluchino et al. 2008). Upon acute inflammatory injuries, such as stroke, neurogenesis is notably increased (Zhang et al. 2004). Conversely, a persistent brain inflammation in chronic inflammatory disorders, such as MS (Pluchino, et al. 2008) has been shown to alter both the proliferative and migratory capacities of NSCs in the SVZ, thus leading to a perpetuating non cell-autonomous dysfunction of the endogenous CNS stem cell compartment.

Both in the globally ischemic and focally demyelinated rat brains, we observed that transplantation of hNSCs can effectively decrease reactive astrogliosis and dampen microglial activation in the injuried areas (Rota Nodari, et al. 2010); unpublished results).

This phenomenon may, in fact, participate in the low immunogenic response that these cells seem to elicit in the CNS, together with the lack of expression of Molecular

Histocompatibility Complex class II components (MHCII) (Imitola et al. 2004a;Imitola, et al. 2004b)(see also Fig 1). Notwithstanding, it is also true that some level of immune surveillance is maintained in the adult brain upon NSC engraftment, which explains the widespread need to use immune suppression (Wennersten, et al. 2006) in experimental and clinical intracerebral transplantation (Bjorklund, et al. 2003;Olstorn, et al. 2007).The successful use of transient immunosuppression proposes a suitable milder approach to immunosuppression for the prospective use of hNSCs for clinical purposes. The fact that the discontinuous treatment with cyclosporine does not affect integration of transplanted cells in most of the brain regions, which to all effects emerge as immunoprivileged when considering hNSCs, is in good accordance with most recent findings (Wennersten, et al. 2006). These evidences are driving the progressive translation of the knowledge "from the bench to the bedside", thus leading to the use of hNSCs as a suitable tool to model transplantation in pre-clinical settings and to the promotion of GMP-grade hNSC for stem cell-mediated therapy of neurodegenerative disorders.

9. Transplanted NSC switch on or off the immune reactivity into host?

Usually, after the cell or tissue transplant into CNS, the intensity and rapidity of the rejection depend on the phylogenetic distance between donor and host (Dymecki et al. 1990;Mason et al. 1986;Pakzaban and Isacson 1994) and the status of the host immune system (Marion et al. 1990), but also from the nature and differentiation state of transplanted cells. Capetian and colleagues (Capetian et al. 2011) demonstrate that murine NSCs derived from newborn C57BL/6, cultured as neurospheres and placed into kidney capsule as a non-immunopriviliged site of BALB/c survived for 28 days without rejection although these 2 strains were been immunologically incompatible. However the graft were readly rejected when the recipient animal was either pre or post sensitized using donor splenocytes.

Also in these example, as well as in our human cells (Figure 1) the murine neural stem cells showed no expression of MHC I or II, in contrast with surrounding tissue or other terminally differentiated cells. This demonstrated that NSCs themselves are not attacked by immune defense mechanisms since they do not sensitize host (so they have a low immunogenicity), but can however be rejected if the host is or becomes sensitized.

In the past there have been concerns that the loss or lack of clinical improvement after neural grafting could be due to immunological rejection processes that compromise neural graft survival and function. However, autopsy findings of patients at long-term follow-up post-transplantation showed little evidence of immunological reactions (Freeman et al. 2000;Kordower et al. 2008;Kordower et al. 1996;Li et al. 2008;Mendez et al. 2005).

According to results of different clinical trials on Huntington Disease where all the patients received adequate immunosuppression for over 1 year, most of the patients developed anti HLA I antibodies but only few showed overt signs of immunological rejection.

Moreover there are accruing evidences (Pluchino, et al. 2009) that NSCs injected into CNS or intravenously in multiple sclerosis animal models are scarcely (if any) prone to differentiate, while they are able to exert a plethora of "healing actions", such as production of pleiotropic factors and cytokines, scavenging of toxic molecules and immunomodulation of the inflammatory environment. In addition Akesson and colleagues (Akesson, et al. 2009) have shown that human Neural stem cells derived from aborted fetuses of 5-12 weeks of gestation were able to inhibit lymphocyte proliferation induced by alloantigen and at NSC:Lymphomonocyte ratio of 1:1 a complete suppression was seen. These effect was clearly specific and mediated by cell-cell interactions as demonstrated by tha fact that the above mentioned proliferation was not affected by presence or absence of supernatants from NSCs cultures.

Moreover, recent evidence has suggested that the majority of the stem cell-mediated therapeutic effects in inflammatory CNS disorders are possibly taking place peripherally, at the level of immune relevant anatomical site, such as secondary lymphoid organs.

On the other hand the surgery could influence "per se" the fate of transplanted cells, albeit stereotactic techniques allow to inject NSCs by a minimally invasive procedure.

There are three main factors to be taken in account that can influence the extent of the host reaction and graft survival in an intraparenchimal cell graft: i) the extent of tissue trauma during injection, ii) cell suspension preparation and iii) the site of implantation.

The intraparenchymal injection lead to breakage of blood brain barrier at least for a couple of weeks facilitating the limphomonocyte patrolling and reaction against the graft. A low viability of cell suspensions could also trigger an immune reaction. Furthermore, the site of implantation can have a considerable effect on the host immune reaction. For example, peri- or intraventricular graft placement can lead to increased rates of immune response in terms of MHC class I expression inside the grafts and lymphocyte invasion (Oertel et al. 2004).

10. Conclusions

Although NSCs cell therapy seem to be a promising development for a number on neurological diseases, transplantation of NSC into the central nervous system is from an immunological viewpoint a true challenge both for the host as well as for the donor cells. Moreover more experiments are necessary to fully elucidate the mechanisms underlining the interactions between stem cells graft and host immune system. In conclusion, the mildest approach for clinical trials on humans is likely a transient immunosuppression regimen.

11. Acknowledgements

We thank Cristina Zalfa for image editing, Giuseppe Lamorte for FACS analysis and Prof. Angelo Vescovi for precious suggestions. This work was supported by Fondazione Borgonovo, Fondazione Neurothon ONLUS, Fondazione Cellule Staminali of Terni, Fondazione Milan.

12. References

Akesson E, Wolmer-Solberg N, Cederarv M, Falci S and Odeberg J. 2009. Human neural stem cells and astrocytes, but not neurons, suppress an allogeneic lymphocyte response. Stem Cell Res 2(1):56-67.

Alvarez-Buylla A and Garcia-Verdugo JM. 2002. Neurogenesis in adult subventricular zone. J Neurosci 22(3):629-34.

Alvarez-Buylla A, Garcia-Verdugo JM and Tramontin AD. 2001. A unified hypothesis on the lineage of neural stem cells. Nat Rev Neurosci 2(4):287-93.

Anderson DJ, Gage FH and Weissman IL. 2001. Can stem cells cross lineage boundaries? Nat Med 7(4):393-5.

Armstrong RC, Harvath L and Dubois-Dalcq ME. 1990. Type 1 astrocytes and oligodendrocyte-type 2 astrocyte glial progenitors migrate toward distinct molecules. J Neurosci Res 27(3):400-7.

Bacigaluppi M, Pluchino S, Peruzzotti Jametti L, Kilic E, Kilic U, Salani G, Brambilla E, West MJ, Comi G, Martino Gand others. 2009. Delayed post-ischaemic neuroprotection following systemic neural stem cell transplantation involves multiple mechanisms. Brain 132(Pt 8):2239-51.

Barker RA and Widner H. 2004. Immune problems in central nervous system cell therapy. NeuroRx 1(4):472-81.

Beers DR, Henkel JS, Xiao Q, Zhao W, Wang J, Yen AA, Siklos L, McKercher SR and Appel SH. 2006. Wild-type microglia extend survival in PU.1 knockout mice with familial amyotrophic lateral sclerosis. Proc Natl Acad Sci U S A 103(43):16021-6.

Behrstock S, Ebert A, McHugh J, Vosberg S, Moore J, Schneider B, Capowski E, Hei D, Kordower J, Aebischer Pand others. 2006. Human neural progenitors deliver glial cell line-derived neurotrophic factor to parkinsonian rodents and aged primates. Gene Ther 13(5):379-88.

Belmadani A, Tran PB, Ren D and Miller RJ. 2006. Chemokines regulate the migration of neural progenitors to sites of neuroinflammation. J Neurosci 26(12):3182-91.

Ben-Hur T. 2008. Immunomodulation by neural stem cells. J Neurol Sci 265(1-2):102-4.

Ben-Hur T, Ben-Menachem O, Furer V, Einstein O, Mizrachi-Kol R and Grigoriadis N. 2003. Effects of proinflammatory cytokines on the growth, fate, and motility of multipotential neural precursor cells. Mol Cell Neurosci 24(3):623-31.

Bjorklund A, Dunnett SB, Brundin P, Stoessl AJ, Freed CR, Breeze RE, Levivier M, Peschanski M, Studer L and Barker R. 2003. Neural transplantation for the treatment of Parkinson's disease. Lancet Neurol 2(7):437-45.

Butovsky O, Ziv Y, Schwartz A, Landa G, Talpalar AE, Pluchino S, Martino G and Schwartz M. 2006. Microglia activated by IL-4 or IFN-gamma differentially induce neurogenesis and oligodendrogenesis from adult stem/progenitor cells. Mol Cell Neurosci 31(1):149-60.

Cao QL, Zhang YP, Howard RM, Walters WM, Tsoulfas P and Whittemore SR. 2001. Pluripotent stem cells engrafted into the normal or lesioned adult rat spinal cord are restricted to a glial lineage. Exp Neurol 167(1):48-58.

Capetian P, Dobrossy M, Winkler C, Prinz M and Nikkhah G. 2011. To be or not to be accepted: the role of immunogenicity of neural stem cells following transplantation into the brain in animal and human studies. Semin Immunopathol.

Centonze D, Muzio L, Rossi S, Furlan R, Bernardi G and Martino G. 2010. The link between inflammation, synaptic transmission and neurodegeneration in multiple sclerosis. Cell Death Differ 17(7):1083-91.

Chu K, Kim M, Park KI, Jeong SW, Park HK, Jung KH, Lee ST, Kang L, Lee K, Park DKand others. 2004. Human neural stem cells improve sensorimotor deficits in the adult rat brain with experimental focal ischemia. Brain Res 1016(2):145-53.

Craig CG, Tropepe V, Morshead CM, Reynolds BA, Weiss S and van der Kooy D. 1996. In vivo growth factor expansion of endogenous subependymal neural precursor cell populations in the adult mouse brain. J Neurosci 16(8):2649-58.

De Filippis L, Ferrari D, Rota Nodari L, Amati B, Snyder E and Vescovi AL. 2008. Immortalization of human neural stem cells with the c-myc mutant T58A. PLoS One 3(10):e3310.

De Filippis L, Lamorte G, Snyder EY, Malgaroli A and Vescovi AL. 2007. A novel, immortal, and multipotent human neural stem cell line generating functional neurons and oligodendrocytes. Stem Cells 25(9):2312-21.

Doetsch F. 2003. A niche for adult neural stem cells. Curr Opin Genet Dev 13(5):543-50.

Dymecki J, Poltorak M and Freed WJ. 1990. The degree of genetic disparity between donor and host correlates with survival of intraventricular substantia nigra grafts. Reg Immunol 3(1):17-22.

Ebert AD, Beres AJ, Barber AE and Svendsen CN. 2008. Human neural progenitor cells over-expressing IGF-1 protect dopamine neurons and restore function in a rat model of Parkinson's disease. Exp Neurol 209(1):213-23.

Emsley JG, Mitchell BD, Magavi SS, Arlotta P and Macklis JD. 2004. The repair of complex neuronal circuitry by transplanted and endogenous precursors. NeuroRx 1(4):452-71.

Freeman TB, Cicchetti F, Hauser RA, Deacon TW, Li XJ, Hersch SM, Nauert GM, Sanberg PR, Kordower JH, Saporta Sand others. 2000. Transplanted fetal striatum in Huntington's disease: phenotypic development and lack of pathology. Proc Natl Acad Sci U S A 97(25):13877-82.

Gage FH. 2000. Mammalian neural stem cells. Science 287(5457):1433-8.

Gage FH, Kempermann G, Palmer TD, Peterson DA and Ray J. 1998. Multipotent progenitor cells in the adult dentate gyrus. J Neurobiol 36(2):249-66.

Garrido RS, Aguado JM, Diaz-Pedroche C, Len O, Montejo M, Moreno A, Gurgui M, Torre-Cisneros J, Pareja F, Segovia Jand others. 2006. A review of critical periods for opportunistic infection in the new transplantation era. Transplantation 82(11):1457-62.

Glass CK, Saijo K, Winner B, Marchetto MC and Gage FH. 2010. Mechanisms underlying inflammation in neurodegeneration. Cell 140(6):918-34.

Glezer I, Simard AR and Rivest S. 2007. Neuroprotective role of the innate immune system by microglia. Neuroscience 147(4):867-83.

Gritti A, Parati EA, Cova L, Frolichsthal P, Galli R, Wanke E, Faravelli L, Morassutti DJ, Roisen F, Nickel DDand others. 1996. Multipotential stem cells from the adult mouse brain proliferate and self-renew in response to basic fibroblast growth factor. J Neurosci 16(3):1091-100.

Guo J, Zeng Y, Liang Y, Wang L, Su H and Wu W. 2007. Cyclosporine affects the proliferation and differentiation of neural stem cells in culture. Neuroreport 18(9):863-8.

Hauben E, Butovsky O, Nevo U, Yoles E, Moalem G, Agranov E, Mor F, Leibowitz-Amit R, Pevsner E, Akselrod Sand others. 2000. Passive or active immunization with myelin basic protein promotes recovery from spinal cord contusion. J Neurosci 20(17):6421-30.

Hofstetter HH, Sewell DL, Liu F, Sandor M, Forsthuber T, Lehmann PV and Fabry Z. 2003. Autoreactive T cells promote post-traumatic healing in the central nervous system. J Neuroimmunol 134(1-2):25-34.

Imitola J, Comabella M, Chandraker AK, Dangond F, Sayegh MH, Snyder EY and Khoury SJ. 2004a. Neural stem/progenitor cells express costimulatory molecules that are differentially regulated by inflammatory and apoptotic stimuli. Am J Pathol 164(5):1615-25.

Imitola J, Raddassi K, Park KI, Mueller FJ, Nieto M, Teng YD, Frenkel D, Li J, Sidman RL, Walsh CAand others. 2004b. Directed migration of neural stem cells to sites of CNS injury by the stromal cell-derived factor 1alpha/CXC chemokine receptor 4 pathway. Proc Natl Acad Sci U S A 101(52):18117-22.

Jiang Q, Zhang ZG, Ding GL, Zhang L, Ewing JR, Wang L, Zhang R, Li L, Lu M, Meng Hand others. 2005. Investigation of neural progenitor cell induced angiogenesis after embolic stroke in rat using MRI. Neuroimage 28(3):698-707.

Kim SU and de Vellis J. 2009. Stem cell-based cell therapy in neurological diseases: a review. J Neurosci Res 87(10):2183-200.

Kordower JH, Chu Y, Hauser RA, Freeman TB and Olanow CW. 2008. Lewy body-like pathology in long-term embryonic nigral transplants in Parkinson's disease. Nat Med 14(5):504-6.

Kordower JH, Rosenstein JM, Collier TJ, Burke MA, Chen EY, Li JM, Martel L, Levey AE, Mufson EJ, Freeman TBand others. 1996. Functional fetal nigral grafts in a patient with Parkinson's disease: chemoanatomic, ultrastructural, and metabolic studies. J Comp Neurol 370(2):203-30.

Kuhn HG, Winkler J, Kempermann G, Thal LJ and Gage FH. 1997. Epidermal growth factor and fibroblast growth factor-2 have different effects on neural progenitors in the adult rat brain. J Neurosci 17(15):5820-9.

Lalive PH, Paglinawan R, Biollaz G, Kappos EA, Leone DP, Malipiero U, Relvas JB, Moransard M, Suter T and Fontana A. 2005. TGF-beta-treated microglia induce oligodendrocyte precursor cell chemotaxis through the HGF-c-Met pathway. Eur J Immunol 35(3):727-37.

Larsson LC, Corbascio M, Pearson TC, Larsen CP, Ekberg H and Widner H. 2003. Induction of operational tolerance to discordant dopaminergic porcine xenografts. Transplantation 75(9):1448-54.

Larsson LC, Corbascio M, Widner H, Pearson TC, Larsen CP and Ekberg H. 2002. Simultaneous inhibition of B7 and LFA-1 signaling prevents rejection of discordant neural xenografts in mice lacking CD40L. Xenotransplantation 9(1):68-76.

Li JY, Englund E, Holton JL, Soulet D, Hagell P, Lees AJ, Lashley T, Quinn NP, Rehncrona S, Bjorklund Aand others. 2008. Lewy bodies in grafted neurons in subjects with Parkinson's disease suggest host-to-graft disease propagation. Nat Med 14(5):501-3.

Lindvall O and Kokaia Z. 2010. Stem cells in human neurodegenerative disorders--time for clinical translation? J Clin Invest 120(1):29-40.

Lindvall O, Kokaia Z and Martinez-Serrano A. 2004. Stem cell therapy for human neurodegenerative disorders-how to make it work. Nat Med 10 Suppl:S42-50.

Madri JA. 2009. Modeling the neurovascular niche: implications for recovery from CNS injury. J Physiol Pharmacol 60 Suppl 4:95-104.

Marion DW, Pollack IF and Lund RD. 1990. Patterns of immune rejection of mouse neocortex transplanted into neonatal rat brain, and effects of host immunosuppression. Brain Res 519(1-2):133-43.

Mason DW, Charlton HM, Jones AJ, Lavy CB, Puklavec M and Simmonds SJ. 1986. The fate of allogeneic and xenogeneic neuronal tissue transplanted into the third ventricle of rodents. Neuroscience 19(3):685-94.

Mendez I, Sanchez-Pernaute R, Cooper O, Vinuela A, Ferrari D, Bjorklund L, Dagher A and Isacson O. 2005. Cell type analysis of functional fetal dopamine cell suspension transplants in the striatum and substantia nigra of patients with Parkinson's disease. Brain 128(Pt 7):1498-510.

Mendez I, Vinuela A, Astradsson A, Mukhida K, Hallett P, Robertson H, Tierney T, Holness R, Dagher A, Trojanowski JQand others. 2008. Dopamine neurons implanted into people with Parkinson's disease survive without pathology for 14 years. Nat Med 14(5):507-9.

Moalem G, Leibowitz-Amit R, Yoles E, Mor F, Cohen IR and Schwartz M. 1999. Autoimmune T cells protect neurons from secondary degeneration after central nervous system axotomy. Nat Med 5(1):49-55.

Neumann J, Gunzer M, Gutzeit HO, Ullrich O, Reymann KG and Dinkel K. 2006. Microglia provide neuroprotection after ischemia. FASEB J 20(6):714-6.

Odeberg J, Piao JH, Samuelsson EB, Falci S and Akesson E. 2005. Low immunogenicity of in vitro-expanded human neural cells despite high MHC expression. J Neuroimmunol 161(1-2):1-11.

Oertel J, Samii M and Walter GF. 2004. Fetal allogeneic dopaminergic cell suspension grafts in the ventricular system of the rat: characterization of transplant morphology and graft-host interactions. Acta Neuropathol 107(5):421-7.

Okura Y, Tanaka R, Ono K, Yoshida S, Tanuma N and Matsumoto Y. 1997. Treatment of rat hemiparkinson model with xenogeneic neural transplantation: tolerance induction by anti-T-cell antibodies. J Neurosci Res 48(5):385-96.

Olstorn H, Moe MC, Roste GK, Bueters T and Langmoen IA. 2007. Transplantation of stem cells from the adult human brain to the adult rat brain. Neurosurgery 60(6):1089-98; discussion 1098-9.

Pakzaban P and Isacson O. 1994. Neural xenotransplantation: reconstruction of neuronal circuitry across species barriers. Neuroscience 62(4):989-1001.

Pastrana E, Cheng LC and Doetsch F. 2009. Simultaneous prospective purification of adult subventricular zone neural stem cells and their progeny. Proc Natl Acad Sci U S A 106(15):6387-92.

Pluchino S, Gritti A, Blezer E, Amadio S, Brambilla E, Borsellino G, Cossetti C, Del Carro U, Comi G, t Hart Band others. 2009. Human neural stem cells ameliorate autoimmune encephalomyelitis in non-human primates. Ann Neurol 66(3):343-54.

Pluchino S, Muzio L, Imitola J, Deleidi M, Alfaro-Cervello C, Salani G, Porcheri C, Brambilla E, Cavasinni F, Bergamaschi Aand others. 2008. Persistent inflammation alters the function of the endogenous brain stem cell compartment. Brain 131(Pt 10):2564-78.

Pluchino S, Quattrini A, Brambilla E, Gritti A, Salani G, Dina G, Galli R, Del Carro U, Amadio S, Bergami Aand others. 2003. Injection of adult neurospheres induces recovery in a chronic model of multiple sclerosis. Nature 422(6933):688-94.

Pluchino S, Zanotti L, Rossi B, Brambilla E, Ottoboni L, Salani G, Martinello M, Cattalini A, Bergami A, Furlan Rand others. 2005. Neurosphere-derived multipotent precursors promote neuroprotection by an immunomodulatory mechanism. Nature 436(7048):266-71.

Popa-Wagner A, Buga AM and Kokaia Z. 2009. Perturbed cellular response to brain injury during aging. Ageing Res Rev.

Reynolds BA and Weiss S. 1992. Generation of neurons and astrocytes from isolated cells of the adult mammalian central nervous system. Science 255(5052):1707-10.

Rezzani R. 2006. Exploring cyclosporine A-side effects and the protective role-played by antioxidants: the morphological and immunohistochemical studies. Histol Histopathol 21(3):301-16.

Romanko MJ, Rola R, Fike JR, Szele FG, Dizon ML, Felling RJ, Brazel CY and Levison SW. 2004. Roles of the mammalian subventricular zone in cell replacement after brain injury. Prog Neurobiol 74(2):77-99.

Rota Nodari L, Ferrari D, Giani F, Bossi M, Rodriguez-Menendez V, Tredici G, Delia D, Vescovi AL and De Filippis L. 2010. Long-Term Survival of Human Neural Stem Cells in the Ischemic Rat Brain upon Transient Immunosuppression. PLoS One 5(11):e14035.

Schwartz M and Moalem G. 2001. Beneficial immune activity after CNS injury: prospects for vaccination. J Neuroimmunol 113(2):185-92.

Shihabuddin LS, Horner PJ, Ray J and Gage FH. 2000. Adult spinal cord stem cells generate neurons after transplantation in the adult dentate gyrus. J Neurosci 20(23):8727-35.

Streit WJ. 2002. Microglia and the response to brain injury. Ernst Schering Res Found Workshop(39):11-24.

Suhonen JO, Peterson DA, Ray J and Gage FH. 1996. Differentiation of adult hippocampus-derived progenitors into olfactory neurons in vivo. Nature 383(6601):624-7.

Temple S. 2001. The development of neural stem cells. Nature 414(6859):112-7.

Temple S and Alvarez-Buylla A. 1999. Stem cells in the adult mammalian central nervous system. Curr Opin Neurobiol 9(1):135-41.

Ubiali F, Nava S, Nessi V, Frigerio S, Parati E, Bernasconi P, Mantegazza R and Baggi F. 2007. Allorecognition of human neural stem cells by peripheral blood lymphocytes despite low expression of MHC molecules: role of TGF-beta in modulating proliferation. Int Immunol 19(9):1063-74.

Weiss S, Reynolds BA, Vescovi AL, Morshead C, Craig CG and van der Kooy D. 1996. Is there a neural stem cell in the mammalian forebrain? Trends Neurosci 19(9):387-93.

Wennersten A, Holmin S, Al Nimer F, Meijer X, Wahlberg LU and Mathiesen T. 2006. Sustained survival of xenografted human neural stem/progenitor cells in experimental brain trauma despite discontinuation of immunosuppression. Exp Neurol 199(2):339-47.

Wood MJ, Sloan DJ, Wood KJ and Charlton HM. 1996. Indefinite survival of neural xenografts induced with anti-CD4 monoclonal antibodies. Neuroscience 70(3):775-89.

Yoles E, Hauben E, Palgi O, Agranov E, Gothilf A, Cohen A, Kuchroo V, Cohen IR, Weiner H and Schwartz M. 2001. Protective autoimmunity is a physiological response to CNS trauma. J Neurosci 21(11):3740-8.

Zhang R, Zhang Z, Wang L, Wang Y, Gousev A, Zhang L, Ho KL, Morshead C and Chopp M. 2004. Activated neural stem cells contribute to stroke-induced neurogenesis and neuroblast migration toward the infarct boundary in adult rats. J Cereb Blood Flow Metab 24(4):441-8.

Ziv Y, Avidan H, Pluchino S, Martino G and Schwartz M. 2006a. Synergy between immune cells and adult neural stem/progenitor cells promotes functional recovery from spinal cord injury. Proc Natl Acad Sci U S A 103(35):13174-9.

Ziv Y, Ron N, Butovsky O, Landa G, Sudai E, Greenberg N, Cohen H, Kipnis J and Schwartz M. 2006b. Immune cells contribute to the maintenance of neurogenesis and spatial learning abilities in adulthood. Nat Neurosci 9(2):268-75.

16

Current Immunosuppression in Abdominal Organ Transplantation

Raffaele Girlanda, Cal S. Matsumoto,
Keith J. Melancon and Thomas M. Fishbein
Transplant Institute, Georgetown University Hospital, Washington DC
USA

1. Introduction

Organ transplantation has saved the lives of thousands of patients beginning from the mid 1950s. At the end of 2007 the Organ Procurement and Transplantation Network (OPTN) database recorded 183,222 people living with a functioning graft in the United States (Wolfe et al., 2010). Over the last two decades survival rates have continued to improve and currently 81-91% of kidney transplant recipients and 74-79% of liver transplant recipients are alive 5 years post-transplant (Wolfe et al., 2010). This success is a dramatic improvement compared to the early era of transplantation and is the result of advances in organ preservation, surgical technique, intensive care and immunosuppression. Particularly, the development of potent immunosuppressive medications has contributed significantly to the success of organ transplantation by reducing the incidence of rejection and graft loss. In recent large studies the incidence of acute rejection is reported as low as 8-15% 1 year after kidney transplant (Ekberg et al., 2009) and graft loss due to acute rejection has now become very uncommon.

Clinical immunosuppression after organ transplantation has come a long way over the last fifty years. It started with total body irradiation, steroids and azathioprine (see Starzl, 2000 for a review on the history of immunosuppression). The rationale behind total body irradiation was to control the immune response to the allograft by ablation of the bone marrow, a similar principle applied today with the use of depleting agents (see below). Other early attempts at controlling the bone marrow and obtain lymphocyte depletion included splenectomy, thymectomy and thoracic duct drainage, but these had limited success. Instead, anti-lymphocyte globulin (ALG), prepared from the serum of horses or rabbits inoculated with human lymphocytes, was introduced in 1966 with the aim of mitigating cellular immunity using heterologous antibodies. (Starzl et al., 1967)

From the early 1960s to 1980s post-transplant immunosuppression consisted of azathioprine, high dose corticosteroids and antilymphocyte globulin. Cyclosporine was introduced in the early 1980s, followed by monoclonal antibodies, then by tacrolimus in the 1990s and lately by mycophenolic acid and sirolimus (see list below). Immunosuppression regimens have changed since the early era of transplantation as a result of the development of new drugs. Furthermore, the number of available drugs continues to increase. This article will describe the immunosuppressive drugs currently used in clinical transplantation and will focus on recent developments. We will also review current organ-specific IMS protocols for kidney, liver, pancreas and intestine transplant to highlight the differences in abdominal organ transplantation that require specific immunosuppressive strategies (ie immunosuppression in the highly sensitized kidney recipient, prevention of disease recurrence after liver transplant, role of induction in intestinal transplantation). Finally, we will highlight current areas of ongoing research and future developments in clinical immunosuppression.

2. Current immunosuppressive agents

There are several immunosuppressive drugs currently used in different combinations in abdominal organ transplantation (see table 1). Most agents target T cell activation and proliferation, given the central role of T lymphocytes in organ rejection. Indeed, the control of T cell-based mechanisms is key to prevent rejection, especially in the early post-transplant period. However, increasing attention is being given to the role of B cells and to the production of alloantibodies in late graft injury and chronic rejection. In addition, components of the innate immune system (neutrophils, complement) are becoming the target for development of new immunosuppressive agents. Here we discuss the immunosuppressive agents currently used in clinical transplantation and present new drugs being investigated in clinical trials.

Antibodies (monoclonal)
Alemtuzumab
Basiliximab
Daclizumab
Muromonab-CD3 (OKT3)
Rituximab
Antibodies (polyclonal)
ALG
Atgam
Thymoglobulin
Azathioprine
Calcineurin inhibitors
Cyclosporine
Tacrolimus
Corticosteroids
mTOR inhibitors
Everolimus
Sirolimus
Mycophenolic acid
Mycophenolate mofetil
Mycophenolate sodium
Others
Belatacept
Bortezomib

Table 1. Immunosuppressive drugs currently used in clinical transplantation

2.1 Corticosteroids

Corticosteroids (prednisone, prednisolone, methylprednisolone) were the first immunosuppressive drugs to be used in transplantation and remain today first line treatment across organs for both prevention and treatment of rejection. The multiple anti-inflammatory and immunomodulatory effects on a wide variety of cells including lymphocytes, granulocytes, macrophages, monocytes and endothelial cells are well known and the molecular mechanisms of action of steroids have been described extensively (Adcock et al., 2000). Briefly, corticosteroids down regulate cytokine gene expression in lymphocytes, antagonize macrophage differentiation, inhibit neutrophil adhesion to endothelial cells thereby decreasing their extravasation to the site of inflammation, decrease circulating eosinophil and basophil counts, inhibit IgE-dependent release of histamine and leukotriene from basophils and inhibit degranulation of mast cells. Additionally, glucocorticoids downregulate endothelial cell function including expression of class II MHC antigen and expression of adhesion molecules.

Based on these multiple effects on different cellular components of the immune response corticosteroids are very effective in preventing and treating acute allograft rejection. Indeed episodes of acute rejection are routinely treated with pulse steroids with generally good response, although there are instances of steroid-resistant rejection episodes.

The multiple side effects of steroids are also well known and include impaired wound healing, increased risk of infection, hypertension, weight gain, hyperglycemia, osteoporosis, fluid retention, hirsutism, acne and cataracts . Side effects may have an important impact especially in the long term and in children (ie growth pattern), therefore multiple trials of steroid withdrawal and steroid-free regimens have been designed in an attempt to limit the side effects of corticosteroids, with variable results (see below specific organs). In addition, several steroid withdrawal protocols have been associated with increased acute rejection (Knight et al., 2010). Corticosteroids still maintain a central role in the armamentarium of immunosuppressive agents currently available in clinical transplantation.

2.2 Azathioprine

Azathioprine was the main immunosuppressive agent, with steroids, for many years in clinical transplantation. It is a nucleotide analogue originally developed during research on new chemotherapy agents for leukemia. The mechanism of action of azathioprine is to incorporate into and to halt DNA replication thus blocking the *de-novo* purine synthesis in lymphocytes. It was originally tested in experimental kidney transplantation in the 1960s (Calne et al., 1961) and it obtained improved graft survival with less toxicity compared to analogue agents such as 6-mercaptopurine. Azathioprine is now very rarely used and it has been replaced by mycophenolic acid (see below) in many transplant programs.

2.3 Calcineurin inhibitors

Calcineurin inhibitors (CNI) are main immunosuppressive agents in use today in virtually every transplant program. Cyclosporine and tacrolimus are the two CNI currently used in clinical transplantation. Their immunosuppressive effect is to block the production of pro-inflammatory cytokines including IL-2, INF-γ, TNF-α and to inhibit T cell activation and proliferation by inactivating calcineurin, an intracellular calcium/calmodulin phosphatase triggered by the engagement of T cell receptor by donor MHC and responsible for de-phosphorilation of nuclear factor for activated T cells (NF-AT) which promotes the transcription of cytokine genes.

Although CNI remain the cornerstone of current immunosuppressive protocols, increasing attention is being devoted to their long term side effects (ie nephrotoxicity). The impact of these side effects and the concomitant introduction of alternative immunosuppressive agents led to the design of trials to reduce CNI exposure. Strategies to limit CNI exposure include CNI minimization, avoidance, and withdrawal (Flechner SM et al., 2008) However, to date trials incorporating mycophenolate mofetil or mTOR inhibitors showed mixed results because of adverse events or lack of efficacy (Larson et al., 2006, Ekberg et al., 2007).

2.3.1 Cyclosporine

Cyclosporine, a metabolite extracted from the soil fungi *Cylindrocarpon lucidum* and *Trichoderma polysporum,* initially was investigated as an antifungal but was also shown to be immunosuppressive in mice models of skin allotransplantation. Its potent anti-lymphocyte properties prolonged the survival of kidney transplants in the dog. The introduction of cyclosporine in the early 1980s has revolutionized clinical transplantation and has remained the cornerstone of immunosuppression for kidney, liver, heart and other organs for many years. The mechanism of action and the immunologic effects of cyclosporine have been reported above. With cyclosporine a dramatic increase in early graft survival was observed in many centers with some programs reporting almost doubling their 1-year graft survival rate from 50% in the late 1970s to 86% in the 1980s (Merion RM et al, 1984). Since the early 1980s triple immunosuppressive therapy with cyclosporine, azathioprine and steroids has been standard protocol for a long time in many centers and has allowed dramatic growth of transplant programs worldwide.

The main side effects of cyclosporine are nephrotoxicity and hypertension. Other side effects include diabetes and cosmetic changes like gingival hyperplasia and hirsutism. With long-term follow-up, it has become apparent that up to 15% to 20% of patients treated with calcineurin inhibitors experience chronic renal insufficiency requiring dialysis and/or renal transplantation (Ojo et al., 2003). The nephrotoxicity of cyclosporine is thought to result from its vasoconstrictor effects on renal blood vessels. Although early toxicity resulting in renal dysfunction may be reversible, the late stages of cyclosporine nephrotoxicity resulting in advanced tubular interstitial fibrosis and scarring may be irreversible. Now cyclosporine is used less frequently since other potent immunosuppressive drugs became available (see below).

2.3.2 Tacrolimus

The introduction of tacrolimus has further improved the remarkable results previously obtained with cyclosporine by reducing rejection rates and improving long term graft function and survival (Busuttil et al., 2004).

Tacrolimus (FK506) is a metabolite of the fungus *Streptomyces tsukubaensis.* The mechanism of action of tacrolimus is identical to that of cyclosporine. Upon entering the cytoplasm, it binds to an immunophilin referred to as FK-binding protein 12 and inhibits calcineurin, preventing the dephosphorylation of the transcription factor NFAT and inhibiting the transcription of cytokines necessary for rejection. Tacrolimus has gradually replaced cyclosporine in many transplant programs since it was found to be much more potent then cyclosporine. Indeed, its first successful use was reported as rescue therapy for rejected liver grafts failing conventional therapy (Starzl et al., 1989). Subsequently, tacrolimus has gradually been included in routine immunosuppression protocols in liver transplantation. Multicenter trials compared the efficacy and safety of tacrolimus with cyclosporine and showed that tacrolimus was associated with significantly fewer episodes of corticosteroid resistant or refractory rejection, although graft survival and patient survival were not significantly different; additional findings included a lower incidence of chronic rejection and infection. (The U.S. Multicenter FK506 Liver Study Group, 1994; European FK506 Multicentre Liver Study Group, 1994)

Since the early 1990s, an increasing number of patients receiving liver, kidney, heart, and heart-lung has been successfully immunosuppressed with tacrolimus-based regimens rather than cyclosporine. In addition, tacrolimus has made a significant impact on the outcomes of intestinal transplantation (see below). As a result, currently many transplant programs worldwide have adopted tacrolimus-based immunosuppressive regimens. However, like for cyclosporine, the toxicity profile of tacrolimus has become evident with studies showing that the use of tacrolimus is associated with higher risk of diabetes post-transplant and with incidence of nephrotoxicity and neurotoxicity comparable or higher than those of cyclosporine (Ekberg et al., 2007).

Tacrolimus is administered twice daily. To improve compliance with the medication a modified-release once daily dose form of tacrolimus has been developed and shown to have equivalent systemic exposure of conventional twice-daily tacrolimus (Cross et al., 2007) and similar efficacy in preventing kidney (Kramer et al., 2010) and liver (Truneka et al., 2010) transplant rejection.

2.4 Mycophenolic acid

Mycophenolate mofetil and mycophenolate sodium are similar pro-drugs both converted to the active compound mycophenolic acid by liver metabolism and they will be discussed together. Mycophenolic acid emerged as a new immunosuppressive agent in the early 1990s with a mechanism of action different from CNI (Mele et al., 2000) (Stewart et al., 2001). Whereas cyclosporine and tacrolimus both inhibit the enzyme calcineurin and the induction of cytokine synthesis soon after T cell activation, mycophenolic acid has no direct effect on the production of cytokines but prevents T and B cell proliferation by inhibiting a pathway required for cell division. Mycophenolic acid is a selective and noncompetitive inhibitor of inosine monophosphate dehydrogenase, which is an important enzyme in the *de novo* pathway of guanine nucleotide synthesis. This results in the inhibition of DNA synthesis in T and B lymphocytes thereby inhibiting cell proliferation and function. Other cell types can use salvage pathways and are not affected, therefore the effects of mycophenolic acid are largely on the immune cells with few effects on the non-immune system. Clinically, mycophenolate acid has largely replaced azathioprine because of its fewer myelotoxic and hepatotoxic side effects. It is usually combined into a regimen including a calcineurin inhibitor and steroids.

Since the 1990s, when large, double-blind, randomized trials in kidney transplant recipients showed the efficacy of mycophenolate acid in preventing early acute rejection in combination with cyclosporine and prednisone, this drug has been used widely as a part of various combination regimens of immunosuppressive agents. Common mycophenolic acid-related side effects comprise gastrointestinal symptoms such as abdominal pain, diarrhea and nausea, infections (cytomegalovirus) and myelosuppression, namely anemia and leucocytopenia, malignancy (post-transplant lymphoproliferative disorders and non melanoma skin cancer).

Mycophenolate sodium is an enteric-coated preparation that allows delayed release of the active drug in the small intestine rather than the stomach. This may help alleviate some of the gastrointestinal side effects of mycophenolate mofetil. There is no significant difference in rejection and side effects in large randomized trial of mycophenolate mofetil versus mycophenolate sodium (Ciancio et al., 2011). The ability of mycophenolic acid to facilitate sparing of other immunosuppressive agents, particularly cyclosporine and its related nephrotoxicity, is promising. By permitting reduction in cyclosporine doses, mycophenolic acid may stabilize or improve renal graft function in patients with cyclosporine-related nephrotoxicity or chronic allograft nephropathy.

2.5 mTOR inhibitors

The mTOR inhibitors sirolimus and everolimus are among the most recently introduced immunosuppressive agents with a mechanism of action different from CNI and from antimetabolites. Sirolimus (or rapamycin) is a macrolide antibiotic, structurally similar to tacrolimus, isolated from the fungus *Streptomyces hygroscopicus* in 1968 and found to have immunosuppressive properties in the late 1980s. Like the calcineurin inhibitors, sirolimus acts by binding to an intracellular immunophilin FKB12. This complex sirolimus-immunophilin inhibits a protein called mammalian target of rapamycin (*mTOR)*. Inhibition of mTOR results in selective inhibition of synthesis of new ribosomal proteins which are essential for progression of the cells from the G1 to the S phase. This results in blockage of T cell activation. In addition, sirolimus has been associated with inhibition of fibroblast growth factors required for tissue repair. This antifibrotic effect has two potentially beneficial effects after transplantation in reducing the progression to fibrosis in post liver transplant hepatitis C recurrence (see below) and in reducing the risk of malignancy in transplant recipients because of its antiangiogenic effects (Geisler et al., 2010).

The half life of sirolimus is 60 hours which allows single daily dose unlike other agents given twice daily and this has an important impact on patient compliance to immunosuppression regimens. Everolimus is a modified form of sirolimus to improve its absoprion. Its half life is shorter and is administred twice daily. Everolimus is currently undergoing clinical trials in liver transplantation. In addition to being used as immunosuppressant, it has been investigated in the treatment of renal cell carcinoma for its proliferation signal inhibition and in drug-coated stents to prevent restenosis of coronary arteries for its antifibrotic effect (Gabardi et al., 2010)

There have been a number of studies investigating the impact of adding sirolimus to low dose CNI regimens in order to reduce nephrotoxicity of CNI after kidney (Schena et al., 2009), liver (Harper et al., 2011) and heart (Raichlin et al., 2007) transplantation. The use of sirolimus with mycophenolate mofetil or azathioprine to avoid *de novo* CNI exposure has improved glomerular filtration rate for at least two years in most studies in kidney transplantation with comparable incidence of rejection, however experience is limited in liver and heart transplantation. However, there have been also reports of an increased risk of nephrotoxicity when combining sirolimus with high doses calcineurin inhibitors (Kahan, 2000)

Sirolimus, unlike calcineurin inhibitors, has been shown to enhance the development and function of regulatory T cells, a subset of CD4(+)CD25(+) lymphocytes with the ability to suppress alloimmune responses in vitro and in vivo. It is therefore being evaluated as a component of strategies to promote tolerance in organ transplant recipients (Knektle 2010).

In intestinal transplant recipients the introduction of sirolimus in tacrolimus-based regimens has significantly delayed the onset and reduced the severity of rejection (see below).

The adverse effects of sirolimus include thrombocytopenia, leukopenia, anemia, arthralgias, hyperlipidemia, pneumonitis, and diarrhea. There have also been reports of wound complications (delayed wound healing, incisional hernia) in the post-transplant period, an affect probably secondary to its antiproliferative effects on fibroblasts. Oral ulcers were seen with the liquid preparation; however, this seems to be less frequent with the use of the pill preparation.

2.6 Antibodies

The use of antibodies as part of the immunosuppression regimen post-transplant dates from the beginning of clinical transplantation when anti-lymphocyte globulin (ALG) prepared from the serum of horses or rabbits inoculated with human lymphocytes was added to azathioprine and steroids. In 1986 muromonab CD3, a monoclonal antibody (mAb) targeting CD3, was first approved for prevention and treatment of renal allograft rejection. Originally, the rationale for the use of antibodies as immunosuppressants was to deplete and block the function of immune competent cells. The purified IgG fraction of polyclonal antibody preparations is directed against cell-surface molecules expressed on T cells, B cells, NK cells and macrophages, causing complement mediated cell lysis, uptake of opsonised cells by the reticulo-endothelial system and modulation of surface receptors of lymphocytes. Infact the administration of polyclonal antibodies results in profound lymphopenia. Polyclonal antibodies are obtained by inoculating rabbits or horses with human lymphocytes or thymocytes. Currently available preparations include Thymoglobulin and Atgam. Monoclonal antibodies are produced in response to a single antigen. These include the mouse monoclonal antibody muromonab (OKT3), which is specific to the CD3 receptor and was the first monoclonal antibody to be used in transplantation to treat acute rejection. Other monoclonal antibodies include the anti-IL-2 receptor antibodies daclizumab and basiliximab, anti CD20 rituximab, antiCD52 alemtuzumab. Other new mAbs are emerging, targeting co-stimulatory signals, cell surface receptors and novel protein constructs.

Antibodies are further classified into lymphocyte-depleting or nondepleting agents (review Klipa et al., 2010) The total lymphocyte counts and CD3 counts are usually measured during therapy to monitor the achievement of effective depletion and to make dose adjustments in case of incomplete depletion.

Currently, antibodies are administered as induction immunosuppression to the majority of kidney, pancreas and intestine transplant recipients in the United States, and less frequently to liver recipients. Induction therapy, as opposed to maintenance immunosuppression, refers to the use of biological agents and high dose steroids to prevent immune engagement and T-cell activation during tissue injury from organ preservation, reperfusion, and alloresponse immediately after transplant. The agents most commonly used are thymoglobulin and alemtuzumab (depleting) and basiliximab, daclizumab and rituximab (non depleting) (review in Aparna et al., 2009).

The benefits of induction therapy include a decreased incidence and delayed onset of acute rejection, and also delayed introduction of or lowering dose of CNI in the early post-transplant period allowing for peri-operative renal dysfunction to recover. Other uses of antibodies are in desensitization protocols in sensitized kidney transplant recipients (see below) and in the treatment of steroid resistant rejection. Rituximab has also been used to treat antibody-mediated rejection in kidney transplant (Kaposztas et al., 2009). In addition to considerable cost, side effects include cytokine release phenomena secondary to cytolysis and characterized by fevers, chills, hypotension. Other side effects are nausea, diarrhea, arthralgias, thrombocytopenia, dyspnea, and seizures. The risk of infection and of posttransplantation lymphoproliferative disease is increased with antibody therapy.

2.7 New immunosuppressive drugs

Different pathways and stages of the immunologic response are the target of strategies to develop new immunosuppressive drugs: cell-surface molecules, signaling mechanisms, T-cell proliferation, cell trafficking and cell recruitment.

New immunosuppressive drugs include mainly proteins targeting T-cell and B-cell surface receptors and non-protein drugs (also called small molecules) targeting intracellular pathways.

Belatacept is a fusion protein composed of the Fc fragment of a human IgG1 immunoglobulin linked to the extracellular domain of CTLA-4. (review Weclawiak et al., 2010) It represents a new class of immunosuppressants. Unlike calcineurin inhibitors that block or diminish the effects of T-cell activation on allografts, belatacept prevents T-cell activation by selectively blocking T-cell costimulation molecules. In the initial trial in kidney transplant recipients it was as effective as cyclosporine in preventing acute rejection but with better preservation of kidney function and reduction of chronic allograft nephropathy (Vincenti et al., 2005) The stability of graft function and the safety profile of belatacept at 5 years has been reported in a subsequent study (Vincenti et al., 2010).

Memory T cells play a crucial role in acute and chronic rejection and are a potent barrier to transplantation tolerance. **Alefacept**, a fusion protein combining Leukocyte Function associated Antigen-3 (LFA3) with IgG currently approved for psoriasis, binds to CD2 on T cells (Ellis et al, 2001). Unlike belatacept that prevents activation of naïve T cells, alefacept targets memory T cells (Weaver et al., 2008) since CD2 is espressed more on memory than naïve T cells.

Efalizumab (Dedrick et al., 2002) is a humanized antiCD11a (LFA1) monoclonal antibody used in patients with chronic plaque psoriasis (Kuschei et al., 2011). It blocks the binding of LFA1 to intracellular adhesion molecule-1 (ICAM-1) causing loss of activation, adhesion and migration of T-cells. Preliminary experience with efalizumab in kidney transplantation showed efficacy in controlling rejection but raised concern of overimmunosuppression since 8% of patients developed post-transplant lymphoproliferative disease (Vincenti et al., 2007).

New non-protein drugs (also identified as small molecules) target intracellular pathways of the immune response to the allograft, such as Janus kinase proteins (JAK), which mediate signal transmission between cell membrane receptors and the nucleus. The immunosuppressive effect of inhibition of JAK3 results from blocking the signaling of the gamma chain subfamily of cytokines (interleukins 2, 4, 7, 9, 15 and 21). **Tofacitinib**, a Janus kinase 1/3 inhibitor developed for the treatment of rheumatoid arthritis (Flanagan et al., 2010) prolonged kidney allograft survival in cynomolgus monkeys without concomitant use of calcineurin inhibitor (Borie et al., 2005). In clinical kidney transplantation it has been used in a calcineurin inhibitor- free regimen (Busque et al., 2009). This study reported comparable acute rejection rates between tofacitinib and tacrolimus-based immunosuppression but raised concern of overimmunosuppression in the form of increased BK virus infection rates.

Two new other biologic agents being developed are **4D11,** a costimulation blockade agent targeting CD40 (Aoyagi et al., 2009) and **natalizumab**, a humanized IgG4 approved for multiple sclerosis and Crohn's disease targeting alpha4 submunit of integrins thus inhibiting leucocyte adhesion (Hutchinson 2010).

Voclosporine (ISA247) is a novel oral semisynthetic structural analogue of cyclosporine that has been modified at the first amino acid residue of the molecule. This drug has been shown to be more potent than cyclosporine in vitro and in vivo in rat heterotopic heart transplantation. The advantage of this cyclosporine-analogue drug is the lack of nephrotoxicity. There is still limited experience with this drug in clinical transplantation.

Preliminary results show non-inferiority to tacrolimus in preventing rejection (Gaber et al., 2008). More data is needed on the efficacy and safety profile in the long term.
Protein kinases (PKC) play a key role in signaling pathways downstream of the T-cell receptor (signal 1) and CD28 (signal 2) and thereby are involved in early T-cell activation. There are several isoforms of PKC. PKCh is largely restricted toT lymphocytes and mediates activation of the transcription factors activator protein-1 and nuclear factor (NF) jB, leading to downstream IL-2 production. The PKCh knockout mice demonstrate impaired T-cell activation. **Sotrastaurin (AEB071)** is a new oral low molecular weight compound that effectively blocks early T-cell activation by selective inhibition of PKC and therefore has a different mechanism of action from that of the CNIs. (Kovarik et al., 2011)
In kidney transplantation the deleterious effects of the humoral (antibody-mediated) component of acute rejection and their impact on long term graft survival are being increasingly recognized. This has prompted the development of more targeted antihumoral therapies. **Bortezomib** is an antineoplastic agent originally developed for the treatment of multiple myeloma. It is a proteasome inhibitor that induces apoptosis in rapidly dividing cells with active protein synthesis like plasma cells. In kidney transplantation it has been reported to revert antibody-mediated rejection (Perry et al., 2009, Walsh et al., 2010). Early antibody-mediated rejection demonstrated increased response to proteasome inhibitors than late AMR (Walsh et al.,2011)

3. Immunosuppression in kidney transplantation

Kidney transplant is the most frequently performed among abdominal organ transplants and in 2010 16,896 patients received a kidney transplant in the United States, 37% of which were from live donor. (unos) (http://optn.transplant.hrsa.gov/latestData/rptData.asp). The advantages of live-donor versus deceased donor kidney transplant are multiple including shorter time on the waiting list, shorter cold ischemia time (ie the interval between organ procurement and transplantantation), less preservation injury and overall better graft function in the short and long term. However, the immunologic risk in live-donor kidney transplant is not inferior to deceased donor, even in case of live-related donor (ie between non-identical siblings). On the contrary, live donor kidney transplant is becoming a bigger immunological challenge than deceased donor with the increasing number of transplants performed in highly sensitized or ABO incompatible recipients (see below).
There are several immunosuppression protocols currently used in kidney transplantation, but the majority include induction with depleting or non-depleting antibodies and maintenance immunosuppression based on a combination of agents (usually triple therapy) including CNI, mycophenolic acid, sirolimus and steroids.
Current acute rejection rate is 10-15% (Gaston et al., 2009) and usually the function of the graft is maintained after treatment of the rejection episode. Immunosuppression regimens currently available are very effective in treating episodes of acute rejection so that graft loss due to acute rejection has now become a rare event. Instead, chronic rejection (or chronic allograft nephropathy) remains a major cause of graft loss, usually a late event (years) after transplant. The causes of chronic allograft nephropathy and graft loss are multiple including repeated episodes of rejection, disease recurrence, CNI toxicity and others. Indeed, one of the main side effects of CNI is nephrotoxicity, affecting up to 16% of non-renal transplant recipients at 3 years and resulting in end stage kidney disease requiring dialysis in 5-20% of patients 5 years after transplant (Ojo et al.,2003). This prompted the design of several trials

of CNI withdrawal, minimization or avoidance in an attempt to limit the impact of CNI nephrotoxicity. However, CNI cannot be avoided completely in kidney transplantation without paying the price of high rejection rate up to 53% within the first year (Vincenti et al., 2001). So another approach would be to reduce CNI (Ekberg et al., 2007).

Increasing attention is being recently devoted to the role of late antibody mediated rejection causing chronic sub-acute immune mediated injury. Chronic antibody mediated injury is being recognized as a cause of late graft loss and is a process that is not controlled by CNI or other current drugs (Colvin 2010, Kirk et al., 2010).

Highly sensitized and ABO-incompatible recipients

Immunologic sensitization in a transplant candidate refers to the presence of pre-formed antibodies and it is measured as PRA (Panel of Reactive Antibodies), which express the percentage of the antigenic repertoire in the general population to which the transplant candidate has developed antibodies (0-100%). The causes of sensitization are multiple and include blood transfusions, previous transplant, pregnancies and infections. Highly sensitized patients have PRA of 80% or higher. These patients are at greater risk of rejection and graft loss than non-sensitized patients. In addition, highly sensitized patients are likely to wait longer for a 0-mismatch kidney graft than non-sensitized patients. This has prompted the development of desensitization protocols to enable highly sensitized patients to receive a successful transplant in a timely manner. The aim of desensitization protocols is to reduce the amount of circulating HLA antibodies and to prevent the formation of new antibodies. Strategies currently adopted to achieve these goals include plasmapheresis to remove HLA antibodies, intravenous immunoglobulins (IvIg) to neutralize circulating antibodies and to inhibit complement activation, rituximab (a chimeric anti CD20 monoclonal antibody) to deplet B cells and, more recently, bortezomib, a proteasome inhibitor that targets plasma cells (see above). The protocol at our Institute also includes mycophenolate sodium started the week before transplant as part of the strategy to control the B cell component of the immune response (Melancon et al., 2011) Current results of desensitization programs demonstrate graft function and graft survival comparable to non-sensitized patients (Montgomery et al., 2010, Melancon et al., 2011, Niederhaus et al., 2011).

Until recently, another barrier to a successful kidney transplant has been ABO-incompatibility between donor and recipient (ie donor blood type is A or B and recipient blood type is O). Over the last decade this barrier has been overcome in some transplant centers by the implementation of programs of paired kidney exchange and antibody reduction therapies in which a number of donor-recipient pairs are entered into a pool and matched according to blood type compatibility (Montgomery et al., 2006) (Melancon et al., 2011). In addition to entering an exchange program, the recipient of an ABO incompatible pair with high isohemoagglutinin titers can also be treated with plasmapheresis and anti-B cell agents to reduce the isohemoagglutinin titer to 1:16 or below, a level considered safe to proceed with ABO incompatible transplant. Since the number of kidneys from deceased donors remains inadequate, living kidney donation has allowed for more patients to be removed from the waiting list. Programs of paired kidney exchange and the implementation of antibody reduction therapies have allowed the use of ABO incompatible donors and also the inclusion of non-directed *good Samaritan* donors, who enter the system with a desire to donate a kidney to someone for purely altruistic purposes. These strategies have all contributed to magnify the opportunities for a successful transplant for patients who otherwise would have had to wait 5-7 years for a matched kidney from deceased donor. In our recent series, all patients received a transplant within 90 days of their initial evaluation for living donor transplantation (Melancon et al., 2011).

4. Immunosuppression in liver transplantation

Liver transplantation has become an established treatment for patients with decompensated cirrhosis and acute liver failure and today the liver is the second most commonly performed abdominal organ transplant. Currently, 6,000 liver transplants are performed in the US yearly (unos). (http://optn.transplant.hrsa.gov/ar2009/Chapter_IV_AR_CD.htm?cp=5#TOC).

In parallel to the success of kidney transplantation, the outcomes of liver transplantation have continued to improve over the last two decades following better surgical techniques and the introduction of more potent immunosuppression. The introduction of cyclosporine first and later tacrolimus has allowed to control the rejection rate and prolong allograft survival ((Starzl et al., 1985, Busuttil et al., 2004). Especially tacrolimus has played an important role in liver transplantation since its introduction by allowing to rescue grafts from cyclosporine resistant rejection (Starzl et al., 1989). As a result, cyclosporine is less commonly used today in liver transplantation and most immunosuppression protocols are based on tacrolimus, associated to mycophenolic acid and steroids (reviewed in Geissler et al., 2009 and Pillai et al., 2009).

Usually liver transplant recipients do not receive antibody-based induction immunosuppression. Rather, high-dose methylprednisolone (500 mg - 1 g) is given intravenously as induction at the time of implantation of the liver and rapidly tapered from the time of surgery to a daily maintenance dose of 5 to 10 mg per day. Many programs taper and discontinue prednisone at 3 to 6 months to avoid the side effects of long-term prednisone use. Prednisone cessation does not seem to have a negative impact on graft function. Indeed, steroid withdrawal trials have demonstrated that corticosteroid-free regimens do not lead to increased rejection rates. However, in patients transplanted for immune-mediated liver disease such as primary biliary cirrhosis, primary sclerosing cholangitis and autoimmune hepatitis it seems prudent to maintain prednisone therapy in the long term, albeit at a low-dose, in order to reduce the risk of disease recurrence.

Corticosteroids are also used in the treatment of episodes of acute cellular rejection: intravenous methylprednisolone is usually given at a dose of 1,000 mg on alternate days for a total of 3 doses, followed by taper.

Acute rejection does not impact on graft function in the long term in the vast majority of cases given the resilience and the regenerative capacity of the liver as opposed to kidney or other solid organs.

An important issue in immunosuppression in liver transplant recipients is the prevention of nephrotoxicity associated with CNI. Chronic renal damage is affecting up to 16% of non-renal transplant recipients treated with CNI (Ojo et al., 2003) and the search for the best renal sparing immunosuppression strategy in liver transplantation is still ongoing. A key factor seems to be the tailoring of the immunosuppression *regimen* to the individual patient. In patients with renal insufficiency at the time of transplant one strategy is to hold calcineurin inhibitors and to use an IL-2 receptor blocker as induction agent. This will obtain effective immunosuppression early post-transplant allowing the introduction of CNI to be delayed until after resolution of peri-operative renal dysfunction. In the event of non-recovery of renal function, the addition of sirolimus may be considered. A number of studies have reported on the use of sirolimus in patients with renal insufficiency after liver transplantation and especially in those with calcineurin inhibitor (CNI)-associated nephrotoxicity. The results of these studies have not been conclusive. A recent meta-analysis showed that conversion to sirolimus from CNIs in LT recipients with renal insufficiency [glomerular filtration rate (GFR) < 60 mL/minute or creatinine level ≥ 1.5 mg/dL] is associated with a non-significant improvement in renal function. In addition, although patient and graft survival were not significantly different, infections, ulcers and discontinuation of therapy were significantly more common in patients treated with sirolimus compared to control (Asrani et al., 2010). This adds to an earlier concern raised by previous randomized studies when sirolimus was first tried in liver transplantation in 1999. One study (Wiesner et al 2002) reported increased risk of hepatic artery thrombosis and death compared to standard immunosuppression. This study was interrupted and led the FDA to issue an alert on the use of sirolimus in liver transplant. (http://www.fda.gov/Drugs/DrugSafety/PostmarketDrugSafetyInformationforPatientsandProviders/DrugSafetyInformationforHeathcareProfessionals/ucm165015.htm).

However, sirolimus is currently being used by transplant programs in selected patients. A recent single center retrospective study on 148 patients converted to sirolimus at any time post-transplant for renal function impairment or for progression of fibrosis in HCV positive recipients documents that sirolimus was safe and effective with low rejection rates (3.4%) and no cases of hepatic artery thrombosis (Harper et al., 2011). Another large single center retrospective study reported on the safety and efficacy of sirolimus in liver transplant with lower incidence of rejection and similar survival rates compared to other regimens (Campsen et al., 2011).

Finally, other recent studies have reported that the antifibrotic and antiangiogenic effects of sirolimus may have a favorable impact in HCV positive recipients and patients transplanted for hepatocellular carcinoma, respectively (see below).

A special consideration has been given over the last few years to immunosuppression regimens used in HCV positive liver transplant recipients. HCV-related cirrhosis is now the most common indication for liver transplantation in the US and HCV recurrence in the graft is a major risk factor for graft loss. To date there is no single best strategy to successfully prevent HCV recurrence post-transplant, although new antivirals are being developed that may have a positive impact. The management of immunosuppression in HCV liver transplant recipients has been the focus of several studies but consensus on the best immunosuppression regimen in HCV recipients is lacking. However, it seems to be now accepted in many centers that the use of steroids, especially high-dose intravenous boluses to treat acute cellular rejection should be considered very carefully in patients with hepatitis C because of the risk of severe recurrence of hepatitis C. (Berenguer 2011). Therefore, the prevention of rejection by obtaining and maintaining adequate levels of tacrolimus from the very early post-operative period is very important. Cyclosporine has been suggested to be superior to tacrolimus in controlling HCV recurrence post-transplant given the antiviral effects of cyclosporine in vitro but clinical trials failed to confirm this expectation and currently there is no evidence that the choice of CNI (cyclosporine or tacrolimus) makes a significant difference in outcome in HCV recipients (Berenguer et al., 2010). Antiviral therapy with interferon and ribavirin is an option in selected transplant recipients with recurrent HCV: progression to cirrhosis is slower, risk of graft decompensation is lower and patient survival is longer in responders to antiviral treatment compared to non-responders (Berenguer et al., 2008). However, the pro-inflammatory effects of interferon increase the risk of acute rejection, chronic rejection and de-novo autoimmune hepatitis post-transplant

(Nazia et al., 2011). Pre-transplant antiviral treatment is poorly tolerated in Child C patients (Melero et al., 2009).

The antifibrotic effect of sirolimus has been considered to have a potential impact on slowing down fibrosis progression in HCV-positive recipients (Wagner et al., 2010). A recent study on 88 patients treated with sirolimus-based immunosuppression reports that, although timing or severity of post-transplant HCV recurrence were not affected, hepatitis activity and fibrosis scores were lower on serial biopsy compared to conventional immunosuppression regimens (Asthana et al., 2011). Further studies will have to confirm the role of sirolimus in HCV-infected grafts.

Liver transplantation is the most radical and successful treatment for selected patients with hepatocellular carcinoma (HCC) who fulfill transplant criteria. Tumor recurrence affects 10-20% of patients within 2 years after transplant and is a major determinant of patient survival. Multiple factors determine the risk of recurrence of HCC after liver transplant, including staging and biologic aggressivity of HCC. Post-transplant immunosuppression increases the risk of tumor recurrence and the choice of the immunosuppression regimen may have an impact on outcomes. Drugs like mTOR inhibitors (sirolimus, see above) effectively reduce cell growth and angiogenesis in animal models of hepatocellular cancer (review in Treiber 2009) and may have a role in reducing the risk of recurrence in patients transplanted for HCC. In a recent study patients transplanted for HCC and treated with sirolimus had lower recurrence rates than patients treated with tacrolimus (Chinnakotla et al., 2009); a subsequent study on registry data confirmed better survival rates in sirolimus patients compared to non-sirolimus (Toso et al., 2010).

New drugs are being developed for the treatment of HCC. Sorafenib is a tyrosine kinase inhibitor shown to increase survival in patients with advanced HCC (Llovet et al., 2008). Trials are ongoing on the use of sorafenib to prevent recurrence after transplant (Villanueva et al., 2011).

Currently, antibodies are not commonly used in liver transplantation. OKT3 has been in the past the most commonly used monoclonal antibody in liver transplantation. It was originally introduced in 1987 for prophylaxis of acute cellular rejection but now it is mainly used in patients with steroid-resistant cellular rejection. The use of OKT3 and of other depleting agents is associated with early and severe recurrences of hepatitis C and must be used with caution in this cohort of patients. (Rosen et al., 1997, Eghtesad et al., 2005)

Two non-depleting IL-2 receptor antibodies, daclizumab and basiliximab, are being used in liver transplantation for induction immunosuppression in patients with renal failure to allow a delayed introduction of CNI (Verna et al., 2011).

Alemtuzumab has been used in tolerance inducing protocols in liver transplantation but is not currently used outside research protocols (Weissenbacher et al., 2010).

5. Immunosuppression in pancreas transplantation

Currently about 1,100 patients receive a pancreas transplant in the US per year. The main indication is to restore normoglycemia in patients with type I diabetes on high insulin regimens to improve or at least to arrest the progression of diabetic nephropathy, retinopathy and neuropathy. The advantages of pancreas transplant versus insulin therapy in obtaining normoglycemia have been well documented (Gremizzi et al., 2010). Hypoglycemia unawareness, a complication of insulin therapy, is also an indication for pancreas transplant. Since the year 2000 islet cell transplant has been introduced as an alternative less invasive treatment for diabetes (Shapiro et al., 2000) with reports of variable success over the years (review in (de Kort et al., 2011)). The long term function of transplanted islets remains an unresolved issue. Recent studies report that pancreas transplant obtains higher rates of and longer lasting insulin independence compared to islet cell transplant, but with higher risk of surgical complications (Vardanyan et al., 2010, Maffi et al., 2011). The immunological aspects and immunosuppression regimens specific to islet transplant have been extensively reviewed (Azzi et al., 2010) and will not be discussed here.

The pancreas is transplanted either simultaneously with the kidney for patients with renal failure due to type 1 diabetes mellitus or as isolated pancreas. In addition, the pancreas is included in the multivisceral graft for selected patients transplanted for intestinal failure (see below). Advances in surgical techniques and immunosuppression management have obtained current pancreas graft survival rates of 86% at 1 year, between 60 and 80% at 3 years and 53% at 10 years, respectively (Gruessner et al., 2010).

Most pancreas transplant recipients receive induction therapy with T-cell-depleting agents thymoglobulin or alemtuzumab and maintenance immunosuppression with a combination of CNI (mostly tacrolimus), mycophenolate mofetil, sirolimus and rapid steroid withdrawal (review in Heilman et al., 2010). The incidence of acute rejection after pancreas transplant is reported between 20 and 35% at 3 years (Farney et al., 2009). Like in kidney transplant, the combination of sirolimus with full dose CNI may accentuate nephrotoxicity. There have been trials of elimination of CNI to avoid nephrotoxicity with similar patient and graft survival at 6 months compared to tacrolimus based regimens, but with higher rates of acute rejection (Gruessner et al 2005). Over the last years, more and more maintenance protocols have avoided the use of steroids (Knight et al., 2010).

6. Immunosuppression in intestinal transplantation

Intestinal transplantation is the newest and most recently developed among abdominal organ transplants. Although it has been attempted experimentally for decades since the pioneering work of Lillehei (Lillehei et al 1959), the first successful intestinal transplant in humans was reported in 1990 (Grant et al., 1990). Over the last decade intestinal transplantation has become clinically established as an effective treatment for patients with intestinal failure and life-threatening complications of parenteral nutrition (Fishbein 2009). In recent years 150-180 intestinal transplants are performed in US per year. (unos) http://optn.transplant.hrsa.gov/latestData/rptData.asp

Rejection has been a formidable obstacle to successful intestinal transplantation. The development of effective immunosuppression together with advanced surgical techniques and improved patient management have significantly contributed to the success of intestinal transplantation. Although initially rejection and mortality rates were high, the outcomes of intestinal transplantation have markedly improved over the last decade and now survival rates are close to other solid organ transplants. However, still transplantation of the intestine remains a greater immunologic challenge compared to other solid organs. The high immunogenicity of the intestinal graft is related to its rich composition in lymphoid tissue (80% of the body immune cells reside in the gut) and also to the presence of a complex innate immune system continuously exposed to intraluminal foreign antigens and microbes. A delicate and fine balance between absorption of nutrients and defense from infection is regulated at the level of the intestinal surface and the interplay between innate and acquired components of the immune response at the level of the intestinal mucosa is being better understood in recent years (see below).

The introduction of tacrolimus in the early 1990 and induction immunotherapy (Reyes et al 2005) have decreased the rejection rate from historical rates of 80 or more to 20-40% in most recent series. Episodes of acute rejection are treated with intravenous pulse steroids and/or thymoglobulin, depending on severity. The severity of rejection episodes has been better controlled with the introduction of sirolimus in addition to tacrolimus-based maintenance immunosuppression (Fishbein et al., 2002, Gupta et al., 2005). Infliximab, an anti-tumor necrosis factor alpha antibody used for Crohn's disease, has been successful in isolated cases as salvage therapy in patients with thymoglobulin resistant rejection (De Greef et al., 2011). Immunosuppression protocols continue to evolve (Abu-Elmagd et al., 2009, Pirenne et al., 2009) and different drug combinations are used with the cornerstone for maintenance immunosuppression being tacrolimus.

New insight in intestine transplant function and on new strategies to control allograft rejection comes from studies on gut microflora and innate immunity. The normal intestinal flora is dominated by anaerobic species Bacteroides and Clostridia. Post-transplant the composition of the gut microflora changes and the microbial community is dominated by Lactobacilli and Enterobacteria, which are facultative anaerobes (Hartman et al., 2009). This represents an inversion of the normal flora. After surgical closure of the ileostomy, which is usually undertaken three months post-transplant, the microbial community reverts to the normal flora. Therefore, the transplanted intestine can function with either of two alternate microbial populations. As in patients with inflammatory bowel disease, the functional impact of alterations in the gut microflora is only recently being recognized and may have implications for the management of intestinal transplant rejection.

The nucleotide-binding oligomerization domain 2 (NOD2) is an intracellular sensor for pathogen/microbe associated molecular patterns that recognizes a component of the bacterial cell wall. NOD2 protein is a critical regulator of bacterial immunity in the intestine and is required for the expression of intestinal anti-microbial peptides. Mutations of NOD2 are highly correlated with Crohn's disease. We found that 35% of intestinal transplant recipients have NOD2 mutations associated with Crohn's disease and that the risk severe rejection and of graft failure were significantly greater in the NOD2 mutant recipients compared with the NOD2 wild-type recipients (Fishbein et al 2008). The presence of a NOD2 polymorphism in the recipient may influence the viability of the allograft by interrupting NOD2- dependent circuits required to maintain intestinal homeostasis with respect to commensal flora: a recipient lacking a functional intestinal microbial-sensing system may be more exposed to allograft damage secondary to rejection than a recipient with an intact system.

7. Future perspectives

Renal function impairment, opportunistic infections (Cytomegalovirus, Epstein-Barr related post-transplant lymphoproliferative disease and others) and metabolic disorders (diabetes and others) are frequent complications of prolonged immunosuppression and remain a major challenge to improve the long term outcomes of transplant recipients. Future strategies to limit the impact of these complications include the development of new non-nephrotoxic agents, the individualization of organ-specific immunosuppression regimens tailored to patient needs and the design of protocols of minimization of immunosuppression and tolerance induction. Studies on gene expression profiling and other methods derived from the -omics approach will further contribute to characterize the rejection process and to monitor the immune response.

The role of B cells and antibodies is increasingly being investigated and recognized as a target for treatment. The presence and persistence of donor-specific antibodies in the long term follow-up of kidney transplant recipients led to the recognition that chronic antibody mediated injury may be responsible for late graft loss. (Colvin 2010). This has prompted interest in new **B-cell** based therapeutic strategies and trials are under way involving agents to control humoral immunity.
The contribution of memory T cells (Lo et al., 2011) and of systemic complement activation (Damman et al., 2011) to the rejection process will also be better characterized by ongoing trials.

8. References

Abu-Elmagd KM, Costa G, Bond GJ, Wu T, Murase N, Zeevi A, et al. (2009). Evolution of the immunosuppressive strategies for the intestinal and multivisceral recipients with special reference to allograft immunity and achievement of partial tolerance. *Transplant International* 22 :96–109.

Adcock IM, Ito K. (2000).Molecular mechanisms of corticosteroid actions. *Monaldi Arch Chest Dis* 55(3):256–66.

Aoyagi T, Yamashita K, Suzuki T, Uno M, Goto R, Taniguchi M, et al. (2009). A human anti-CD40 monoclonal antibody, 4D11, for kidney transplantation in cynomolgus monkeys: induction and maintenance therapy. *Am J Transplant.* 9(8):1732-41.

Aparna P, Augustine JJ, Hricik DE. (2009).Induction Antibody Therapy in Kidney Transplantation. *Am J Kidney Dis* 54:935-944.

Asrani SK, Leise MD, West CP, Murad MH, Pedersen RA, Erwin PJ, Tian J, Wiesner RH, Kim WR (2010). Use of sirolimus in liver transplant recipients with renal insufficiency: a systematic review and meta-analysis. *Hepatology.* 52(4):1360-70.

Asthana S, Toso C, Meeberg G (2011). The impact of sirolimus on hepatitis C recurrence after liver transplantation. *Can J Gastroenterol,* 25(1):28-34.

Azzi J, Geara AS, El-Sayegh S, Abdi R. (2010).Immunological aspects of pancreatic islet cell transplantation. *Expert Rev Clin Immunol.* 6(1):111-24.

Berenguer M, Palau A, Aguilera V, Rayón JM, Juan FS, Prieto M. (2008).Clinical benefits of antiviral therapy in patients with recurrent hepatitis C following liver transplantation. *Am J Transplant.* 8(3):679-87.

Berenguer M, Aguilera V, San Juan F, Benlloch S, Rubin A, López-Andujar R, Moya A, Pareja E, Montalva E, Yago M, de Juan M, Mir J, Prieto M. (2010). Effect of calcineurin inhibitors in the outcome of liver transplantation in hepatitis C virus-positive recipients. *Transplantation.* 90(11):1204-9.

Berenguer M. (2011).Hot topic debate on HCV: The type of immunosuppression does not matter. *Liver Transpl.* Jun 1. doi: 10.1002/lt.22347. [Epub ahead of print]

Borie DC, Changelian PS, Larson MJ et al.(2005). Immunosuppression by the JAK3 inhibitor CP-690,550 delays rejection and significantly prolongs kidney allograft survival in nonhuman primates. *Transplantation* 79: 791–801

Busque S, Leventhal J, Brennan DC, Steinberg S, Klintmalm G, Shah T, Mulgaonkar S, Bromberg JS, Vincenti F, Hariharan S, Slakey D, Peddi VR, Fisher RA, Lawendy N, Wang C, Chan G.(2009). Calcineurin-inhibitor-free immunosuppression based on the JAK inhibitor CP-690,550: a pilot study in de novo kidney allograft recipients. *Am J Transplant.* 9(8):1936-45

Busuttil RW, Lake JR.(2004). Role of tacrolimus in the evolution of liver transplantation. *Transplantation*. 77(9 Suppl):S44-51.

Calne RY (1961) Inhibition of the rejection of renal homografts in dogs by purine analogues. *Transpl Bull* 28(2):445-461

Campsen J, Zimmerman MA, Mandell S, Kaplan M, Kam I. (2011). A Decade of Experience Using mTor Inhibitors in Liver Transplantation. *J Transplant*. 2011;2011:913094. Epub 2011 Mar 15.

Chinnakotla S, Davis GL, Vasani S.(2009). Impact of sirolimus on the recurrence of hepatocellular carcinoma after liver transplantation. *Liver Transpl*, 15(12): 1834-42.

Ciancio G, Gaynor JJ, Zarak A, Sageshima J, Guerra G, Roth D, Brown R, Kupin W, Chen L, Tueros L, Hanson L, Ruiz P, Burke GW 3rd.(2011) Randomized trial of mycophenolate mofetil versus enteric-coated mycophenolate sodium in primary renal transplantation with tacrolimus and steroid avoidance: four-year analysis. *Transplantation*. 91(11):1198-1205.

Colvin RB, Hirohashi T, Farris AB, Minnei F, Collins AB, Smith RN. (2010). Emerging role of B cells in chronic allograft dysfunction. *Kidney Int Suppl*. 119:S13-7.

Colvin RB. (2010). Dimensions of antibody-mediated rejection. *Am J Transplant*. 10(7):1509-10.

Cross SA, Perry CM. (2007).Tacrolimus once-daily formulation in the prophylaxis of transplant rejection in renal or liver allograft recipients. *Drugs*. 67(13):1931-43.

Damman J, Seelen MA, Moers C, Daha MR, Rahmel A, Leuvenink HG, Paul A, Pirenne J, Ploeg RJ. (2011) Systemic Complement Activation in Deceased Donors Is Associated With Acute Rejection After Renal Transplantation in the Recipient. *Transplantation*. 92(2):163-169.

Dedrick RL, Walickeb P, Garovoya M. (2002). Anti-adhesion antibodies. Efalizumab, a humanized anti-CD11a monoclonal antibody. *Transplant Immunology* 9: 181–186.

De Greef E, Avitzur Y, Grant D, De-Angelis M, Ng V, Jones N, Ngan B, Shapiro R, Steinberg R, Gana JC. (2011). The Successful Use of Infliximab as Salvage Therapy in Pediatric Intestinal Transplant Patients with Steroid and Thymoglobulin Resistant Late Acute Rejection. *J Pediatr Gastroenterol Nutr*. [Epub ahead of print]

de Kort H, de Koning EJ, Rabelink TJ, Bruijn JA, Bajema IM (2011). Islet transplantation in type 1 diabetes. *BMJ*.;342:d217. doi: 10.1136/bmj.d217.

Eghtesad B, Fung JJ, Demetris AJ, Murase N, Ness R, Bass DC, Gray EA, Shakil O, Flynn B, Marcos A, Starzl TE (2005). Immunosuppression for liver transplantation in HCV-infected patients: mechanism-based principles. *Liver Transpl*. 11(11):1343-52.

Ellis CN, Krueger GG; Alefacept Clinical Study Group.(2001).Treatment of chronic plaque psoriasis by selective targeting of memory effector T lymphocytes. *N Engl J Med*. 345(4):248-55

Ekberg H, Tedesco-Silva H, Demirbas A, Vítko S, Nashan B, Gürkan A, Margreiter R, Hugo C, Grinyó JM, Frei U, Vanrenterghem Y, Daloze P, Halloran PF; ELITE-Symphony Study. (2007) Reduced exposure to calcineurin inhibitors in renal transplantation. *N Engl J Med*. 357(25):2562-75

Ekberg H, Grinyó J, Nashan B, Vanrenterghem Y, Vincenti F, Voulgari A, Truman M, Nasmyth-Miller C, Rashford M. (2007) Cyclosporine sparing with mycophenolate mofetil, daclizumab and corticosteroids in renal allograft recipients: the CAESAR Study. *Am J Transplant*. 7(3):560-70.

Ekberg H, Bernasconi C, Tedesco-Silva H, Vítko S, Hugo C, Demirbas A, Acevedo RR, Grinyó J, Frei U, Vanrenterghem Y, Daloze P, Halloran P. (2009). Calcineurin inhibitor minimization in the Symphony study: observational results 3 years after transplantation. *Am J Transplant.* 9(8):1876-85.

European FK506 Multicentre Liver Study Group.(1994) Randomised trial comparing tacrolimus (FK506) and cyclosporin in prevention of liver allograft rejection. *Lancet.* 344(8920):423-8

Farney AC, Doares W, Rogers J, Singh R, Hartmann E, Hart L, Ashcraft E, Reeves-Daniels A, Gautreaux M, Iskandar SS, Moore P, Adams PL, and Stratta RJ.(2009) A Randomized Trial of Alemtuzumab Versus Antithymocyte Globulin Induction in Renal and Pancreas Transplantation.*Transplantation* 88: 810–819.

Fishbein TM, Florman S, Gondolesi G, Schiano T, LeLeiko N, Tschernia A, Kaufman S. (2002). Intestinal transplantation before and after the introduction of sirolimus. *Transplantation.* 73(10):1538-42

Fishbein T, Novitskiy G, Mishra L, Matsumoto C, Kaufman S, Goyal S, Shetty K, Johnson L, Lu A, Wang A, Hu F, Kallakury B, Lough D, Zasloff M (2008). NOD2-expressing bone marrow-derived cells appear to regulate epithelial innate immunity of the transplanted human small intestine. *Gut.* 57(3):323-30.

Fishbein TM.(2009) Intestinal transplantation. *N Engl J Med.* 361(10):998-1008.

Flanagan ME, Blumenkopf TA,Brissette WH,Brown MF, Casavant JM, Shang-Poa C, Doty JL,Elliott EA, Fisher MB, Hines M, Kent C,Kudlacz EM, Lillie BM, Magnuson KS, McCurdy SP,Munchhof MJ,Perry BD, Sawyer PS, Strelevitz TJ, Subramanyam C,Sun J,Whipple DA, Changelian PS (2010). Discovery of CP-690,550: A Potent and Selective Janus Kinase (JAK) Inhibitor for the Treatment of Autoimmune Diseases and Organ Transplant Rejection *J. Med. Chem.* 53: 8468–8484.

Flechner SM, Kobashigawa J, Klintmalm G.(2008) Calcineurin inhibitor-sparing regimens in solid organ transplantation: focus on improving renal function and nephrotoxicity. *Clin Transplant.* 22(1):1-15.

Gabardi S, Baroletti SA. (2010) Everolimus: a proliferation signal inhibitor with clinical applications in organ transplantation, oncology, and cardiology. *Pharmacotherapy.* 30(10):1044-56.

Gaber AO, Busque S, Mulgaonkar S, Gaston R, Jevnikar A,Meier-Kriesche H-U. (2008) ISA247: A phase IIB multicenter, open label,concentration-controlled trial in de novo renal transplantation. *Am J Transplant* 8(Suppl 2): 336.

Gaston RS, Kaplan B, Shah T, Cibrik D, Shaw LM, Angelis M, Mulgaonkar S, Meier-Kriesche HU, Patel D, Bloom RD. (2009) Fixed- or controlled-dose mycophenolate mofetil with standard- or reduced-dose calcineurin inhibitors: the Opticept trial. *Am J Transplant.*9(7):1607-19.

Geissler EK, Schlitt HJ.(2009) Immunosuppression for liver transplantation. *Gut* 58: 452-463

Geissler EK, Schlitt HJ.(2010) The potential benefits of rapamycin on renal function, tolerance, fibrosis, and malignancy following transplantation. *Kidney Int.* 78(11):1075-9.

Grant D, Wall W, Mimeault R, Zhong R, Ghent C, Garcia B, (1990) Successful small-bowel/liver transplantation. *Lancet* 335(8683):181-4.

Gremizzi C, Vergani A, Paloschi V, Secchi A.(2010) Impact of pancreas transplantation on type 1 diabetes-related complications. *Curr Opin Organ Transplant.* 15(1):119-23.

Gruessner RW, Kandaswamy R, Humar A, Gruessner AC, Sutherland DE.(2005) Calcineurin inhibitor- and steroid-free immunosuppression in pancreas-kidney and solitary pancreas transplantation. *Transplantation* 79:1184–1189.

Gruessner AC, Sutherland DE, Gruessner RW (2010) Pancreas transplantation in the United States: a review. *Curr Opin Organ Transplant.* 15(1):93-101.

Gupta P, Kaufman S, Fishbein TM.(2005) Sirolimus for solid organ transplantation in children. *Pediatr Transplant.* 9(3):269-76

Harper SJ, Gelson W, Harper IG, Alexander GJ, Gibbs P.(2011) Switching to sirolimus-based immune suppression after liver transplantation is safe and effective: a single-center experience. *Transplantation.* 91(1):128-32.

Hartman A, Denver ML, Barupal DK, Fiehn O, Fishbein T, Zasloff M and Eisen JA (2009) Human gut microbiome adopts an alternative state following small bowel transplantation *PNAS* 106(40):17187–17192

Heilman RL, Mazur MJ, Reddy KS. (2010) Immunosuppression in Simultaneous Pancreas-Kidney Transplantation. Progress to Date . *Drugs* 70 (7): 793-804

(http://optn.transplant.hrsa.gov/ar2009/Chapter_III_AR_CD.htm?cp=4#1)

Hutchinson M (2010) Natalizumab therapy of multiple sclerosis. *J Interferon Cytokine Res.* 30(10):787-9.

Kahan BD.(2000) Efficacy of sirolimus compared with azathioprine for reduction of acute renal allograft rejection: a randomized multicentre study. The Rapamune US Study Group. *Lancet* 356(15):194.

Kaposztas Z, Podder H, Mauiyyedi S, Illoh O, Kerman R, Reyes M, Pollard V, Kahan BD.(2009) Impact of rituximab therapy for treatment of acute humoral rejection. *Clin Transplant.* 23(1):63-73.

Kirk AD, Turgeon NA, Iwakoshi NN (2010). B cells and transplantation tolerance. *Nat Rev Nephrol.* 6(10):584-93.

Klipa D, Mahmud N, Ahsan N.(2010) Antibody immunosuppressive therapy in solid organ transplant: Part II. *MAbs.* 2(6):607-12.

Knechtle SJ. (2010) Immunoregulation and tolerance. *Transplant Proc.* 42(9 Suppl):S13-5.

Knight RJ, Podder H, Kerman RH, Lawless A, Katz SM,Van Buren CT, Gaber AO, Kahan BD.(2010) Comparing an early corticosteroid/late calcineurin-free immunosuppression protocol to a sirolimus-, cyclosporine A-, and prednisone based regimen for pancreas-kidney transplantation. *Transplantation* 89:727–732.

Kovarik JM, Steiger JU, Grinyo JM, Rostaing L, Arns W, Dantal J, Proot P, Budde K, Sotrastaurin Renal Transplant Study Group (2011). Pharmacokinetics of sotrastaurin combined with tacrolimus or mycophenolic acid in de novo kidney transplant recipients. *Transplantation.* 91(3):317-22.

Krämer BK, Charpentier B, Bäckman L, Silva HT Jr, Mondragon-Ramirez G, Cassuto-Viguier E, Mourad G, Sola R, Rigotti P, Mirete JO; Tacrolimus Prolonged Release Renal Study Group.(2010) Tacrolimus once daily (ADVAGRAF) versus twice daily (PROGRAF) in de novo renal transplantation: a randomized phase III study. *Am J Transplant.* 10(12):2632-43.

Kuschei WM, Leitner J, Majdic O, Pickl WF, Zlabinger GJ, Grabmeier-Pfistershammer K, Steinberger P.(2011) Costimulatory signals potently modulate the T cell inhibitory capacity of the therapeutic CD11a antibody Efalizumab. *Clin Immunol.* 139(2):199-207.

Larson TS, Dean PG, Stegall MD, Griffin MD, Textor SC, Schwab TR, Gloor TM, Cosio FG, Lund WJ, Kremers WK, Nyberg SL, Ishitani MB, Prieto M, Velosa JA

(2006).Complete Avoidance of Calcineurin Inhibitors in Renal Transplantation: A Randomized Trial Comparing Sirolimus and Tacrolimus. *Am J Transpl* 6:514–522

Lillehei RC, Goot B, Miller FA.(1959) The physiological response of the small bowel of the dog to ischemia including prolonged in vitro preservation of the bowel with successful replacement and survival. *Ann Surg* 150(4): 543-560

Llovet JM, Ricci S, Mazzaferro V(2008). Sorafenib in advanced hepatocellular carcinoma. *N Engl J Med* 359(8):378–390.

Lo DJ, Weaver TA, Stempora L, Mehta AK, Ford ML, Larsen CP, Kirk AD (2011). Selective targeting of human alloresponsive CD8+ effector memory T cells based on CD2 expression. *Am J Transplant.* 11(1):22-33.

Maffi P, Scavini M, Socci C, Piemonti L, Caldara R, Gremizzi C, Melzi R, Nano R, Orsenigo E, Venturini M, Staudacher C, Del Maschio A, Secchi A. (2011). Risks and benefits of transplantation in the cure of type 1 diabetes: whole pancreas versus islet transplantation. A single center study. *Rev Diabet Stud.* 8(1):44-50.

Melancon JK, Cummings LS, Graham J, Rosen-Bronson S, Light J, Desai CS, Girlanda R, Ghasemian S, Africa J, Johnson LB.(2011). Paired kidney donor exchanges and antibody reduction therapy: novel methods to ameliorate disparate access to living donor kidney transplantation in ethnic minorities. *J Am Coll Surg.* 212(4):740-5.

Mele TS, Halloran PF.(2000) The use of mycophenolate mofetil in transplant recipients. *Immunopharmacology* 47:215–245.

Melero J, Berenguer M. (2009).Antiviral therapy in patients with HCV-cirrhosis. *Ann Hepatol.* 8(4):292-7.

Merion RM, White DJ, Thiru S, Evans DB, Calne RY.(1984). Cyclosporine: five years' experience in cadaveric renal transplantation. *N Engl J Med.* 310(3):148-54

Montgomery RA, Gentry SE,Marks WH. (2006). Domino paired kidney donation: a strategy to make best use of live non-directed donation. *Lancet* 368:419–421.

Montgomery RA. (2010) Renal transplantation across HLA and ABO antibody barriers: integrating paired donation into desensitization protocols. *Am J Transplant* 10:449–457.

Nazia S, Guindi M, Renner EL, Berenguer M. (2011). Immune-mediated complications of the graft in interferon-treated hepatitis C positive liver transplant recipients. *J of Hepatol* 55: 207–217

Niederhaus SV, Muth B, Lorentzen DF, Wai P, Pirsch JD, Samaniego-Picota M, Leverson GE, D'alessandro AM, Sollinger HW, Djamali A. (2011) Luminex-based desensitization protocols: the university of wisconsin initial experience. *Transplantation.* 92(1):12-7.

Ojo AO, Held PJ, Port FK, Wolfe RA, Leichtman AB, Young EW, Arndorfer J, Christensen L, Merion RM.(2003) Chronic renal failure after transplantation of a nonrenal organ. *N Engl J Med.* 349(10):931-40

Perry DK, Burns JM, Pollinger HS, Amiot BP, Gloor JM, Gores GJ, Stegall MD. (2009). Proteasome Inhibition Causes Apoptosis of Normal Human Plasma Cells Preventing Alloantibody Production. *Am J Transpl* 9(1) 201-209.

Pillai AA, Levitsky J.(2009) Overview of immunosuppression in liver transplantation. *World J Gastroenterol.* 15(34):4225-33.

Pirenne J, Kawai M.(2009). Intestinal transplantation: evolution in immunosuppression protocols. *Current Opinion in Organ Transplantation* 14:250–255

Raichlin E, Khalpey Z, Kremers W, Frantz RP, Rodeheffer RJ, Clavell AL, Edwards BS, Kushwaha SS. (2007). Replacement of calcineurin-inhibitors with sirolimus as primary immunosuppression in stable cardiac transplant recipients.*Transplantation.* 84(4):467-74.

Reyes J, Mazariegos GV, Abu-Elmagd K, Macedo C, Bond GJ, Murase N, Peters J, Sindhi R, Starzl TE. (2005). Intestinal transplantation under tacrolimus monotherapy after perioperative lymphoid depletion with rabbit anti-thymocyte globulin (thymoglobulin). *Am J Transplant.* 5(6):1430-6.

Rosen HR, Shackleton CR, Higa L, Gralnek IM, Farmer DA, McDiarmid SV, Holt C, Lewin KJ, Busuttil RW, Martin P.(1997) Use of OKT3 is associated with early and severe recurrence of hepatitis C after liver transplantation. *Am J Gastroenterol.* 92(9):1453-7

Schena FP, Pascoe MD, Alberu J, del Carmen Rial M, Oberbauer R, Brennan DC, Campistol JM, Racusen L, Polinsky MS, Goldberg-Alberts R.(2009). Conversion from calcineurin inhibitors to sirolimus maintenance therapy in renal allograft recipients: 24-month efficacy and safety results from the CONVERT trial. *Transplantation.* 87(2):233-42.

Shapiro AMJ, Lakey JRT, Ryan EA, Korbutt GS, Toth E, Warnock GL.(2000) Islet transplantation in seven patients with type 1 diabetes mellitus using a glucocorticoid-free immunosuppressive regimen. *N Engl J Med* 343:230-8.

Starzl TE, Marchioro TL, Hutchinson DE, Porter KA, Cerilli GJ, Brettschneider L.(1967) The clinical use of antilymphocyte globulin in renal homotransplantation. *Transplantation.* 5(4):Suppl:1100-5.

Starzl TE.(2000) History of clinical transplantation. *World J Surg.* 24(7):759-82.

Starzl TE, Iwatsuki S, Shaw BW Jr, Gordon RD, Esquivel CO (1985) Immunosuppression and other nonsurgical factors in the improved results of liver transplantation. *Semin Liver Dis.* 5(4):334-43.

Starzl TE, Todo S, Fung J, Demetris AJ, Venkataramman R, Jain A (1989). FK 506 for liver, kidney, and pancreas transplantation. *Lancet.* 8670 (2):1000-4.

Stewart SF, Hudson M, Talbot D, Manas D, Day CP.(2001) Mycophenolate mofetil monotherapy in liver transplantation. *Lancet* 357: 609-610

The U.S. Multicenter FK506 Liver Study Group.(1994) A comparison of tacrolimus (FK 506) and cyclosporine for immunosuppression in liver transplantation. *N Engl J Med.* 331(17):1110-5.

Toso C, Merani S, Bigam DL.(2010). Sirolimus-based immunosuppression is associated with increased survival after liver transplantation for hepatocellular carcinoma. *Hepatology*, 51(4): 1237-43.

Treiber G.(2009) mTOR inhibitors for hepatocellular cancer: a forward-moving target. *Expert Rev Anticancer Ther.* 9(2):247-61.

Trunečka P, Boillot O, Seehofer D, Pinna AD, Fischer L, Ericzon BG, Troisi RI, Baccarani U, Ortiz de Urbina J, Wall W.(2010). Once-daily prolonged-release tacrolimus (ADVAGRAF) versus twice-daily tacrolimus (PROGRAF) in liver transplantation. Tacrolimus Prolonged Release Liver Study Group. *Am J Transplant.* 10(10):2313-23.

Vardanyan M, Parkin E, Gruessner C, Rodriguez Rilo HL. (2010) Pancreas vs. islet transplantation: a call on the future. *Curr Opin Organ Transplant.* 15(1):124-30.

Verna EC, Farrand ED, Elnaggar AS, Pichardo EM, Balducci A, Emond JC, Guarrera JV,Brown RS (2011). Basiliximab Induction and Delayed Calcineurin Inhibitor Initiation in Liver Transplant Recipients With Renal Insufficiency. *Transplantation* 91: 1254–1260.

Villanueva A, Llovet JM.(2011) Targeted therapies for hepatocellular carcinoma. *Gastroenterology*. 140(5):1410-26.

Vincenti F, Ramos E, Brattstrom C, Cho S, Ekberg H, Grinyo J, Johnson R, Kuypers D, Stuart F, Khanna A, Navarro M, Nashan B.(2001) Multicenter trial exploring calcineurin inhibitors avoidance in renal transplantation.*Transplantation*. 71(9):1282-7.

Vincenti F, Larsen C, Durrbach A, Wekerle T, Nashan B, Blancho G, Lang P, Grinyo J, Halloran PF, Solez K, Hagerty D, Levy E, Zhou W, Natarajan K, Charpentier B for the Belatacept Study Group (2005). Costimulation Blockade with Belatacept in Renal Transplantation. *N Engl J Med* 353:770-781

Vincenti F, Mendez R, Pescovitz M, Rajagopalan PR, Wilkinson AH, Butt K, Laskow D, Slakey DP, Lorber MI, Garg JP, Garovoy M (2007) A phase I/II randomized open-label multicenter trial of efalizumab, a humanized anti-CD11a, anti-LFA-1 in renal transplantation. *Am J Transplant*. 7(7):1770-7.

Vincenti F, Blancho G, Durrbach A, Friend P, Grinyo J, Halloran PF, Klempnauer J, Lang P, Larsen CP, Mühlbacher F, Nashan B, Soulillou JP, Vanrenterghem Y, Wekerle T, Agarwal M, Gujrathi S, Shen J, Shi R, Townsend R, Charpentier B. (2010). Five-year safety and efficacy of belatacept in renal transplantation. *J Am Soc Nephrol*. 21(9):1587-96.

Wagner D, Kniepeiss D, Schaffellner S. (2010). Sirolimus has a potential to influent viral recurrence in HCV positive liver transplant candidates. *Int Immunopharmacol*, 10(8):990-3.

Walsh RC, Everly JJ, Brailey P, Rike AH, Arend LJ, Mogilishetty G, Govil A, Roy-Chaudhury P, Alloway RR, Woodle ES. (2010). Proteasome inhibitor-based primary therapy for antibody-mediated renal allograft rejection. *Transplantation*. 89(3):277-84.

Walsh RC, Brailey P, Girnita A, Alloway RR, Shields AR, Wall GE, Sadaka BH, Cardi M, Tevar A, Govil A, Mogilishetty G, Roy-Chaudhury P, Woodle ES.(2011). Early and late acute antibody-mediated rejection differ immunologically and in response to proteasome inhibition. *Transplantation*. 91(11):1218-26

Weaver TA, Charafeddine AH, Agarwal A,1 Leopardi F, Kampen R, Starost MF,Larsen CP, Kirk AD.(2008) Targeting of Costimulation Blockade Resistant T Effector Memory (TEM) Cells in Non-Human Primate Renal Transplantation withLFA-3-Ig (Alefacept) Prolongs Allograft Survival. *Am J Transpl* 8(suppl2):204

Wéclawiak H, Kamar N, Ould-Mohamed A, Cardeau-Desangles I, Rostaing L.(2010) Biological agents in kidney transplantation: belatacept is entering the field. *Expert Opin Biol Ther*. 10(10):1501-8.

Weissenbacher A, Boesmueller C, Brandacher G, Oellinger R, Pratschke J, Schneeberger S.(2010) Alemtuzumab in solid organ transplantation and in composite tissue allotransplantation. *Immunotherapy*. 2(6):783-90.

Wiesner, R, for the Rapamune Liver Transplant Study Group (2002) The safety and efficacy of sirolimus and low-dose tacrolimus vs. tacrolimus in de novo orthotopic liver transplant recipients: results from a pilot study. *Hepatology*, 36: 208A.

Wolfe RA, Roys EC, Merion RM. (2010) Trends in organ donation and transplantation in the United States, 1999-2008. *Am J Transplant*. 10(4 Pt 2):961-72.

17

Induction Therapy in Renal Transplant Recipients

Cheguevara Afaneh, Meredith J. Aull, Sandip Kapur and David B. Leeser
Department of Surgery, Division of Transplant Surgery
New York-Presbyterian Hospital- Weill Cornell Medical College, New York, NY
USA

1. Introduction

1.1 Historical overview

Renal transplantation remains the most effective treatment modality for end-stage renal disease. The initial results with renal transplantation were plagued with significant perioperative morbidity and high rates of immunological events. At the time, the transplant physician's armamentarium consisted of glucocorticoids and azathioprine. As modifications and improvements in surgical technique reduced morbidity, immunological events remained formidable foes to the transplant physician. Significant efforts were undertaken to elucidate the components and mechanisms of these immunological events, ultimately leading to the discovery of lymphocytes as the primary culprits in acute rejection. Early preclinical trials demonstrated that lymphocyte-specific antibodies could be induced in animal models by injecting them with lymphocytes. The serum could then be isolated and re-injected in other animals to decrease the lymphocyte count. Thus, these experiments lead to the earliest forms of antilymphocyte antibody formulations, including antithymocyte globulin, antilymphocyte serum, and antilymphocyte globulin (Bishop et al., 1975; Cosimi et al., 1976). These initial medications had little specificity and broad effects, but their potent ability to treat acute rejection episodes led to their widespread use in the 1970's (Cosimi, 1981a).

The extensive use of these formulations exposed their various drawbacks. Because of nonspecific binding, cross-reactivity with various hematopoietic cells revealed dose-limiting side effects including thrombocytopenia, anemia, and neutropenia (Henricsson et al., 1977; Rosenberg, 1975). Additionally, the method of preparation was not standardized, thus leading to dosing variations. Because these formulations were typically made in rabbits or horses, the proteins had potential antigenic properties leading to the development of serum sickness, cytokine release syndrome, or even anaphylaxis (Niblack et al., 1987; Prin Mathieu et al., 1997; Tatum et al., 1984).

The development of specific, monoclonal antibodies by Kohler and Milstein circumvented many of the drawbacks of polyclonal formulations, including lack of specificity and variability in preparation (Kohler & Milstein, 1975). Muromonab, or OKT3, was the first monoclonal antibody prepared from mouse, which is specific for cluster of differentiation 3 (CD3) (Cosimi et al, 1981b). OKT3 was effective at specifically depleting T cells from the circulation, and became widely used as a valuable tool to combat acute rejection episodes (Ortho Multicenter Transplant Study Group, 1985; Ponticelli et al., 1987). Nevertheless, these monoclonal formulations still maintained some of the similar side effect profile of the polyclonal formulations, including cytokine release syndrome and human antigenic response to animal proteins, which lead to limited dosing in some patients (Jaffers et al., 1986).

The 1980's marked an important era in transplantation with new advances in genetic engineering. Monoclonal antibodies became more sophisticated, targeting specific T cell populations and allowing blockade of T cell activation, such as the interleukin-2 receptor (IL-2R) or CD25 (Vincenti et al., 1997). Moreover, the ability to avoid antigenic proteins by encoding genetic sequences of DNA binding sites of animal proteins onto human antibodies led to the development of chimeric monoclonal antibodies (Boulianne et al., 1984; Jones et al., 1986; Morrison et al., 1984). Using these techniques, soluble fusion proteins can be formed by merging nonantibody receptors with the Fc portion of antibodies.

1.2 Antibodies

Comprehension of the structure and function of antibodies is critical to understanding the efficacy of antibody induction therapy. Antibodies are composed of two identical heavy chains (either μ, γ, α, ε, or δ) and two identical light chains (either κ or λ). The heavy and light chain portions create two identical antigen binding sites (Fab fragment) which are held together by the common region, termed the Fc portion (Capra & Edmundson, 1977). The type of heavy chain differentiates the immunoglobulin type as IgM, IgG, IgA, IgE, and IgD. In clinical transplantation, the IgG molecule is typically utilized, as it's readily produced and structurally feasible to manipulate with ease (Fig. 1).

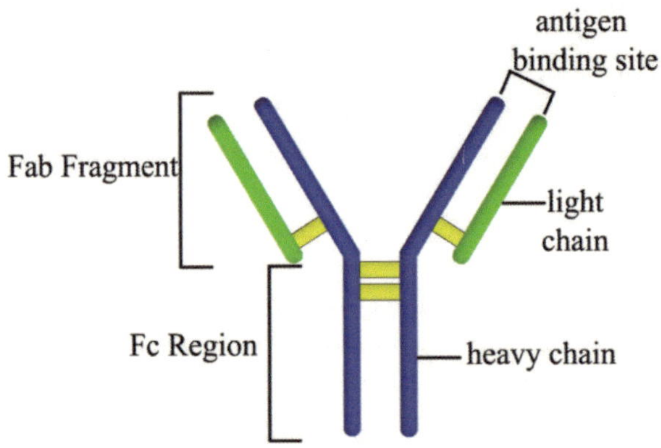

Fig. 1. Basic antibody structure. Depicted is a standard IgG molecule. The heavy chains are colored in blue, while the light chains are colored in green. The yellow lines signify the disulfide bonds

Antibodies are present on the surface of B cells. Upon secretion into the serum, antibodies are able to neutralize circulating antigens. Antibodies maintain their effector functions irrespective of species, which make them useful in early studies of antibody therapies in transplantation. Antibodies are capable of various functions, including mimicking activating ligands of receptors and serving as receptor inhibitors by blocking the ligand binding site

(Tite et al., 1986; Wong et al., 1990). In some instances, antibody binding can lead to both activation and inhibition by inducing surface molecule internalization, whereby the molecule is removed from the surface of the cell (Kerr & Atkins, 1989). This results in a negligible net effect. A major limitation of antibody use is the inability to directly bind intracellular molecules.

Antibodies have the ability to deplete target cells through two fundamental mechanisms. First, antibodies have the capability to activate the complement system resulting in complement-mediated lysis of target cells. Second, certain cells with Fc region receptors have the ability to phagocytose cells covered with antibodies through a mechanism termed antibody-dependent cellular cytotoxicity (ADCC)(Fig.2). The efficacy with which this occurs depends upon the Fab fragment and the Fc region (Ferrant et al., 2004). It is important to note that cells which have significantly matured, or memory cells, are somewhat resistant to antibody-dependent depletion mechanisms, possibly due to increased expression of antiapoptotic or complement regulatory genes (Pearl et al, 2005).

The vast properties of antibodies make them suitable for therapeutic indications. Nevertheless, even minor changes in antibody structure can significantly alter function. Additionally, the interplay of the complement system and ADCC properties further complicates the predicted function of various antibody-depleting therapies.

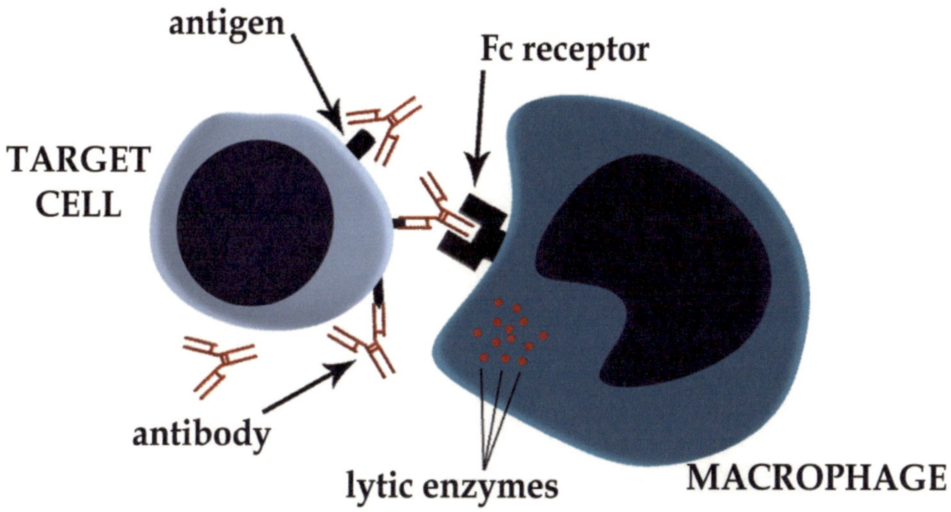

Fig. 2. Antibody-dependent cellular cytotoxicity (ADCC). The Fc receptor on the machrophage is used to bind the constant Fc portion of antibodies to facilitate engulfment of cells coated with antibodies

1.3 Clinical classification of induction agents

Induction immunosuppressive medications can be classified into two groups: depleting agents and non-depleting agents. The categorization is based on the ability of the medication to target specific antigens or cells, leading to a decrease in the total expression or cell count. Most depleting agents are relatively potent with potential for toxicity with prolonged administration. Non-depleting agents are generally well-tolerated. Depleting agents are also used for severe or refractory cases of acute rejection and have proven to be more effective than glucocorticoids in treating episodes of acute rejection (Webster et al., 2006). In addition, the use of induction agents has decreased the rates of acute rejection in the first 6 months compared to no induction therapy (Szczech et al., 1997). Although these short-term benefits appear promising, long-term outcomes, including patient and graft survival rates, have not been shown to be altered by the use of induction therapy. This is possibly related to the effects of long-term maintenance immunosuppressive therapy or patient co-morbidities.

The overall success of a transplanted renal allograft is contingent on both surgical prowess and the use of potent immunosuppressive medications. Although induction therapy has not affected surgical morbidity, the rate of allograft thrombosis has been shown to be reduced in children with the use of induction agents (Humar et al., 2001; Singh et al., 1997). However, not all medications used are FDA-approved for induction therapy. Moreover, it is important to note that these medications are not without definite risks, including serious infectious complications and the development of post-transplant lymphoproliferative disorder (PTLD), which has been well-described with the use of OKT3 and maintenance immunosuppression (Bustami et al., 2004; Jamil et al., 1999). Because of the effects of depleting agents on T cells, appropriate prophylactic therapies should be administered to all transplant recipients. Duration of therapy is typically contingent on the donor and recipient immunological history. Thus, tailoring the immunosuppressive regimen to each patient is critical to avoiding complications.

In 1995 induction therapy was used in less than half of all kidney transplants in the United States, while 10 years later, approximately 70% of all kidney transplant recipients received induction therapy (Meier-Kriesche et al., 2006). Given the availability of various potent, specific induction agents in modern transplantation, the clinical dilemma lies in selecting the most appropriate agent for a given patient, taking into account co-morbidities, donor quality, immunological status, and planned maintenance therapy.

2. Depleting agents

2.1 Antithymocyte globulin

2.1.1 Mechanism

Various polyclonal depleting agents are available; however, this discussion will focus on rabbit antithymocyte globulin (rATG). In rATG, the polyclonal heterologous antibody formulation is produced from immunizing rabbits with human thymocytes, which serve as the immunogens (Fig. 3) (Hardinger, 2006). The rabbit serum is then gathered and purified to remove antibodies with potentially detrimental effects and only the IgG isotypes are collected. Despite these purification techniques, it is possible that the majority of antibodies in these formulations serve no therapeutic purpose (Bonnefoy-Berard et al., 1991). When administered to humans, the rATG antibody formulations bind all antigens that the rabbits were exposed to during the immunization process.

Rabbit ATG binds multiple T cell surface antigens and receptors involved in antigen recognition, adhesion and costimulation. These include CD2, CD3, CD4, CD5, CD8, CD28, CD45, and CD40L. In addition, rATG may also bind non-T cell molecules such as CD16, CD20, CD56, and the major histocompatibility molecules (class I and II) (Bonnefoy-Berard et al., 1991; Hardinger, 2006). The depleting effect of rATG occurs within 24 hours of administration and can persist with a prolonged serum half-life of several weeks (Bunn et al., 1996; Guttmann et al., 1997). The effects of lymphocyte depletion are persists for years following administration, as evidenced by selectively low $CD4^{+}$ T cell counts (Brennan et al., 1999; Hardinger et al., 2004).

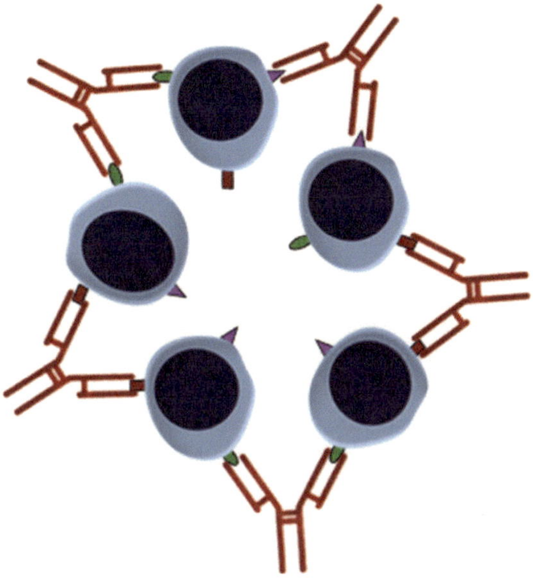

Fig. 3. Polyclonal antibodies. Polyclonal antibodies are non-specific and bind multiple antigens as shown in the figure

2.1.2 Applications

Rabbit ATG has been approved for use as an induction agent and for the treatment of acute rejection in Europe since 1984 (IMTIX-SangStat, 2003). However, in the United States, rATG is indicated only for the treatment of acute rejection (as of 1998). Nevertheless, it is routinely administered as induction therapy in many centers in the United States. Early studies demonstrated an increased risk of infectious complications and post-transplant malignancy when administered in conjunction with cyclosporine (Merion et al., 1984). With a better understanding of PTLD, improved infectious prophylaxis protocols, and experience using lower doses of rATG, the use of rATG as an induction agent has increased.

The most effective use of rATG depends on timing of administration. Ideally, the first dose should be given before the vascular anastomosis at the time of transplantation (typical dose 1.5mg/kg/dose for a total of 4.5 to 7.5 mg/kg). This may minimize ischemia-reperfusion injury and potentially prevent the development of delayed graft function (Shoskes & Halloran, 1996). Delayed graft function is known to portend poorer outcomes in kidney transplant recipients, thus rATG has been used in patients at higher risk of developing this delayed graft function, including recipients of donation after cardiac death donors, and recipients of extended criteria donors (Beiras-Fernandez et al., 2006; Cecka et al., 1993; Shield et al., 1997). It is also administered in patients at higher risk of developing acute rejection in the perioperative period, such as retransplants and patients who may have prolonged avoidance of calcineurin inhibitors as well as to minimize maintenance therapies such as facilitating early corticosteroid withdrawl (Schaffer et al., 2003; Shield et al., 1997).

The use of rATG to treat severe or refractory acute cellular rejection episodes has been well-established. Refractory acute cellular rejection is defined as failure to respond to 3 consecutive days of bolus methylprednisolone (i.e. 500 mg per day) treatment. rATG is superior to glucocorticoids in treating acute cellular rejection episodes. Compared to other polyclonal antibody formulations, rATG has proven to be superior in reversing steroid-resistant rejection and prolonging rejection-free events (Gaber et al., 1998). Patient or graft survival, however, have not been shown to be affected. Given the potency of rATG, it is typically used as supplemental agent to corticosteroids for the treatment of severe or refractory episodes of acute rejection. Additionally, recurrent episodes of acute rejection may be treated with multiple courses of rATG as long as preformed antirabbit antibodies are not present (Bock et al., 1995).

2.1.3 Adverse effects

Patients treated with rATG may experience a variety of side effects. It has been associated with a phenomenon called cytokine release syndrome (Fig. 4), which is common to many polyclonal antibody formulations. Patients may experience mild flu-like symptoms, such as fever, chills, nausea, urticaria, rash, and headache (Guttmann et al., 1997). This occurs as a result of increased production of tumor necrosis factor-α, IL-1, and IL-6 from antibody binding to cell surface receptors and ensuing cell lysis (Debets et al., 1989; Guttmann et al., 1997; Hardinger, 2006). Premedication with corticosteroids, antipyretics, and antihistamines can prevent and/or treat the flu-like symptoms that can occur in a subset of kidney transplant recipients. In some cases, patients may develop more severe shock-like reactions, such as dyspnea, severe hypotension, pulmonary edema, or even anaphylaxis. Although patients frequently experience the mild flu-like symptoms and not the more severe reactions, recipient co-morbid conditions, such as cardiac or pulmonary disease, should be considered when selecting rATG as an induction agent. Serum sickness has also been associated with rATG administration in up to 7-10% of patients (Buchler et al., 2003; Mourad et al., 2001).

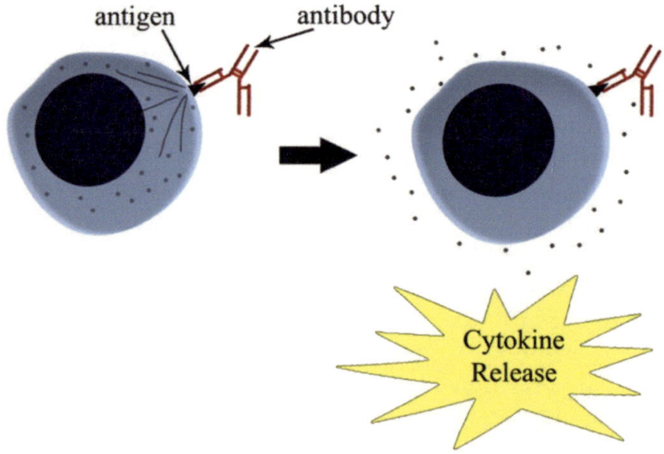

Fig. 4. Antibody activation and cytokine release. Antibodies can bind antigens resulting in activation of the cell and cytokine release as illustrated in the figure

Hematological adverse events may occur, including leucopenia and thrombocytopenia. It is important to monitor white blood cell, lymphocyte, and platelet counts for patients receiving rATG. Not surprisingly, these events may lead to an increase in infectious complications, including cytomegalovirus (CMV), herpes simplex virus, Epstein-Barr virus (EBV), and varicella (Abott et al., 2002; Gourishankar et al., 2004).

2.2 Muromonab (OKT3)

2.2.1 Mechanism

Muromonab, or OKT3, is a monoclonal antibody. It is an IgG2 mouse antibody known to bind the epsilon component of human CD3. The CD3 complex is a T cell receptor intimately involved in T cell signaling and activation via a calcineurin-dependent pathway (Ortho Multicenter Transplant Study Group, 1985). Once the antibody binds the target cell, complement is activated leading to cell lysis and ADCC (Vallhonrat et al., 1999). By this method, most T cells are effectively removed from the peripheral circulation. However, the T cell binding also results in T cell activation before clearance, leading to systemic cytokine release. When OKT3 binds the T cell receptor, the CD3 complex is internalized (Fig. 5) to prevent further activation by persistent antigen presence (Chatenoud et al., 1990). Effectively, T cells that fail to be cleared are unable to be activated by the CD3 complex.

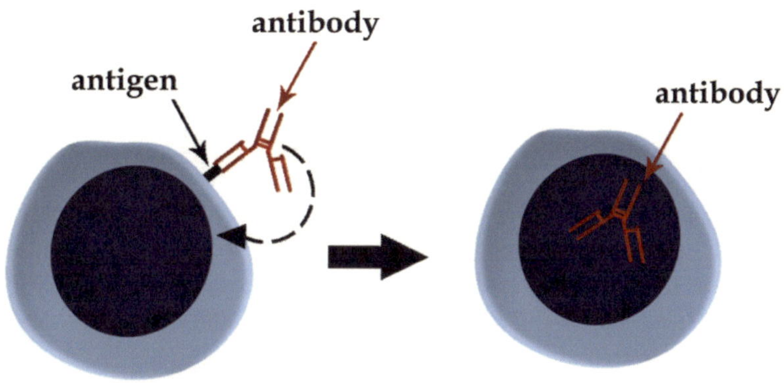

Fig. 5. Internalization of an antibody. This figure is an example of internalization of the antigen-antibody complex after activation to prevent further stimulation by persistently low level of antibody in the peripheral circulation (i.e. OKT3 binding)

2.2.2 Applications

Early studies demonstrated the efficacy of OKT3 as an induction agent in kidney transplantation in conjunction with maintenance immunosuppression (Debure et al., 1988; Norman et al., 1988; Vigeral et al., 1986). Efficacy relies on serum availability, thus once administration of OKT3 ceases, maintenance immunosuppressive therapy is required. Typical dosing is 5 to 10 mg/dose through a peripheral or central line. Premedication with methylprednisolone, acetaminophen, and diphenhydramine can significantly lower the amount of cytokine release associated with first infusion (Chatenoud et al., 1991). Additionally, slower administration rates are helpful in blunting the cytokine response. Dosing can be continued for up to 14 days for a total dose of 70 mg. Patients with significant sensitization have especially benefitted from OKT3 (Opelz, 1995). In addition, recipients of renal allografts experiencing delayed graft function benefit from OKT3 infusion, as calcineurin inhibitor therapy can be delayed, avoiding added renal toxicity (Benvenisty et al., 1990).

Early studies of OKT3 demonstrated a reduction in acute rejection rates and time to first rejection episodes; however, overall patient and graft survival rates were not changed (Henry et al., 2001; Norman et al., 1993). Its use has been linked to various infectious and malignant morbidities. Aseptic meningitis has also been linked to its use (Martin et al., 2002). Moreover, PTLD rates are significantly increased, especially in EBV negative recipients receiving EBV positive allografts (Thistlethwaite et al., 1988; Cherikh et al., 2003). The significant side effect profile and immunogenicity of OKT3 has lead to a decline in its use as an induction agent.

OKT3 remains an effective treatment for severe episodes of acute cellular rejection, or those refractory to steroid therapy and rATG. In the majority of cases of vigorous rejection, OKT3 has proven efficacious (Cosimi et al., 1981b; Ortho Multicenter Transplant Study Group, 1985; Thistlethwaite et al., 1987). The efficacy of OKT3 is maintained even if prior lymphocyte depleting agents have been used (Ponticelli et al., 1987). However, timing of therapy is important, as a delay in treatment following the 3 days of high-dose methylprednisolone therapy for steroid-resistant acute rejection is associated with decreased success (Tesi et al., 1993). OKT3 has also been used to treat vascular rejection episodes (Banff grade 2 or 3) (Kamath et al., 1997).

2.2.3 Adverse effects

As a monoclonal antibody, OKT3 selectively targets T cells, avoiding the leucopenia and thrombocytopenia associated with rATG. Similar to rATG, OKT3 is associated with cytokine release syndrome. With respect to OKT3, this is more pronounced, especially with the first dose as the T cells may be in a more activated state (i.e. acute cellular rejection). The cytokine release syndrome with OKT3 results in severe flu-like symptoms, including fever, chills, malaise, nausea, vomiting, and even rigors (Thistlethwaite et al., 1988). As vascular permeability increases, patients may experience pulmonary edema, hypotension, and volume overload. If there is renal dysfunction present, patients should undergo hemodialysis prior to first infusion to avoid volume-related complications. Patients should be closely monitored, especially during the initial infusions for cardiac or pulmonary complications.

The utilization of OKT3 is clearly associated with antimouse antibodies in at least 30% of patients, depending on the immunosuppression regimens used at the time (Colvin & Preffer, 1991; Schroeder et al., 1990). The antibodies form against the mouse IgG molecule. If there is antibody formation, OKT3 is typically not reused, although higher doses may overcome this. This can be documented by laboratory evidence of antimouse antibody (Chatenoud et al., 1986; Legendre et al., 1992).

2.3 Alemtuzumab

2.3.1 Mechanism

Alemtuzumab, or Campath-1H, is a monoclonal antibody to rat antihuman CD52 (Fig. 6). It is an IgG1 humanized molecule (Hale et al., 1986). CD52 is present in high abundance on most lymphocytes, including T cell, B cells, and monocytes, but not hematopoietic precursors (Hale, 2001). It effectively depletes T cells, and some B cells and monocytes in the circulation as well as the allograft (Kirk et al., 2003).

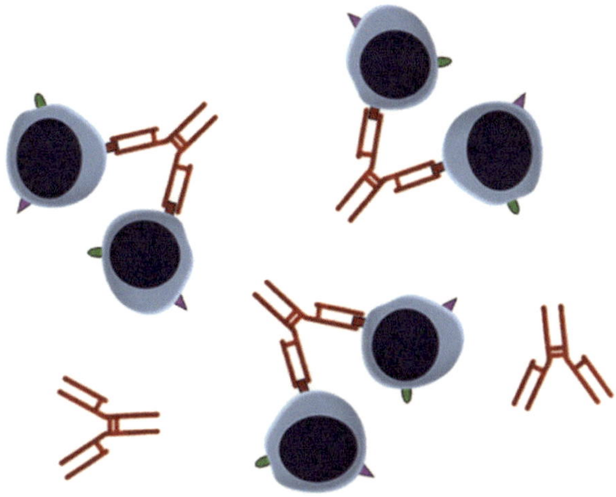

Fig. 6. Monoclonal antibodies. Monoclonal antibodies are specific and bind a single antigen as shown in the figure

2.3.2 Applications

Alemtuzumab has not been approved for use as an induction agent; however, this is a common off-label use. Currently, it is only approved to treat lymphogenous malignancies. As an off-label induction agent, it's been used with various immunosuppression regimens, including steroid-sparing regimens. Effectively, it depletes lymphocytes at the time of transplantation and last for several months to a year before the immune system is reconstituted (Gabardi et al., 2011). Alemtuzumab is given at a dose of 30 mg or 0.3 mg/kg through a peripheral line over 3 hours. Sometimes 2 doses are given, although T cells are expectedly removed within 1 hour of initial administration (Kirk et al., 2003; Pearl et al., 2005).

Alemtuzumab depletes all T cell subsets, but has a predilection for more naïve T cells (Pearl et al., 2005). Memory T cell subsets may not be depleted with this therapy, but these cell types are especially susceptible to calcineurin inhibitors. Because of the prompt and intense depletion, alemtuzumab is especially appealing to use in patients with delayed graft function, as calcineurin inhibitor therapy can be withheld to avoid concomitant calcineurin-induced renal insults.

Early studies of alemtuzumab demonstrated its efficacy as a treatment therapy for acute rejection; however, it was associated with significant infectious morbidity and mortality (Hale et al., 1986). Patients were significantly over-immunosuppressed, especially on a triple maintenance therapy. More recent literature has been small studies or anecdotal data (Clatworthy et al., 2009; Csapo et al., 2005; Jirasiritham et al., 2010). Because its efficacy is greatest against naïve T cells, its use in sensitized patients may-be limited.

In a recent study, alemtuzumab was prospectively compared to basiliximab and rATG as an induction agent in patients on a steroid-sparing immunosuppressive regimen (Hanaway et al., 2011). Alemtuzumab demonstrated lower short-term rates of acute rejection compared to basiliximab in patients at low-risk of developing acute rejection. At 3-years, however, the rates of acute rejection were no different between alemtuzumab and rATG. Additionally, patients receiving alemtuzumab did not experience an increased incidence of adverse events.

2.3.3 Adverse effects

Similar to other depleting agents (rATG and OKT3), alemtuzumab is also associated with cytokine release syndrome, albeit to a lesser extent. If properly premedicated with methylprednisolone, acetaminophen, and diphenhydramine, the cytokine release is blunted. Urticaria and rash manifestations are common, while anaphylaxis and hypotension have also been reported. It has not been associated with antibody formation, as in the case of OKT3. It has been linked to the development of autoimmune thyroiditis in patients treated with alemtuzumab for multiple sclerosis (Coles et al., 1999). This has also been reported in a renal transplant recipient treated with alemetuzumab (Kirk et al., 2006).

3. Non-depleting agents

3.1 Basiliximab

3.1.1 Mechanism

Basiliximab is a chimeric mouse-human monoclonal IgG1 antibody to CD25. CD25 is the α-subunit of the IL-2 receptor, which is a binding site of IL-2. Basiliximab inhibition of IL-2 binding occurs through steric hindrance (Fig.7). In this case, the effect is not depletional, but rather, preventative of early T cell activation (Gabardi et al., 2011).

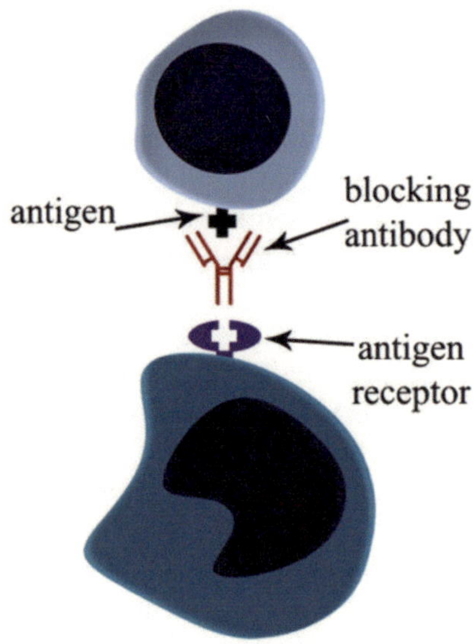

Fig. 7. Antibody blockade. In this figure the antibody functions by blocking the antigen from binding to the receptor

3.1.2 Applications

Basiliximab's biological bias for naïve T cells has limited its role to an induction agent. One dose is typically administered on the day of transplant as well as one dose on postoperative day 4 (20 mg per dose) through a peripheral line. Its use has been associated with decreased rates of acute cellular rejection compared to no formal induction agent (besides methylprednisolone) on triple or double drug immunosuppression regimens (Kahan et al., 1999; Nashan et al., 1997). Additional studies comparing basiliximab induction to polyclonal antibody depleting induction agents in the setting of triple maintenance immunosuppression regimens have shown similar outcomes, including acute rejection rates and delayed graft function (Lebranchu et al., 2002; Mourad et al., 2004). Basiliximab induction has also been used in steroid avoidance immunosuppression regimens (Afaneh et al., 2010). In the setting of monotherapy or calcineurin inhibitor free regimens, basiliximab has not been shown to be useful (Parrott et al., 2005; Vincenti et al., 2001). In some instances of excellent allograft human leukocyte antigen (HLA)-matching (i.e. 2-haplotype matches), it's been used as an effective induction agent with steroid-sparing immunosuppressive regimens (Afaneh et al., 2010). Given the relatively mild side effect profile, basiliximab is well-tolerated in all patients, even those with significant cardiac or pulmonary co-morbidities. It has no role in the treatment of acute rejection episodes as a rescue agent.

3.1.3 Adverse effects

Because of the mechanism of action of basiliximab, the side effect profile is relatively mild (Kahan et al., 1999; Nashan et al., 1997). Cytokine release syndrome does not occur, as T cells are not activated or stimulated. The most serious adverse event is hypersensitivity, which is rare (<1%)(Gabardi et al., 2011). There is no increased risk of infectious complications or PTLD compared to no induction therapy (Cherikh et al., 2003).

3.2 Daclizumab

3.2.1 Mechanism

Similar to basiliximab, daclizumab is an antagonist to CD25; however, it is a humanized IgG1 antibody. The CD25 molecule was the first humanized monoclonal antibody to be successfully targeted in the field of transplantation (Kirkman et al., 1991). The mechanism of action of daclizumab essentially duplicates that of other IL-2 receptor antagonists.

3.2.2 Applications

Like basiliximab, daclizumab has been shown to decrease the incidence of acute cellular rejection when administered as an induction agent (Hershberger et al., 2005; Nashan et al., 1999). Given the favorable side effect profile, it is tolerated well in recipients, irrespective of co-morbid conditions. The main disadvantage of daclizumab, as compared to basiliximab, is that it is more costly and requires repeated administrations (Gabardi et al., 2011). Because the demand for the medication has been relatively low, it has been discontinued by the manufacturer. It has no role as a rescue agent for acute rejection.

3.2.3 Adverse effects

The side effect profile is similar to that of basiliximab and generally favorable. Cytokine release is not typically associated with this agent (Hershberger et al., 2005; Nashan et al., 1999). Like other IL-2 receptor antagonists, the risk of PTLD is not significantly increased with use (Cherikh et al., 2003).

4. Desensitizing agents

4.1 Rituximab

4.1.1 Mechanism

Rituximab is a monoclonal chimeric antibody to the CD20 molecule. CD20 is a glycoprotein on the cell surface of circulating, mature B cells. Rituximab effectively depletes $CD20^+$ cells from the circulation by inducing apoptosis (Deans et al., 2002). These cells are precursors to antibody-producing plasma cells, and their role in transplantation is only partially characterized. They may play a role in acute rejection, as B cells can act as antigen-presenting cells.

4.1.2 Applications

Rituximab is approved for use in various lymphomas, leukemias, PTLD, and rheumatoid arthritis (Gabardi et al., 2011; Grillo-Lopez et al., 1999). Peripheral veins can be used for administration and dosing is dependent on the indication. A recent study examining the role of rituximab as an induction agent found no benefit compared to placebo (Tyden et al., 2009). However, it does play a role as a desensitizing agent in patients with preformed donor specific antibodies (DSA), in conjunction with total plasmapheresis and/or intravenous immunoglobulin (IVIG)(Fuchinoue et al., 2011; Sonnenday et al., 2004). Additionally, it has been used to aid in transplanting across blood group barriers in donor recipient pairs and in patients with positive crossmatches following antibody elimination. Rituximab is increasingly being used to treat episodes of vascular rejection and antibody-mediated rejections (Y.T. Becker et al., 2006; Fehr et al., 2009). Finally, rituximab is a proven and effective agent in the treatment of PTLD (Svoboda et al., 2006). Administration does not replace immunosuppression reduction or chemotherapy, but rather supplements the other modalities.

4.1.3 Adverse effects

Rituximab is generally well-tolerated with minimal side effects. Anaphylaxis remains a theoretical concern, as is the case with most agents. Reports on infectious complications related to rituximab have been variable (Grim et al., 2007; Kamar et al., 2010; Nishida et al., 2009). In some instances there was no difference in bacterial, viral, or fungal infections in kidney transplant recipients treated with rituximab, however, this remains controversial.

4.2 Bortezomib

4.2.1 Mechanism

Bortezomib is a proteasomal inhibitor that causes apoptosis of plasma cells. It binds the 26S subunit of the proteasome (Bonvini et al., 2007). Proteasome inhibition ultimately leads to apoptosis during mitosis. Bortezomib selectively causes apoptosis in $CD138^+$ plasma cells (Perry et al., 2009). Additionally, Bortezomib may block T cell cycling and decrease the number of circulating B cells by reducing bone marrow levels of IL-6 (San Miguel et al., 2008).

4.2.2 Applications

Bortezomib has not been approved for use in kidney transplantation; however, it has been used in sensitized patients (Perry et al., 2009). Bortezomib has been successfully used to decrease DSA levels, which may play a role in acute antibody-mediated rejection (AMR)

(Trivedi et al., 2009). Furthermore, in vivo data has demonstrated a decrease in the percentage of bone marrow plasma cells, antibody production, and allospecificities of plasma cells in bone marrow aspirates of patients treated with bortezomib i in the setting of AMR (Perry et al., 2009).

4.2.3 Adverse events

Bortezomib has been associated with various side effects. Although gastrointestinal side effects are the most common, peripheral neuropathy has also been reported, especially in patients with a pre-existing history of neuropathy (Bonvini et al., 2007). Moreover, myelosuppression and shingles has been reported.

4.3 Intravenous Immunoglobulin (IVIG)

4.3.1 Mechanism

Intravenous immunoglobulin, or IVIG, is pooled polyclonal antibodies from different human donors. These are high-dose human IgG fractions with a wide range of specificities. These are non-T cell specific formulations and have no specific cell targets (Jordan et al., 2011). It is able to bind activated complement components or even inhibit complement activation (Jordan et al., 2009). IVIG may also modulate the alloimmune response by binding to the Fc receptor of antigen-presenting cells, effectively quelling the alloimmune response (Kazatchkine & Kaveri, 2001).

4.3.2 Applications

Despite the inability to deplete T cells, IVIG is an effective treatment of acute cellular rejection. Early studies showed that IVIG was as effective as OKT3 in reversing steroid-resistant acute rejection episodes (Casadei et al., 2001). In the setting of antibody-mediated rejection, IVIG has been shown to be beneficial when used in conjunction with plasmapheresis and/or rituximab (Lefaucher et al., 2009; Shehata et al., 2010). As a desensitization agent alone, no study has demonstrated a clear benefit (Pisani et al., 1999; Shehata et al., 2010). Definitive reduction of antibody was not shown and a survival advantage was not evident.

4.3.3 Adverse effects

The side-effect profile of IVIG increases with dosing. High-dose IVIG is associated with more infusion-related complications, such as headache, thrombotic incidents, hemolysis, bronchospasms, osmotic nephropathy, or even aseptic meningitis (Jordan et al., 2011; Kahwaji et al., 2009). Sucrose-based and high osmolality products have a higher risk of developing osmotic nephropathy as opposed to other preparation. Nevertheless, it is typically well-tolerated, especially at lower doses and most patients report only headache.

5. Experimental agents

5.1 Siplizumab (MEDI-507)

Originally described as BTI-322, siplizumab is a monoclonal humanized antibody to CD2. It is an IgG1k molecule derived from rat (Pruett et al., 2009). CD2, or lymphocyte function-associated antigen-2 (LFA-2), is an important T cell adhesion molecule that binds to CD58, or LFA-3. This is a transmembrane signal transduction molecule that facilitates T cell receptor binding. Early studies examined the use of siplizumab as an induction agent and treatment modality for acute rejection in solid organ transplantation as well as graft-versus-host disease (Pruett et al., 2009; Squifflet et al., 1997). The first human study of siplizumab demonstrated the safety and feasibility in kidney transplantation, as compared to placebo; however, current endeavors are focused on investigating its use in nonmyeloablative conditioning regimens to achieve mixed chimerism (Kawai et al., 2008; Pruett et al., 2009; Spitzer et al., 2003). In addition, it is being investigated for the treatment of plaque psoriasis (Langley et al., 2010).

5.2 Alefacept

Alefaept is a dimeric fusion protein (Fig.8) constituted from LFA-3 and the human Fc portion of IgG1. Studies have demonstrated inhibition of T cell proliferation and depletion of effector memory T cells (Ellis & Krueger, 2001; Gordon et al., 2003). Currently, alefacept is approved to treat plaque psoriasis. Preclinical studies in nonhuman primates have demonstrated a survival benefit of alefacept, when used in conjunction with costimulatory blockade, but not alone; however in human trials have never shown a benefit (Weaver et al., 2009).

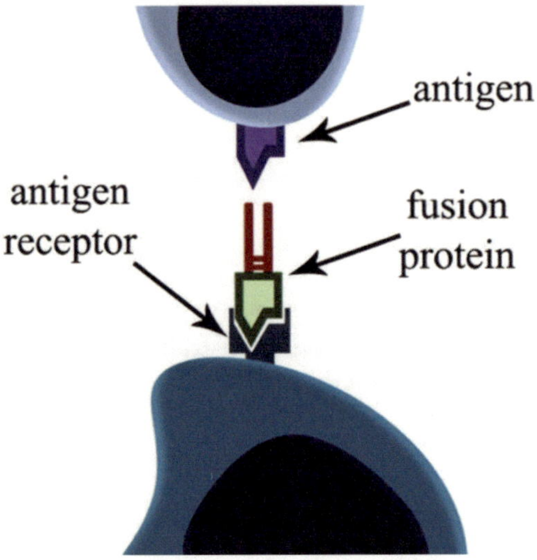

Fig. 8. Mimicry. In this figure, the antibody is fused with a protein structural similar to the intended antigen, which can serve as activating or inhibitory

5.3 Costimulatory blockade

5.3.1 Abatacept

Abatacept is a recombinant cytotoxic T-lymphocyte antigen 4 (CTLA4) fused with the Fc portion of IgG1 (Lenschow et al., 1992; Turka et al., 1992). Animal models demonstrated its ability to delay or even prevent the onset of allograft rejection, which is comparable to basiliximab and some polyclonal antibody therapies (Kirk et al., 1997; Lenschow et al., 1992; Turka et al., 1992). It has been approved for treatment of rheumatoid arthiritis (Genovese et al., 2005; Nogid & Pham, 2006). Further investigations of this medication are not currently under development.

5.3.2 Belatacept

Belatacept is the improved version of abatacept, providing selective blockade of T cell activation as a fusion protein. Two amino acids have been changed to improve dissociation rates when binding to CD80 and CD86 (Vincenti et al., 2005, 2010). In the phase II trial comparing belatacept to cyclosporine, acute rejection rates were similar, while allograft function was significantly improved in patients receiving belatacept (Vincenti et al., 2005). In the phase III trial of kidney transplantation, patients receiving belatacept experienced improved allograft function at 12 months; however, acute rejection rates and severity of acute rejection episodes were significantly higher in the belatacept arm of the study. Additionally, the incidence of PTLD was greater in patients receiving belatacept (Vincenti et al., 2010). An additional study investigating the efficacy of belatacept in kidney transplantation of extended criteria donors demonstrated similar results, with a predilection towards central nervous system (CNS) forms of PTLD (Durrbach et al., 2010). The novelty of costimulation blockade is the ability to avoid calcineurin inhibitors, especially in allografts at increased risk of delayed graft function. Belatacept has recently been approved for the prophylaxis of organ rejection in adult patients receiving a kidney transplant, in combination with basiliximab induction, mycophenolate mofetil, and corticosteroids (Bristol-Myers Squibb Company 2011). Current recommendations include using it only in patients who are EBV seropositive; however, patients should be monitored for an increased risk of infectious complications and Progressive Multifocal Leukoencephalopathy.

5.3.3 CD7 antagonism

SDZCHH380 is a monoclonal antibody targeting CD7. This IgG1 chimeric mouse antibody was initially studied in kidney transplantation (Lazarovits et al., 1993; Sharma et al., 1997). The CD7 molecule is expressed on T cells and natural killer cells during early differentiation, functioning as a costimulatory molecule. Early studies of SDZCHH380 as an induction agent in kidney transplantation demonstrated comparable short and long-term outcomes to OKT3 induction (Sharma et al., 1997). Despite favorable results up to 4 years following administration, further investigative endeavors were not pursued in solid organ transplantation.

5.3.4 T cell receptor antagonism

T10B9, or Medi-500, is a monoclonal antibody to the T cell receptor. Specifically, this is a murine IgMκ molecule to the αβ heterodimer region of the CD3 complex (Brown et al., 1996; Waid et al., 1992, 2009). Because it does not bind directly to the Fc receptor, there is reduced immune stimulation and occurrence of cytokine release syndrome. The end result is T cell depletion. Early studies demonstrated the efficacy of this agent as induction therapy and a treatment modality for acute rejection in solid organ transplantation, as compared to OKT3 (Waid et al., 1997a, 1997b). However, given the efficacy of similar humanized monoclonal antibodies, further investigations in solid organ transplantation were not pursued.

6. Special considerations

6.1 High risk donor kidneys & recipients

Marginal donor kidneys are defined as expanded criteria donors (ECD) or donation after cardiac death donors (DCD). These allografts are at higher risk of developing delayed graft function, which has been shown to decrease overall allograft survival and increase the incidence of acute rejection (Deroure et al., 2010; Rudich et al., 2002). There was a large prospective, international, randomized controlled trial examining the efficacy of rATG versus basiliximab in patients at high risk of delayed graft function (Brennan et al., 2006). Patients were maintained on a cyclosporine-based triple drug immunosuppression regimen and eligibility criteria included ECD or DCD allografts, standard criteria donors (SCD) with greater than 24 hours of cold ischemia time, repeat transplants, panel-reactive antibody value exceeding 20% before transplantation, donors with acute tubular necrosis (ATN), recipient black race, or one or more HLA mismatches. The incidence of delayed graft function was not significantly different between patients receiving rATG and basiliximab induction. However, the incidence of biopsy-proven acute rejection was significantly lower in patients receiving rATG. Additionally, severe rejection episodes requiring antibody therapy were less frequent in the rATG group. Interestingly, the overall incidence of infection was significantly lower in the basiliximab group, yet the incidence of CMV was lower in the rATG group.

6.2 Sensitization & incompatibility

Sensitization to HLA antigen typically occurs as a result of blood transfusions, pregnancy, or previous transplantation (Marfo et al., 2011). These patients are more likely develop circulating DSA and have a positive cross-match during transplantation evaluation. Sensitized patients wait considerable longer on the deceased donor waitlist.

Various modalities have been developed to combat sensitization. Antibodies can be removed by plasmapheresis and immunoadsorption techniques; however anti-HLA antibodies generally rebound and return to baseline (Hakim et al., 1990). As discussed earlier, rituximab has also been used with varying success, as B cells recovery occurs 6 to 12 months following administration. Bortezomib has been used in sensitized patients (Perry et al., 2009). Recently, a new medication called eculizumab has emerged as a humanized monoclonal antibody to complement component 5 (C5) to mediate complement-mediated injury, which may have potential in desensitization protocols (Larrea et al., 2010). IVIG has also been used in sensitized patients to acutely decrease PRA levels, especially in ABO-incompatible patients. Finally, splenectomy has also been used in desensitization protocols of ABO-incompatible patients (Kaplan et al., 2007).

Despite these numerous combinations of these therapies with acceptable short-term outcomes, intermediate-term outcomes have been modest at best. Some have reported graft survival rates at 3 years to be 78% (Haririan et al., 2009) and 4-year graft survival of only 66% (Lefaucher et al., 2007). Additionally, higher rates of clinical and subclinical antibody-mediated rejection have been reported (Haas et al, 2007; Loupy et al., 2009).

6.3 Older recipients

Several considerations should be examined when choosing induction therapy in older recipients. Older patients may have lower rates of acute rejection as a result of diminished immune activity (B.N. Becker 1996; Friedman et al., 2004). There is also a higher rate of infectious complications as well as malignancies (Meier-Kriesche et al., 2001; Stratta et al., 2008). Thus, less intense induction and immunosuppression appear sufficient. However, if significant HLA-mismatch is present, higher rates of acute rejection have been described (Frei et al., 2008; Fritsche et al., 2003; Giessing et al., 2003). Nevertheless, the safety profile of

IL-2 receptor antibodies in patients with considerable comorbidities, such as the older recipients, may be preferred.

7. Acknowledgements

The authors gratefully acknowledge the expert assistance of Ms. Johanna Martin in creating all figures depicted in the chapter.

8. References

Abott, K.C.; Hypolite, I.O.; Viola, R., et al. (2002). Hospitalizations for cytomegalovirus disease after renal transplantation in the United States. *Ann Epidemiol*, Vol.12, No.6, (August 2002), pp. 402-409, ISSN 1047-2797.

Afaneh, C.; Halpern, J.; Cheng, E., et al. (2010). Steroid avoidance in two-haplotype-matched living donor renal transplants with basiliximab induction therapy. *Transplant Proc*, Vol.42, No.10, (December 2010), pp. 4526-9, ISSN 0041-1345.

Becker, B.N.; Ismail, N.; Becker, Y.T., et al. (1996). Renal transplantation in the older end stage renal disease patient. *Semin Nephrol*, Vol.16, No.4, (July 2006), pp. 353-62, ISSN 0720-9295.

Becker, Y.T.; Samaniego-Picota, M., & Sollinger, H.W. (2006). The emerging role of rituximab in organ transplantation. *Transpl Int*, Vol.19, No.8, (August 2006), pp. 621-8, ISSN 0934-0874.

Beiras-Fernandez, A.; Chappell, D.; Hammer, C., et al. (2006). Influence of polyclonal anti-thymocyte globulins upon ischemia reperfusion injury in a non-human primate model. *Transpl Immunol*, Vol.15, No.4, (April 2006), pp. 273-9, ISSN 0966-3274.

Benvenisty, A.I.; Cohen, D.; Stegall, M.D., et al. (1990). Improved results using OKT3 as induction immunosuppression in renal allograft recipients with delayed graft function. *Transplantation*, Vol.49, No.2, (February 1990), pp. 321-7, ISSN 0041-1337.

Bishop, G.; Cosimi, A.B.; Voynow, N.K., et al. (1975). Effect of immunosuppressive therapy for renal allografts on the number of circulating sheep red blood cells rosetting cells. *Transplantation*, Vol.20, No.2, (Augusut 1975), pp. 123-9, ISSN 0041-1337.

Bock, H.A.; Gallati, H.; Zurcher, R.M., et al. (1995). A randomized prospecitve trial of prophylactic immunosuppression with ATG-Fresenius versus OKT3 after renal transplantation. *Transplantation*, Vol.59, No.6, (March 1995), pp. 830-40, ISSN 0041-1337.

Bonnefoy-Berard, N.; Vincent, C., & Revillard, J. (1991). Antibodies against the functional leukocyte surface molecules in polyclonal antilymphocyte and antithymocyte globulins. *Transplantation*, Vol.51, No.3, (March 1991), pp. 669-73, ISSN 0041-1337.

Bonvini, P.; Zorzi, E.; Basso, G., et al. (2007). Bortezomib-mediated 26S proteasome inhibition causes cell-cycle arrest and induces apoptosis in CD-30+ anaplastic large cell lymphoma. *Leukemia*, Vol.21, No.4 (April 2007), pp. 838–42, ISSN 0887-6924.

Boulianne, G.L.; Hozumi, N.; Shulman, M.J., et al. (1984). Production of functional chimaeric mouse/human antibody. *Nature*, Vol.312, No.5995, (December 1984), pp. 643-6, ISSN 0028-0836.

Brennan, D.C.; Flavin, K.; Lowell, J.A., et al. (1999). A randomized,double-blinded comparison of thymoglobulin versus Atgam for induction immunosuppressive therapy in adult renal transplant recipients. *Transplantation*, Vol.67, No.7, (April 1999), pp. 1011-8, ISSN 0041-1337.

Brennan, D.C.; Daller, J.A.; Lake, K.D., et al. (2006). Rabbit antithymocyte globulin versus basiliximab in renal transplantation. *N Engl J Med*, Vol.355, No.19, (November 2006), pp. 1967-77, ISSN 0028-4793.

Bristol-Myers Squibb Company. (2011). Nulojix® (belatacept) prescribing information. Princeton, New Jersey, USA; (2011).

Brown, S.A.; Lucas, B.A.; Waid, T.H., et al. (1996). T10B9 (MEDI-500) mediated immunosuppression: studies on the mechanism of action. *Clin Transplant*, Vol.10, No.6, (December 1996), pp. 607-13, ISSN 0902-0063.

Buchler, M.; Hurault de Ligny, B.; Madec, C., et al. (2003). Induction therapy by anti-thymocyte globulin (rabbit) in renal transplantation: a 1-yr follow-up of safety and efficacy. *Clin Transplant*, Vol.17, No.6, (December 2003), pp. 539-45, ISSN 0902-0063.

Bunn, D.; Lea, C.K.; Bevan, D.J., et al. (1996). The pharmacokinetics of anti-thymocyte globulin (ATG) following intravenous infusion in man. *Clin Nephrol*, Vol.45, No.1, (January 1996), pp. 29-32, ISSN 0301-0430.

Bustami, R.T.; Ojo, A.O.; Wolfe, R.A., et al. (2004). Immunosuppression and the risk of post-transplant malignancy among cadaveric first kidney transplant recipients. *Am J Transplant*, Vol.4, No.1, (January 2004), pp. 87-93, ISSN 1600-6135.

Capra, J.D., & Edmundson, A.B. (1977). The antibody combining site. *Sci Am*, Vol.236, No.1, (January 1977), pp. 50-9, ISSN 0036-8733.

Casadei, D.H.; del C Rial, M.; Opelz, G., et al. (2001). A randomized and prospective study comparing treatment with high-dose intravenous immunoglobulin with monoclonal antibodies for rescue of kidney grafts with steroid-resistant rejection. *Transplantation*, Vol.71, No.1, (January 2001), pp. 53-8, ISSN 0041-1337.

Cecka, J.M.; Gjertson, D., & Terasaki, P. (1993). Do prophylactic antilymphocyte globulins (ALG and OKT3) improve renal transplant in recipient and donor high-risk groups? *Transplant Proc*, Vol.25, No.1, (February 1993), pp. 548-9, ISSN 0041-1345.

Chatenoud, L.; Jonker, M.; Villemain, F., et al. (1986). The human immune response to the OKT3 monoclonal antibody is oligoclonal. *Science*, Vol.232, No.4756), (June 1986), pp. 1406-8, ISSN 0036-8075.

Chatenoud, L.; Ferran, C.; Legendre, C., et al. (1990). In vivo cell activation following OKT3 administration: systemic cytokine release and modulation by corticosteroids. *Transplantation*, Vol.49, No.4, (April 1990), pp. 697-702, ISSN 0041-1337.

Chatenoud, L.; Legendre, C.; Ferran, C., et al. (1991). Corticosteroid inhibition of the OKT3-induced cytokine-related syndrome- dosage and kinetics prerequisites. *Transplantation*, Vol.51, No.2, (February 1991), pp. 334-8, ISSN 0041-1337.

Cherikh, W.S.; Kauffman, H.M.; McBride, M.A., et al. (2003). Association of the type of induction immunosuppression with posttransplant lymphoproliferative disorder, graft survival, and patient survival after primary kidney transplantation. *Transplantation*, Vol.76, No.9, (Novemeber 2003), pp. 1289-93, ISSN 0041-1337.

Clatworthy, M.R.; Friend, P.J.; Calne, R.Y., et al. (2009). Alemtuzumab (CAMPATH-1H) for the treatment of acute rejection in kidney transplant recipients: long-term follow-up. *Transplantation*, Vol.87, No.7, (April 2009), pp. 1092-5, ISSN 0041-1337.

Coles, A.J.; Wing, M.; Smith, S., et al. (1999). Pulsed monoclonal antibody treatment and autoimmune thyroid disease in multiple sclerosis. *Lancet*, Vol.354, No.9191, (Novemeber 1999), pp. 1691-5, ISSN 0140-6736.

Colvin, R.B., & Preffer, F.I. (1991). Laboratory monitoring of therapy with OKT3 and other murine monoclonal antibodies. *Clin Lab Med*, Vol.11, No.3, (September 1991), pp. 693-714, ISSN 0272-2712.

Cosimi, A.B.; Wortis, H.H.; Delmonico, F.L., et al. (1976). Randomized clinical trial of antilthymocyte globulin in cadaver renal allograft recipients: importance of T cell monitoring. *Surgery*, Vol.80, No.2, (August 1976), pp. 155-63, ISSN 0039-6060.

Cosimi, A.B. (1981a). The clinical value of antilymphocyte antibodies. *Transplant Proc*, Vol.13, No.1, (March 1981), pp. 462-8, ISSN 0041-1345.

Cosimi, A.B.; Burton, R.C.; Colvin, R.B., et al. (1981b). Treatment of acute renal allograft rejection with OKT3 monoclonal antibody. *Transplantation*, Vol.32, No.6, (December 1981), pp. 535-9, ISSN 0041-1337.

Csapo, Z.; Benavides-Viveros, C.; Podder, H., et al. (2005). Campath-1H as rescue therapy for the treatment of acute rejection in kidney transplant patients. *Transplant Proc*, Vol.37, No.5, (June 2005), pp. 2032-6, ISSN 0041-1345.

Deans, J.P.; Li, H.; Polyak, M.J., et al. (2002). CD20-mediated apoptosis: signaling through lipid rafts. *Immunology*, Vol.107, No.2, (October 2002), pp. 176-82, ISSN 0019-2805.

Debets, J.M.H.; Leunissen, K.M.L.; van Hooff, H.J., et al. (1989). Evidene of involvement of tumor necrosis factor in adverse reactions during treatment of kidney allograft rejection with antithymocyte globulin. *Transplantation*, Vol.47, No.3, (March 1989), pp. 487-92, ISSN 0041-1337.

Debure, A.; Chekoff, N.; Chatenoud, L., et al. (1988). One-month prophylactic use of OKT3 in cadaver kidney transplant recipients. *Transplantation*, Vol.45, No.3, (March 1988), pp. 546-53, ISSN 0041-1337.

Deroure, B.; Kamar, N.; Depreneuf, H., et al. (2010). Expanding the criteria of renal kidneys for transplantation: use of donors with acute renal failure. *Nephrol Dial Transplant*, Vol.25, No.6, (June 2010), pp. 1980-6, ISSN 0931-0509.

Durrbach, A.; Pestana, J.M.; Pearson, T., et al. (2010). A phase III study of belatacept versus cyclosporine in kidney transplants from extended criteria donors (BENEFIT-EXT study). *Am J Transplant*, Vol.10, No.3, (March 2010), pp. 547-57, ISSN 1600-6135.

Ellis, C.N.; Krueger, G.G. & Alefacept Clinical Study Group. (2001). Treatment of chronic plaque psoriasis by selective targeting of memory effector T lymphocytes. *N Engl J Med*, Vol.345, No.4, (July 2001), pp. *248-55*, ISSN 0028-4793.

Fehr, T.; Rüsi, B.; Fischer, A., et al. (2009). Rituximab and intravenous immunoglobulin treatment of chronic antibody-mediated kidney allograft rejection. *Transplantation*, Vol.87, No.12, (June 2009), pp. 1837-41, ISSN 0041-1337.

Ferrant, J.L.; Benjamin, C.D.; Cutler, A.H., et al. (2004). The contribution of the Fc effector mechanisms in the efficacy of anti-CD154 immunotherapy depends on the nature of the immune challenge. *Int Immunol*, Vol.16, No.11, (Novemeber 2004), pp. 1583-94, ISSN 0953-8178.

Frei, U.; Noeldeke, J.; Machold-Fabrizii, V., et al. (2008). Prospective age-matching in elderly kidney transplant recipients – a 5-year analysis of the Eurotransplant Senior Program. *Am J Transplant*, Vol.8, No.1, (January 2007), pp. 50-7, ISSN 1600-6135.

Friedman, A.L.; Goker, O.; Kalish, M.A., et al. (2004). Renal transplant recipients over aged 60 have diminished immune activity and a low risk of rejection. *Int Urol Nephrol*, Vol.36, No.3, (2004), pp. 451-6, ISSN 0301-1623.

Fritsche, L.; Horstrup, J.; Budde, K., et al. (2003). Old-for-old kidney allocation allows successful expansion of the donor and recipient pool. *Am J Transplant*, Vol.3, No.11, (November 2003), pp. 1434-9, ISSN 1600-6135.

Fuchinoue, S.; Ishii, Y.; Sawada, T., et al. (2011). The 5-year outcome of ABO-incompatible kidney transplantation with rituximab induction. *Transplantation*, Vol.91, No.18, (April 2011), pp. 853-7, ISSN 0041-1337.

Gabardi, S.; Martin, S.T.; Roberts, K.L., et al. (2011). Induction immunosuppressive therapies in renal transplantation. *Am J Health Syst Pharm*, Vol.68, No.3, (February 2011), pp. 211-8, ISSN 1079-2082.

Gaber, A.O.; First, M.R.; Tesi, R.J., et al. (1998). Results of the double-blind, randomized, multicenter, phase III clinical trial of Thymoglobulin versus Atgam in the treatment of acute graft rejection episodes after renal transplantation. *Transplantation*, Vol.66, No.1, (July 1998), pp. 29-37, ISSN 0041-1337.

Genovese, M.C.; Becker, J.C.; Schiff, M., et al. (2005). Abatacept for rheumatoid arthritis refractory to tumor necrosis alpha inhibition. *N Engl J Med*, Vol.353, No.11, pp. 1114-23, ISSN 0028-4793.

Genzyme Corporation. (2005).. Thymoglobulin (rabbit antithymocyte globulin) prescribing information. Cambridge, MA; 2005.

Giessing, M.; Budde, K.; Fritsche, L., et al. (2003). 'Old-for-old' cadaveric renal transplantation: surgical findings, perioperative complications and outcome. *Eur Urol*, Vol.44, No.6, (December 2003), pp. 701-8, ISSN 0302-2838.

Gordon, K.B.; Vaishnaw, A.K.; O'Gorman, J., et al. (2003). Treatment of psoriasis with alefacept: correlation of clinical improvement with reductions of memory T-cell counts. *Arch Dermatol*, Vol.139, No.12, (December 2003), pp. 1563-70, ISSN 0003-987X.

Gourishankar, S.; McDermid, J.C.; Jhangri, G.S., et al. (2004). Herpes zoster infection following solid organ transplantation: incidence, risk factors and outomes in the current immunosuppressive era. *Am J Transplant*, Vol.4, No.1, (January 2004), pp. 108-15, ISSN 1600-6135.

Grillo-Lopez, A.J.; White, C.A.; Varns, C., et al. (1999). Overview of the clinical development of rituximab: first monoclonal antibody approved for the treatment of lymphoma. *Semin Oncol*, Vol.26, No.5, (October 1999), pp. 66-73, ISSN 0093-7754.

Grim, S.A.; Pham, T.; Thielke, J., et al. (2007). Infectious complications associated with the use of rituximab for ABO-incompatible and positive cross-match renal transplant recipients. *Clin Transplant*, Vol.21, No.5, (September 2007), pp. 628-32, ISSN 0902-0063.

Guttmann, R.D.; Caudrelier, P.; Alberici, G., et al. (1997). Pharmacokinetics, foreign protein immune response, cytokine release, and lymphocyte subsets in patients receiving thymoglobuline and immunosuppression. *Transplant Proc*, Vol.29, No.7A, pp. 24S–6, ISSN 0041-1345.

Haas, M.; Montgomery, R.A.; Segev, D.L., et al. (2007). Subclinical acute antibody-mediated rejection in positive crossmatch renal allografts. *Am J Transplant*, Vol.7, No.3, (January 2007), pp. 576-85, ISSN 1600-6135.

Hakim, R.M.; Milford, E.; Himmelfarb, J., et al. (1990). Extracorporeal removal of anti-HLA antibodies in transplant candidates. *Am J Kidney Dis,* Vol.16, No.5, (November 1990), pp. 423-31, ISSN 0272-6386.

Hale, G.; Waldmann, H.; Friend, P., et al. (1986). Pilot study of CAMPATH-1, a rat monoclonal antibody that fixes human complement, as an immunosuppressant in organ transplantation. *Transplantation,* Vol.42, No.3, (September 1986), pp. 308-11, ISSN 0041-1337.

Hale, G. (2001). The CD52 antigen and development of the CAMPATH antibodies. *Cytotherapy,* Vol.3, No.3, (2001), pp. 137-43, ISSN 1465-3249.

Hanaway, M.J.; Woodle, E.S.; Mulgaonkar, S., et al. (2011). Alemtuzumab induction in renal transplantation. *N Engl J Med,* Vol. 364, No.20, (May 2011), pp. 1909-19, ISSN 0028-4793.

Hardinger, K.L.; Schnitzler, M.A.; Miller, B., et al. (2004). Five-year follow up of thymoglobulin versus ATGAM induction in adult renal transplantation. *Transplantation* 2004; 78: 136, ISSN 0041-1337.

Hardinger, K.L. (2006). Rabbit antithymocyte globulin induction therapy in adult renal transplantation. *Pharmacotherpay,* Vol.26, No.12, (December 2006), pp. 1771-83, ISSN 0277-0008.

Haririan, A.; Nogueira, J.; Kukuruga, D., et al. (2009). Positive cross-match living donor kidney transplantation: Longer-term outcomes. *Am J Transplant,* Vol.9, No.3, (February 2009), pp. 536-42, ISSN 1600-6135.

Henricsson, A.; Husberg, B., & Bergentz, S.E. (1977). The mechanism behind the effect of ALG on platelets in vivo. *Clin Exp Immunol,* Vol.29, No.3, (September 1977), pp. 515-22, ISSN 0009-9104.

Henry, M.L.; Pelletier, R.P.; Elkhammas, E.A., et al. (2001). A randomized prospective trial of OKT3 induction in the current immunosuppression era. *Clin Transplant,* Vol.15, No.6, (December 2001), pp. 410-4, ISSN 0902-0063.

Hershberger, R.E.; Starling, R.C.; Eisen, H.J., et al. (2005). Daclizumab to prevent rejection after cardiac transplantation. *N Engl J Med,* Vol.352, No.26, (June 2005), pp. 2705-13, ISSN 0028-4793.

Humar, A.; Ramcharan, T.; Denny, R., et al. (2001). Are wound complications after a kidney transplant more common with modern immunosuppression? *Transplantation,* Vol.72, No.12, (December 2001), pp. 1920-3, ISSN 0041-1337.

IMTIX-SangStat. (2003). Thymoglobuline (rabbit antithymocyte globulin) prescribing information. Lyon, France; 2003.

Jaffers, G.J.; Fuller, T.C.; Cosimi, A.B., et al. (1986). Monoclonal antibody therapy: anti-idiotype and non-anti-idiotype antibodies to OKT3 arising despite intense immunosuppression. *Transplantation,* Vol.41, No.5, (May 1986), pp. 572-8, ISSN 0041-1337.

Jamil, B.; Nicholls, K.; Becker, G.J., et al. (1999). Impact of acute rejection therapy on infections and malignancies in renal transplant recipients. *Transplantation,* Vol.68, No.10, (November 1999), pp. 1597-603, ISSN 0041-1337.

Jirasiritham, S.; Khunprakant, R.; Techawathanawanna, N., et al. Treatment of simultaneous acute antibody-mediated rejection and acute cellular rejection with alemtuzumab in kidney transplantation: a case report. *Transplant Proc,* Vol.42, No.3, (April 2010), pp. 987-9, ISSN 0041-1345.

Jones, P.T.; Dear, P.H.; Foote, et al. (1986). Replacing the complementarity-determining regions in human antibody with those from a mouse. *Nature,* Vol.321, No.6069, (May 1986), pp. 522-5, ISSN 0028-0836.

Jordan, S.C.; Toyoda, M., & Vo, A.A. (2009). Intravenous immunoglobulin a natural regulator of immunity and inflammation. *Transplantation,* Vol.88, No.1, (July 2009), pp. 1-6, ISSN 0041-1337.

Jordan, S.C.; Toyoda, M.; Kahwaji, J., et al. (2011). Clinical Aspects of Intravenous Immunoglobulin Use in Solid Organ Transplant Recipients. *Am J Transplant,* Vol.11, No.2, (January 2011), pp. 196-202, ISSN 1600-6135.

Kahan, B.D.; Rajagopalan, P.R. & Hall, M. (1999). Reduction of the occurrence of acute cellular rejection among renal allograft recipients treated with basiliximab, a chimeric anti-interleukin-2-receptor monoclonal antibody. *Transplantation,* Vol.67, No.2, pp. 276-84, ISSN 0041-1337.

Kahwaji, J.; Barker, E.; Pepkowitz, S., et al. (2009). Acute hemolysis after high dose IVIG therapy in highly HLA sensitized patients. *Clin J Am Soc Nephrol,* Vol.4, No.12, (October 2009), pp. 1993-7, ISSN 1555-9041.

Kamar, N.; Milioto, O.; Puissant-Lubrano, B., et al. (2010). Incidence and predictive factors for infectious disease after rituximab therapy in kidney-transplant patients. *Am J Transplant,* Vol.10, No.1, (July 2009), pp. 89-98, ISSN 1600-6135.

Kamath, S.; Dean, D.; Peddi, V.R., et al. (1997). Efficacy of OKT3 as primary therapy for histologically confirmed acute renal allograft rejection. *Transplantation,* Vol.64, No.10, (November 1997), pp. 1428-32, ISSN 0041-1337.

Kaplan, B.; Gangemi, A.; Thielke, J., et al. (2007). Successful rescue of refractory severe antibody mediated rejection with splenectomy. *Transplantion,* Vol.83, No.1, (January 2007), pp. 99-100, ISSN 0041-1337.

Kawai, T.; Cosimi, A.B.; Spitzer, T.R., et al. (2008). HLA-mismatched renal transplantation without maintenance immunosuppression. *N Engl J Med,* Vol.358, No..4, (January 2008), pp. 353-61, ISSN 0028-4793.

Kazatchkine, M.D. & Kaveri, S.V. (2001). Immunomodulation of autoimmune and inflammatory disease with intravenous immune globulin. *N Engl J Med,* Vol.345, No.10, (September 2001), pp. 747-55, ISSN 0028-4793.

Kerr, P.G. & Atkins, R.C. (1989). The effects of OKT3 therapy on infiltrating lymphocytes in rejecting renal allografts. *Transplantation,* Vol.48, No.1, (July 1989), pp. 33-6, ISSN 0041-1337.

Kirk, A.D.; Harlan, D.M.; Armstrong, N.N., et al. (1997). CTLA4-Ig and anti-CD40 ligand prevent renal allograft rejection in primates. *Proc Natl Acad Sci U S A,* Vol.94, No.16, (August 1997), pp. 8789-94, ISSN 0027-8424.

Kirk, A.D.; Hale, D.A.; Mannon, R.B., et al. (2003). Results from a human renal allograft tolerance trial evaluating the humanized CD52-specific monoclonal antibody alemtuzumab (CAMPATH-1H). *Transplantation,* Vol.76, No.1, (July 2003), pp. 120-9, ISSN 0041-1337.

Kirk, A.D.; Hale, D.A.; Swanson, S.J., et al. (2006). Autoimmune thyroid disease after renal transplantation using depletional induction with alemtuzumab. *Am J Transplant,* Vol.6, No.5, (May 2006), pp. 1084-5, ISSN 1600-6135.

Kirkman, R.L.; Shapiro, M.E.; Carpenter, C.B., et al. (1991). A randomized prospective trial of anti-Tac monoclonal antibody in human renal transplantation. *Transplantation*, Vol.51, No.1, (January 1991), pp. 107-13, ISSN 0041-1337.

Kohler, G. & Milstein, C. (1975). Continuous cultures of fused cells secreting antibody of predefined specificity. *Nature*, Vol.256, No.5517, (August 1975), pp. 495-7, ISSN 0028-0836.

Langley, R.G.; Papp, K.; Bissonnette, R., et al. (2010). Safety profile of intravenous and subcutaneous siplizumab, an anti-CD2 monoclonal antibody, for the treatment of plaque psoriasis: results of two randomized, double-blind, placebo-controlled studies. *Int J Dermatol*, Vol.49, No.7, (July 2010), pp. 818-28, ISSN 0011-9059.

Larrea, C.F.; Cofan, F.; Oppenheimer, F., et al. (2010). Efficacy of eculizumab in the treatment of recurrent atypical hemolytic-uremic syndrome after renal transplantation. *Transplantation*, Vol.89, No.7, (April 2010), pp. 903-4, ISSN 0041-1337.

Lazarovits, A.I.; Rochon, J.; Banks, L., et al. (1993). Human mouse chimeric CD7 monoclonal antibody for the prophylaxis of kidney transplant rejection. *J Immunol*, Vol.150, No.11, (June 1993), pp. 5163-74, ISSN 0022-1767.

Lebranchu, Y.; Bridoux, F.; Buchler, M., et al. (2002). Immunoprophylaxis with basiliximab compared with antithymocyte globulin in renal transplant patients receiving MMF-containing triple therapy. *Am J Transplant*, Vol.2, No.1, pp. 48-56, ISSN 1600-6135.

Lefaucheur, C.; Nochy, D.; Hill, G.S., et al. (2007). Determinants of poor graft outcome in patients with antibody-mediated acute rejection. *Am J Transplant*, Vol.7, No.4, (April 2007), pp. 832-41, ISSN 1600-6135.

Lefaucheur, C.; Nochy, D.; Andrade, J., et al. (2009). Comparison of combination plasmapheresis/IVIG/Anti-CD20 versus high dose IVIG in the treatment of antibody-mediated rejection. *Am J Transplant*, Vol.9, No.5, (May 2009), pp. 1099-107, ISSN 1600-6135.

Legendre, C.; Kreis, H.; Bach, J., et al. (1992). Prediction of successful allograft rejection retreatment with OKT3. *Transplantation*, Vol.53, No.1, (January 1992), pp. 87-90, ISSN 0041-1337.

Lenschow, D.J.; Zeng, Y.; Thistlethwaite, J.R., et al. (1992). Long-term survival of xenogeneic pancreatic islet grafts induced with CTLA4Ig. *Science*, Vol.257, No.5071, (August 1992), pp. 789-92, ISSN 0036-8075.

Loupy, A.; Suberbielle-Boissel, C.; Hill, G.S., et al. (2009). Outcome of subclinical antibody-mediated rejection in kidney transplant recipients with preformed donor-specific antibodies. *Am J Transplant*, Vol.9, No.11, (September 2009), pp. 2561-70, ISSN 1600-6135.

Marfo, K.; Lu, A.; Ling, M., et al. (2011). Desensitization protocols and their outcome. *Clin J Am Soc Nephrol*, Vol.6, No.4, (March 2011), pp. 922-36, ISSN 1555-9041.

Martin, M.A.; Massanari, M.; Nghiem, D.D., et al. (1988). Nosocomial aseptic meningitis associated with administration of OKT3. *JAMA*, Vol.259, No.13, (April 1988), pp. 2002-5, ISSN 0002-9955.

Meier-Kriesche, H.U.; Ojo, A.O.; Hanson, J.A., & Kaplan, B. (2001). Exponentially increased risk of infectious death in older renal transplant recipients. *Kidney Int*, Vol.59, No.4, (April 2001), pp. 1539-43, ISSN 0085-2538.

Meier-Kriesche, H.U.; Li, S.; Gruessner, R.W., et al. (2006). Immunosuppression: evolution in practice and trends, 1994-2004. *Am J Transplant*, Vol.6, No.5, (2006), pp. 1111-31, ISSN 1600-6135.

Merion, R.; White, D.J.; Thiru, S., et al. (1984). Cyclosporine: five years experience in cadaveric renal transplantation. *N Engl J Med*, Vol.310, No.3, (January 1984), pp. 148-54, ISSN 0028-4793.

Morrison, S.L.; Johnson, M.J.; Herzenberg, L.A., et al. (1984). Chimeric human antibody molecules: mouse antigen-binding domains with human constant region domains. *Proc Natl Acad Sci U S A*, Vol.81, No.21, (November 1984), pp. 6851-5, ISSN 0027-8424.

Mourad, G.; Garrigue, V.; Squifflet, J.P., et al. (2001). Induction versus noninduction in renal transplant recipients with tacrolimus-based immunosuppression. *Transplantation*, Vol.72, No.6, (September 2001), pp. 1050-5, ISSN 0041-1337.

Mourad, G.; Rostaing, L.; Legendre, C., et al. (2004). Sequential protocols using basiliximab versus antithymocyte globulins in renal-transplant patients receiving mycophenolate mofetil and steroids. *Transplantation*, Vol.78, No.4, (August 2004), pp. 584-90, ISSN 0041-1337.

Nashan, B.; Moore, R.; Amlot, P., et al. (1997). Randomized trial of basiliximab versus placebo for control of acute cellular rejection in renal allograft recipients. CHIB201 International Study Group. *Lancet*, Vol.350, No.9086, (October 1997), pp. 1193-8, ISSN 0140-6736.

Nashan, B.; Light, S.; Hardie, I.R., et al. (1999). Reduction of acute renal allograft rejection by daclizumab. *Transplantation*, Vol.67, No.1, (January 1999), pp. 110-5, ISSN 0041-1337.

Niblack, G.; Johnson, K.; Williams, T., et al. (1987). Antibody formation following administration of antilymphocyte serum. *Transplant Proc*, Vol.19, No.1, (February 1987), pp. 1896-7, ISSN 0041-1345.

Nishida, H.; Ishida, H.; Tanaka, T., et al. (2009). Cytomegalovirus infection following renal transplantation in patients administered low-dose rituximab induction therapy, *Transpl Int*, Vol.22, No.10, (July 2009), pp. 961-9, ISSN 0934-0874.

Nogid, A. & Pham, D.Q. (2006). Role of abatacept in the management of rheumatoid arthritis.*Clin Ther*, Vol.28, No.11, (November 2006), pp. 1764-78, ISSN 0149-2918.

Norman, D.J.; Shield, C.F. III; Barry, J., et al. (1988). Early use of OKT3 monoclonal antibody in renal transplantation to prevent acute rejection. *Am J Kidney Dis*, Vol.11, No.2, (February 1988), pp. 107-10, ISSN 0272-6386.

Norman, D.J.; Kahana, L.; Stuart, F.P. Jr., et al. (1993). A randomized clinical trial of induction therapy with OKT3 in kidney transplantation. *Transplantation*, Vol.55, No.1, (January 1993), pp. 44-50, ISSN 0041-1337.

Opelz, G. (1995). Efficacy of rejection prophylaxis with OKT3 in renal transplantation. Collaborative Transplant Study. *Transplantation*, Vol.60, No.11, (December 1995), pp. 1220-4, ISSN 0041-1337.

Ortho Multicenter Transplant Study Group. (1985). A randomized clinical trial of OKT3 monoclonal antibody for acute rejection of cadaveric renal transplants. *N Engl J Med*, Vol. 313, No.6, (August 1985), pp. 337-42, ISSN 0028-4793.

Parrott, N.R.; Hammad, A.Q.; Watson, C.J., et al. (2005). Multicenter, randomized study of the effectiveness of basiliximab in avoiding addition of steroids to cyclosporine a monotherapy in renal transplant recipients. *Transplantation*, Vol.79, No.3, (February 2005), pp. 344-8, ISSN 0041-1337.

Pearl, J.P.; Parris, J.; Hale, D.A., et al. (2005). Immunocompetent T-cells with a memory-like phenotype are the dominant cell type following antibody-mediated T-cell depletion. *Am J Transplant*, Vol.5, No.3, (March 2005), pp. 465-74, ISSN 1600-6135.

Perry, D.K.; Burns, J.M.; Pollinger, H.S., et al. (2009). Proteasome inhibition causes apoptosis of normal human plasma cells preventing alloantibody production. *Am J Transplant*, Vol.9, No.1, (January 2009), pp. 201-9, ISSN 1600-6135.

Pisani, B.A.; Mullen, G.M.; Malinowska, K., et al. (1999). Plasma- pheresis with intravenous immunoglobulin G is effective in patients with elevated panel reactive antibody prior to cardiac transplantation. *J Heart Lung Transplant*, Vol.18, No.7, (July 1999), pp. 701-6, ISSN 1053-2498.

Ponticelli, C.; Rivolta, E.; Tarantino, A., et al. (1987). Treatment of severe rejection of kidney transplant with OKT3.PAN. *Transplant Proc*, Vol.1, No.1, (February 1987), pp. 1908-9, ISSN 0041-1345.

Prin Mathieu, C.; Renoult, E.; Kennel De March, A., et al. (1997). Serum anti-rabiit and anti-horse IgG, IgA, and IgM in kidney transplant recipients. *Nephrol Dial Transplant*, Vol.12, No.10, (October 1997), pp. 2133-9, ISSN 0931-0509.

Pruett, T.L.; McGory, R.W.; Wright, F.H., et al. (2009). Safety profile, pharmacokinetics, and pharmacodynamics of siplizumab, a humanized anti-CD2 monoclonal antibody, in renal allograft recipients. *Transplant Proc*, Vol.41, No.9, (November 2009), pp. 3655-61, ISSN 0041-1345.

Rosenberg, J.C.; Lekas, N.; Lysz, K., et al. (1975). Effect of antithymocyte globulin and other immune reactants on human platelets. *Surgery*, Vol.77, No.4, (April 1975), pp. 520-9, ISSN 0039-6060.

Rudich, S.M.; Kaplan, B.; Magee, J.C., et al. (2002). Renal transplantations performed using non-heart-beating organ donors: going back to the future? *Transplantation*, Vol.74, No.12, (December 2002), pp. 1715-20, ISSN 0041-1337.

San Miguel, J.F.; Schlag, R.; Khuageva, N.K., et al. (2008). Bortezomib plus melphalan and prednisone for initial treatment of multiple myeloma. *N Engl J Med*, Vol.359, No.9, (August 2008), pp. 906-17, ISSN 0028-4793.

Schaffer, D.; Langone, A.; Nylander, W.A., et al. (2003). A pilot protocol of a calcineurin-inhibitor free regimen of kidney transplant recipients of marginal donor kidneys or with delayed graft function. *Clin Transplant*, Vol.17, No.9, (2003), pp. 31-4, ISSN 0902-0063.

Schroeder, T.J.; First, M.R.; Mansour, M.E., et al. (1990). Antimurine antibody formation following OKT3 therapy. *Transplantation*, Vol.49, No.1, pp. 48-51, ISSN 0041-1337.

Sharma, L.C.; Muirhead, N., & Lazarovits, A.I. (1997). Human mouse chimeric CD7 monoclonal antibody (SDZCHH380) for the prophylaxis of kidney transplant rejection: analysis beyond 4 years. *Transplant Proc*, Vol.29, No.1-2, (February 1997), pp. 323-4, ISSN 0041-1345.

Shehata, N.; Palda, V.; Meyer, R., et al. (2010). The use of immunoglobulin therapy for patients undergoing solid organ transplantation: an evidence -based practice guideline. *Transf Med Rev*, Vol.24, No.1, (January 2010), pp. S7-27, ISSN 0887-7963.

Shield, C.F.; Edwards, E.B.; Davies, D.B., et al. (1997). Antilymphocyte induction therapy in cadaver renal transplantation. *Transplantation*, Vol.63, No.9, (May 1997), pp. 125763 ISSN 0041-1337.

Shoskes, D.A. & Halloran, P.F. (1996). Delayed graft function in renal transplantation: etiology, management and long-term significance. *J Urol*, Vol.155, No.6, (June 1996), pp. 1831-40, ISSN 0022-5347.

Singh, A.; Stablein, D., & Tejani, A. (1997). Risk factors for vascular thrombosis in pediatric renal transplantation: a special report of the North American Pediatric Renal Transplant Cooperative Study. *Transplantation*, Vol.63, No.9, (May 1997), pp. 1263-7, ISSN 0041-1337.

Sonnenday, C.J.; Warren, D.S.; Cooper, M., et al. (2004). Plasmapheresis, CMV, hyperimmune globulin, and anti-CD20 allow ABO-incompatible renal transplantation without splenectomy. *Am J Transplant*, Vol.4, No.8, (August 2004), pp. 1315-22, ISSN 1600-6135.

Spitzer, T.R.; McAfee, S.L.; Dey, B.R., et al. (2003). Nonmyeloablative haploidentical stem-cell transplantation using anti-CD2 monoclonal antibody (MEDI-507)-based conditioning for refractory hematologic malignancies. *Transplantation*, Vol.75, No.10, (May 2003), pp. 1748-51, ISSN 0041-1337.

Squifflet, J.P.; Besse, T.; Malaise, J., et al. (1997). BTI-322 for induction therapy after renal transplantation: a randomized study. *Transplant Proc*, Vol.29, No.1-2, (February 1997), pp. 317-9, ISSN 0041-1345.

Stratta, P.; Morellini, V.; Musetti, C., et al. (2008). Malignancy after kidney transplantation: results of 400 patients from a single center. *Clin Transplant*, Vol.22, No.4, (February 2008), pp. 424-7, ISSN 0902-0063.

Svoboda, J.; Kotloff, R., & Tsai, D.E. (2006). Management of patients with post-transplant lymphoproliferative disorder: the role of rituximab. *Transpl Int*, Vol.19, No.4, (April 2006), pp. 259-69, ISSN 0934-0874.

Szczech, L.A.; Berlin, J.A.; Aradhye, S., et al. (1997). Effect of anti-lymphocyte induction therapy on renal allograft survival: a meta-analysis. *J Am Soc Nephrol*, Vol.8, No.11, (November 1997), pp. 1771-7, ISSN 1046-6673.

Tatum, A.H.; Bollinger, R.R., & Sanfilippo, F. (1984). Rapid serological diagnosis of serum sickness from antilymphocyte globulin therapy using enzyme immunoassay. *Transplantation*, Vol.38, No.6, (December 1984), pp. 582-6, ISSN 0041-1337.

Tesi, R.J.; Elkhammas, E.A.; Henry, M.L., et al. (1993). OKT3 for primary therapy of the first rejection episode in kidney transplants. *Transplantation*, Vol.55, No.5, (May 1993), pp. 1023-9, ISSN 0041-1337.

Thistlethwaite, J.R. Jr; Gaber, A.O.; Haag, B.W., et al. (1987). OKT3 treatment of steroid-resistant renal allograft rejection. *Transplantation*, Vol.43, No.2, (February 1987), pp. 176-84, ISSN 0041-1337.

Thistlethwaite, J.R. Jr; Stuart, J.K.; Mayes, J.T., et al. (1988). Complications and monitoring of OKT3 therapy. *Am J Kidney Dis*, Vol.11, No.2, (February 1988), pp. 112-9, ISSN 0272-6386.

Tite, J.P.; Sloan, A.; Janeway, C.J. (1986). The role of L3T4 in T cell activation: L3T4 may be both an Ia-binding protein and a receptor that transduces a negative signal. *J Mol Cell Immunol*, Vol.2, No.4, (1986), pp. 179-90, ISSN 0724-6803.

Trivedi, H.L.; Terasaki, P.I.; Feroz, A., et al. (2009). Abrogation of anti-HLA antibodies via proteasome inhibition. *Transplantation*, Vol.87, No.10, (May 2009), pp.1555-61, ISSN 0041-1337.

Turka, L.A.; Linsley, P.S.; Lin, H., et al. (1992). T-cell activation by the CD28 ligand B7 is required for cardiac allograft rejection in vivo. *Proc Natl Acad Sci U S A*, Vol.89, No.22, (November 1992), pp. 11102-5, ISSN 0027-8424.

Tyden, G.; Genberg, H.; Tollemar, J., et al. (2009). A randomized, double-blind, placebo-controlled, study of single-dose rituximab as induction in renal transplantation. *Transplantationl*, Vol.87, No.9, (May 2009), pp. 1325-9, ISSN 0041-1337.

Vallhonrat, H.; Williams, W.W.; Cosimi, A.B., et al. (1999). In vivo generation of C4b, Bb, iC3b, and SC5b-9 after OKT3 administration in kidney and lung transplant recipients. *Transplantation*, Vol.67, No.2, (January 1999), pp. 253-8, ISSN 0041-1337.

Vigeral, P.; Chkoff, N.; Chatenoud, L., et al. (1986). Prophylactic use of OKT3 monoclonal antibody in cadaveric kidney recipients: utilization of OKT3 as the sole immunosuppressive agent. *Transplantation*, Vol.41, No.6, (June 1986), pp. 730-3, ISSN 0041-1337.

Vincenti, F.; Lantz, M.; Birnbaum, J., et al. (1997). A phase I trial of humanized anti-interleukin 2 receptor antibody in renal transplantation. *Transplantation*, Vol.63, No.1, (January 1997), pp. 33-8, ISSN 0041-1337.

Vincenti, F.; Ramos, E.; Brattstrom, C., et al. (2001). Multicenter trial exploring calcineurin inhibitors avoidance in renal transplantation. *Transplantation*, Vol.71, No.9, (May 2011), pp. 1282-7, ISSN 0041-1337.

Vincenti, F.; Larsen, C.; Durrbach, A., et al. (2005). Costimulation blockade with belatacept in renal transplantation. *N Engl J Med*, Vol.353, No.8, (August 2005), pp. 770-81, ISSN 0028-4793.

Vincenti, F.; Charpentier, B.; Vanrenterghem, Y., et al. (2010). A phase III study of belatacept-based immunosuppression regimens versus cyclosporine in renal transplant recipients (BENEFIT study). *Am J Transplant*, Vol.10, No.3, (March 2010), pp. 535-46, ISSN 1600-6135.

Waid, T.H.; Lucas, B.A.; Thompson, J.S., et al. (1992). Treatment of acute cellular rejection with T10B9.1A-31 or OKT3 in renal allograft recipients. *Transplantation*, Vol.53, No.1, (January 1992), pp. 80-6, ISSN 0041-1337.

Waid, T.H.; Lucas, B.A.; Thompson, J.S, et al. (1997a). Treatment of renal allograft rejection with T10B9.1A-31 or OKT3: Final analysis of a phase 2 clinical trial. *Transplantation*, Vol.64, No.2, (July 1997), pp. 274-81, ISSN 0041-1337.

Waid, T.H.; Thompson, J.S.; McKeown, J.W., et al. (1997b). Induction immunotherapy in heart transplantation with T10B9.1A-31: a phase I study. *J Heart Lung Transplant*, Vol.16, No.9, (September 1997), pp. 913-6, ISSN 1053-2498.

Waid, T.H.; Thompson, J.S.; Siemionow, M., et al. (2009). T10B9 monoclonal antibody: a short-acting nonstimulating monoclonal antibody that spares gammadelta T-cells and treats and prevents cellular rejection. *Drug Des Devel Ther*, Vol.3, (Septemeber 2009), pp. 205-12 ISSN 1177-8881.

Weaver, T.A.; Charafeddine, A.H.; Agarwal, A., et al. (2009). Alefacept promotes co-stimulation blockade based allograft survival in nonhuman primates. *Nat Med*, Vol.15, No.7, (July 2009), pp. 746-9, ISSN 1078-8956.

Webster, A; Pankhurst, T.; Rinaldi, F., et al. (2006). Polyclonal and monoclonal antibodies for treating acute rejection episodes in kidney transplant recipients. *Cochrane Database Syst Rev*, Vol.19, No.2, (April 2006), pp. CD004756, ISSN 1469-493X.

Wong, J.T.; Eylath, A.A.; Ghobrial, I., et al. (1990). The mechanism of anti-CD3 monoclonal antibodies: mediation of cytolysis by inter-T cell bridging. *Transplantation*, Vol.50, No.4, (October 1990), pp. 683-9, ISSN 0041-1337.

18

Radiotherapy and Immunity – A Mini Review

Rosangela Correa Villar
Department of Radiation Oncology, University of Sao Paulo, Medicine School
Brasil

1. Introduction

Slavin *et al.* in [1976], were the first to found that rejection of skin and heart allograft was greatly delayed in rodents treated with Total Lymphoid Irradiation (TLI). Since 1980, the immunosupression of TLI has been applied in transplants and autoimmune diseases. However, the development of immunosuppressive drugs decreased the use of radiotherapy for immunosuppressive finality except for the use of total body irradiation (TBI) or TLI as myeloablative treatment before bone marrow transplantation

The mechanism by which TLI-treated patients have a graft prolongation is not entirely understood. During many years of its use many changes has been observed specially in lymphocytes counts. The majority of the studies, however, were done without modern techniques to characterize the fate of different subtypes of lymphocytes and is difficult to compare the results. The majority of the studies has been done *in vitro* and in regimes using TBI and bone marrow transplants. There is some evidence that suppressor T-cells might be involved in the long term maintenance of allografts in these patients [Gray et al, 1989]. TLI provokes a more pronounced impairment of T-dependent immunological functions, as measured with phytohemaglutinin- (PHA), concanavalin A- (Con A), and pokeveed-induced (PWM) blastogenesis than does conventional immunosuppression. The more profound changes in the balance between T helper and T suppressor cells after TLI are also associated with a more pronounced suppressor cell activity, as measured with different functional suppressor cell assays. [Fergunson et al, 1981; Waer et al, 1987]. The TLI seems to produce an "amnesic state" and the autoantigens cannot be recognized by the host anymore.

In the past, radiation therapy had traditionally been viewed as immunosuppressive (Cole, 1986; James et al., 1989; Wasserman et al., 1989). Lymphocyte radiosensitivity is well established and remains the dominant explanation for this effect. However, substantial evidence suggests more varied effects of radiation on the immune system, prompting the re-characterization of radiation as 'immunomodulatory' rather than immunosuppressive (McBride et al., 2004).

Ionising radiation induces diverse effects on cell survival, apoptosis, proliferation and differentiation depending on the dosage and target cell (Jonathan et al. 1999). High dose of radiation often results in massive DNA damage that involves double-strand breaks and subsequent cell death. Low dose of irradiation induces reactive oxygen species (ROS) and the activation of specific intracellular signaling pathways and transcription factors leading to proliferation and differentiation of target cells (Kasid et al. 1996, Lander et al. 1997, Finkel 1998). Therefore, irradiation can modulate immune response via its variable effects on immune cell survival and differentiation (Shankar et al. 1999, Rho et al. 2004, Liu 2007, Shan et al.2007).

The immune system responds to ionizing radiation with distinct characteristics depending on multiple factors such as dose and dose rate, tissue and cell types. Overall, immune cells are susceptible to radiation-induced damage and readily undergo apoptosis in response to small doses of radiation. Cellular apoptosis is critically regulated by various intracellular and extracellular signaling mechanisms. CD95 (Apo-1/Fas) is a homotrimeric tumour necrosis factor receptor (TNFR) family member characterised by the presence of a death domain in its cytoplasmic tail. CD95-mediated apoptosis is an important process with enormous physiological and pathophysiological impact and cell-type-specific features. CD95 molecules have been implicated in the maintenance of self-tolerance and T-cell homeostasis by transmitting apoptotic signals to repeatedly activated antigen-specific T cells, as well as to antigen-presenting dendritic cells (DCs) and activated B cells. (Schu¨ tze et al. 2008). For example, It has been described that Treg maintain immunological tolerance by suppression of autoreactive T cells but it was also shown that low dose total body irradiation (LTBI) selectively decreased the proportion and absolute number of Treg and enhanced antitumor immunity in murine model. It occurs because Treg displaying much higher apoptotic baseline and apoptosis-related proteins are more radiosensitive than its effector counterpart CD4pCD257T cells (Mendge et al, 2011) An important finding to help explain the immune 'stimulating' effect of low dose irradiation is the differential impact on Treg vs. CD4þ CD257 cell population. These relevant findings appoint to the hypotheses that the net balance for the immune system may be a relative decrease in Treg-mediated suppression and a net increase in effector T cell activity. Similar effect was confirmed in in-vivo that LTBI is a very attractive adjuvant strategy to enhance overall cancer immunotherapy or vaccine responses (Liu et al.2010). Other possible mechanisms of immune enhancement are elimination of suppressor cells as Treg and myeloid suppressor cells and augmentation of the immune response including natural killer (NK) cells, B cells and T cells activation, costimulatory molecules upregulation, IFNg and IL-2 production and release, and enhanced proliferative activity of lymphocytes to mitogenic stimuli (Belka et al, 1999; Hashimoto et al, 1999; Safwat 2000a; 2000b; Liu et al, 2001; Kipnis et al, 2004; Jin et al, 2007; Shan et al, 2007)

Although the effects of radiation on the survival of lymphocytes have been extensively studied *in vitro*, a correlation of the frequency of radiation-induced apoptosis in human peripheral blood lymphocytes during TLI have not previously been performed. In 2008 we published the clinical results of a protocol using TLI plus immunosuppressive agents to prevent recurrence after renal transplant in patients with focal and segmental glomerulosclerosis (FSGS) (Villar et al, 2008). This disease presents with early recurrence after renal transplants and an involvement of the immune system has been implicated in its pathogenesis. During the study the purpose was also to investigate the changes in peripheral blood monocyte and lymphocyte subpopulations and the role of the *in vivo* induction of apoptosis in patients undergoing TLI pre renal transplant (TX) (unpublished data). It was a very rare opportunity to study *in vivo* the immunosuppressant effect caused by TLI during each week of the treatement in patients that had not received any immunosuppressive drug or chemotherapy before. We studied 9 patients and they were treated with aggressive immunosuppressive treatment associating TLI with the drugs mycophenolate mofetil (MMF), prednisone (PRED) and cyclosporine (CsA) commonly used in conventional immunosuppressive treatments. TLI were performed as described in Villar et al, 2008. Immunophenotyped peripheral blood T and B lymphocyte subsets and monocytes were performed before treatment (control) and followed during each week of

TLI (after each 9 Gy), on TX´s day and after TX (30, 60 and 90 days) using flow cytometry. The percentages of T-helper, T-suppressor, B-lymphocytes and monocytes/macrophages cells, were determined on the cells in the lymphogate. Mitogen stimulation tests in lymphocytes culture using phytohemaglutinin (PHA) and pokeweed mitogen (PWM) were performed before and after completion of TLI, at the TX day and at 1 month interval up to three months post-transplantation.

1.1 Isolation of lymphocytes and detection of apoptosis

The *in vivo* radiation-induced apoptosis in lymphocytes was investigated in blood samples of 9 patients before TLI, pre and pos-hemodyalisis (controls 1 and 2) and 6h and 24h after the first and the second fraction of TLI and 6h after each 9 Gy until the end of TLI. The observation of apoptosis on freshly blood samples (2 patients) were insignificant then in the others (7 patients), we decided to observe the commitment to apoptosis of the lymphocytes irradiated *in vivo* after 72h in cell culture with and without mitogen (PHA) using an *ex vivo* test. After the cells were kept in culture they were assessed for binding of Annexin by resuspending 2 x10^5 cel/100µl and subsequently by incubating with 10µl Annexin V-FITC for 30min. In order to distinguish between apoptotic (Annexin V+/PI-) and secondary necrotic (Annexin V +/PI+) cells, 10µl of propidiun iodeto (PI) (2µg/ml) was also added before analyzing on a Coulter Epics XL-MCL flow cytometer. Two-colour flow-cytometric analyses were performed on a FACSort. A gate was put on Annexin V + (green) cells and a backgating performed on the scatter plot in order to discriminate optimally platelets and debris from smaller apoptotic cells with exclusion of monocytes (increased side scatter). In cells with a damaged membrane PI cannot be excluded anymore and a red fluorescent signal was observed indicating secondary necrotic cells. The results were expressed as percentage of apoptotic cells in 10.000 cells counted in the pre-determined window. All the results were expressed as the percentage of the pre-treatment value. Statistical analysis was performed comparing the values before and after treatment (Friedman`s ANOVA - $p \leq 0.05$). We observed significant reduction of all parameters analysed after treatment. Leukocytes decreased 55%, lymphocytes had a reduction of 60%, 70 % and 97 % for CD3/CD4, CD8 and CD19, respectively, at the transplant's day (p<0,05) The statistical analysis showed a significant decrease since the first week of TLI (p<0,05). The steep decrease for T cells was not significantly different between CD4 and CD8, but the decrease of B-cells was significantly more important than T-cells (**fig.1**). The decrease observed in CD14 cells was not significant (p=0,569). Lymphocytes proliferative activity decrease 60% (with PHA) and 67% (with PWM) after TLI. The PWM response was less expressive (p = 0,09), statistical analysis showed reduction significantly maintained after TX only with PHA (p=0,009) **(fig 2,3).**

There was significant increase of apoptosis *in vivo* in peripheral blood lymphocytes (PBL) in the beginning of TLI, (6h after first fraction of TLI) and necrosis at the end of TLI (10 and 15 fractions of TLI) **(fig. 4,5)**. The phenomenon (apoptosis) was significantly increased by PHA stimulus **(fig.6)**.

In our experience TLI provide important immunosuppresion with a significant fall in T and B lymphocytes and functional response to PHA. The B lymphocytes were the more radiosensitive and the monocyte the most radioresistant cells. No significant differences between T-helper and T-supressor/cytotoxic cells were observed.TLI induced significant increase of apoptosis *in vivo* in PBL after low doses and necrosis after high doses of TLI.

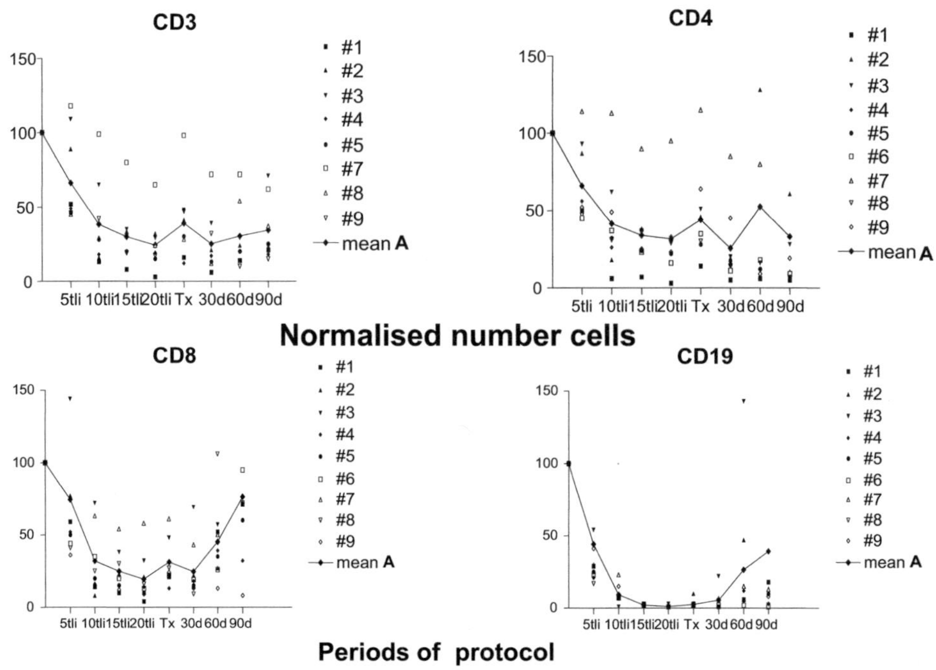

Fig. 1. Response of CD3, CD4, CD8, CD19 lymphocytes during radiotherapy and after transplant. The results were normalized to the values obtained before the treatment and plotted against the equivalent period of evaluation. A mean time-response curve resulting from statistical analyse to the data of all patients (mean A). Individual patients results are indicated on the figures

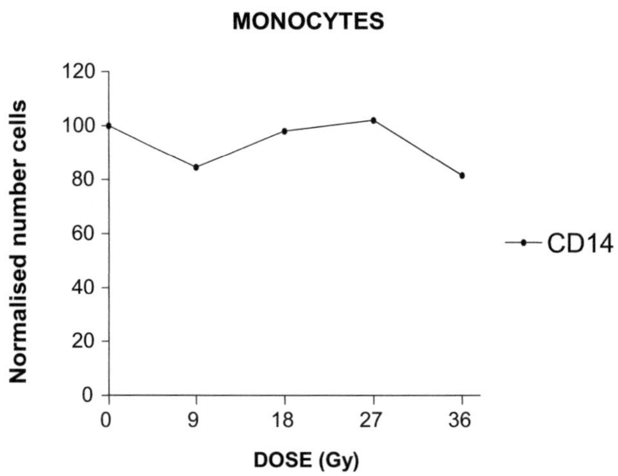

Fig. 2. Response of monocytes (CD14) with dose (Gy) in the nine (9) patients. The results were normalised to the values obtained before the start of the TLI and plotted against the equivalent period of the irradiation (first to fourth week).

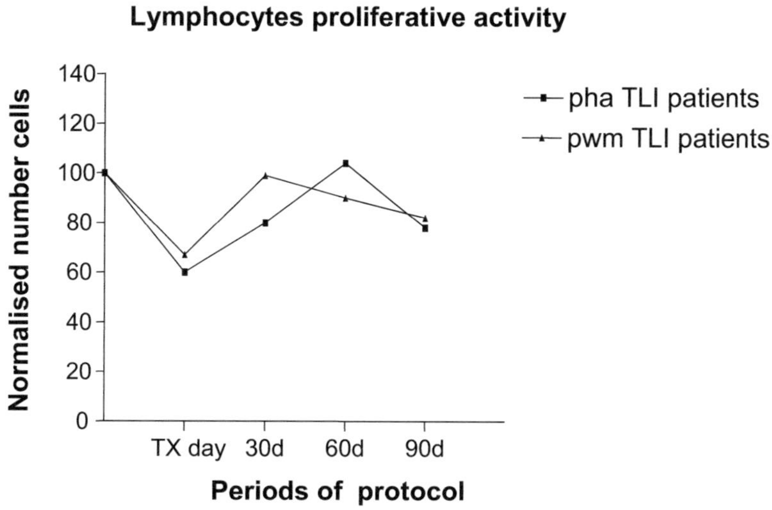

Fig. 3. Lymphoproliferative activity of 9 patients during the periods of protocol: control, after TLI (day of TX), 30, 60 and 90 days after TX. PHA = lymphocytes culture with phitohemaglutinin mitogen stimulation. PWM = lymphocytes culture with pokeweed mitogen stimulation

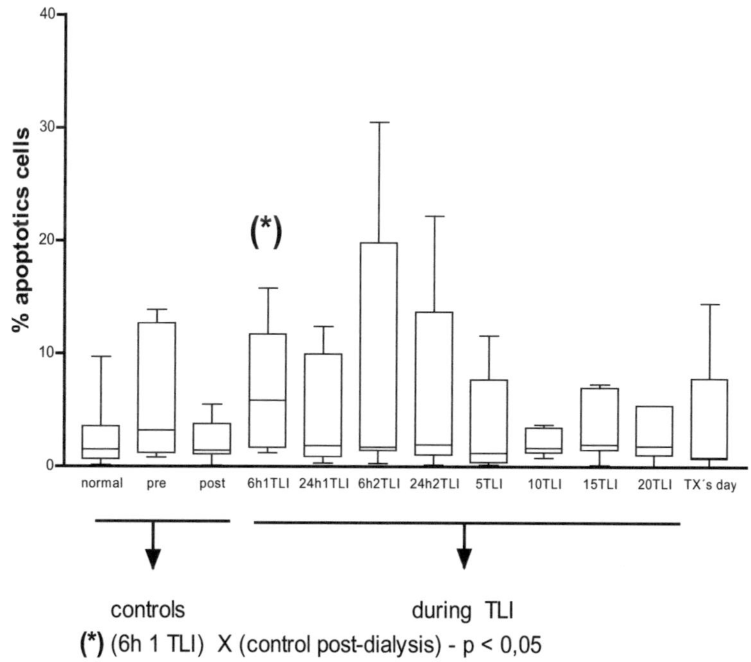

Fig. 4. Percentagem of apoptotic cells (Annexin+) observed in culture of lymphocytes without PHA. Results of controls (normal subjects, patients pre and post-dialysis and before TLI) , patients during TLI and on TX´s day

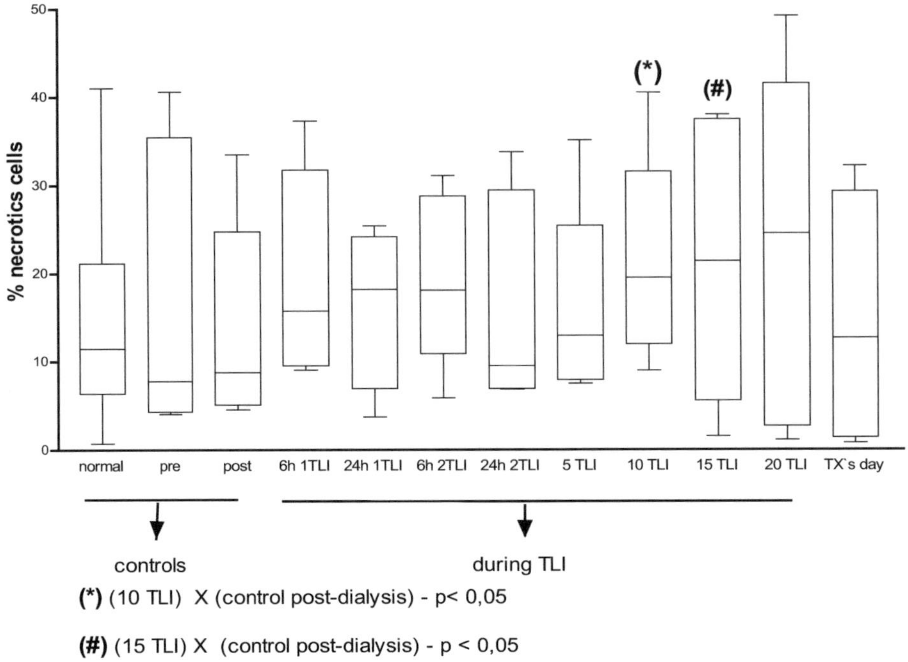

Fig. 5. Percentagem of necrotic cells (Pi +) observed in culture of lymphocytes without PHA. Results of controls (normal subjects, patients pre and post-dialysis and before TLI) , patients during TLI and on TX´s day. Necrotics cells increased at the end of TLI

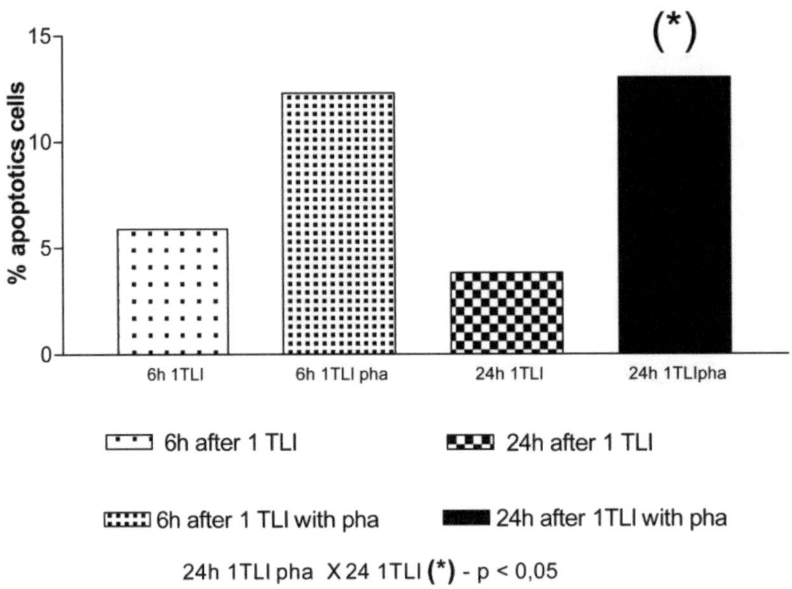

Fig. 6. Comparative analyse of percentagem of apoptotics cells observed in the periods of 6h and 24h after first fraction of TLI in culture of lymphocites with and without PHA.The percentagem of apoptosis was higher in the presence of PHA

2. Mini review

Lymphocyte radiosensitivity is well established and remains the dominant explanation for the immunosuppressive effect of radiotherapy. However, substantial evidence suggests more varied effects of radiation on the immune system, prompting the re-characterization of radiation as 'immunomodulatory' rather than immunosuppressive (McBride et al., 2004). The effect of radiotherapy in microenviroment, cytokines, gene expressions and the importance of the dose in the immunossuprressive effect has emerging as new and important concepts. The use of the immunomodulatory effect of radiation in oncology has been pointed as a new perspective and its participation has again increasing in transplants tolerance and in treatment of autoimmune diseases. In the next pages we describe the new and important concepts recently acquired in radiotherapy and immunity

2.1 The role of radiation

2.1.1 Immunomodulatory effects of radiation

Increased expression of proinflammatory cytokines, including TNF-a and IL-1b following radiation has been reported by some authors (Hallahan et al.,1989; Ishihara et al., 1995; Nemoto et al., 1995). These observations suggest a potential role for radiation in signaling 'danger' and, perhaps, in the activation of antigen presenting cells (McBride et al., 2004). However, studies aimed at determining the effects of radiation on antigen-presenting cell phenotype, cytokine expression and function have been contradictory. While alterations in dendritic cells (DC) phenotype have been demonstrated infrequently (Cao et al.,2004), a number of investigators have noted changes in the cytokine secretory profile and function of DCs following irradiation. For example, Shigematsu et al. (2007), reported enhanced expression of IL-2, IL-12 and IFN-g by irradiated DCs and it was correlated with greater T-cell proliferation compared to non-irradiated DCs. In contrast, Merrick et al. (2005) reported decreased IL-12 production and impaired naive T-cell priming by irradiated compared to non-irradiated DCs. These contradictory findings may be attributable to the different irradiation strategies and models utilized in these studies. The effect of radiation on DC antigen presentation also remains controversial with a number of studies suggesting significant modulation of, or no effect on, T-cell stimulatory capacity. Interestingly, Liao et al. (2004) reported impaired T-cell priming against endogenously processed antigen and enhanced priming against exogenous peptide pointing to a more complex interplay between radiation and DC function. A number of factors may explain why the consistent characterization of immune responses to radiation remains elusive including differences in radiosensitivity or reactivity of different cell and tissue types, and dose-dependent effects. For example, the dose effect has been explored in a number of studies, some of which suggesting that lower doses of radiation have a greater potential to enhance immune responses (Hashimoto et al., 1999; Cao et al., 2002; Shigematsu et al., 2007)

3. Irradiation and transplants

Recently, the approach of combined organ and hematopoietic cell transplantation has been successfully applied to tolerance induction in humans (Fudaba el al., 2006; Scandling et al., 2008; Kawai et al., 2008). Conditioning regimens used to achieve mixed chimerism and tolerance include lethal and sublethal total body irradiation (TBI) with or without thymic irradiation and anti-T cell antibodies (Ildstad & Sachs 1984; Kawai et al., 2002; Stykes 2001),

TLI with and without anti-T cell antibodies (Slavin et al., 1976; Slavin et al., 1978; Slavin et al, 1977; Scandling et al., 2008 ;Hayamizu et al, 1999; Lan et al, 2000; Higuchi et al, 2002), costimulatory blockade with or without rapamycin therapy or cytoreduction (Wekerle et al, 2000; Durhan et al, 2000; Lambert et al., 2002;Graca et al., 2006), injection of naturally occurring CD4+CD25+ Treg (nTreg) cells combined with radiation cytoreduction (Golshayn et al., 2007; Wood & Sakaguchi, 2003), and chemical cytoreduction combined with thymic irradiation, and anti-T cell antibodies (Fudaba et al, 2006; Kawai et al 2008,).

Although central and peripheral clonal deletion in chimeras can explain the lack of reactivity of host immune cells to donor alloantigens (Stikes 2001; Wekerle et al, 1998), host regulatory T cells that remain after cytoreduction or that are injected after cytoreduction can also play an important role in the engraftment of the donor organ and hematopoietic cells (Higushi 2002, Golshayn et al, 2007; Wood & Sakaguchi 2003).

In the mixed chimera and tolerance induction model with TLI, anti-thymocyte serum (ATS),and bone marrow transplantation, tolerance is dependent on the residual host natural killer (NK) T cells . However,CD4 regulatory T cells, (Tregs) and nTregs induced from CD4+CD25- T cell precursors (iTregs) have been shown to play an important role in promoting tolerance to allografts in both chimeric and non-chimeric mouse models (Lambert et al., 2002,Chai et al, 2005,Graca et al., 2002, Sakaguchi, 2005, Kang et al, 2007). Nador et al, 2010 has been studying the role of residual host Tregs in the mixed chimera model using TLI and ATS conditioning. They demonstrated the requirement for host Tregs selectively depleting these cells pretransplant with a single injection of anti-CD25 mAb. The experiment results showed that deficiency in either NK T cell or Tregs prevents chimerism and tolerance in the TLI and ATS model. This lymphodepletive-conditioning regimen facilitated tolerance by altering the balance of host T cell subsets to markedly favor the NKT cells and Tregs over alloreactive host naïve (CD62LhiCD44lo) T cells. Therefore, the changes in the balance of regulatory and naïve T cell subsets and their contributions to graft acceptance or rejection using a TLI and ATS conditioning regimen is the responsible to induce mixed chimerism and tolerance after combined heart and bone marrow transplantation (Hayamizu et al., 1999; Lan et al., 2000; Higuchi et al., 2002).

It was demonstrated that one day after the completion of TLI and ATS conditioning (time point of donor bone marrow infusion) there was a marked increase in the ratio of CD4+ CD25+Foxp3+ Treg cells and NKT cells to naïve conventional T cells. The change in the balance of T cell subsets is best explained by their differential resistance to radiation induced cell death due to differential expression of the anti-apoptotic protein, Bcl-2, as reported previously (Yao et al., 2009). Nador et al, 2010 showed thatp53-/- mice had no change in the balance after TLI. T cell proliferation and thymic generation of T cells play a minimal role whereas the p53/Bcl-2 apoptotic pathway plays the dominant role in the changes (Yao et al, 2009). The considerable resistance of Treg cells to apoptosis induced by ATS as compared to conventional T cells has been reported to be due to high levels of expression of the anti-apoptotic protein, BCLXL (Ninamimura et al, 2006). It is of interest that the altered balance of T cell subsets favoring Treg and NKT cells returned to normal about 6 weeks after conditioning, and by that time the stable mixed chimeras are tolerant to the heart allografts due to clonal deletion (Higuchi et al, 2002).

The relationship between NKT cells and Tregs in responses to alloantigens has been reported recently (Pillai et al, 2009). Naïve but not memory phenotype CD4+ T cells from untreated mice show alloreactivity in the MLR, and alloreactivity by conventional T cells in the MLR is suppressed by Treg cells at a 1:1 ratio (Dutt et al., 2007; Schiopu, A. & Wood, 2008). The changed ratio of these cells on day 1 was likely to have prevented the hosts from rejecting bone marrow and heart allografts acutely. In another experiment, the ability of naïve and memory phenotype T cells from untreated BALB/c mice to reject C57BL/6 heart allografts was compared by transferring equal numbers of sorted cells to immunodeficient RAG-2-/- BALB/ c hosts bearing the grafts. Whereas the naïve cell injection resulted in rejection of all grafts, the memory phenotype cell injection obtained from donors that had not been exposed to alloantigens resulted in no rejection over a 100-day observation period. In conclusion, the TLI and ATS tolerance induction model requires both regulatory NKT cells and Tregs for graft acceptance. Tolerance is promoted by profound but transient changes in the balance of regulatory and naive T cells of host origin favoring the regulatory cells. (Nador et al, 2010)

4. Irradiation and self-reactive immune response

CD4 regulatory T cells (Tregs) are the main effectors of immunological tolerance in adult life. Several studies have indicated that quantitative and qualitative abnormalities of regulatory Tregs contribute to the pathogenesis of autoimmune diseases as collagen-induced disease arthritis (CIA) (Morgan et al, 2003; Morgan et al, 2005) and in a spontaneous model of Rheumatoid Arthritis (RA).(Sakaguchi et al, 2003) There is evidence that the local proinflammatory environment is fundamental in imparting a Treg defect, because the treatment with anti-tumour necrosis factor (TNF)α may restore their function by generating transforming growth factor (TGF)β producing Tregs.(Nadkarmi et al, 2007). Therefore, generating functionally effective Tregs may provide an effective approach for the treatment of collagen-induced disease.

The adoptive transfer of Tregs can be efficacious in the treatment of autoimmune diseases in preclinical models,(Tang Q, 2004) but the major limitation of such a strategy is that, in order to obtain a dose sufficient for clinical use, Tregs need to be expanded in vitro with implications on their functionality (Hoffman et al, 2009). An alternative strategy is to increase the number of Tregs by exploiting the selective advantage of Tregs over conventional T cells during homeostatic reconstitution following cell ablative treatments (Cox et al., 2005; Nadal et al., 2007). It was previously reported that even non-myeloablative doses of irradiation are sufficient to determine a selective retention/expansion of Tregs capable of producing an immunosuppressive activity against donor haematopoietic antigens, thus facilitating their engraftment (Weng et al, 2007). Therefore, one very possible hypothesis is that partial myeloablation could also generate the conditions to control autoimmune diseases.

Myeloablative regimens have successfully been used for the treatment of severe forms of autoimmune arthritis (Dazzi et al.; 2007) whereby the consequent haematopoietic reconstitution is associated with a comprehensive renewal of the T cell repertoire (Murano et al, 2005). The major drawback of these approaches is toxicity. Mild myeloablation appears to be sufficient to modulate pathogenic immune responses and produce beneficial effects on CIA (Nakatsukasa et al, 2008) but the mechanisms remain to be clarified.

Weng et al., 2010 demonstrated that low-dose irradiation ameliorates CIA at the time of disease induction and if used when clinical signs of the disease are detectable. They established a causative relationship between the therapeutic efficacy of irradiation and Treg mediated tolerance. Irradiation induced immune tolerance to the immunizing collagen through modalities that require the presence of Tregs. The therapeutic activity is associated with the development of Treg immunosuppressive activity and the in vivo depletion of Tregs prevents the beneficial effects of irradiation.

Tregs selectively survive myeloablative regimens and undergo a marked expansion while retaining their functional activity (Bayer et al., 2009). The same mechanisms might account for the therapeutic efficacy of autologous BM transplantation in autoimmune arthritis (Roord et al., 2008). In a proteoglycan-induced arthritis, the conditioning of recipient mice with a lethal irradiation dose (7.5 cGy) and subsequent syngeneic BM transplantation significantly reduced the severity of arthritis. This study observed an increment in the proportion of CD4CD25 T cells and the clinical improvement was prevented if recipient mice received anti-CD25 depleting antibodies 1 week after the transplant. In contrast to other results, the investigators did not observe any effect if anti-CD25 antibodies were given on the day of the transplant. The disparity should be ascribed to the different intensity of the conditioning regimen (7.5 cGy vs 4 cGy) that delayed Treg homeostatic reconstitution as demonstrated by the delayed peak of Treg expansion following the myeloablative dose (Bayer et al, 2009).

The transient nature of the therapeutic effect induced by low-dose irradiation in the CIA model can result from the contribution of various factors. Firstly, the Tregs that are proportionally expanded following the non-myeloablative regimen are of recipient origin and, because of the rapid expansion kinetics, of the memory type. Their effect could be less durable and/or less potent than the naive Tregs that are generated at a later stage during the haematopoietic reconstitution following full myeloablation (Roord et al., 2008). However, to our knowledge there is no evidence of such at difference in the activity of different Treg subtypes and it is more likely that the magnitude of myeloablation differently influences the duration and thus the efficacy of the Tregs proportional increment (Weng et al., 2007; Laylor et al, 2005). The quantization of CD4CD25FoxP3+ following low-dose irradiation indicated that the percentage of Tregs increased at 12 days and, although less so, also remained elevated a week later. However, when we enumerated the absolute values, the numbers of CD4CD25FoxP3+ were much reduced as compared to CIA controls. Since the absolute number of CD4FoxP3−T cells, which contain the fraction responsible for mediating the disease, was equally reduced, it is the resulting change in the ratio between effectors and Tregs that should account for the therapeutic effect. The characterization of the effector cells in treated mice suggests that the dose of irradiation used did not affect the proportion of IL17 producing T cells. Since IL17 has been suggested to play an important role in RA and CIA (Fugimoto et al, 2008), it appears that neither irradiation nor the proportional Treg expansion is sufficient to interfere with IL17 production. Although this could justify the incomplete therapeutic effect, the levels of T helper 17 cells (Th17) in peripheral lymphoid tissues do not correlate with their levels in the injured tissues. It has been reported that anti-TNFα treatment, despite its ability to prevent Th17 in the joints increases their numbers in draining LNs.(Notley et al., 2008) We also observed that the numbers of IFNγ-producing cells are reduced in the irradiated animals. While reducing the inflammatory activity, the inhibition of IFNγ production also limits the potential to convert effector to FoxP3+ cells.(Xiao et al., 2008) The interpretation of the data is complicated by the fact that the pathogenic or protective effects of these cytokines are dependent on the timing of their production.(Lohr et al., 2006) The evidence provided the rationale to exploit the selective Treg activation induced by partial immunoablation for the treatment of autoimmune diseases. Further studies are however warranted to improve the duration of the therapeutic efficacy (Weng et al., 2010).

5. Radiotherapy and immunomodulation in cancer

Radiation is commonly used as a method of decreasing lymphocyte numbers via cytotoxicity for the purpose of bone marrow transplantation (BMT). CD25þCD4þ regulatory T cells (Treg) comprise 5–10% of the circulating CD4þ T cell population and suppress immune responses. A large body of experimental data suggests an essential role played by these cells in self-tolerance, transplantation, allergy and tumor/microbial immunity (Wing et al. 2006). Currently, many investigators are pursuing strategies to modulate the function or the number of Treg, which may offer a means to regulate host immunity for therapeutic effect in autoimmune diseases and cancers (Zou 2006). However, previous investigators have also suggested that low-dose whole-body irradiation (LTBI) results in immune enhancement in the treatment of chronic lymphocytic leukemia (CLL) and lymphoma (Safwat 2000a, 2000b). Accumulating evidence shows that irradiation influences the phenotype and function of immune cells (Cao et al. 2004, 2009, Reuben et al. 2004, Merrick et al. 2005). For example, Cao et al, showed that irradiation inhibited proliferation and suppressive ability of Treg with dose-dependent decrease of FOXP3 expression (Cao et al. 2009). A differential radiosensitivity and apoptosis-related proteins expression exist at varying doses of radiation between human Treg and effector T cells. LTBI is successful in inducing long-term remissions and has been shown to be as effective as the chemotherapy to which it has been compared in lymphoma (Safwat 2000a). However, the mechanism of this effect is unknown. The efficacy of LTBI could be partly attributed to a radiation-induced immune enhancement rather than to direct killing of tumor cells by radiation. This type of immune enhancement could be induced by two mechanisms: a differential elimination of the suppressive T subset of lymphocytes or an augmentation of the immune response through direct and/or indirect stimulation of T lymphocytes. RT can also theoretically enhance anti-tumor immunity via increasing the expression of tumor-associated antigens, inducing immune-mediated targeting of the tumor stroma, and diminishing regulatory T cell activity. Recent evidence suggests that RT may also activate effectors of innate immunity through Toll-like receptor (TLR)-dependent mechanisms, thereby augmenting the adaptive immune response to cancer (Roses et al. 2008). Thus RT can be better-characterized as having immunomodulatory properties that can allow its use as adjunct to immunotherapy (McBride et al. 2004).

6. Enhancement of antitumor effectors mechanisms

The efficacy of radiation therapy in the treatment of many tumor types is well established. While radiation induced tumor regression is largely the result of directed damage to radiosensitive tumor cells, evidence points to a number of additional immune-mediated mechanisms. Suppressor populations of T cells may be more radiosensitive than their effector counterparts and, conversely, tumor-specific effector T cells may be relatively radio-resistant (North, 1986; Dunn and North, 1991). This notion, as it relates to contemporary definitions of regulatory T cells (Tregs), has not been extensively explored. However, one recent study implicated Treg depletion in the enhanced efficacy of adoptive T-cell immunotherapy for transplanted melanomas following whole-body irradiation in a murine model (Antony et al., 2005). Enhanced functionality of adoptively transferred T cells following radiation induced lympho-depletion has also been linked to increased availability of homeostatic cytokines (Wrzesinski et al., 2007). A number of studies have measured the effects of low-dose total-body irradiation on the relative size of T-cell subpopulations and expression of cytokines associated with T-cell activation. In one report, low dose irradiation following transplantation of a hepatoma cell line in a rat model resulted in an increased proportion of CD8-positive splenocytes, increased numbers of tumor infiltrating lymphocytes, increased TNF-a and IFN-g expression and decreased TGF-b expression This response correlated with a reduction in metastases (Hashimoto et al., 1999). Another study demonstrated an increased CD4:CD8 T cell ratio, and decreased expression of TGF-b and VEGF following low-dose total body-irradiation, which correlated with delayed tumor growth in mice transplanted with the Lewis lung carcinoma cell line (Miller et al., 2003). The so-called 'abscopal effect', whereby radiation results in reduced tumor growth outside the direct radiation field, suggests radiation-induced immune-mediated mechanisms. The fact that this effect may be enhanced with Fms-like tyrosine kinase receptor 3 ligand (Flt-3L), a stem cell mobilizing factor that augments the number of circulating DC precursors, in immunocompetent mice and abrogated in T-cell-deficient mice lends additional support to this contention (Demaria et al., 2004).

7. Stromal effects

Radiation may induce immune-mediated targeting of tumor stroma. Antigen released following tumor irradiation may be presented by stromal cells for subsequent destruction by CTLs. This mechanism was recently demonstrated by Zhang et al. (2007) in experiments utilizing immunodeficient mice given tumor transplants. Only the combination of irradiation and adoptive transfer of CTLs resulted in tumor regression. This regression correlated with increased expression of tumor-specific peptide-MHC complexes as delineated using a tumor antigen/MHC complex-specific TCR tetramer. Direct effects of radiation on the stroma may play a role in enhancing immune-mediated tumor regression as well. Induced modulation of the expression of adhesion molecules, such as accumulation of P-selectin in the lumen of tumor vasculature, may enhance infiltration of immune effectors into the tumor stroma (Hallahan et al., 1998; Hallahan and Virudachalam, 1999). Enhancement of tumor antigen recognition Induction of antitumor immunity by radiation may result from enhanced tumor antigen recognition. Irradiation induces tumor cell apoptosis, or necrosis secondary to vascular injury (Acker et al., 1998). Subsequent phagocytosis of apoptotic bodies by DCs and initiation of antitumor T-cell responses through cross presentation may ensue if DC maturation signals are concomitantly present. A number of studies have suggested that necrosis, but not apoptosis, is associated with DC maturation signals (Basu et al., 2000; Sauter et al., 2000) However, more recently evidence that some apoptotic pathways do induce DC maturation and antitumor immunity has emerged (Scheffer et al., 2003). Sublethal irradiation of tumors may also result in enhanced expression of surface molecules recognized or targeted by immune effectors, as is suggested by studies demonstrating increased expression of the MHC class I antigen, H-2D, by melanoma cells (Hauser et al., 1993) and tumor associated antigens including carcinoembryonic antigen by gastric adenocarcinoma cells (Hareyama et al., 1991). Increased expression of the death receptor Fas following radiation has also been demonstrated in a transgenic carcinoembryonic antigen-expressing tumor model and associated with greater susceptibility to CTL mediated tumor cell lysis (Chakraborty et al., 2003). Combining immunotherapy and radiation building upon the hypothesis that radiation can enhance anti-tumor immunity, investigators have begun to combine radiation therapy with immunotherapies as was recently reviewed (Demaria et al., 2005a). Generally, such efforts employ radiation to induce tumor cell apoptosis or necrosis with resultant antigen release for subsequent presentation by DCs. Several investigators have studied combinations of intra-tumoral or peri-tumoral DC administration (Nikitina and), or administration of Flt-3L (Chakravarty et al., 1999, 2006; Demaria et al., 2004) combined with irradiation, yielding promising results. Administration of a recombinant viral vaccine-expressing tumor-associated antigen(s) and costimulatory molecules in combination with tumor irradiation may capitalize on the capacity of radiation to enhance immune recognition of antigen-expressing tumor cells. Such an effect was recently demonstrated and linked to radiation induced up regulation of Fas on tumor cells (Chakraborty et al., 2004). A number of investigators have explored combinations of cytokine therapy and irradiation; studied cytokines include IL-3 (Chiang et al., 2000), IL-12 (Seetharam et al., 1999; Lohr et al., 2000) and TNFa (Weichselbaum et al., 1994). Local radiation therapy in combination with CTLA-4 blockade is an additional novel approach for overcoming mechanisms of tumor tolerance. This combination was recently demonstrated to induce anti-tumor CD8 T cells in a poorly immunogenic murine adenocarcinoma model, whereas CTLA-4 blockade alone did not (Demaria et al., 2005b). Collectively, these studies encourage optimism regarding the potential of combined immunotherapy and radiotherapy.

The 'innate' components of the mammalian immune system has been reviewed and new concepts introduced; the discovery of Toll-like receptors (TLRs) is a notable example. These receptors recognize highly conserved molecular patterns common to pathogens, termed pathogen-associated molecular patterns (Janeway and Medzhitov, 2002). Examples of pathogen-associated molecular patterns and corresponding TLRs include:doublestranded RNA, which is recognized by TLR3 (Alexopoulou et al., 2001), Lipopolysaccharide (LPS), which is recognized by TLR4 (Poltorak et al., 1998) and many others (Roses et al., 2008).

An extensive investigation into the molecular basis of TLR function has been undertaken in recent years (Akira and Takeda, 2004). Though considerable overlap exists between implicated pathways, signaling through the various TLRs may initiate discreet downstream molecular events. Most TLRs act through the myeloid differentiation primary response protein 88 (MyD88) and tumor necrosis factor receptor-associated factor 6 to activate nuclear factor kB (NF-kB) and mitogen-activated protein kinases and induce gene transcription. At the cellular level, TLR binding results not only in the activation of effectors of innate immunity, but also in the induction of adaptive responses. Ligation of TLRs expressed by antigen presenting cells may result in the expression of co-stimulatory molecules (for example, CD80 and CD86) and cytokines (for example, IL-6 and IL-12) (Macagno et al., 2007). Moreover, TLR-primed dendritic cells induce antigen-specific high avidity CD8 (Xu et al., 2003, 2006) and type-I polarized CD4 T-cell responses (Wesa et al., 2007). These findings have provided a foundation for immunotherapeutic strategies targeting tumor-associated antigens for the treatment of malignancies

Through the induction of antigen-presenting cell maturation and secretion of proinflammatory chemokines and cytokines, TLRs provide a link between innate and adaptive immunity, which may be exploited to induce robust immune responses against specific antigens, the therapeutic potential of TLR-targeted therapies. Conversely, TLR-targeted therapy may enhance subsequent responses to chemotherapy. Such combinations have been explored in a number of preclinical studies, sometimes with promising results (Lake and Robinson, 2005; Bourquin et al., 2006; Shi et al., 2007). While radiation therapy has not been explored as extensively, it too is emerging as a potentially powerful tool when combined with immunotherapies.

8. Radiation-induced TLR signaling

Investigations into the function TLRs have provided mechanistic insight into the actions of several established cancer therapies. Recent evidence suggests that TLR-dependent mechanisms contribute to the therapeutic effects of radiation as well. It has been widely hypothesized that tumor irradiation activates effectors of innate immunity through the induction of tumor cell apoptosis and the release of endogenous TLR agonists. The observation that such ubiquitous factors heat-shock proteins and uric acid can act through TLRs and induce DC maturation (Gallucci et al., 1999) supports this mechanism as does the demonstration that immature DCs, when administered into irradiated tumors, induce antitumor immunity (Kim et al., 2004).Most recently, the high-mobility-group box 1 alarmin protein, released by dying tumor cells, was shown to act on TLR4 expressed by DCs. Moreover, binding of TLR4 was demonstrated to increase the efficiency of tumor antigen processing and presentation (Apetoh et al., 2007). TLR dependent mechanisms may play a role in systemic therapies as well. Whole body irradiation was recently shown to increase bacterial translocation and circulating levels of the TLR 4 agonist lipopolysaccharide. This phenomenon was associated with enhanced anti-tumor immunity in an adoptive transfer model (Paulos et al., 2007). When considered together, such evidence provides a strong rationale for the use of radiation therapy as an immune intervention; a paradigm shift from the traditional view of radiation therapy as a cytotoxic therapy. The capacity of radiation to elicit the expression of TLR ligands systemically after gastrointestinal tract irradiation, or locally after tumor irradiation, may prove valuable in conjunction with other immunotherapies.

Potentiating anti-tumor immunity with radiation therapy and TLR agonists

Few investigators have directly studied the combination of radiation and TLR-targeted therapies; this despite recognition that the therapeutic effects of radiation maybe dependent upon TLR signaling. Mason et al. (2005) recently demonstrated a markedly enhanced tumor response to radiation therapy following peri- and intratumoral injections of the TLR agonist, CpG, in a murine fibrosarcoma model (Milas et al., 2004). In light of the recently elucidated role of TLRs in radiation induced responses, this effect may reflect synergy at the level of TLR signaling. Further investigations are required to determine the applicability of such approaches but potential implications of these findings are broad. TLR-targeted therapy may sensitize a wide range of tumor types to radiation therapy and result in a reduction of the radiation dose necessary to achieve a therapeutic effect. Such approaches may become increasingly important as new TLR-targeted therapies emerge.

9. Conclusions

Definitely, radiotherapy has been seen now as a immunomodulatory treatment. Many concepts has been changing during the past few years. A role for novel neoadjuvant immunotherapies is emerging and will result in opportunities to study their interplay with conventional treatments, such as chemotherapy and radiation and immunosuppressive drugs. Radiation therapy may be an important adjunct to immunotherapies with the potential to enhance the antigenicity of tumors and promote stromal targeting. Perhaps more importantly, radiation therapy may activate effectors of innate immunity through TLR-dependent mechanisms. The relative contributions of these distinct radiation-induced mechanisms remain unclear. As we learn more about the immune-mediated mechanisms we will be better able to utilize these modalities and emerging immunotherapies in combination (Roses et al, 2008).

10. References

Acker, J.C.; Marks, L.B.; Spencer, D.P.; et al. (1998). Serial in vivo observations of cerebral vasculature after treatment with a large single fraction of radiation. Radiat Res 149:350–359.

Akira, S. & Takeda, K. (2004). Toll-like receptor signalling. Nat Rev Immunol 4:499–511.

Alexopoulou, L.; Holt, A.C.; Medzhitov, R; et al. (2001). Recognition of double-stranded RNA and activation of NF-kappaB by Toll-like receptor 3. Nature 413:732–738.

Antony, P.A; Piccirillo, C.A; Akpinarli, A, et al. (2005). CD8+ T cell immunity against a tumor/self-antigen is augmented by CD4+ T helper cells and hindered by naturally occurring T regulatory cells. J Immunol 174: 2591-2601.

Apetoh, L.; Ghiringhelli, F; Tesniere, A.; et al. (2007). Toll-like receptor 4-dependent contribution of the immune system to anticancer chemotherapy and radiotherapy. Nat Med 13:1050–1059.

Basu, S.; Binder R.J.; Suto, R.;et al. (2000). Necrotic but not apoptotic cell death releases heat shock proteins, which deliver a partial maturation signal to dendritic cells and activate the NF-kappa B pathway. Int Immunol 12:1539–1546.

Bayer, A.L.; Jones, M.; Chirinos, J.; et al. (2009) Host CD4+CD25+ T cells can expand and comprise a major component of the Treg compartment after experimental HCT. Blood; 113:733–43.

Bourquin, C.; Schreiber, S.; Beck, S. ; et al. (2006). Immunotherapy with dendritic cells and CpG oligonucleotides can be combined with chemotherapy without loss of efficacy in a mouse model of colon cancer. Int J Cancer 118:2790–2795.

Belka, C.; Ottinger, H.; Kreuzfelder, E.; et al. (1999). Impact of localized radiotherapy on blood immune cells counts and function in humans. Radiotherapy & Oncology, 50:199–204.

Cao, M.D.; Chen, Z.D.; Xing, Y. (2004). Gamma irradiation of human dendritic cells influences proliferation and cytokine profile of T cells in autologous mixed lymphocyte reaction. Cell Biol Int 28:223–228.

Cao, Z.A.; Daniel, D.; Hanahan D. (2002). Sub-lethal radiation enhances anti-tumor immunotherapy in a transgenic mouse model of pancreatic cancer. BMC Cancer 2:11.

Cao, M.; Cabrera, R.; Xu, Y; et al. (2009). Gamma irradiation alters phenotypes and function of CD4þCD25þ regulatory T cells. Cell Biology International 33:565–571.

Chai, J.G.; Xue, S.A.; Coe D.; et al. (2005) Regulatory T cells, derived from naiveCD4+CD25- T cells by in vitro Foxp3 gene transfer, can induce transplantation tolerance. Transplantation; 79(10):1310–1316.

Chakraborty, M.; Abrams, S.I.; Camphausen, K.; et al. (2003). Irradiation of tumor cells up-regulates Fas and enhances CTL lytic activity and CTL adoptive immunotherapy. J Immunol 170:6338–6347.

Chakravarty, P.K.; Alfieri, A.; Thomas, E.K.; et al. (1999). Flt3-ligand administration after radiation therapy prolongs survival in a murine model of metastatic lung cancer. Cancer Res 59:6028–6032.

Chakravarty, P.K.; Guha, C.; Alfieri, A. et al. (2006). Flt3L therapy following localized tumor irradiation generates long-term protective immune response in metastatic lung cancer:its implication in designing a vaccination strategy. Oncology 70:245–254.

Chiang, C.S.; Hong, J.H.; Wu, Y.C.; et al. (2000). Combining radiation therapy with interleukin-3 gene immunotherapy. Cancer Gene Ther 7:1172–1178.

Cole, S. (1986). Long-term effects of local ionizing radiation treatment on Langerhans cells in mouse footpad epidermis. J Invest Dermatol, 87:608–612.

Cox, A.L., Thompson, S.A., Jones, J.L., et al. (2005) Lymphocyte homeostasis following therapeutic lymphocyte depletion in multiple sclerosis. Eur J Immunol ;35:3332–3342.

Dazzi, F.; van Laar J.M.; Cope, A.; et al. (2007) Cell therapy for autoimmune diseases. Arthritis Res Ther 2007;9:206.

Demaria, S.; Ng B.; Devitt, M.L.; et al. (2004). Ionizing radiation inhibition of distant untreated tumors (abscopal effect) is immune mediated. Int J Radiat Oncol Biol Phys 58:862–870.

Demaria, S.; Bhardwaj, N.; McBride, W.H.; et al. (2005a). Combining radiotherapy and immunotherapy:a revived partnership. Int J Radiat Oncol Biol Phys 63:655–666.

Demaria, S.; Kawashima, N.; Yang, A.M.; et al. (2005b). Immune-mediated inhibition of metastases after treatment with local radiation and CTLA-4 blockade in a mouse model of breast cancer. Clin Cancer Res 11:728–734.

Dunn, P.L. & North RJ. (1991). Selective radiation resistance of immunologically induced T cells as the basis for irradiationinduced T-cell-mediated regression of immunogenic tumor. J Leukoc Biol 49:388–396.

Durham, M.M.; Bingaman, A.W.; Adams, A.B.; et al.(2000) Cutting edge: administration of anti-CD40 ligand and donor bone marrow leads to hemopoietic chimerism and donor-specific tolerance without cytoreductive conditioning. J Immunol;165(1):1–4.

Dutt, S.; Tseng, D.; Ermann, J.; et al.(2007) Naive and memory T cells induce different types of graft-versus-host disease. J Immunol 2007;179(10):6547–6554.

Ferguson, R.M.; Sutherland D.E.R.; Kim, T., et al (1981) The in vitro assessment of the immunosuppressive effect of fractionated total lymphoid irradiation in renal allotransplantation. Transplant Proc, 3:1673-1675.

Finkel, T. (1998). Oxygen radicals and signaling. Current Opinion in Cell Biology, 10:248–253.

Fudaba, Y.; Spitzer ,T.R.; Shaffer, J., et al.(2006) Myeloma responses and tolerance following combined kidney and nonmyeloablative marrow transplantation: in vivo and in vitro analyses. Am J Transplant ;6(9):2121–2133.

Fujimoto M, Serada S, Mihara M, et al (2008) Interleukin-6 blockade suppresses autoimmune arthritis in mice by the inhibition of infl ammatory Th17 responses. Arthritis Rheum; 58:3710–9.

Gallucci, S. ; Lolkema, M. ; Matzinger, P. (1999). Natural adjuvants:endogenous activators of dendritic cells. Nat Med 5:1249–1255.

Golshayan, D.; Jiang, S.; Tsang, J.; et al.(2007) In vitro-expanded donor alloantigenspecific CD4+CD25+ regulatory T cells promote experimental transplantation tolerance. Blood;109(2):827–835.

Graca L, Cobbold SP, Waldmann H. (2002) Identification of regulatory T cells in tolerated allografts. J Exp Med ;195(12):1641–1646.

Graca, L., Daley, S., Fairchild, P.J.,et al. (2006) . Co-receptor and co-stimulation blockade for mixed chimerism and tolerance without myelosuppressive conditioning. BMC Immunol;7:9.

Gray, C.M; Smit Jam; Myburgh J.A (1989): Function and Numbers of natural killer (NK) cells in patients conditioned with total lymphoid irradiation (TLI). Tranplant Proc; 21(1):1980-1981.

Hallahan, D.E. & Virudachalam, S. (1999). Accumulation of P-selectin in the lumen of irradiated blood vessels. Radiat Res 152:6–13.

Hallahan, D.E.; Spriggs, D.R.; Beckett, M.A et al. (1989). Increased tumor necrosis factor alpha mRNA after cellular exposure to ionizing radiation. Proc Natl Acad Sci USA 86:10104–10107.

Hashimoto, S.; Shirato, H.; Hosokawa, M.; et al. (1999). The suppression of metastases and the change in host immune response after low-dose total-body irradiation in tumor-bearing rats. Radiation Research, 151:717–724.

Hauser SH, Calorini L, Wazer DE; et al. (1993). Radiation-enhanced expression of major histocompatibility complex class I antigen H-2Db in B16 melanoma cells. Cancer Res 53:1952–1955.

Hayamizu, K.; Lan, F.; Huie, P., Sibley,R.K.; et al. (1999) Comparison of chimeric acid and non-chimeric tolerance using posttransplant total lymphoid irradiation: cytokine expression and chronic rejection.Transplantation ;68(7):1036–1044.

Higuchi, M.; Zeng, D.; Shizuru, J.; et al. (2002). Immune tolerance to combined organ and bone marrow transplants after fractionated lymphoid irradiation involves regulatory NK T cells and clonal deletion. J Immunol 2002;169(10):5564–5570.

Hoffmann P, Boeld TJ, Eder R, et al. (2009) Loss of FOXP3 expression in natural human CD4+CD25+ regulatory T cells upon repetitive in vitro stimulation. Eur J Immunol ;39:1088–97.

Ildstad ST, Sachs DH (1984). Reconstitution with syngeneic plus allogeneic or xenogeneic bone marrow Leads to specific acceptance of allografts orxenografts. Nature;307(5947):168–170.

Ishihara, H., Tanaka, I.; Nemoto, K.; et al. (1995). Immediate-early, transient induction of the interleukin-1 beta gene in mouse spleen macrophages by ionizing radiation. J Radiat Res (Tokyo) 36:112–124.

Janeway Jr, C.A. & Medzhitov, R. (2002). Innate immune recognition. Annu Rev Immunol 20:197–216.

James,R.F.; Lake, S.P.; Chamberlain J., et al. (1989). Gamma irradiation of isolated rat islets pretransplantation produces indefinite allograft survival in cyclosporine-treatedrecipients. Transplantation, 47:929–933.

Jin, S.Z.; Pan, X.N.; Wu N.; et al. (2007). Whole-body low dose irradiation promotes the efficacy of conventional radiotherapy for cancer and possible mechanisms. Dose Response 5:349–358.

Jonathan, E.C.; Bernhard, E.J; McKenna, W.G. (1999). How does radiation kill cells? Current Opinion in Chemical Biology, 3:77–83.

Kang,S.M.; Tang, Q.; Bluestone, J.A. (2007)CD4+CD25+ regulatory T cells in transplantation: progress, challenges and prospects. Am J Transplant ;7(6):1457–1463.

Kasid, U.; Suy, S.; Dent, P., et al. (1996). Activation of Raf by ionizing radiation. Nature, 382:813–816.

Kawai, T.; Cosimi, A.B; Wee, S.L.; et al. (2002). Effect of mixed hematopoietic chimerism on cardiac allograft survival in cynomolgus monkeys.Transplantation ; 73(11):1757–1764.

Kawai T.; Cosimi A.B.; Spitzer, T.R.; et al (2008). HLA mismatchedrenal transplantation without maintenance immunosuppression. N Engl J Med 2008;358 (4):353–361.

Kim, K.W.; Kim, S.H.; Shin, J.G.; et al. (2004). Direct injection of immature dendritic cells into irradiated tumor induces efficient antitumor immunity. Int J Cancer 109:685–690.

Kipnis, J.; Avidan, H.; Markovich, Y.; et al. (2004). Low-dose gamma-irradiation promotes survival of injured neurons in the central nervous system via homeostasis-driven proliferation of T cells. European Journal of Neuroscience 19:1191–1198.

Lake, R.A. & Robinson, B. W. (2005). Immunotherapy and chemotherapy—a practical partnership. Nat Rev Cancer 5: 397–405.

Lambert, J.F., Colvin, G.A.; Zhong S., et al (2002). H2-mismatched transplantation with repetitive cell infusions and CD40 ligand antibody infusions without myeloablation. Br J Haematol ;119(1):155–163.

Lan F, Hayamizu K, Strober S (2000). Cyclosporine facilitates chimeric and inhibits nonchimeric tolerance after posttransplant total lymphoid irradiation. Transplantation;69(4):649–655.

Lander, H.M.; Tauras, J.M.; Ogiste, J.S., et al(1997). Activation of the receptor for advanced glycation end products triggers a p21(ras)-dependent mitogen-activated protein kinase pathway regulated by oxidant stress. Journal of Biological Chemistry, 272:17810–17814.

Laylor R, Dewchand H, Simpson E, et al. (2005). Engraftment of allogeneic hematopoietic stem cells requires both inhibition of host-versus-graft responses and 'space' for homeostatic expansion. Transplantation;79:1484–91.

Liao , Y.P.; Wang, C.C.; Butterfield, L.H.; et al. (2004). Ionizing radiation affects human MART-1 melanoma antigen processing and presentation by dendritic cells. J Immunol 173:2462–2469.

Liu, R.; Xiong, S.; Zhang, L.; et al.(2010). Enhancement of antitumor immunity by low-dose total body irradiationis associated with selectively decreasing the proportion and number of T regulatory cells. Cellular & Molecular Immunology, 7:157–162.

Liu, S.Z.; Jin, S.Z;, Liu, X.D.; et al. (2001). Role of CD28/B7 costimulation and IL-12/IL-10 interaction in the radiationinduced immune changes. BMC Immunology 2:8.

Lohr, F.; Hu, K.; Haroon Z.; et al. (2000). Combination treatment of murine tumors by adenovirus-mediated local B7/IL12 immunotherapy and radiotherapy. Mol Ther 2:195–203.

Lohr, J.; Knoechel, B.; Wang, J.J.; et al (2006). Role of IL-17 and regulatory T lymphocytes in a systemic autoimmune disease. J Exp Med ;203:2785–91.

Macagno, A.; Napolitani, G.; Lanzavecchia, A. ; et al., (2007). Duration, combination and timing:the signal integration model of dendritic cell activation. Trends Immunol 28:227–233.

Mason, K.A.; Ariga, H. ; Neal, R. ; et al. (2005). Targeting toll-like receptor 9 with CpG oligodeoxynucleotides enhances tumor response to fractionated radiotherapy. Clin Cancer Res 11:361–369.

Mcbride, W.H.; Chiang, C.S.; Olson, J.L, et al (2004). A sense of danger from radiation. Radiat Res 2004, 162:1-19.

Mengde, C., et al. (2011). Different radiosensitivity of CD4þCD25þ regulatory T cells and effector T cells to low dose gamma irradiation in vitro. Int. J. Radiat. Biol., 87(1) : 71–80.

Merrick, A.; Errington, F.; Milward, K.; et al. (2005). Immunosuppressive effects of radiation on human dendritic cells:reduced IL-12 production on activation and impairment of naive T-cellpriming. Br J Cancer 92:1450–1458.

Milas, L.; Mason, K.A.; Ariga, H. ; et al. (2004). CpG oligodeoxynucleotide enhances tumor response to radiation. Cancer Res 64:5074–5077.

Miller GM, Kim DW, Andres ML; et al. (2003). Changes in the activation and reconstitution of lymphocytes resulting from total-body irradiation correlate with slowed tumor growth. Oncology 65:229–241.

Minamimura, K., Gao, W., Maki, T. (2006) CD4+ regulatory T cells are spared from deletion by antilymphocyteserum, a polyclonal anti-T cell antibody.J Immunol;176(7):4125–4132.

Morgan ME, Sutmuller RP, Witteveen HJ, et al.(2003) CD25+ cell depletion hastens the onset of severe disease in collagen-induced arthritis. Arthritis Rheum ;48:1452–60.

Morgan ME, Flierman R, van Duivenvoorde LM, et al. (2005) Effective treatment of collageninduced arthritis by adoptive transfer of CD25+ regulatory T cells. Arthritis Rheum 52:2212–21.

Muraro, P.A., Douek, D.C., Packer, A.; et al (2005). Thymic output generates a new and diverse TCR repertoire after autologous stem cell transplantation in multiple sclerosis patients. J Exp Med 2005;201:805–16.

Nadal E, Garin M, Kaeda J, et al (2007) Increased frequencies of CD4(+)CD25(high) T(regs) correlate with disease relapse after allogeneic stem cell transplantation for chronic myeloid leukemia. Leukemia ;21:472–9.

Nadkarni S, Mauri C, Ehrenstein MR.(2007) Anti-TNF-alpha therapy induces a distinct regulatory T cell population in patients with rheumatoid arthritis via TGF-beta. J Exp Med;204:33–9.

Nador, R.G; Hongo, D; Yao, Z et al.; (2010) The Changed Balance of Regulatory and Naive T Cells Promotes Tolerance After TLI and Anti-T Cell Antibody Conditioning. Am J Transplant.; 10(2): 262–272.

Nakatsukasa H, Tsukimoto M, Ohshima Y, et al. (2008) Suppressing effect of low-dose gamma-ray irradiation on collagen-induced arthritis. J Radiat Res 2008;49:381–389.

Nemoto K, Ishihara, H., Tanaka, I.; et al. (1995). Expression of IL-1 beta mRNA in mice after whole body X-irradiation. J Radiat Res (Tokyo) 36:125–133.

Nikitina EY, Gabrilovich DI. (2001). Combination of gammairradiation and dendritic cell administration induces apotent antitumor response in tumor-bearing mice:approach to treatment of advanced stage cancer. Int J Cancer 94: 825–833.

North RJ. (1986). Radiation-induced, immunologicallymediated regression of an established tumor as an example of successful therapeutic immunomanipulation Preferential elimination of suppressor T cells allows sustained production of effector T cells. J Exp Med 164: 1652–1666.

Notley CA, Inglis JJ, Alzabin S, et al. (2008). Blockade of tumor necrosis factor in collageninduced arthritis reveals a novel immunoregulatory pathway for Th1 and Th17 cells. J Exp Med;205:2491–2497.

Paulos, C.M.; Wrzesinski, C.; Kaiser, A., et al. (2007). Microbial translocation augments the function of adoptively transferred self/tumor-specific CD8 T cells via TLR4 signaling. J Clin Invest 117: 2197–2204.

Pillai, A.B.; George, T.I., Dutt, S.; et al. (2009) Host natural killer T cells induce an IL-4 dependent expansion of donor CD4+CD25+Foxp3+ Tregs that protects against graft-versus-host disease. Blood.

Poltorak, A.; He, X.; Smirnova, I.; et al. (1998). Defective LPS signaling in C3H/HeJ and C57BL/10ScCr mice:mutations in Tlr4 gene. Science 282: 2085–2088.

Reuben JM; Korbling M; Gao H, et al.; (2004). The effect of low dose gamma irradiation on the differentiation and maturationof monocyte derived dendritic cells. Journal of Gravitational Physiology 11:P49–52.

Rho, H.S.; Park S.S.; Lee, C.E. (2004). Gamma irradiation up-regulatesexpression of B cell differentiation molecule CD23 by NFkappaB activation. Journal of Biochemistry and Molecular Biology 37:507–514.

Roord ST, de Jager W, Boon L, et al.(2008) Autologous bone marrow transplantation in autoimmune arthritis restores immune homeostasis through CD4+CD25+Foxp3+ regulatory T cells. Blood;111:5233–41.

Roses R E; Xu M; Koski GK; et al. (2008). Radiation therapy and Toll-like receptor signaling: Implications for the treatment of cancer. Oncogene 27:200–207.

Safwat A. (2000a). The immunobiology of low-dose total-body irradiation: More questions than answers. Radiation Research 153(5 Pt 1):599–604.

Safwat A.(2000b). The role of low-dose total body irradiation in treatment of non-hodgkin's lymphoma: A new look at an old method. Radiotherapy & Oncology 56:1–8.

Sakaguchi N, Takahashi T, Hata H, et al. (2003) Altered thymic T-cell selection due to a mutation of the ZAP-70 gene causes autoimmune arthritis in mice. Nature;426:454–60.

Sakaguchi S. (2005) Naturally arising Foxp3-expressing CD25+CD4+ regulatory T cells in immunological tolerance to self and non-self. Nat Immunol 2005;6(4):345–352.

Sauter B, Albert ML, Francisco L.; et al. (2000). Consequences of cell death:exposureto necrotic tumor cells, but not primary tissue cells orapoptotic cells, induces the maturation of immunostimulatory dendritic cells. J Exp Med 191:423–434.

Seetharam, S.; Staba, M.J.; Schumm, L.P. ; et al. (1999). Enhanced eradication of local and distant tumors by genetically produced interleukin-12 and radiation. Int J Oncol 15:769–773.

Scandling, J.D.; Busque S.; Dejbakhsh-Jones S.; et al (2008). Tolerance and chimerism after renal and hematopoietic-cell transplantation. N Engl J Med 2008;358(4):362–368.

Scheffer SR, Nave H, Korangy F, et al. (2003). Apoptotic, but not necrotic, tumor cell vaccines induce a potent immune response in vivo. Int J Cancer 103:205–211.

Schiopu, A. & Wood, K.J. (2008) Regulatory T cells: hypes and limitations. Curr Opin Organ Transplant 2008;13 (4):333–338.

Schu¨ tze S.; Tchikov, V.; Schneider-Brachert, W. (2008). Regulation of TNFR1 and CD95 signalling by receptor compartmentalization. Nature Reviews. Molecular Cell Biology 9:655–662.

Shan, Y.X.; Jin, S.Z.; Liu, X.D.; et al. (2007). Ionizing radiation stimulates secretion of pro-inflammatory cytokines: Dose response relationship, mechanisms and implications.Radiation and Environmental Biophysics 46:21-29.

Shankar, B.; Premachandran, S.; Bharambe, S.D.; et al. (1999). Modification of immune response by low dose ionizing radiation: Role of apoptosis. Immunology Letters 68:237–245.

Shi, Y.; White, D.; He, L. ; et al.; (2007). Toll-like receptor-7 tolerizes malignant B cells and enhances killing by cytotoxic agents. Cancer Res 67:1823–1831.

Shigematsu, A., Adachi, Y., Koike-Kiriyama, N., et al. (2007). Effects of low- dose irradiation on enhancement of immunity by dendritic cells. J Radiat Res (Tokyo) 48:51–55.

Slavin S, Strober S, Fuks Z (1977), et al. Induction of specific tissue transplantation tolerance using fractionated total lymphoid irradiation in adult mice: long-term survival of allogeneic bone marrow and skin grafts. J Exp Med;146(1):34–48.

Slavin, S.; Reitz, B.; Bieber, C.P.; et al (1978). Transplantation tolerance in adult rats using total lymphoid irradiation: permanent survival of skin, heart, and marrow allografts. J Exp Med;147(3):700–707.

Slavin, S.; Strober, S.; Fuks, Z.; Kapla, H.S. (1976). Long-term survival of skin allografts in mice treated with fractionated total lymphoid irradiation. Science ;193(4259):1252–1254.

Sykes M. (2001) Mixed chimerism and transplant tolerance. Immunity 2001;14(4):417–42.

Tang Q, Henriksen KJ, Bi M, et al. In vitro-expanded antigen-specifi c regulatory T cells suppress autoimmune diabetes. J Exp Med 2004;199:1455–65.

Villar, R.C.; Chocair, P.R.; Nadalin, W.; et al (2008). Total Lymphoid Irradiation for pretransplant immunossuppression and reccurrence of focal segmental glomerulosclerosis Transpl Int., Mar;21(3):286-9.

Waer, M.; Vanrenterghen, E.; Van der schueren, E., et al (1987). Identification and function of a major OKT3, OKT8, Leu-7, posiitve lymphocyte subpopulation in renal transplant recipients treated with total lymphoid irradiation. Transplant Proc 19(1):1570-1571.

Wasserman, J.; Blomgren, H; Rotstein, S; et al. (1989). Immunosuppression in irradiated breastcancer patients: in vitro effect of cyclooxygenase inhibitors. Bull N Y Acad Med, 65:36–44.

Wekerle T.; Sayegh, M.H.;Hill J.; et al.(1998) Extrathymic T cell deletion and allogeneic stem cell engraftment induced with costimulatory blockade is followed by central T cell tolerance. J Exp Med 187(12):2037–2044.

Wekerle, T.; Kurtz, J.; Ito, H.; et al. (2000) Allogeneic bone marrow transplantation with co-stimulatory blockade induces macrochimerism and tolerance without cytoreductive host treatment. Nat Med 2000;6(4):464–469.

Weng L, Dyson J, Dazzi F. (2007) Low-intensity transplant regimens facilitate recruitment of donor- specific regulatory T cells that promote hematopoietic engraftment. Proc Natl Acad Sci USA;104:8415–20.

Weng, L.; Willians, O.S.; Vieira, P.L. et al., (2010). The therapeutic activity of low-dose irradiation on experimental arthritis depends on the induction of endogenous regulatory T cell activity Ann Rheum Dis 2010;69:1519–1526.

Weichselbaum, R.R.; Hallahan, D. E.; Beckett, M.A. ; et al. (1994). Gene therapy targeted by radiation preferentially radiosensitizes tumor cells. Cancer Res 54:4266–4269.

Wesa, A.; Kalinski, P.; Kirkwood, J.M. , et al. (2007). Polarized type-1 dendritic cells (DC1) producing high levels of IL-12 family members rescue patient TH1-type antimelanoma CD4+ T cell responses in vitro. J Immunother 30:75- 82.

Wing K, Fehervari Z, Sakaguchi S. (2006). Emerging possibilities in the development and function of regulatory T cells. International Immunology 18:991–1000.

Wood,K.J.; Sakaguchi, S. (2003). Regulatory T cells in transplantation tolerance. Nat Rev Immunol 2003;3(3):199–210.

Wrzesinski C, Paulos CM, Gattinoni L et al. (2007). Hematopoietic stem cells promote the expansion and function of adoptively transferred antitumor CD8 T cells. J Clin Invest 117:492–501.

Xiao X, Kroemer A, Gao W, et al. (2008) OX40/OX40L costimulation affects induction of Foxp3+ regulatory T cells in part by expanding memory T cells in vivo. J Immunol;181:3193–201.

Xu, S.; Koski, G. K. ; Maeurer, M.; et al. (2003). Rapid high efficiency sensitization of CD8+ T cells to tumor antigens by dendritic cells leads to enhanced functional avidity and direct tumor recognition through an IL-12-dependent mechanism. J Immunol 171:2251–2261.

Yao, Z.; Liu, Y.; Jones, J.; Strober, S. (2009). Differences in Bcl-2 expression by T-cell subsets alter their balance after in vivo irradiation to favor CD4+Bcl-2hi NKT cells. Eur J Immunol;39(3):763–775.

Zhang, B.; Bowerman, N. A., Salama, J.K., et al. (2007). Induced sensitization of tumor stroma leads to eradication of established cancer by T cells. J Exp Med 204:49–55.

Zou W. (2006) . Regulatory T cells, tumour immunity and immunotherapy. Nature Reviews. Immunology 6:295–307.

19

The Role of Cyclosporine A in the Treatment of Prosthetic Vascular Graft Infections with the Use of Arterial Homografts

Artur Pupka and Tomasz Płonek
Wroclaw Medical University
Poland

1. Introduction

Infections of prosthetic grafts in vascular surgery are the cause of many serious postoperative complications including death (Bahnini et al.,1991; Callow,1996; Wilson,2001; Yeager&Porter,1992). Encouraging results were obtained when cold-preserved fresh arterial homografts and other biologic grafts were used to replace infected prosthetic grafts (Chiesa et al.,1998, 2002). Cooling down the grafts only to 4°C allows preservation of the arterial endothelium. However, the endothelium is immunogenic, and thus immunosuppression is needed (Cerilli et al.,1985; Methe et al.,2007; Paul et al.,1985; Pober et al.,1984). Moreover, organ donors should be selected with respect to histocompatibility and blood group types (Gabriel et al.,2002; Mirelli et al.,1998, 1999; Scolari et al.,1998). Experimental studies show that immunosuppressive treatment is helpful after the implantation of cold-preserved fresh arterial homografts (Azuma et al.,1999; Gabriel&Fandrich,2002). On the other hand, there is a concern that immunosuppressive drugs can exacerbate the infection. There are no clinical studies examining the need to use immunosuppression after the transplantation of fresh arterial homografts in prosthetic graft infections (Mirelli et al.,1999). We assumed that administration of Cyclosporine A with a concomitant antibiotic therapy may improve the viability of the fresh arterial homografts and improve the patients' condition.

One of the diagnostic methods used to detect infections in vascular surgery is scintigraphy with the use of Technetium-99m labeled leucocytes. Leucocytes migrate and accumulate in the infected area allowing for the area of accumulation to be estimated (Plissonnier et al.,1995). Objective monitoring of the infection after an arterial graft implantation facilitates the decision of choosing the right treatment, especially for patients treated with immunosuppressive drugs.

The aim of our study was to assess the influence of Cyclosporine A administration on the outcome of patients who underwent fresh arterial homograft transplantation in the treatment of prosthetic graft infections.

2. Materials and methods

2.1 Study design

We carried out a prospective, non-randomized observational study. 79 patients were admitted to our clinic between March 2001 and January 2009 due to a prosthetic graft infection. In all cases we observed infection of the prosthetic graft with purulent fistulas, fluid spaces around the prostheses and bleeding from the vascular anastomoses. All patients that could not wait for the fresh arterial homograft had the prosthesis replaced with a silver coated prosthesis (27 patients). 52 patients who could wait for the arterial homograft were put on a waiting list and were treated with antibiotics and local disinfectants until they had the infected prosthesis replaced with an arterial homograft. According to the protocol approved by the Ethics Committee of the University of Medicine of Wroclaw, patients decided whether they wanted to take Cyclosporine A after obtaining detailed information about the possible benefits and risks of taking this medication. We defined early and late postoperative periods as ≤30 days and >30days respectively. The patients were divided into 2 groups: Group 1 - consisting of 26 patients who received 1-3 mg/kg of Cyclosporine A per day with dose adjustments to maintain a serum concentration of 120-140 mg/ml and group 2 - consisting of 26 patients who were treated without immunosuppressive drugs (Table 1). All patients with positive cross-match were assigned to group 1 (3 patients).

Characteristics of homograft recipients	Group 1 (N=26)	Group 2 (N=26)
Age (years, mean+-SD)	42-68 (57±1)	50-71 (59±5)
Male	25	24
Female	1	2
Additional illnesses		
Diabetes	8 (30%)	8 (31%)
Ischemic heart disease	15 (58%)	14 (54%)
Renal failure	4 (15%)	4 (15%)
Leg necrosis	7 (27%)	6 (23%)
Graft-duodenal fistula	6 (23%)	5 (19%)

Table 1. Characteristics of homografts recipients

In each case, the infection was confirmed with Duplex- Doppler Ultrasound, CT and scintigpraphy using Technetium-99m labeled leucocytes. The patients received antibiotics (vancomycin, ciprofloxacin, imipenem) according to the antibiogram, usually for a period of up to 30 days after the operation.

All of the homografts were evaluated before the implantation using scanning electron microscopy. In each case, the examination revealed a non-damaged arterial wall and the presence of the endothelium.

Immunological characteristics of patients qualified for an arterial transplantation		
Homograft	Group 1 (N=26)	Group 2 (N=26)
ABO compatibility	26 (100%)	26 (100%)
Negative cross-match	23 (88%)	26 (100%)
Number of incompatibilities in HLA (average+-SD)	3.7±1.8	3.7±1.5
Negative virological examination in donor	26 (100%)	26 (100%)
Time of graft's preservation (hrs, average+-SD)	6-24 (15.2±4.8)	8-22 (14.4±4.9)

Table 2. Immunological characteristics of patients qualified for an arterial transplantation

2.2 Patients

2.2.1 Group 1

The administration of Cyclosporine A (Sandimmun®; Novartis Pharma GmbH) began intraoperatively after revascularization. In this group, 21 Y-shaped, 4 ilio-femoral and 1 aorto-femoral cold-preserved fresh arterial grafts were implanted. The time of simple hypothermia preservation of aortic allografts did not exceed 24 hours. 3 patients from this group had slightly positive cross-match results with the donors' lymphocytes. Microbiological cultures from the specimens from the groin, retroperitoneal space and the infected prosthesis revealed MRSA (24 patients; 92 %), *Staphylococcus epidermidis* (10; 38%) and *Pseudomonas aeruginosa* (7; 27%) infections.

2.2.2 Group 2

In group 2, 22 bifurcated and 4 ilio-femoral arterial allografts were implanted. The time of homograft preservation did not exceed 22 hours. Bacteriological cultures confirmed the infection with MRSA (21 patients; 81%), *S.epidermidis* (9; 35%) and *P.aeruginosa* (5; 19%).

2.3 Homografts

There was no statistical difference in tissue histocompatibility between both groups (Table 2). Arterial homografts were collected from dead donors with a confirmed brain death. During this procedure, a fragment of an artery was taken for a microbiological and microscopic evaluation. Homografts were preserved in the UW (University of Wisconsin) fluid. Just before the operation, the tissues surrounding the allograft were removed and smaller arterial branches were tied up using monofilament sutures.

2.4 Methods

The postoperative treatment (the course of infection and the effects of the therapy), was monitored using scintigraphy. Before and after the operation, computed tomography (CT), duplex-doppler ultrasound, and in some cases, angiography were performed. Microbiological examination, tissue histocompatibility (A and B locus from class I HLA and D locus from class II HLA), ABO compatibility and cross-matches were carried out in every patient. The activity of CD3+, CD4+ and CD8+ lymphocytes was measured before and after the vascular procedure on the 1st, 3rd, 7th day, and in the 1st, 3rd, 6th, 12th, 18th and 24th month after the operation. Virological and serological examinations were performed in each donor (anty-HIV, HBs-Ag, anty-HBc, anty-HCV, anty-EBV, Hbe-Ag, anty-CMV, VDRL test).

The primary endpoint was the recurrence of infection confirmed by clinical and laboratory examinations or by scintigraphy. Secondary endpoints were early and late postoperative mortality and morbidity, amputations, graft patency, rupture of the graft and presence of the graft aneurysm.

2.5 Statistical analysis

Statistical analysis was performed with the use of Statistica 9,0 software. The results were analyzed by parametrical and non-parametrical tests such as chi-square, chi-square analysis of variance (ANOVA) and the U test of Mann-Whitney. Statistical significance was assumed at $p<0.05$.

2.6 Ethical approval for research

The protocol of this study was approved by the Ethics Committee of the University of Medicine of Wroclaw.

3. Results

52 patients were enrolled into the study. The mean ± standard deviation (SD) follow-up was 23.3 ± 6.1 months in group 1 and 19.2 ± 10.7 months in group 2. A long-term follow up was completed for 15 patients from group 1 and 14 from group 2.

3.1 Postoperative morbidity and mortality

3.1.1 Postoperative mortality

In group 1, one (4%) patient with an aorto-duodenal fistula died 14 days after the operation due to septic shock and one (4%) died 11 months after the operation due to a cerebrovascular accident. In group 2, four (15%) patients died in the early postoperative period. Two patients (8%) died due to a graft-duodenal fistula on the 5th and 19th postoperative day, one (4%) in the course of septic shock (3rd day) and one (4%) due to myocardial infarction (7th day). Two (8%) patients died in the late postoperative period due to rupture of the allograft (4th and 5th postoperative month) (Table 3, Fig.1). The mortality was higher in group 2 (23%) than in group 1 (8%), but this difference failed to reach statistical significance (p>0.05).

Postoperative mortality	Group 1 (N=26)	Group 2 (N=26)
Early<30 days		
Septic shock	1 (4%)	1 (4%)
Graft-duodenal fistula	-	2 (8%)
Myocardial infarction	-	1 (4%)
	1 (4%)	**4 (15%)**
Late>30 days		
Rupture of graft	-	2 (8%)
Cerebrovascular accident	1 (4%)	-
	1 (4%)	**2 (8%)**

Table 3. Postoperative mortality

3.1.2 Postoperative morbidity

In the group treated with cyclosporine, three (12%) early complications (graft thrombosis, wound dehiscene with evisceration, a hematoma in the inquinal area) and three (12%) late complications (symptoms of bowel ischemia, lower extremity ischemia, tibial arteries occlusion) were observed. Graft aneurysms or late thrombosis of the transplanted artery were not detected in this group. In the group treated without immunosuppression, there were no early complications and 9 (35%) late complications (MRSA inferction of the homograft, 5 cases of homograft aneurysms of which 3 ruptured and 3 femoral amputations due to graft thrombosis) (Table 4). The incidence of late postoperative complications was statistically greater in group 2 than in group 1 (p=0.030). There was no statistically significant difference between group 1 and 2 in the occurrence of early postoperative complications and in the number of both early and late complications.

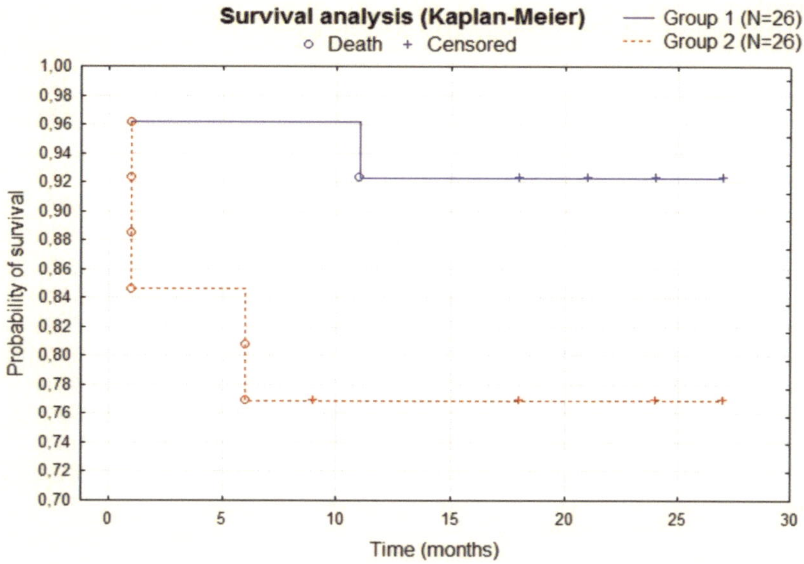

Fig. 1. Kapalan-Meier survival analysis of the patients

Postoperative morbidity	Group 1 (N=26)	Group 2 (N=26)
Early<30 days		
Infection of postoperative wound	1 (4%)	-
Graft thrombosis	1 (4%)	-
Hematoma	1 (4%)	-
	3 (12%)	**0 (0%)**
Late>30 days		
Graft infection	-	1 (4%)
Graft thrombosis - amputation	-	3 (12%)
Low extremity ischemia	2 (8%)	-
Graft aneurysm	-	2 (8%)
Symptoms of bowel ischemia	1 (4%)	-
Rupture of graft	-	3 (12%)
	3 (12%)	**9 (35%)**

Table 4. Postoperative morbidity

3.2 Laboratory and radiological examinations

In both groups, laboratory and radiological examinations confirmed the regression of the infection after the arterial graft implantation. Acute phase proteins were within normal range. The ultrasound examination showed no evidence of fluid spaces around the homografts. Scintigraphy revealed the statistically significant ($p=0.011$) decrease of accumulation of the Tc-99m labeled leucocytes around the allograft in both groups during the whole observation period of 27 months. The biggest drop in the area of accumulated leucocytes was in the 6th postoperative month in both groups. The rate of the decrease was slightly greater in the group without immunosuppression, but this difference did not reach statistical significance.

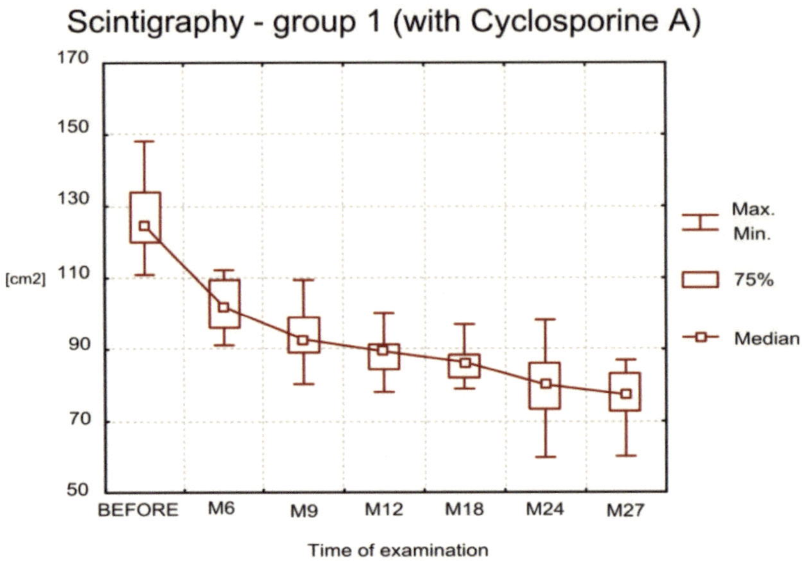

Fig. 2. The reduction of the area of accumulation of Tc99-labelled lymphocytes in patients from group 1 (with Cyclosporine A)

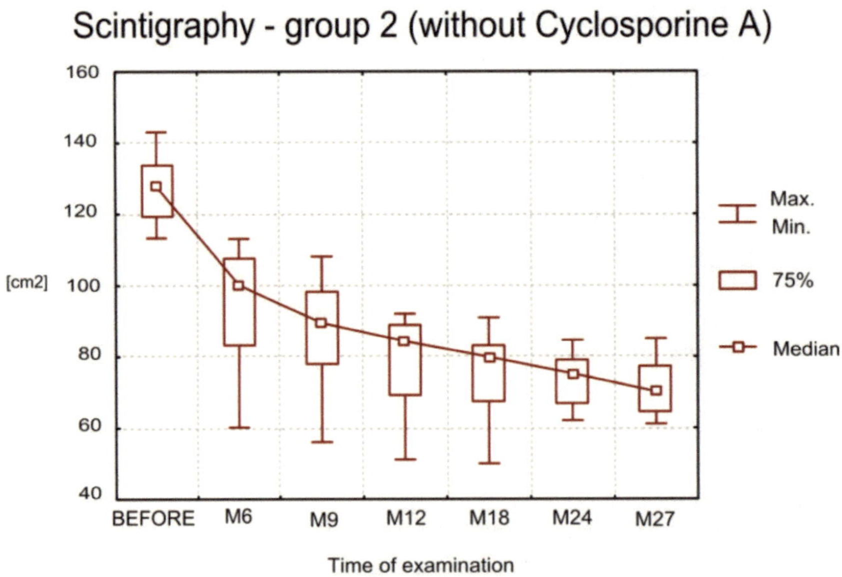

Fig. 3. The reduction of the area of accumulation of Tc99-labelled lymphocytes in patients from group 2 (without Cyclosporine A)

The total reduction of the area of accumulation of the Tc-99m labeled leucocytes during the postoperative period was 35% in group 1 and 44% in group 2 (Fig. 2,3). The statistically significant (p=0.016) difference between both groups in the area of accumulation was observed 18 months after the operation, and it was bigger in group 2.
When there was an increase or no decrease of the leucocytes accumulation, antibiotics were administered according to the antibiogram. This took place 4 times in group 1 (15%) and 3 times in group 2 (12%). The antibacterial treatment resulted in the reduction of the leucocytes accumulation and there were no further clinical signs of reinfection.

3.3 The activity of CD3+, CD4+ and CD8+ lymphocytes in blood

The analysis of the immunological response in both examined groups revealed an increase in the activity of CD3+ and CD4+ lymphocytes and a decrease in the activity of CD8+ lymphocytes. The increase in activity of CD3+ lymphocytes in group 1 was observed from the first postoperative day and it was statistically significant (p=0.04). The increase in activity of CD3+ lymphocytes was greater in group 2 than in group 1, and reached its maximal value on the 7th postoperative day (Fig.4,5). This difference in activity was also statistically significant (p=0.038). Statistical differences in CD3+ lymphocyte activity between both groups began in the sixth postoperative month and lasted until the 24th month (p=0.027).

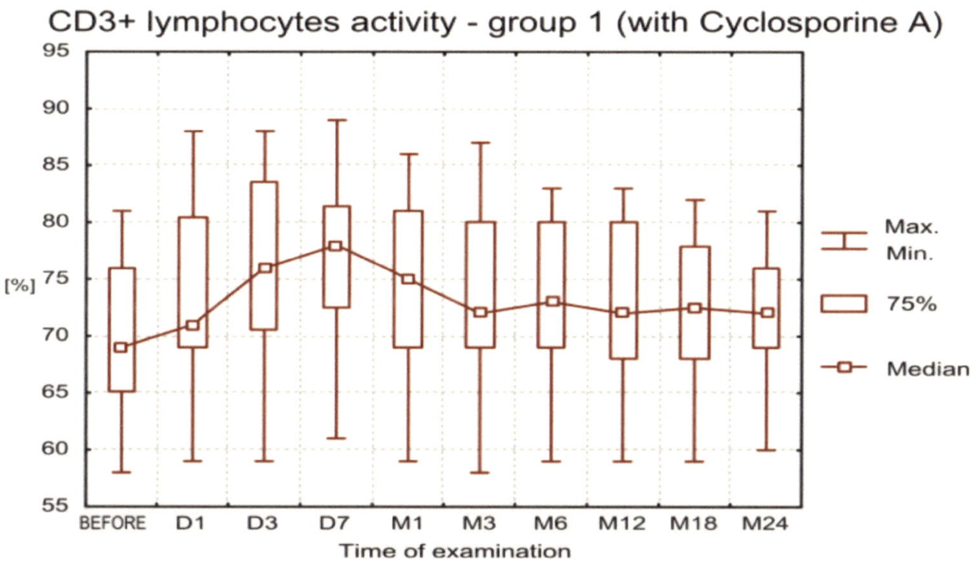

Fig. 4. The CD3+ lymphocytes' activity in patients from group 1 (with Cyclosporine)

The increase in activity of CD4+ lymphocytes was larger in group 2 than in group 1 (Fig. 6,7). The change in activity of CD4+ lymphocytes in both groups was statistically significant (p=0.035). The maximum activity was noted on the 7th postoperative day. A statistically significant difference in activity of CD4+ lymphocytes between both groups was seen on the first day (p=0.032) and in the third month after the arterial graft implantation (p=0.041).

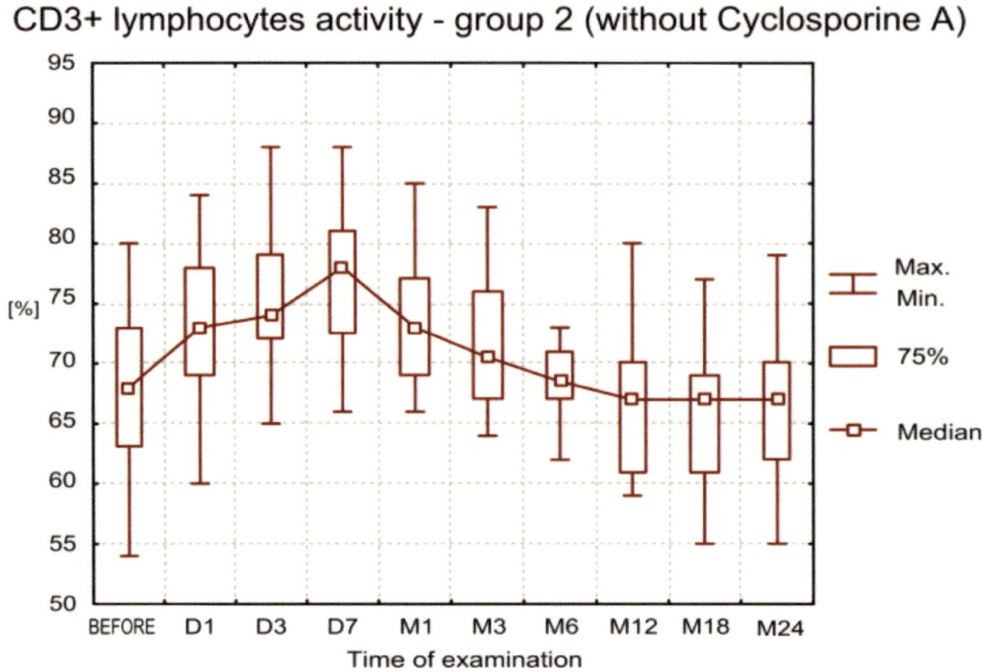

Fig. 5. The CD3+ lymphocytes' activity in patients from group 2 (without Cyclosporine)

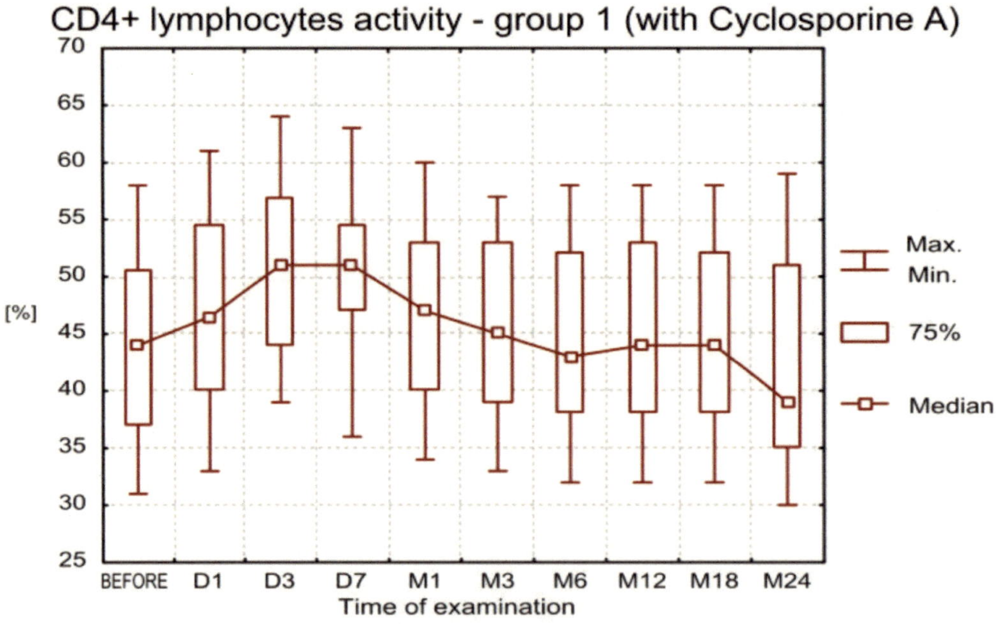

Fig. 6. The CD4+ lymphocytes' activity in patients from group 1 (with Cyclosporine)

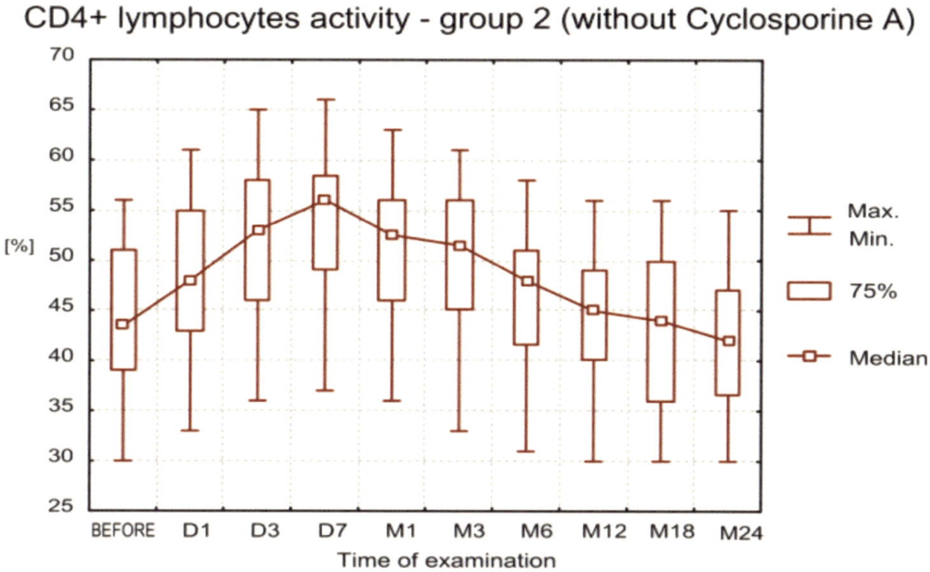

Fig. 7. The CD4+ lymphocytes' activity in patients from group 2 (without Cyclosporine)

The decrease in activity of CD8+ lymphocytes was at its maximum on the 7th day in group 1 and in the 1st month in group 2 after the operation (Fig. 8,9). This decrease was statistically significant (p=0.02) in both examined groups. The difference in activity of these leucocytes between group 1 and 2 was statistically significant (p=0.016) in the 18th month of the observation and was greater in group 2.

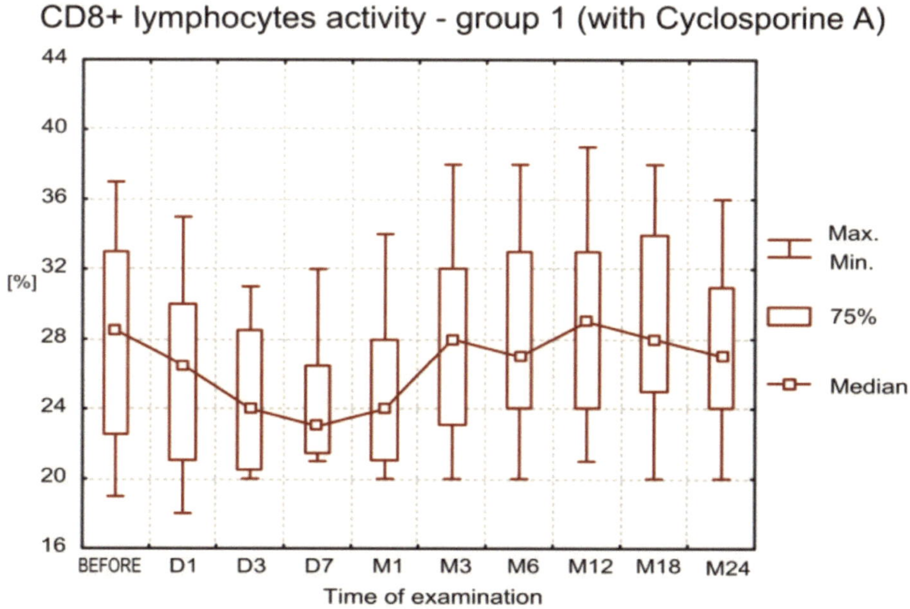

Fig. 8. The CD8+ lymphocytes' activity in patients from group 1 (with Cyclosporine)

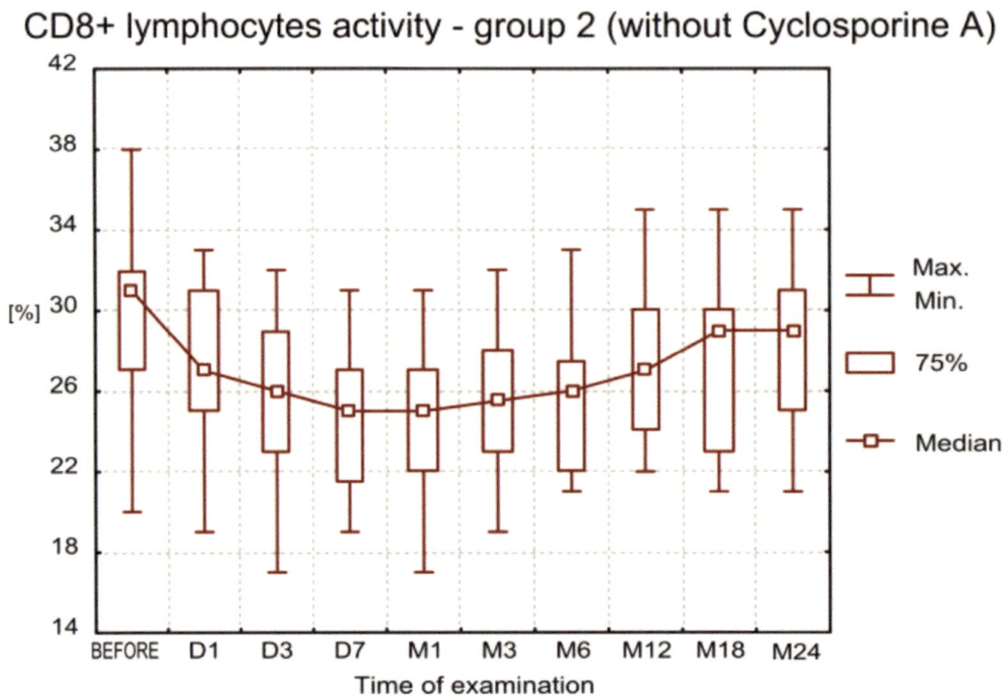

Fig. 9. The CD8+ lymphocytes' activity in patients from group 2 (without Cyclosporine)

3.4 Scanning electron microscopy

Scanning electron microscopy examinations were performed in two patients. One patient from group 1 and another one from group 2 had the arterial homografts removed due to late postoperative complications. The tissue specimens were prepared in the usual manner and assessed by an experienced histologist.

9 months after the transplantation, we collected a fragment of the ilio-femoral homograft from a patient from group 2, who had the transplanted artery removed due to an MRSA infection and rupture of the graft. Scanning electron microscopy (SEM) revealed a complete destruction of the homograft's wall - absence of the endothelium, single, damaged cells and cell fragments of the medial membrane (Fig.11).

We collected a fragment of the artery from a patient from group 1, who was operated on 13 months after the homograft implantation due to an arterial embolism. SEM showed the presence of the endothelial cells (which were mechanically detached), the intimal wall with thickened elastic lamina, a large amount of elastic and collagen fibres, fibrin inclusions, active myoblasts and myofibroblasts (Fig.10). The above mentioned patient stopped taking prescribed immunosuppressive drugs and was admitted to the hospital 12 months after the previous embolectomy. He suffered from lower extremity ischemia in the course of an arterial homograft embolism. Thrombectomy was carried out but this procedure did not improve the blood supply to the leg. Consequently, an amputation was performed. During this operation, a fragment of the arterial homograft's wall was collected. SEM revealed the absence of endothelial cells and the presence of cell apoptosis.

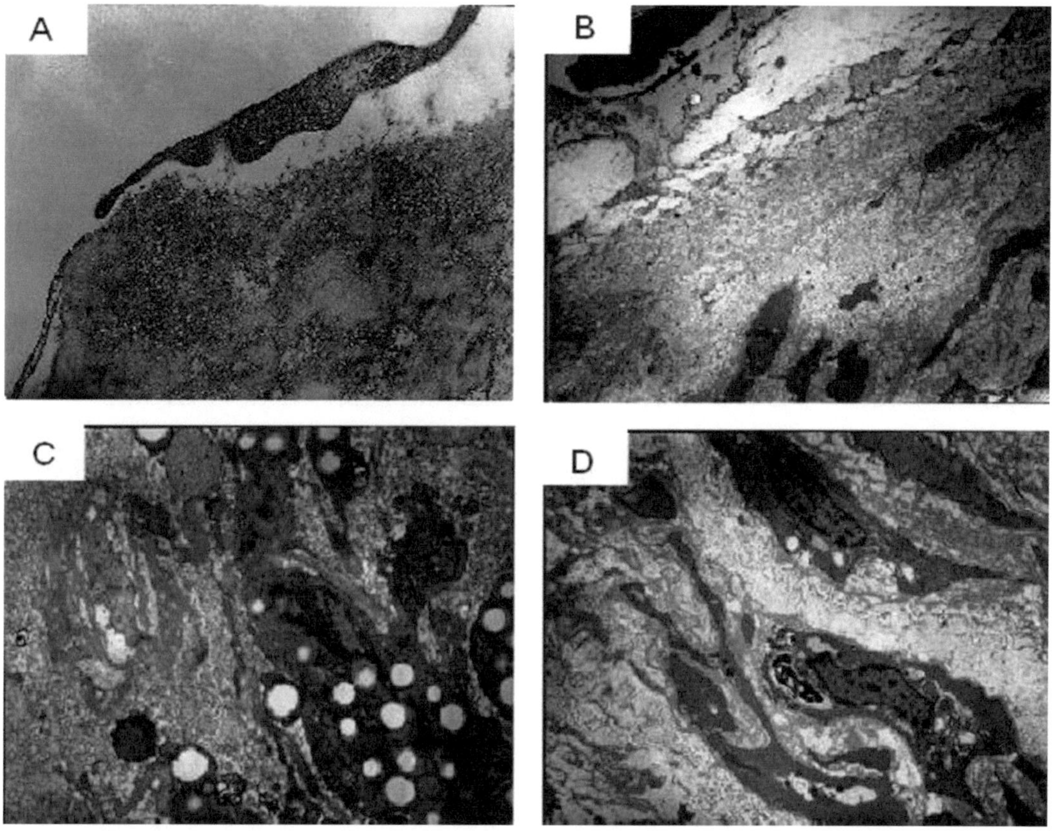

Fig. 10. Scanning electron microscope image - homograft with immunosuppression. A) Endothelial cells. B) Thickened elastic lamina of the intimal wall. C) Active myofibroblasts fagocyting lipids. D) Active myofibroblasts producing collagen

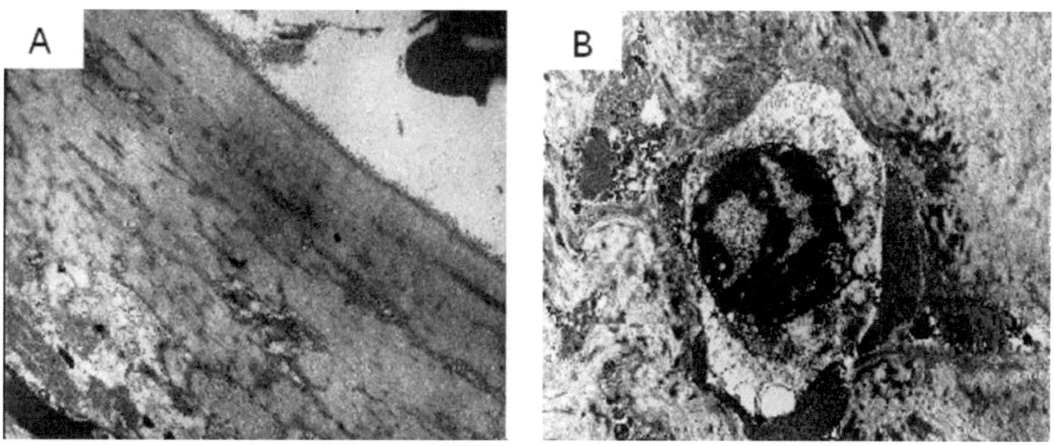

Fig. 11. Scanning electron microscope image - homograft without immunosuppression. A) Absence of endothelium. B) Apoptosis

4. Discussion

The infections of synthetic prostheses in our study were classified as third degree, according to the Szilagy scale, and fifth degree according to the Samson scale (Samson et al.,1988; Szilagyi et al.,1972). The replacement of the infected prosthesis with an arterial allograft was a reasonable solution in these life threatening conditions. We chose cold-preserved fresh arterial homografts because we believed the deep-freeze method was more likely to decrease long-term viability of the arterial wall and less likely to cause the degradation of the endothelium (Bujan et al.,2000; Desgranges et al.,1998; Manaa et al.,2003; Pascual et al.,2001, 2002; Vischjager et al., 1996a, 1996b).

Some scientists claim that the arterial homograft is characterized by low immunogenity and maintain that the graft rejection process is inconsiderable and does not cause an impaired functioning and survivability of the graft (Mirelli et al.,1998, 1999). This is why some vascular surgery centers transplant the arteries without the selection of ABO and HLA compatible donors. There are also numerous research studies showing that the usage of fresh arterial homografts with a preserved endothelium is associated with the immunological response of the graft recipient. This suggests the importance of the selection of donors of the same blood type and similar HLA histocompatibility when fresh arterial allografts are to be used (Chiesa et al.,1998; da Gama et al.,1994; Mirelli et al.,1998, 1999; Prager et al.,2002). We believe that in life threatening infections, the transplantation of the artery despite a slightly positive cross-match is acceptable. In this situation, the usage of immunosuppressive drugs is reasonable. However, we agree that the ABO compatibility is essential (Bracale et al.,1999; Chiesa et al.,1998; Prager et al.,2002).

Clinical trials show that there are changes in an arterial homograft's wall typical for a chronic rejection process (Allaire et al.,1994; Bandyk et al.,2001; Mirelli et al.,1999; Ruotolo et al.,1997). Immunosuppressive treatment can help to stop the degradation of the arterial wall and prolong its viability (Vischjager et al.,1996a, 1996b). However, there is still a question of whether or not to use these drugs in the presence of the infection.

Prolonged functioning of the arterial graft in patients treated with the immunosuppressive drugs was confirmed in some experimental trails (Deaton et al.,1992; Miller et al.,1993; Vermassen et al.,1991; Vischjager et al.,1996). In his experimental trial, Azuma et al. observed that lack or discontinuation of the intake of immunosuppressive medications caused the degradation of the arterial graft's wall and loss of the endothelial cells (Azuma et al.,1999). It was also proven that insufficient dosages of these drugs caused an impaired functioning of the transplanted artery (Gabriel et al.,2002; Geerling et al.,1994; Stoltenberg et al.,1995).

In our study, the increase in activity of CD3+ and CD4+ lymphocytes and the decrease in activity of CD8+ lymphocytes (probably caused by the increase of the infiltration of the homograft's wall by these cells) in transplanted patients suggest arterial allograft's antigenicity.A larger decrease in CD3+ and CD4+ lymphocyte activity and a smaller decrease in CD8+ lymphocyte activity were observed in patients treated with Cyclosporine A than in those treated without immunosuppression. We assume that this was caused by the reduced immunological response of T helper lymphocytes (CD4+) and a smaller infiltration of the allograft by cytotoxic lymphocytes (CD8+). We also believe that this mechanism could help to keep the arterial wall undamaged (Mirelli et al.,1998, 1999).

One month of an antibiotic therapy and the replacement of the infected prosthesis with an arterial homograft lead to the remission of the infection despite the immunosuppressive treatment in almost all patients. This was confirmed with radiological examinations, mainly scintigraphy, using Technetium-99m labeled leucocytes. The maintenance of a small accumulation of the labeled leucocytes around the homograft can be regarded as a chronic reaction against the foreign tissue. We stopped administering the antibiotics according to the scintigraphy results. Prolonged antibiotic and cyclosporine A therapy did not cause any complications associated with decreased immunity. We assume that the application of immunosuppressive drugs reduced the immunological response of the patients against transplanted grafts.

In patients who received immunosuppressive drugs no graft aneurysms were observed compared to 5 cases (19%) of this complication in patients without this therapy. Cyclosporine A may have helped to stop the degradation process of the arterial wall and thus prevented its aneurismal dilatation. The number of cases of postoperative infections was even smaller in those who received immunosuppressive medications. Our study suggests that profits from reasonable immunosuppression outweigh the risk of potential infection in patients with an arterial homograft implanted due to infection of a vascular prosthesis.

5. Conclusions

We believe that Cyclosporine A helped to stop the processes of damaging the graft's wall. Patients treated with this drug had fewer late postoperative complications. Our study suggests that cyclosporine A can be used in patients with an infection of a synthetic vascular prosthesis, undergoing the implantation of a fresh arterial allograft. We found out that fresh arterial homografts may be immunogenic in an extent which leads to its chronic rejection by the patient's immunological system. The results support the hypothesis that Cyclosporine A may prevent the autoimmunologic response of the patient and reduce the risk of damaging the arterial homograft.

Our study was carried out on a relatively small group of patients and it could be the reason why some of the differences between both examined groups of patients failed to reach statistical significance. Therefore, a multicentre randomized trial is needed to definitively establish the role of immunosuppression in the treatment of prosthetic vascular graft infections with the use of arterial homografts.

6. References

Allaire, E., Guettier, C., Bruneval, P., Plissonnier, D.&Michel, J. B. (1994). Cell-free arterial grafts: morphologic characteristics of aortic isografts, allografts, and xenografts in rats. *J Vasc Surg,* 19, 3, (Mar), 446-456, 0741-5214 (Print)

Azuma, N., Sasajima, T.&Kubo, Y. (1999). Immunosuppression with FK506 in rat arterial allografts: fate of allogeneic endothelial cells. *J Vasc Surg,* 29, 4, (Apr), 694-702, 0741-5214 (Print)

Bahnini, A., Ruotolo, C., Koskas, F.&Kieffer, E. (1991). In situ fresh allograft replacement of an infected aortic prosthetic graft: eighteen months' follow-up. *J Vasc Surg,* 14, 1, (Jul), 98-102, 0741-5214 (Print)

Bandyk, D. F., Novotney, M. L., Back, M. R., Johnson, B. L.&Schmacht, D. C. (2001). Expanded application of in situ replacement for prosthetic graft infection. *J Vasc Surg,* 34, 3, (Sep), 411-419; discussion 419-420, 0741-5214 (Print)

Bracale, G. C., Porcellini, M., Bernardo, B., Bauleo, A.&Capasso, R. (1999). Arterial homografts in the management of infected axillofemoral prosthetic grafts. *J Cardiovasc Surg (Torino),* 40, 2, (Apr), 271-274, 0021-9509 (Print)

Bujan, J., Pascual, G., Garcia-Honduvilla, N., Gimeno, M. J., Jurado, F., Carrera-San Martin, A.&Bellon, J. M. (2000). Rapid thawing increases the fragility of the cryopreserved arterial wall. *Eur J Vasc Endovasc Surg,* 20, 1, (Jul), 13-20, 1078-5884 (Print)

Callow, A. D. (1996). Arterial homografts. *Eur J Vasc Endovasc Surg,* 12, 3, (Oct), 272-281, 1078-5884 (Print)

Cerilli, J., Brasile, L., Galouzis, T., Lempert, N.&Clarke, J. (1985). The vascular endothelial cell antigen system. *Transplantation,* 39, 3, (Mar), 286-289, 0041-1337 (Print)

Chiesa, R., Astore, D., Piccolo, G., Melissano, G., Jannello, A., Frigerio, D., Agrifoglio, G., Bonalumi, F., Corsi, G., Costantini Brancadoro, S., Novali, C., Locati, P., Odero, A., Pirrelli, S., Cugnasca, M., Biglioli, P., Sala, A., Polvani, G., Guarino, A., Biasi, G. M., Mingazzini, P., Scalamogna, M., Mantero, S., Spina, G., Prestipino, F.&et al. (1998). Fresh and cryopreserved arterial homografts in the treatment of prosthetic graft infections: experience of the Italian Collaborative Vascular Homograft Group. *Ann Vasc Surg,* 12, 5, (Sep), 457-462, 0890-5096 (Print)

Chiesa, R., Astore, D., Frigerio, S., Garriboli, L., Piccolo, G., Castellano, R., Scalamogna, M., Odero, A., Pirrelli, S., Biasi, G., Mingazzini, P., Biglioli, P., Polvani, G., Guarino, A., Agrifoglio, G., Tori, A.&Spina, G. (2002). Vascular prosthetic graft infection: epidemiology, bacteriology, pathogenesis and treatment. *Acta Chir Belg,* 102, 4, (Aug), 238-247, 0001-5458 (Print)

da Gama, A. D., Sarmento, C., Vieira, T.&do Carmo, G. X. (1994). The use of arterial allografts for vascular reconstruction in patients receiving immunosuppression for organ transplantation. *J Vasc Surg,* 20, 2, (Aug), 271-278, 0741-5214 (Print)

Deaton, D. W., Stephens, J. K., Karp, R. B., Gamliel, H., Rocco, F., Perelman, M. J., Liddicoat, J. R., Glick, D. B.&Watkins, C. W. (1992). Evaluation of cryopreserved allograft venous conduits in dogs. *J Thorac Cardiovasc Surg,* 103, 1, (Jan), 153-162, 0022-5223 (Print)

Desgranges, P., Beaujan, F., Brunet, S., Cavillon, A., Qvarfordt, P., Melliere, D.&Becquemin, J. P. (1998). Cryopreserved arterial allografts used for the treatment of infected vascular grafts. *Ann Vasc Surg,* 12, 6, (Nov), 583-588, 0890-5096 (Print)

Gabriel, M.&Fandrich, F. (2002). Estimation of graft arteriosclerosis after allogeneic fresh and cryopreserved aortic transplantation in the rat. *Transplant Proc,* 34, 2, (Mar), 711-712, 0041-1345 (Print)

Gabriel, M., Kostrzewa, A.&Sobieska, M. (2002). Immune response after cryopreserved aortic allograft replacement for major vascular infection. *Transplant Proc,* 34, 2, (Mar), 713-714, 0041-1345 (Print)

Geerling, R. A., de Bruin, R. W., Scheringa, M., Bonthuis, F., Jeekel, J., Ijzermans, J. N.&Marquet, R. L. (1994). Suppression of acute rejection prevents graft arteriosclerosis after allogeneic aorta transplantation in the rat. *Transplantation,* 58, 11, (Dec 15), 1258-1263, 0041-1337 (Print)

Manaa, J., Sraieb, T., Khayat, O., Ben Romdhane, N., Hamida, J.&Amor, A. (2003). [The effect of cryopreservation on the structural and functional properties of human vascular allografts]. *Tunis Med,* 81 Suppl 8, 645-651, 0041-4131 (Print)

Methe, H., Hess, S.&Edelman, E. R. (2007). Endothelial immunogenicity--a matter of matrix microarchitecture. *Thromb Haemost*, 98, 2, (Aug), 278-282, 0340-6245 (Print)

Miller, V. M., Bergman, R. T., Gloviczki, P.&Brockbank, K. G. (1993). Cryopreserved venous allografts: effects of immunosuppression and antiplatelet therapy on patency and function. *J Vasc Surg*, 18, 2, (Aug), 216-226, 0741-5214 (Print)

Mirelli, M., Nanni-Costa, A., Scolari, M. P., Iannelli, S., Buscaroli, A., Ridolfi, L., Petrini, F., Stella, A., DeSanctis, L., Borgnino, L. C., Stefoni, S., D'Addato, M.&Bonomini, V. (1998). Mismatch-specific anti-HLA antibody production following aorta transplants. *Transpl Int*, 11 Suppl 1, S444-447, 0934-0874 (Print)

Mirelli, M., Stella, A., Faggioli, G. L., Scolari, M. P., Iannelli, S., Freyrie, A., Buscaroli, A., De Santis, L., Resta, F., Bonomini, V.&D'Addato, M. (1999). Immune response following fresh arterial homograft replacement for aortoiliac graft infection. *Eur J Vasc Endovasc Surg*, 18, 5, (Nov), 424-429, 1078-5884 (Print)

Pascual, G., Garcia-Honduvilla, N., Rodriguez, M., Turegano, F., Bujan, J.&Bellon, J. M. (2001). Effect of the thawing process on cryopreserved arteries. *Ann Vasc Surg*, 15, 6, (Nov), 619-627, 0890-5096 (Print)

Pascual, G., Jurado, F., Rodriguez, M., Corrales, C., Lopez-Hervas, P., Bellon, J. M.&Bujan, J. (2002). The use of ischaemic vessels as prostheses or tissue engineering scaffolds after cryopreservation. *Eur J Vasc Endovasc Surg*, 24, 1, (Jul), 23-30, 1078-5884 (Print)

Paul, L. C., Baldwin, W. M., 3rd&van Es, L. A. (1985). Vascular endothelial alloantigens in renal transplantation. *Transplantation*, 40, 2, (Aug), 117-123, 0041-1337 (Print)

Plissonnier, D., Nochy, D., Poncet, P., Mandet, C., Hinglais, N., Bariety, J.&Michel, J. B. (1995). Sequential immunological targeting of chronic experimental arterial allograft. *Transplantation*, 60, 5, (Sep 15), 414-424, 0041-1337 (Print)

Pober, J. S., Gimbrone, M. A., Jr., Collins, T., Cotran, R. S., Ault, K. A., Fiers, W., Krensky, A. M., Clayberger, C., Reiss, C. S.&Burakoff, S. J. (1984). Interactions of T lymphocytes with human vascular endothelial cells: role of endothelial cells surface antigens. *Immunobiology*, 168, 3-5, (Dec), 483-494, 0171-2985 (Print)

Prager, M., Holzenbein, T., Aslim, E., Domenig, C., Muhlbacher, F.&Kretschmer, G. (2002). Fresh arterial homograft transplantation: a novel concept for critical limb ischaemia. *Eur J Vasc Endovasc Surg*, 24, 4, (Oct), 314-321, 1078-5884 (Print)

Ruotolo, C., Plissonnier, D., Bahnini, A., Koskas, F.&Kieffer, E. (1997). In situ arterial allografts: a new treatment for aortic prosthetic infection. *Eur J Vasc Endovasc Surg*, 14 Suppl A, (Dec), 102-107, 1078-5884 (Print)

Samson, R. H., Veith, F. J., Janko, G. S., Gupta, S. K.&Scher, L. A. (1988). A modified classification and approach to the management of infections involving peripheral arterial prosthetic grafts. *J Vasc Surg*, 8, 2, (Aug), 147-153, 0741-5214 (Print)

Scolari, M. P., De Sanctis, L. B., Iannelli, S., Bonomini, V., D'Addato, M., Stella, A.&Mirelli, M. (1998). Aorta transplantation in man: clinical and immunological studies. *Int J Artif Organs*, 21, 8, (Aug), 483-488, 0391-3988 (Print)

Stoltenberg, R. L., Geraghty, J., Steele, D. M., Kennedy, E., Hullett, D. A.&Sollinger, H. W. (1995). Inhibition of intimal hyperplasia in rat aortic allografts with cyclosporine. *Transplantation*, 60, 9, (Nov 15), 993-998, 0041-1337 (Print)

Szilagyi, D. E., Smith, R. F., Elliott, J. P.&Vrandecic, M. P. (1972). Infection in arterial reconstruction with synthetic grafts. *Ann Surg*, 176, 3, (Sep), 321-333, 0003-4932 (Print)

Vermassen, F., Degrieck, N., De Kock, L., Goubeau, J., Van Landuyt, K., Noens, L.&Derom, F. (1991). Immunosuppressive treatment of venous allografts. *Eur J Vasc Surg,* 5, 6, (Dec), 669-675, 0950-821X (Print)

Vischjager, M., Van Gulik, T. M., De Kleine, R. H., Van Marle, J., Pfaffendorf, M., Klopper, P. J.&Jacobs, M. J. (1996). Experimental arterial allografting under low and therapeutic dosages of cyclosporine for immunosuppression. *Transplantation,* 61, 8, (Apr 27), 1138-1142, 0041-1337 (Print)

Vischjager, M., Van Gulik, T. M., Van Marle, J., Pfaffendorf, M.&Jacobs, M. J. (1996). Function of cryopreserved arterial allografts under immunosuppressive protection with cyclosporine A. *J Vasc Surg,* 24, 5, (Nov), 876-882, 0741-5214 (Print)

Wilson, S. E. (2001). New alternatives in management of the infected vascular prosthesis. *Surg Infect (Larchmt),* 2, 2, (Summer), 171-175; discussion 175-177, 1096-2964 (Print)

Yeager, R. A.&Porter, J. M. (1992). Arterial and prosthetic graft infection. *Ann Vasc Surg,* 6, 5, (Sep), 485-491, 0890-5096 (Print)

20

Clinical Immunosuppression in Solid Organ and Composite Tissue Allotransplantation

Barbara Kern and Robert Sucher
Department of Visceral-, Transplant- and Thoracic Surgery, Medical University Innsbruck Austria

1. Introduction

Although organ and tissue transplantation has been a fantasy for centuries, the epidemic of discovery in transplantation has taken place primarily during the past 55 years. In 1954, Dr J. Murray was presented with the unique opportunity to transplant a human kidney between identical twins without facing the challenges of acute or chronic allograft rejection as well as side effects of long-term immunosuppression (1, 2). Adding to scientific knowledge through basic research helped us to perform complex vascularized composite allotransplants (VCA) like the hand and face today and vascularized tissues recovered from a different individual will soon be extended to all reconstructive transplant procedures currently requiring autologous tissues (3-5).

The development of novel surgical techniques and the discovery of potent immunosuppressive drugs in the second half of the 20th century propelled the clinical development of organ transplantation(6). The combination of corticosteroids and azathioprine, which was the primary immunosuppressive regimen, used from the late 1960's until 1980 culminated in one-year survival rates of only 40% - 50%. Most notably, the discovery of cyclosporine A and tacrolimus in the 1970's and 1980's represented another major milestone in solid organ transplantation resulting in excellent short-term and acceptable long-term survival rates. With current immunosuppressive regimens mainly consisting of the triple combination of corticosteroids, mycophenolate mofetil, and tacrolimus the overall graft and patient survival has improved substantially and reached one-year graft survival rates of 80%-95% leading to consider organ and tissue transplantation as treatment modality of choice for patients with end-stage organ failure or severe tissue defects due to trauma or burn. Despite significant improvements in acute rejection rates, long-term solid organ allograft survival remained unchanged for the last 15 years (7). The major causes for late graft loss include chronic allograft rejection and death with a functioning graft (8, 9).

Since the immunologic graft-loss-rate seemed to be highest within the first months after transplantation, it became the rule that heightened immunosuppression is required early, with progressive reduction over time, leading to the definition of three distinct periods of immunosuppression after transplantation: The perioperative "induction period", where immunosuppressants are initially given at high doses, the "early maintenance period", which is characterized by progressive taper of the individual drugs, and the "chronic

maintenance period", characterized by the combination of different immunosuppressants used at their lowest effective doses.
At the end of 20th century, vascularized composite allotransplantation (VCA) like the hand and face has been performed in humans with success using the same immunosuppressive medications and therapeutic principles used for solid organ transplantation (10). However, since hand and face transplants must be considered as non life-saving operative procedures, novel immunosuppressive treatment protocols for these types of transplants must be developed not only to minimize graft rejection, but also to avoid complications related to adverse effects. Several challenges seem to impede the pharmaceutical industry in bringing novel immunosuppressive agents to the clinic. However, new powerful immunosuppressants are urgently in demand to enable the transplantation of highly immunogenic tissues like the skin and at the same time reduce the incidence of drug-induced toxicity. This goal can only be achieved by either combining synergistic immunosuppressive medications to maximize efficacy and minimize toxicity or by developing minimization protocols where conventional immunosuppression is tapered or even withdrawn shortly after transplantation.

2. Maintenance immunosuppression regimens

Maintenance immunosuppression remains the mainstay of therapy for successful outcomes after solid organ transplantation. Over the past decades, immunosuppressive regimens tried to target multiple immune pathways aiming to decrease acute and chronic allograft rejection and maintain long–term graft survival. Although current maintenance therapy after solid organ transplantation typically includes calcineurin inhibitors, antimetabolites, and corticosteroids, newer therapeutic options including induction therapy with biological agents, mTOR inhibitors, and cellular based therapies have emerged as alternative immunosuppressive strategies. The following paragraph will discuss immunosuppressants that are currently employed in solid organ transplantation.

2.1 Calcineurin-Inhibitors – Backbone of current immunosuppressive regimens

Cyclosporine A

The discovery of cyclosporine A (CsA) still has to be considered as one of the most important breakthroughs in transplantation medicine. CsA was initially discovered in 1968 as a product of *Tolypocladium inflatum gams* and isolated from the soil of the Norwegian plain of Hardanger Vidda (11, 12). At the same time, it was retrieved from fungi imperfecti native to Wisconsin. Almost a decade later, in 1976, Jean-Francois Borel described the immunosuppressive effects for the first time and hence, the first clinical use in a cadaveric kidney transplantation was reported two years later in 1978. Since then, CsA represents the backbone of a multitude of maintenance immunosuppressive protocols used in solid organ transplantation.
The immunosuppressive effects of CsA are based on the inhibition of proliferating CD4+ T cells by interfering with the IL-2 pathway. In other words, CsA was observed to form a complex with cyclophilin that furthermore engages the calcium/calmodulin dependent protein phosphatase calcineurin, which in a further step activates "the nuclear factor of activated T cells" (NFAT) in cell nucleoli to ultimately upregulate interleukin-2 (IL-2)

expression. Based on this IL-2 inhibiton, CsA halts T cell growth and T cell differentiation and thereby acts immunosuppressive (13).

Tacrolimus

Since the early 1990's, tacrolimus (FK 506), a macrolide antibiotic, which has been isolated from *Streptomyces tsukubaensis*, represents a mainstay in immunosuppression. Similar to CsA, tacrolimus blocks T cell activation and proliferation by interfering with the IL-2 pathway. FK 506 has been shown to bind the FK-binding protein 12 (FKBP12), which ultimately results in the inhibition of the calcineurin pathway leading to decreased IL-2 mediated T cell proliferation. The binding potency of FK 506 is 10 to 100 times stronger when compared to CsA, which results in decreased dosage demand by nonetheless retaining it's immunosuppressive capacity (14, 15).

Tacrolimus and cyclosporine A have both similar interactions with other medications, because of their common metabolism occurring in the liver by the cytochrome P-450 family. In addition, they also have a similar side effect profile such as acute and chronic renal insufficiency, dyslipidemia, hypertension, electrolyte disturbances, and post transplant diabetes. Furthermore, tacrolimus is more strongly associated with neurological complications including, seizures, headaches, and tremors.

2.2 Mycophenolate mofetil – A powerful substitute for azathioprine in antiproliferative immunosuppressive therapy

Mycophenolate Mofetil (MMF) is an antimetabolite immunosuppressant whose active component, mycophenolic acid (MPA), inhibits the key enzyme in the purine synthesis pathway, inosine monophosphate dehydrogenase (16). The discovery of this antiproliferative agent dates back to 1896, when it was first isolated from cultures of *Penicillium brevicompactum.* Initial analyses and studies to proof the immunosuppressive competence of MMF were conducted in the early 1980's. MMF has been shown to inhibit B and T cells proliferation, and induce apoptosis of activated T cells. It furthermore limits the expression of adhesion molecules on lymphocytes, which results in a decrease of nitric oxide production and hence, decreases the recruitment of inflammatory cells (17). Nevertheless, it took 15 more years until the Food and Drug Administration (FDA) approved this drug for the prevention of renal allograft rejection in 1995 (18).

Several clinical trials in the recent past pointed out that the combination of MMF with calcineurin inhibitors results in enhanced patient and graft survival and reduces events of acute and chronic rejection (19). MMF furthermore might be an alternative drug for patients developing drug-induced nephrotoxicity due to other immunosuppressive treatment (20). Besides bone marrow suppression and subsequent leucopenia, diarrhea, and GI distress are the most notable side effects of this immunosuppressant. However, recently a new " enteric coated" formulation of MMF has been developed, which has been shown to improve the mycophenolate exposure and hence, decreases GI side effects. In addition, MMF replaced azathioprine after 5 decades of its successful utilization as an antiproliferative immunosuppressive agent in the area of solid organ transplantation.

2.3 Azathioprine

Azathioprine has a long history of use in the field of solid organ transplantation (21). As an antimetabolite, azathioprine exerts its immunosuppressive properties by halting DNA replication of T and B cells, as well as by interfering with costimulatory signals, which ultimately results in lymphocyte depletion (22). Before the discovery of CsA, the combination of azathioprine and steroids represented the standard treatment of choice in solid organ transplantation, however, like most immunosuppressive agents, azathioprine has multiple drug interactions and side effects. If co-administered with allopurinol for the treatment of gout or hyperuricemia due to a decrease in drug metabolism of both agents, azathioprine should only be dosed at 20% to 30% of normal dosage (23). The main toxicity associated with azathioprine is a dose dependent myelosuppression resulting in leucopenia, thrombocytopenia, and macrocytic anemia. Additionally, hepatotoxcicity and an increased incidence in malignancies have been reported. Today, azathioprine has widely been replaced by mycophenolate mofetil.

2.4 mTOR-Inhibitors

Another powerful class of immunosuppressive drugs comprises inhibitors of the mammalian target of rapamycin (mTOR), a key signaling kinase that affects broad aspects of cellular function like cell growth, as well as protein synthesis, and transcription (24, 25). The first mTOR inhibiting substance, sirolimus (Rapamycin), was isolated from soil obtained on Easter Island (Rapa Nui) and was initially identified as a potent antifungal metabolite (26).

However, this macrolide produced by *Streptomyces hygroscopicus* also turned out to inhibit cell proliferation and thereby produced antitumor and immunosuppressive activity. Finally, in 1999 sirolimus got its FDA approval for the prevention of kidney allograft rejection. Initially, the implementation of sirolimus was supposed to potentiate the therapy with CsA, but the combination controversially increased nephrotoxicity, hypertension, as well as the incidence of hemolytic-uremic syndrome. Hence, a controlled trial in kidney transplantation confirmed increased nephrotoxicity and hypertension in the treatment group of sirolimus combined with tacrolimus, which has been compared to the combined use of mycophenolate mofetil and tacrolimus.

The synthetic derivate of sirolimus, everolimus, showed an increased bioavailability, but there were no affects in interaction with CsA compared to sirolimus observed. Severe side effects of both lipophilic macrolides have been reported including hyperlipidemia, thrombocytopenia, aggravation of proteinuria, mouth ulcers, skin lesions, as well as pneumonitis, and impaired wound healing (27). Especially in kidney grafts, delayed recovery from acute tubular necrosis was observed.

2.5 Corticosteroids

From the early beginnings of solid organ transplantation, corticosteroids have played a key role in maintenance immunosuppression as well as treatment of acute rejection episodes. Today, most immunosuppressive protocols contain high doses of methylprednisolone perioperatively with a subsequent tapering to approximately 5 to 7.5mg per day over the ensuing months.

Although it has been shown that corticosteroids have anti-inflammatory and immunosuppressive properties due to their suppression of prostaglandin synthesis, their stabilization of lysosomal membranes, and subsequently their reduction of histamine and bradykinin, the exact mechanism of action remains incompletely understood (18). Experimental data provide evidence that a continuous corticosteroid treatment due to the presence of glucocorticoid receptors on T cells, results in steroid mediated T regulatory FOXP3 expression and thus suppressor activity (28, 29).

In addition to their therapeutic immunosuppressive effects, corticosteroids have several severe side effects, especially when administered for a long time, which limit their applicability in post-transplant therapy (30). These sequels include inter alia: diabetes, hypertension, obesity, cushingoid features, osteoporosis, poor wound heeling, and adrenal suppression (31). However, despite many transplant clinicians search out steroid-sparing or even steroid-free regimens due to their deleterious side effects, especially induction therapy regimens still continue to include steroids in their treatment regimens.

3. Induction therapy

Many transplant centers in the United States and Europe are currently preferring to apply intense therapy at the time of transplantation with the goal to deplete the recipient's immune system in the immediate post-transplant period to decrease early deleterious interactions between the recipient's immune system and the donor allograft to ultimately induce a tolerogenic state (32). It has been widely accepted that early alloreactivity not only leads to an increase in acute rejection episodes, but also promotes chronic rejection which ultimately leads to poor long-term graft survival. While current induction immunosuppression agents have reduced the incidence of acute rejection, the goal of transplant tolerance has not been realized.

3.1 Antibodies

OKT3

Antibody mediated immunosuppressants have been used as induction therapy to suppress the recipient's immune system immediately after transplantation. There are both, polyclonal as well as monoclonal, antibodies available. OKT3 is a murine monoclonal antibody, which targets the T cell receptor CD3 complex resulting in a decrease of T cell activation (33). As a side effect OKT3 treatment commonly causes a "cytokine release syndrom" with fevers, chills, headaches and myalgias. As a consequence, patients are premedicated with steroids, acetaminophen, and diphenhydramine as a prophylaxis against this inflammatory response. Other less frequent side effects include pulmonary edema, seizures, aseptic meningitis, and renal insufficiency (34).

Basiliximab (Simulect)

Basiliximab is another antibody, commonly used as an induction agent, which interferes with the alpha subunit (CD25) of the IL-2 receptor (35). This monoclonal antibody of chimeric human-murine origin formidably decreases T cell proliferation and differentiation without T cell depletion. It is preferentially used in patients with the risk of low to moderate rejection episodes and it's currently approved for dosing 20mg on the first and fourth day after transplant (36). Being humanized, there were only minimal toxic effects reported, although basiliximab has been associated with pulmonary edema and ARDS-like symptoms (37).

Alemtuzumab (Campath)

Alemtuzumab is a humanized-rat monoclonal antibody directed against CD52, which is present on the surface of mature lymphocytes (38). Originally prescribed in lymphocytic leukemia and lymphoma, alemtuzumab is currently also used as a potent induction agent in solid organ and vascularized composite allografts. Although the function of CD52 remains incompletely understood, it is present on the cell surface of B and T cells, as well as macrophages, and NK cells which get depleted upon binding of alemtuzumab. Although alemtuzumab has a half-life of about 2 weeks, different cells have different rates of recovery after therapy. Additionally, alemtuzumab has been shown to deplete T cells inhomogenously, with a relative sparing of memory T cells and T regulatory cells. In terms of side effects, alemtuzumab has been associated with neutropenia, anemia, pancytopenia, first-dose reactions, and autoimmunity (37).

Antithymocyte Globulin

Anthithymocyte globulin (ATG) is a polyclonal antibody derived from animals that have been immunized with human lymphocytes. As a result, ATG is nonspecifically directed against human lymphocytes, which upon treatment get depleted through multiple mechanisms including complement-mediated lysis and opsonisation. In addition, ATG might induce alloantigen specific immunological tolerance as ATG binds lymphocyte costimulatory molecules and similar to OKT3 and alemtuzumab expands T regulatory cells *in vitro and in vivo* (39). Polyclonal antithymocyte globulin is preferrably used as an agent in steroid-free regimes due to its positive effects in the treatment of steroid-resistant rejection episodes. However, ATG treatment frequently induces an acute reaction to initial administration consisting of fever, rigors and anaphylaxis with some patients developing leucopenia and thrombocytopenia.

3.2 Fusion proteins

CTLA4-Ig (Abatacept, Belatacept)

Full T cell activation depends on two signals. The first signal is generated upon MHC-antigen - T cell receptor (TCR) interaction. The costimulation pathway, or signal two, is activated when accessory molecules bind to their ligands. Specifically the CD28/B7 pathway (CD80 and CD86) has proven itself to be relevant for sustained naïve T cell activation. Interfering with these pathways has been one of the most intensively investigated areas in immunology, particularly when considering therapeutic interventions.

After 25 years of research, the fusion receptor protein CTLA4-Ig (abatacept), a competitive antagonist for CD80/CD86 binding, was finally approved for the therapy of rheumatoid arthritis. For the specific use in solid organ transplantation, where an even more robust immunosuppression is required, a second-generation fusion protein called belatacept was developed. Belatacept has proven efficient in prolonging renal allograft survival alone or in combination therapies with basiliximab or MMF and prednisone (40).

3.3 Immunosuppression in Vascularized Composite Allotransplantation

Immunosuppression in vascularized composite allotransplantation (VCA) remains a difficult issue, since the treatment with conventional immunosuppression used in solid organ transplantation is associated with life-threatening infectious complications (41) and metabolic side effects, which seem to be intolerable for non life-saving procedures like hand and face transplantation (42, 43). As a consequence, reconstructive surgeons and immunologists more than ever seek to establish stable donor antigen specific immunological tolerance to vascularized composite allografts, a state that impairs the immune system not to mount responses against a specific allograft, but at the same time facilitates natural defenses

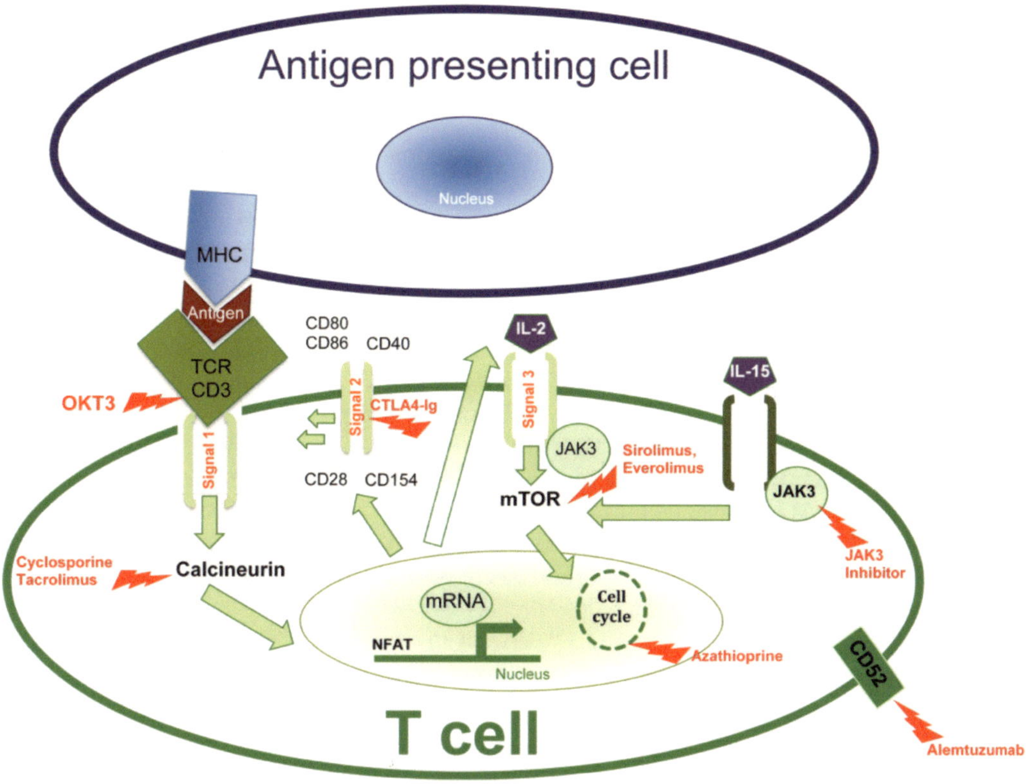

Fig. 1. Immunosuppressive drugs currently used in solid organ transplantation

against viral and bacterial infections. However, in the early days of reconstructive transplantation, immunosuppressive regimens consisted of initial high-dose induction therapy, mainly ATG, or alemtuzumab, which in most cases was followed by a conventional triple combination of corticosteroids, calcineurin inhibitors, and mycophenolate mofetil (44). Exceptions to this conventional immunosuppressive treatment include some recent cases in hand transplantation, where patients received induction therapy with alemtuzumab followed by maintenance immunosuppression with tacrolimus and mycophenolate mofetil (Louisville) or tacrolimus and prednisone (Innsbruck). More recently, the "Pittsburgh Protocol" consisting of an induction therapy with alemtuzumab and a donor specific bonemarrow cell transfusion within 2 weeks after transplantation proofed that maintenance immunosuppression with tacrolimus alone can successfully be achieved in VCA. The idea of donor cell infusion for either the induction of chimerism or the intensification of clonal exhaustion or deletion of alloreactive T cells is appealing, however, the combination of such a concept with high-dose multi drug immunosuppression might be counterproductive, because such phenomena may require the persistence of a certain degree of immune response to be effective. Recent innovative immunosuppressive protocols proofed to be effective in weaning patients off immunosuppression or at least in allowing a reduction of immunosuppression to a minimum level (45, 46). Nevertheless, from the current clinical point of view in reconstructive transplantation, it is difficult to conclude the superiority from one immunosuppressive regimen over another and it seems mandatory to pursue multicenter prospective trials despite the limited number of patients that are currently eligible to be enrolled in such trials.

4. References

[1] Murray JE. The first successful organ transplants in man. J Am Coll Surg. 2005 Jan;200(1):5-9.
[2] Murray JE. The Nobel Lectures in Immunology. The Nobel Prize for Physiology or Medicine, 1990. The first successful organ transplants in man. Scand J Immunol. 1994 Jan;39(1):1-11.
[3] Dubernard JM, Owen E, Herzberg G, Lanzetta M, Martin X, Kapila H, et al. Human hand allograft: report on first 6 months. Lancet. 1999 Apr 17;353(9161):1315-20.
[4] Devauchelle B, Badet L, Lengele B, Morelon E, Testelin S, Michallet M, et al. First human face allograft: early report. Lancet. 2006 Jul 15;368(9531):203-9.
[5] Schneeberger S, Ninkovic M, Gabl M, Hussl H, Rieger M, Loescher W, et al. First forearm transplantation: outcome at 3 years. Am J Transplant. 2007 Jul;7(7):1753-62.
[6] Vincenti F, Kirk AD. What's next in the pipeline. Am J Transplant. 2008 Oct;8(10):1972-81.
[7] Meier-Kriesche HU, Schold JD, Srinivas TR, Kaplan B. Lack of improvement in renal allograft survival despite a marked decrease in acute rejection rates over the most recent era. Am J Transplant. 2004 Mar;4(3):378-83.
[8] Nankivell BJ, Borrows RJ, Fung CL, O'Connell PJ, Allen RD, Chapman JR. The natural history of chronic allograft nephropathy. N Engl J Med. 2003 Dec 11;349(24):2326-33.
[9] Gaston RS, Cecka JM, Kasiske BL, Fieberg AM, Leduc R, Cosio FC, et al. Evidence for antibody-mediated injury as a major determinant of late kidney allograft failure. Transplantation. Jul 15;90(1):68-74.
[10] Sucher R, Hautz T, Brandacher G, Lee WP, Margreiter R, Schneeberger S. [Immunosuppression in hand transplantation: state of the art and future perspectives]. Handchir Mikrochir Plast Chir. 2009 Aug;41(4):217-23.
[11] Kahan BD. The era of cyclosporine: twenty years forward, twenty years back. Transplant Proc. 2004 Mar;36(2 Suppl):5S-6S.
[12] Kostakis A. Early experience with cyclosporine: a historic perspective. Transplant Proc. 2004 Mar;36(2 Suppl):22S-4S.
[13] Morris PJ. Cyclosporine, FK-506 and other drugs in organ transplantation. Curr Opin Immunol. 1991 Oct;3(5):748-51.
[14] Reichenspurner H. Overview of tacrolimus-based immunosuppression after heart or lung transplantation. J Heart Lung Transplant. 2005 Feb;24(2):119-30.
[15] Sigal NH, Dumont FJ. Cyclosporin A, FK-506, and rapamycin: pharmacologic probes of lymphocyte signal transduction. Annu Rev Immunol. 1992;10:519-60.
[16] Allison AC, Eugui EM. Mechanisms of action of mycophenolate mofetil in preventing acute and chronic allograft rejection. Transplantation. 2005 Oct 15;80(2 Suppl):S181-90.
[17] Allison AC, Eugui EM. Mycophenolate mofetil and its mechanisms of action. Immunopharmacology. 2000 May;47(2-3):85-118.
[18] Bhorade SM, Stern E. Immunosuppression for lung transplantation. Proc Am Thorac Soc. 2009 Jan 15;6(1):47-53.

[19] Sollinger HW. Mycophenolates in transplantation. Clin Transplant. 2004 Oct;18(5):485-92.
[20] Hirose R, Vincenti F. Immunosuppression: today, tomorrow, and withdrawal. Semin Liver Dis. 2006 Aug;26(3):201-10.
[21] Taylor AL, Watson CJ, Bradley JA. Immunosuppressive agents in solid organ transplantation: Mechanisms of action and therapeutic efficacy. Crit Rev Oncol Hematol. 2005 Oct;56(1):23-46.
[22] Maltzman JS, Koretzky GA. Azathioprine: old drug, new actions. J Clin Invest. 2003 Apr;111(8):1122-4.
[23] Brooks RJ, Dorr RT, Durie BG. Interaction of allopurinol with 6-mercaptopurine and azathioprine. Biomed Pharmacother. 1982;36(4):217-22.
[24] Brown EJ, Albers MW, Shin TB, Ichikawa K, Keith CT, Lane WS, et al. A mammalian protein targeted by G1-arresting rapamycin-receptor complex. Nature. 1994 Jun 30;369(6483):756-8.
[25] Hay N, Sonenberg N. Upstream and downstream of mTOR. Genes Dev. 2004 Aug 15;18(16):1926-45.
[26] Saunders RN, Metcalfe MS, Nicholson ML. Rapamycin in transplantation: a review of the evidence. Kidney Int. 2001 Jan;59(1):3-16.
[27] Chhajed PN, Dickenmann M, Bubendorf L, Mayr M, Steiger J, Tamm M. Patterns of pulmonary complications associated with sirolimus. Respiration. 2006;73(3):367-74.
[28] Chen X, Murakami T, Oppenheim JJ, Howard OM. Differential response of murine CD4+CD25+ and CD4+CD25- T cells to dexamethasone-induced cell death. Eur J Immunol. 2004 Mar;34(3):859-69.
[29] Demirkiran A, Hendrikx TK, Baan CC, van der Laan LJ. Impact of immunosuppressive drugs on CD4+CD25+FOXP3+ regulatory T cells: does in vitro evidence translate to the clinical setting? Transplantation. 2008 Mar 27;85(6):783-9.
[30] Bodziak KA, Hricik DE. New-onset diabetes mellitus after solid organ transplantation. Transpl Int. 2009 May;22(5):519-30.
[31] Compston JE. Osteoporosis after liver transplantation. Liver Transpl. 2003 Apr;9(4):321-30.
[32] Krischock L, Marks SD. Induction therapy: why, when, and which agent? Pediatr Transplant. May;14(3):298-313.
[33] Chatenoud L, Bluestone JA. CD3-specific antibodies: a portal to the treatment of autoimmunity. Nat Rev Immunol. 2007 Aug;7(8):622-32.
[34] Hong JC, Kahan BD. Immunosuppressive agents in organ transplantation: past, present, and future. Semin Nephrol. 2000 Mar;20(2):108-25.
[35] Gabardi S, Martin ST, Roberts KL, Grafals M. Induction immunosuppressive therapies in renal transplantation. Am J Health Syst Pharm. Feb 1;68(3):211-8.
[36] Delgado JF, Vaqueriza D, Sanchez V, Escribano P, Ruiz-Cano MJ, Renes E, et al. Induction treatment with monoclonal antibodies for heart transplantation. Transplant Rev (Orlando). Jan;25(1):21-6.
[37] Tang IY, Meier-Kriesche HU, Kaplan B. Immunosuppressive strategies to improve outcomes of kidney transplantation. Semin Nephrol. 2007 Jul;27(4):377-92.
[38] Weaver TA, Kirk AD. Alemtuzumab. Transplantation. 2007 Dec 27;84(12):1545-7.
[39] Merion RM, Howell T, Bromberg JS. Partial T-cell activation and anergy induction by polyclonal antithymocyte globulin. Transplantation. 1998 Jun 15;65(11):1481-9.

[40] Larsen CP, Pearson TC, Adams AB, Tso P, Shirasugi N, Strobert E, et al. Rational development of LEA29Y (belatacept), a high-affinity variant of CTLA4-Ig with potent immunosuppressive properties. Am J Transplant. 2005 Mar;5(3):443-53.
[41] Schneeberger S, Lucchina S, Lanzetta M, Brandacher G, Bosmuller C, Steurer W, et al. Cytomegalovirus-related complications in human hand transplantation. Transplantation. 2005 Aug 27;80(4):441-7.
[42] Bonatti H, Brandacher G, Margreiter R, Schneeberger S. Infectious complications in three double hand recipients: experience from a single center. Transplant Proc. 2009 Mar;41(2):517-20.
[43] Schneeberger S, Kreczy A, Brandacher G, Steurer W, Margreiter R. Steroid- and ATG-resistant rejection after double forearm transplantation responds to Campath-1H. Am J Transplant. 2004 Aug;4(8):1372-4.
[44] Schneeberger S, Landin L, Kaufmann C, Gorantla VS, Brandacher G, Cavadas P, et al. Alemtuzumab: key for minimization of maintenance immunosuppression in reconstructive transplantation? Transplant Proc. 2009 Mar;41(2):499-502.
[45] Kirk AD, Mannon RB, Swanson SJ, Hale DA. Strategies for minimizing immunosuppression in kidney transplantation. Transpl Int. 2005 Jan;18(1):2-14.
[46] Schneeberger S, Landin L, Jableki J, Butler P, Hoehnke C, Brandacher G, et al. Achievements and challenges in composite tissue allotransplantation. Transpl Int. Aug;24(8):760-9.

21

HIV/AIDS Associated Malignant Disorders: Role of Highly Active Antiretroviral Therapy

Angel Mayor, Yelitza Ruiz, Diana Fernández and Robert Hunter-Mellado
Retrovirus Research Center, Universidad Central del Caribe School of Medicine, Bayamón
Puerto Rico

1. Introduction

Persons infected with the human immunodeficiency virus (HIV) have an elevated risk for the development of Cancer. Some of the malignant processes are intrinsic to the immunological impact of the HIV infection; others are more often related to the risk scenarios associated to the viral inoculum and subsequent development of the infection. In general terms, malignant transformation is fundamentally caused by genetic alterations to individual cells, which allow the presence of the disorganized autonomous growth of cells and the development of properties associated to the survival of the cancer cells. Properties associated to successful growth of the cancer include the capacity for relative autonomous growth, evasion of the normal regulatory process present within bodies, capacity of tissue invasion, spread to other organs and disruption of the normal organ homeostasis. Predisposing conditions that lead to an increased risk for the malignant transformation include chronic inflammatory states, congenital or acquired genetic mutations, autoimmune diseases, and exposure to environmental factors. The presence of HIV infection, particularly in the context of a deteriorated immune system is associated to an increased risk for the development of Kaposi's sarcoma, high-grade non-Hodgkin's lymphomas, central nervous system lymphoma and invasive uterine cervical cancer. Collectively these entities may be the initial manifestation of HIV infection and are intimately associated to the deteriorated immune system associated to the infection. As such they are considered AIDS defining conditions. The spectrum of HIV associated malignant disorders also includes non-AIDS defining cancers. Non-AIDS defining malignancies are often seen in patients who are at younger age than usual, are associated to a more aggressive behavior and tend to be diagnosed at a more advanced stage. The most common non-AIDS defining malignancies include Hodgkin's lymphomas, non-small cell lung cancer, head and neck cancer, ano-genital cancer, hepatic cancer and possibly multiple myeloma. The role of the HIV virus in triggering the malignant transformation of cells appears to be a direct effect by promoting cancer growth, and indirect in others by disrupting the human regulatory symbiosis provided by the immune system. The introduction of multiple spectrum antiretroviral therapy (ART) and the availability of highly active antiretroviral therapy (HAART) have caused a dramatic improvement in the immunological function of infected subjects with an associated increment in the overall survival of these patients. The use of HAART has been intimately associated to a dramatic decrease in not only AIDS defining opportunistic infections but in some of the AIDS defining tumors particularly Kaposi's sarcoma and non

Hodgkin's lymphomas. Nevertheless changes in the incidence of invasive cervical carcinoma and non-AIDS defining cancers have not been so remarkable. HIV infection has become a chronic condition associated to a longer lifespan of patients and the introduction of an evolving list of co-morbid conditions, including cancer. Under this scenario, understanding the trends on cancer development in this population of patients has become of marked importance, since they represent the next boundary that is limiting the survival of the HIV infected patient. In this chapter we describe the changing trends in the incidence of malignant disorders which affect the HIV infected patients with a particular emphasis on the role of HAART in the expression of these malignant conditions (Bedimo et al, 2004; Bonne et al., 2008; Bower et al, 2006; Caceres et al., 2010; Crum-Clanflone et al, 2009; Engels et al., 2008; Gurlich et al., 2002; Long et al., 2008;Mitsuyasy et al., 2011; Newcomb-Fernandez et al., 2003; Patel et al., 2008; Simard et al., 2010) .

2. Cancer

Hereditary or acquired genetic mutations, autoimmune disorders, and exposure to certain environmental agents may singly or in a combined synergistic fashion, predispose to the development of neoplasms. The role of HIV in inducing the malignant transformation of cells appears to be an indirect effect by disrupting the human immune regulatory process. Immunological deficiency induced by HIV causes a progressive impairment of the cellular immunity responsible for the control of viral growth and the immune recognition against virus-infected or altered cells in the different stages of malignant transformation. HIV induced cytokine deregulation disrupts the host's capacity to control oncogenic viral reactivation and replication, ultimately increasing the risk for malignant transformation. Oncogenic viruses, including the Ebstein-Barr virus (EBV), human herpesvirus 8 (HHV 8), certain subtypes of the human papilloma virus, hepatitis B virus (HBV), and hepatitis C virus (HCV) have all been causally related to the increasing prevalence of cancer development in these patients. In addition the presence of certain risky lifestyle behaviors often present in the HIV infected patients such as smoking, alcohol use, use of illegal drugs and sexual promiscuity may contribute and accelerate the risk of malignant transformation in these subjects. HIV associated severe immunosuppression may be interrupted or partially restored with the use of ART. Improvement or partial restoration of the cell-mediated immunity and the suppression of the HIV viral load will not only improve the patients' immunological status but will improve the overall clinical status with an improvement in overall survival. An increment in the survival of the HIV infected patient leads to an aging patient cohort with a higher likelihood of oncogenic viruses exposure. These elements alter the clinical course of the HIV infection with the development of new morbidity patterns such as altered toxicity profiles of medications, development of metabolic disorders, long lasting co-infections (including HPV, HHV, HCV, HBV and EBV), development of an increased risk of cardiovascular diseases and non-AIDS defining neoplasms. Even though, for many of the tumors described in this chapter, there are no specific prevention guidelines, other than the need to diagnose early and institute therapy as early as possible.

2.1 AIDS defining malignances

Kaposi's sarcoma, high-grade non-Hodgkin's lymphomas, including the high-grade immunoblastic or diffuse large cell lymphoma, the small noncleaved (Burkitt, Burkitt-like or non-Burkitt) lymphoma, primary central nervous system lymphoma (PCNSL), and invasive cervical cancer are neoplasms included as AIDS defining conditions. With the introduction of HAART the spectrum of these cancers has changed, with a dramatic reduction in the incidence of Kaposi's sarcoma and non-Hodgkin's lymphomas. However, the impact of HAART in the invasive cervical cancer had not been significant. It is relevant to mention that in spite of HAART, the risk for AIDS defining cancers continues to be significantly higher as compared to the non HIV infected general population (Simard et al., 2010).

2.1.1 Kaposi's sarcoma

Kaposi's sarcoma is an angio-proliferative disease characterized by tumors composed of new blood vessel (angiogenesis), endothelial spindle cell growth, inflammatory cell infiltration and edema. Kaposi's sarcoma is classified in four epidemiologic variants: the classic, the African endemic, the iatrogenic, and the epidemic AIDS-related. The clinical manifestation of this sarcoma in patients with AIDS is variable but usually presents as a multiple, small, innocuous pigmented cutaneous or oral-pharyngeal lesions. These may grow and spread causing symptom-producing visceral disease. Alternatively it may develop in a multifocal fashion in several sites at the same time. In both cases it may result in a life-threatening process with the need of aggressive therapy.

2.1.1.1 Pathophysiology

The pathogenesis of the condition was clarified in 1994 when human herpes virus-8 (HHV-8) also known as Kaposi's sarcoma -associated herpes virus (KSHV) was described and detected in all forms of Kaposi's sarcoma. HHV-8 is a transmissible DNA virus with a seroprevalence in the United States between 1%-5%. The pathogenesis of AIDS related Kaposi's sarcoma is multifactorial and includes HHV-8 infection, HIV induced cytokine malfunction, and stimulation transactivating transduction (TAT) protein by HIV. HHV-8 is an oncogenic virus transmitted both sexually and through body fluids such as saliva and blood, which encodes a cell protein involved in signal transduction, cell cycle regulation and inhibition of apoptosis. HHV-8 is critical in the pathogenesis of this AIDS related sarcoma, but by itself is not sufficient to cause the cancer. The risk of this cancer is directly related to the degree of immune suppression in the host and can remain in a latent phase for many years. The interaction between HIV-TAT protein and the immune suppressed state of the host allows the activation of the virus resulting in an abnormal inflammatory response and the promotion of angiogenesis by inducing lymphatic reprogramming of the vascular endothelium.

2.1.1.2 Clinical manifestation and diagnosis

The clinical presentation of Kaposi's sarcoma ranges from irregular reddish discrete lesions to violaceous or brown nodules, macules, patches, or plaques. The lesions are usually painless, do not blanch under pressure and may be associated with edema, lymph node or visceral involvement. Pathologic confirmation is required to establish a diagnosis of Kaposi's sarcoma since bacillary angiomatosis can mimic this malignancy even for the seasoned clinician. The lesions may occur in any part of the body, including the face, chest, oral mucosa, penis or scrotum, rectum, and conjunctiva. The oral cavity can be extensively involved resulting in airway obstruction. The gastrointestinal tract is a common site of the disease. These lesions are often asymptomatic but can be associated with abdominal pain, gastro-intestinal bleeding, diarrhea, abdominal cramps, and weight loss. Visceral involvement occurs in over 50% of the cases. Pulmonary involvement is the second most common extra-cutaneous location and may present with life threatening manifestations. Pulmonary involvement is often associated with obstructive respiratory symptoms, hemoptysis and chest pain. The clinical course of this sarcoma is variable with the presence of slowly progressive lesions over the course of many years, or it may have a rapid progression over a course of weeks or months. The external appearance of the cutaneous lesions may lead to emotional distress and stigmatization. The use of corticosteroid therapy has been associated with the induction or exacerbation of this cancer in the context of the HIV infected individual (Bellan et al, 2003; Dezube, 2007).

2.1.1.3 Therapy

The decision to institute therapy needs to consider the extent, location and rate of tumor growth as well as the patient's symptoms, and immune system condition. Optimization of HAART therapy is critical in all patients with Kaposi's sarcoma since this tumor is intrinsically linked to the degree of immunosuppression and the fact that up to 91% of lesions regress with HAART. Immune reconstitution is a primordial therapeutic goal in every patient. For limited skin lesions, the application of topical therapy with liquid nitrogen, vinblastine or retinoic acid may be appropriate. External beam radiotherapy is also an option in certain cases. Interferon-α is an immunomodulator with antiviral and anti-angiogenic effect that has been used with some success in patients with the cutanous form of the disease. Its widespread use has been hampered by its toxicity profile, which is often moderate to severe in nature. For patients with edema, extensive mucocutaneous disease, or symptomatic pulmonary or gastrointestinal involvement, the administration of systemic chemotherapy is recommended. Several single agent drugs are active in this AIDS related sarcoma. These include vincristine, vinblastine, etoposide, anthracyclines, bleomycin and taxol with an overall response rate of 76%. The administration of combination chemotherapy has been utilized since early 1991 for rapidly progressive mucocutaneous or visceral disease. The most common drug combination has been doxorubicin, bleomycin and vincristine (ABV) or bleomycin and vincristine (BV). The use of liposomal anthracyclines is currently considered the optimal first line therapy for the treatment of advanced Kaposi's sarcoma. This single agent therapy has been reported to have similar or improved response rates to other drugs but less toxicity. Paclitaxel (taxol) is the most recent introduction to the systemic chemotherapeutic agents available for these patients. Its use is often prescribed as second line therapy for patients with refractory disease. The response rate with paclitaxel is between 59-71%. Additional drugs that have variable rate of success in this disease include inhibitors of angiogenesis such as thalidomide, inhibitors of tyrosine kinase or mammalian rapamycin pathways such as imatinib and sunitinib. The response rate after standard chemotherapy is usually very good, but they tend to be short lasting. The high incidence of opportunistic infections associated to the administration of chemotherapy along with the chemotherapy associated cytopenias, are major issues in the management of these patients (Berretta et al, 2003; Dezube, 2007).

2.1.1.4 Epidemiology

Kaposi's sarcoma is a rare condition in the HIV negative population; however, it is the most common malignancy associated with HIV infection. This cancer had been more often detected in HIV-positive persons with more advanced immunosuppression ($CD4^+$ T lymphocyte counts of <200 cells/μL), and especially in men who have sex with men (MSM). Among MSM the transition of the HHV-8 is predominately by deep kissing. In these individuals the HHV-8 prevalence that is associated with their number of homosexual partners is considerably greater when compare to the other HIV risk behavior groups. The probability of developing Kaposi's sarcoma in HIV infected persons who are infected with HHV-8 is significantly high. The overall incidence of this cancer was as high as 20% among patients with AIDS before the advent of effective ART. However the incidence decreases dramatically since the introduction of HAART and remains low (Bedimo et al., 2004). The HIV/AIDS Cancer Match Study of 263.254 AIDS cases followed in 15 States of the United States between 1980 and 2008 reveals a significant reduction of this sarcoma incidence of 80% (RR, 0.2: 95% CI, 0.2%-0,2%) in the HAART era (Simard et al, 2010). This study concord with previous studies performed in United States and Puerto Rican's HIV cohorts that reported a significant reduction in the incidence or prevalence of this cancer after the antiretroviral therapies era (Engel et al., 2008; Crum-Cianflone et al., 2009; Mayor et al., 2008b). Despite the significant incidence reduction of Kaposi's sarcoma the risk of this cancer in HIV infected persons remains significantly elevated in the HAART era, when compare to the general population (Simard et al., 2010; Engels et al., 2008; Patel et al., 2008).

2.1.1.5 Prevention

Routine screening for HHV-8 by PCR or serologic testing is not indicated for HIV-infected persons. It has been advocated that HAART therapy will reduce the incidence of Kaposi's sarcoma by improving the immunological state and preventing tumor growth. Thus opportune antiretroviral therapy is an effective preventive strategy for patients who qualify.

2.1.2 Non Hodgkin's lymphoma

Non-Hodgkin's lymphomas represent a diverse group of malignant conditions of the immune system. These tumors are 60-100 times more common in the HIV infected patient as compared to the general population. There are three histological subtypes that are responsible for the majority of non-Hodgkin's lymphomas diagnosed in HIV patients and they include small non-cleaved lymphomas (Burkitts and non Burkitts like), high grade large cell, and the immunoblastic lymphomas, commonly present with the brain as primary site. With the institution of HAART the incidence of lymphomas in these patients has decreased but the decrement is much less as compared to the other AIDS defining conditions. The risk of developing non-Hodgkin's lymphomas has decreased from 1,226 to 306 per 100,000 person years after the introduction of HARRT (Simard et al., 2010). However, the prevalence of these lymphomas in HIV persons after HAART remains high when compare to HIV negative population (Engels et al., 2008; Simard et al., 2010; Bierman et al., 2004; Doweiko, 2007b).

2.1.2.1 Pathophysiology

The pathogenesis of AIDS related non-Hodgkin's lymphomas are fundamentally related to repeated stimulation and proliferation of B cells in the setting of a T-cell immunodeficiency. This results in the loss of immune surveillance and the continued proliferation of aberrant B cell clones. Etiologic agents implicated in the abnormal B cell proliferative response include HIV, Ebstein Barr virus and other infections. The presence of HIV induces the expression of cytokines (IL-6, IL-10 and TNF-α), which also contribute to B cell activation and proliferation. The process of B cell expansion results in lymph node enlargement and is usually accompanied by polyclonal hypergammaglobulinemia. The enhanced proliferative response of B cells increases the opportunity of genetic error, which may result in the dysregulation of suppressor genes (p53) and/or activation of proto-oncogenes (c-myc, BCL-6 or ras). The majority of AIDS-related non-Hodgkin's lymphomas (75%) carry alterations in at least one proto-oncogene and more than 90% have alterations in at least one of the suppression genes. The presence of activation cytokines such as IL-6 and IL-10 contribute to the chronic B cell stimulation resulting in continued growth. Specifically, IL-6 activity that increases early in the course of HIV infection is predictive of the likelihood of lymphoma developing over time. IL10 is an autocrine growth factor for lymphoma and an inhibitor of cellular immune response. Elevated levels of IL-10 are associated to a worse prognosis in AIDS related non-Hodgkin's lymphomas (Bellan et al, 2003; Doweiko, 2007b).

2.1.2.2 Clinical manifestation and diagnosis

The presence of constitutional symptoms (fever, weight loss and night sweats) is seen in 80-90% of patients with AIDS-related non-Hodgkin's lymphomas. It is vital to exclude the presence of opportunistic infections in these patients prior to instituting antineoplastic therapy. Most patients initially present with advanced stage of lymphoma with 80% presenting as a stage IV. Common sites of extra-nodal involvement include central nervous system (30%), gastrointestinal tract (25%), bone marrow (25%) and liver (17%). Nevertheless any site of the body may be involved with AIDS-related non-Hodgkin's lymphomas including the rectum, soft tissue, oral cavity, lungs and heart. Bone marrow and leptomeningeal involvement are more often associated with small, non cleaved (Burkitt-like) lymphoma. Patients with gastrointestinal involvement may present with pain, weight loss, bleeding, obstruction and perforation in 40% of the cases. The prognosis of this group of patients tends to be better; they respond very well to therapy and have a longer survival. Patients with primary central nervous system lymphoma often present with focal neurologic deficits, seizures, and or altered mental status. A diagnosis of non-Hodgkin's lymphomas requires histological confirmation by biopsy with immunephenotypic and molecular rearrangement studies. A complete staging evaluation must be done once a diagnosis is made utilizing body imaging studies of the brain, bone marrow aspiration and biopsy, liver function studies and spinal fluids analysis if clinically indicated. The presence of Ebstein Barr virus DNA in cerebrospinal fluid by polymerase chain reaction is a high specific and sensitive diagnosis criterion for primary central nervous system lymphoma.

The majority of in HIV related non-Hodgkin's lymphomas are associated with one of three histological subtypes mentioned above. The presence of small non-cleaved lymphomas (Burkitts and non Burkitts like) accounts for 40% of them and is usually seen in patients with a higher CD4 counts than other types. They often express an abnormal p53 and c-myc or ras oncogenes. The high-grade large cell histology is seen in 40% of patients and is associated with an abnormal expression of BCL-6 in 40% of the cases. One of the particular presentations of this histology is primary effusion lymphoma. Primary effusion lymphoma occurs as a late manifestation of HIV infection and has a poor clinical outcome and a shorter 6 months survival as compared to other sites of this histology. This high-grade lymphoma originates in the pleura, pericardium, peritoneum, serosal surface or rarely in the meninges. The etiologic cause of this lymphoma is related to herpes virus-8 infection of the tumor clone. A previous history of Kaposi sarcoma increases the risk of developing primary effusion lymphoma, and often genomic material containing the imprint of KSHV/HHV8 genes is found in the malignant clone of cells. The remaining 30% of AIDS-related non-Hodgkin's lymphomas are inmunoblastic plasmocytoid lymphomas and are considered to be related to EBV infection. The most important presentation of this histology is the primary central nervous system lymphoma, which accounts for 20% of all AIDS related lymphomas. This histology is seen in advanced stage AIDS with CD4 cell counts below 30 cells/mm, and they rarely occur outside the brain. The incidence of primary central nervous system lymphoma has decreased with the introduction of HAART but remains a disease with poor outcome. This type of lymphomas is the second most common brain space-occupying lesion in patients with AIDS after toxoplasmosis. The most common location for primary central nervous system lymphomas is cerebral hemispheres, following by basal ganglia, cerebellum, and brain stem, with less than 10% involving posterior fossa. Unlike primary central nervous system lymphoma in the general population, these tumors can have ring-enhancement due to their rapid growth. The tumors usually measure at least 3 cm and may present with central necrosis. Management of this primary lymphoma consists of radiation therapy, the use of corticosteroids and alkylating agents. This therapy will increase length of survival but they rarely induce lasting remissions (Bierman et al., 2004; Doweiko, 2007b).

2.1.2.3 Treatment

The mainstay of therapy for patients with AIDS related non-Hodgkin's lymphomas are systemic chemotherapy. The common used regimens include R-CHOP, m-BACOP, EPOCH although no regimen appears superior to the other. System prophylaxis with intrathecal cytarabine (ARA-C 50 mg) or methotrexate (10-12 mg) every week for four weeks has been shown to reduce central nervous system relapse in the high risk group of patients. The major complication of chemotherapy is myelosuppression with its associated morbidities. Several studies have shown that co-administration with hematopoietic growth factors may enhance the chemotherapy toleration. In addition, prophylaxis with trimethropim/sulfa, azithromycin, fluconazole, ciprofloxacin, and valgancyclovir can reduce the risk of infection during intensive chemotherapy regimen. Refractory or relapse systemic lymphomas have a very poor prognosis with no satisfactory second line therapy available. An important factor in the management of AIDS related non-Hodgkin's lymphomas is the use of HAART to reduce the viral load and enhance the immune system management of the malignant clone.

2.1.2.4 Epidemiology

In the United States, 3% of the AIDS cases present with lymphoma. The major risk factors include older age, magnitude and duration of the immunosuppression, no prior HAART use or insufficient immunologic or virologic response to HAART. The types of risky practices associated to HIV infections are not associated to the presence of lymphoma. AIDS related non-Hodgkin's lymphomas are seen more frequent in men than in women and is seen more often in whites than in blacks. The standardized incidence rate of AIDS associated lymphoma is significantly higher than in the general population (Grulich et al., 2007). Most of the AIDS related non-Hodgkin's lymphomas (75%) have advanced HIV disease, however 25 % of patients develop the disease when the viral load is undetectable. Different studies had reported a significant reduction in the incidence of these lymphomas with the availability of effective antiretroviral therapies, particularly HAART (Bedimo et al., 2004). For example the HIV/AIDS Cancer Match Study of Simard et al, reported a 70% decline in their incidence (RR, 0.3: 95% CI, 0.2%-0.3%) as compared to the pre-HAART era (Simard, et al., 2010). The study found significant reduction in the diffuse large B cell and in the CNS Hodgkin's lymphomas NHL, but no differences were seen in the Burkitt-like histological lymphomas. Similar findings were documented in the other United States and Puerto Rican AIDS cohorts (Engels et al., 2008; Mayor et al., 2008b). Despite this significant reduction, non-Hodgkin's lymphomas risk remained significantly higher in HIV infected persons after HAART when compared to the general population as reported by Patle et al, Simard et al. and Engels et al.

2.1.2.5 Prevention

The risk of developing non-Hodgkin's lymphoma is directly proportional to the disruption of the immune system. The appropriate and opportune use of antiretroviral therapy (HAART) is necessary to reduce this risk. There are no specific prevention guidelines, other than the need to diagnose early and institute therapy as early as possible.

2.1.3 Invasive cervical cancer

Cervical cancer is a malignant proliferation of the squamous epithelium of the ectocervix causing squamous cell carcinoma. Malignant proliferation of the glandular lining of the endocervix carries histology of adenocarcinoma. More than 95% of cervical tumors have squamous cell histology and infection with the Human papilloma virus (HPV) is a necessary factor for the malignant transformation in the majority of these patients. Several subtypes of the HPV have delineated as responsible for the development of cervical dysplasia, which represents the usual histological antecedent to invasive tumors of the ectocervix. A higher incidence of HPV-related dysplasia, more advanced stages of cervical dysplasia and refractoriness to standard therapy is characteristic of this disease in females who also have HIV infection. The similarities in risk profiles and transmission modes between HIV and HPV explain the common and widespread presence of HPV in this group of patients. The higher risk of developing cervical dysplasia in HIV infected women initially promoted the inclusion of cervical cancer as one of the AIDS defining condition in 1993. The presence of HIV associated immunosuppression contributes to an impaired HPV clearance, facilitating progression of early stage to more advanced forms of dysplasia. The role of HIV in the ultimate transformation to cervical carcinoma is not so clearly defined. Cervical cancer is a tumor, which can be prevented and clearly curable if diagnosed at an early stage. Aggressive prevention strategies have significantly decreased the incidence and prevalence of this tumor in developed countries (Molpus &Jone, 2004; Powrie & Cu-Uvin, 2007).

2.1.3.1 Pathophysiology

The majority of squamous cell carcinomas of the cervix are preceded by a premalignant epithelial dysplasia known as cervical intraepithelial neoplasia and squamous intraepithelial lesions. These lesions slowly progress to the invasive form of cervical cancer. HPV infection has an important role in the genesis of this dysplasia and in the progression to an invasive state. This is in large part due to the chronic inflammatory insult induced by this oncogenic virus. HPV infection is the most common sexually transmitted infection in the US with an increasing prevalence seen among HIV infected individuals. HPV Types 16, 18, and 31 are the major virus associated with cervical cancer. Type 16 is more frequently associated with squamous cell histology and type 18 with adenocarcinoma. Other factors associated to the increase incidence of the cervical cancer in these patients include, the use of tobacco, younger age of first intercourse, higher number of sexual partners, immunosuppression, multiple pregnancies, use of hormonal medications, and to a lesser degree family antecedents (Molpus &Jone, 2004; Powrie & Cu-Uvin, 2007).

2.1.3.2 Clinical manifestation and diagnosis

Cervical cancer is asymptomatic in its early stage and is most often seen in patients over the age of 30 years. As the cancer progresses some patients may present with non-menstrual vaginal bleeding, post coital bleeding, postmenopausal bleeding, pain during the sexual intercourse or abnormal vaginal discharges. With more advanced stages of the cancer, the presence of back and pelvic pain, bowel and bladder malfunction, lymph nodes enlargement or urinary obstruction may be present. Cervical intraepithelial neoplasia (CIN) also knows as cervical dysplasia, and invasive stage cancer is diagnosed by histological changes, usually based on cytologic examination of the cervical cells. The Pap smear cervical cytology is the established screening test to evaluate for dysplasia or cancer. A single Pap smear has a sensitivity of 50% and a specificity of 81% when compared to a biopsy of the area. Consecutive Pap smears increase the sensitivity to 99%. In situations where the Pap smears suggests an intraepithelial lesion or the presence of carcinoma, a colposcopy and directed biopsy is usually diagnostic. Any suspicious visible lesion in this anatomic area requires a biopsy.

2.1.3.3 Therapy

The management of cervical dysplasia among HIV-infected patients does not differ from the general guidelines used for the general population. Observation without specific intervention is usually recommended for low degree of cervical dysplasia (CIN 1) unless the lesion persists over a period of 18-24 month. If the lesions evolve to a more advanced degree of dysplasia, or if there is poor adherence to routine monitoring, immediate intervention is necessary. Conventional therapies used for treatment of CIN 2 or 3 dysplasia stage include cryotherapy, laser therapy, cone biopsy, and a loop electrosurgical excision procedure (LEEP). In patients with CIN 1 that have not been treated with one of the outlined interventions, Pap smears or colposcopy should be repeated every 4-6 months to monitor for persistence or progression of lesions. Recurrence rates of 40%-60% after therapy has been reported among HIV-1 infected women undergoing these procedures. Very early stage of cervical cancer with a depth of invasion of less than 3 mm can be treated with hysterectomy or cervical conization. Lager tumors require radical hysterectomy with pelvic lymphadenectomy or pelvic radiation therapy. For advanced stages, therapy with radiation or cisplatin-based chemotherapy is indicated in a palliative or neo-adjuvant basis. Since recurrence of CIN and cervical cancer after conventional therapy is increased in the HIV-infected populations, these patients need careful and repeated follow up examinations with frequent cytologic screening and colposcopic examination if necessary.

2.1.3.4 Epidemiology

Cervical carcinoma is the second most common cause of cancer related mortality in the world. The prevalence of this tumor is much higher in countries in which primary and secondary prevention strategies are not fully implemented. It is estimated that over 12,800 new cases are diagnosed annually in the United States with an associated yearly mortality of 4,600 patients. With the introduction of cervical cytologic screening, the incidence of invasive cancer and mortality associated to this condition has decreased dramatically. Nevertheless the incidence of cervical carcinoma in HIV infected women (16 per 100.000 women) continues to be higher than in the general women population (7 per 100,000) in United States for the year 2004. Contrary to the other AIDS defining malignancies; the incidence of cervical cancer incidence has not changed (RR, 0.8: 95%CI (0.5-1.2) with the introduction of HAART (Bedimo et al.,2004). The standardized incidence ratio (SIR) of cervical cancer continues to be significantly higher in HIV infected females when compared to the general female population (Simard et al., 2010; Engels et al., 2008; Patel et al., 2008). The immunosuppressive effects of the HIV appear to have a lesser role in the pathogenesis of this tumor as compared to the oncogenic effects of HPV. The oncogenic effects of HPV are not interrupted with HAART, limiting the impact of antiretroviral therapy on the overall incidence of cervical cancer in this population of patients. Nevertheless continued immunosupression is associated to a more aggressive disease once invasive carcinoma is present.

2.1.3.5 Prevention

Primary and secondary prevention are essential in order to reduce the incidence of invasive cervical carcinoma in HIV infected women. Early detection of dysplastic changes in the cervical cells and the use of the recently available HPV vaccine are preventive methods directed to reduce the incidence of invasive cancer. HIV infected women need to have a Pap smear on initial evaluation and six months after the initial evaluation. If both tests are negative then follow up exams every year is suggested. If there is cervical dysplasia, a history of a cervical lesion or if the patient is positive for HPV, the Pap smear should be repeated every 4 to 6 months. Some Gynecologists advocate the use of HPV DNA assays as a screening modality in HIV infected females to identify women with a higher risk of dysplasia. Other assays to detect the HPV mRNA of E6 or E7 protein are also used with similar reasons. If a Pap smear demonstrates dysplasia or atypia, colposcopic directed biopsy of the cervix is indicated. HPV vaccine is now available for the active immunization against some of the most common HPV oncogenic virus. This vaccine does not immunize against all oncogenic HPV viruses, thus repeated screening through Pap smear continue to be relevant in the immunized patient. HPV vaccine will provide immunization in females prior to the infection, thus the vaccine is recommended prior to sexual activity usually ages of 9 and 26 years. The efficacy of the vaccine in inducing an effective immune response in the HIV infected host is unknown at this time. Educational interventions on cervical cancer along with its relation with HIV and HPV infections need to be reinforced amongst all health workers and patients.

2.2 Non AIDS defining malignancies (HIV-related)

There are several malignancies that are not AIDS defining, which has a higher prevalence amongst HIV infected individuals. These HIV associated malignancies include, Hodgkin's lymphoma, non-small cell lung cancer, head and neck cancer, anal cancer, liver cancer, multiple myeloma, and central nervous system malignances (Engels, et al., 2008; Simard et al, 2010; Nguyen et al,2010). Most of these malignant conditions can be attributed to persistent infection with oncogenic viruses and are not directly associated to the HIV induced immunodeficiency. The enhanced life expectancy of HIV infected patients with the use of HAART has allowed an increased period of vulnerability where the patients can be exposed to oncogenic viruses. An increase in the period of viral latency also accompanies an increase in survival. Nevertheless, the immunological deficiency associated to HIV contributes to the progressive impairment of cellular immunity against oncogenic viruses and virus-infected tumor cells. HIV infection elicits a cytokine deregulation, which disrupts the host capacity to control the reactivation and replication of oncogenic viruses, increasing the risk of malignant transformation.

2.2.1 Hodgkin's lymphoma

Hodgkin lymphoma is one of the most common non-AIDS defining malignancy in HIV positive patients with an incidence which is 18 times more frequent than in the general population. This lymphoma is characterized by the orderly spread of disease from one lymph node group to another and by the present of systemic symptoms. This histology has been associated to intravenous drug use, but the occurrence of this lymphoma is not exclusively restricted to this risk profile. The diagnosis of Hodgkin lymphoma is usually established late in the course of the HIV infection, when patients present a CD4+ T cell count of 300 cells per mm^3 or less.

2.2.1.1 Pathophysiology

The histology presentation of Hodgkin lymphoma among HIV positive patients tends to be more unfavorable as compared to the general population. The mixed cellularity and the lymphocyte-depleted histology subtypes are more frequently found in HIV infected persons when compared to the general population. Contrary, the nodular sclerosis type is less frequent in HIV persons. The general population with Hodgkin lymphoma demonstrates tumor with an extensive infiltrate of T lymphocytes as compared with the HIV patient in which the malignant cellular infiltrate is substantially depleted of T lymphocytes. These variations in histology convey a more aggressive course for the Hodgkin lymphoma in HIV infected patient. Epstein Barr virus (EBV) is associated with Hodgkin lymphoma, and may play an important role in the pathogenesis of this disorder since 80%-90% of patients with HIV related Hodgkin lymphoma have EBV genome integrated within Reed-Sternberg cells (RSC). This proportion is higher than the one detected in the general population. The RSCs are the malignant cells seen in Hodgkin lymphoma and their presence is essential for the diagnosis of this disorder. The survival of the RSC depends on the antiapoptotic nuclear factor (NF) κB pathways. The activation of this pathway relies on the recruitment of inflammatory cells to the tumor mileu, which provide essential signals that stimulates the proliferation and inhibits the apoptosis of the RSC. In advanced AIDS stages, the incidence of Hodgkin lymphoma may decrease due to inability of the tumor mileu to recruit lymphocytes and other inflammatory cells essential for the survival of the RSC. The latent expression of EBV-associated transforming protein on the surface of the RSC may also help the proliferation of malignant cells. This latent protein mimics the activated CD40 receptor and allows the constitutive activation of the NF κB pathways, resulting in inhibition of the RSC apoptosis. Thus EBV can potentially promote oncogenesis independent of the availability of inflammatory and activated CD4 T cells. The nodular sclerosing histology appears to be less associated to EBV infection and is more likely to be seen in patients with a higher CD4 cell count. All patients with Hodgkin lymphoma require complete staging with total body imaging studies and bone marrow examinations (Portlock & Yahalom, 2004; Doweiko, 2007b).

2.2.1.2 Clinical manifestation and diagnosis

The clinical manifestations of Hodgkin lymphoma in HIV infected patients differ from the presentation seen in the general population. HIV associated Hodgkin lymphoma is more aggressive in nature, usually presents in advanced stages of the disease with more than 75% having stage III or IV at diagnosis. Liver and spleen involvement is seen in 65% of patients and bone marrow involvement in 50%. More than 80% of these patients present constitutional symptoms such as unexplained fever, night sweats, or significant weight loss. The overall survival of HIV related Hodgkin lymphoma prior to the introduction of HAART was around 18 months. This high mortality was associated to an increased vulnerability of infections after systemic chemotherapy and the short disease free interval often associated with this cancer. The introduction of HAART has improved the survival of patients with HIV related Hodgkin lymphoma, decreasing the incidence of opportunistic infections, and allowing greater tolerance to the antineoplastic drugs.

2.2.1.3 Therapy

The therapy of Hodgkin lymphoma depends of the stage of disease at initial presentation. The therapy of this lymphoma is multidisciplinary in nature with external beam radiation therapy, chemotherapy or a combination of both. Surgical interventions have a limited role. Radiation therapy or chemotherapy is an effective treatment for stage I and II of the Hodgkin lymphoma. For more advanced stages, the use of combination chemotherapy with the ABVD regimen (adriamycin, bleomycin, vinblastine and dacarbazine) along with involved field radiation in selected patients is recommended. A rate of 80% of complete remission is associated with this regimen.

2.2.1.4 Epidemiology

Hodgkin's lymphoma accounts for less than 1% of all the tumors in the US and is more common in men than in women. There are two incidence peaks between the ages of 15 to 34 and in those over the age of 55 years. Hereditary factors, infection with Epstein-Barr virus, and T-lymphocyte immune dysfunction, are associated with this type of cancer. The risk for Hodgkin's lymphoma is significantly higher in the HIV/AIDS population with a standardized incidence rates between 5.6 and 16.2 in relation to the general population (Grulich et al., 2007). This type of lymphoma has a more aggressive debut in HIV infected persons, than in the general population. When evaluating the effect of antiretroviral therapies in the incidence of Hodgkin's lymphoma a great majority of the studies reported a significant increment of this type of cancer in the HIV population after the availability of HAART (Bedimo et al., 2004). Standardized incidence rates of Hodgkin's lymphoma that in the pre HAART era was around 2.0 increased beyond 6.0 in the HAART era (Simard et al, 2010; Engels et al., 2008).

2.2.1.5 Prevention

There are not specific measures to prevent this type of lymphoma.

2.2.2 Lung cancer

Lung cancer is one of the most frequent tumors seen in the general population and is the leading cause of cancer related mortality in the United States. Around 90% of the genesis of this neoplasm is directly associated to the use of tobacco. Passive smokers have a small but significant risk of developing lung cancer when compared to non-smoking population (Miller, 2004). Other risk factors for lung cancer include a genetic predisposition, exposure to environmental toxins, the presence of chronic pulmonary infections, and the presence of an immunosuppressive state. This later risk factor has been confirmed in the organ transplanted populations of patients, which require prolonged use of immunosuppressant therapy (Grulich et al., 2007). The incidence of lung cancer is increased in HIV infected individuals and is often diagnosed in younger age individuals with a history of smoking. The implementation of HAART has not resulted in a significant change in the lung cancer incidence in these patients (Bonnet & Chene, 2008).

2.2.2.1 Pathophysiology

The majority of malignant tumors of the lung originate from the bronchial epithelium. These bronchogenic carcinomas are histologically divided into small cell lung cancers and non-small cell lung cancers. The non-small cell lung cancers are subdivided into adenocarcinoma, squamous cell carcinoma and large cell carcinoma. The adenocarcinoma is the most frequent histological subtype found in HIV infected patients. The presence of small cell lung cancers tends to be less common in HIV infected persons. The management of small cell lung cancers is generally chemotherapy and for early stages of non-small cell lung cancers, the use of surgery or radiotherapy is usually employed. The process of malignant transformation towards lung cancer is associated to a multistep accumulation of genetic mutations, which regulate growth, and apoptosis of the respiratory epithelium. Premalignant lesions including squamous dysplasia and atypical alveolar hyperplasia have been associated with some chromosomal mutations including chromosomes 3p, 2p, and 9p. Bronchogenic carcinomas have been related to alterations in chromosomes 3p, 5q, 9p, 11p, 13q and 17P. The majority of the genetic alterations in these tumors involve deletions of tumor suppressor genes that are essential for the proliferation of tumor cells. Other than genetic mutations, an increase in cellular proliferation may be the result of autocrine growth through factors that include neuropeptide growth factors, insulin like growth factors, transforming growth factor alpha, stem cell growth factor, and heregulins. The precise mechanisms behind the increased incidence of HIV associated lung cancer remains unknown. Immunological damage induced by the virus, pulmonary epithelium damage induced by recurrent infections, the use of tobacco and other drugs are synergistic factors which could contribute to the development of this cancer in the HIV population.

2.2.2.2 Clinical manifestation and diagnosis

Lung cancer is usually asymptomatic when it is detected in its early stages. It is not unusual to have an abnormal routine chest radiograph as the initial test, which leads to the diagnosis. In late stages the presence of pulmonary related symptoms is common. Common symptoms and findings in these patients include cough, changes in frequency and intensity of a chronic cough, hemoptysis, airways obstruction, chest pain, disnea, postobstructive pneumonia, fever and pleural effusion. Symptoms related to direct organ invasion to the heart, great vessels of the upper mediastinum, brain, bone, adrenal glands and liver may be present (Miller, 2004). In metastatic cancer, cervical and supraclavicular lymphadenopathy may be present. HIV associated lung cancer is usually diagnosed in the late stages and as a consequence is associated to a worse prognosis (James, 2006). A diagnosis of lung cancer can be made by examination of sputum cytology or histological evaluation of tissue biopsy. Positron- emission tomography scanning or contrast nodule enhancement CT is occasionally used as a non-invasive alternative to discriminate between a malignant and a non-malignant pulmonary lesion. This technique is associated to a high number of false negative and false positive results.

2.2.2.3 Therapy

Surgery is the most appropriate treatment in non-small cell lung cancer for patients that have potentially resectable disease. It is imperative that patients in whom a pulmonary resection is being considered, the baseline pulmonary function tests are adequate to tolerate the resection and that the general medical condition is optimal to minimize surgical complications. Immunological status is not a very important prognostic variable to preclude surgical cure for these patients. Radiation therapy is also an effective treatment for the non-small cell lung cancer, especially when combined with chemotherapy. In advanced stages of the disease, palliative chemotherapy in the form of cisplatin, carboplatin, paclitaxel, mitomycin, vinca alkaloids, gemcitabine, vinorelbine, ifosfamide and etoside may be used. The therapeutic interventions available for HIV positive patients are similar to their HIV negative counterparts.

2.2.2.4 Epidemiology

Lung cancer is one of the most frequent tumors in the US and is the leading cause of cancer related mortality. In 2007, the incidence in the United States was of 65.5 per 100,000. Lung cancer is the most frequent non- AIDS defining tumor in the HIV infected patient. The standardized incidence ratio (SIR) of this tumor is higher in the HIV infected population, as compared to the general population (Simard et al., 2010; Engels et al., 2008; Bonnet et al., 2008; Patel et al., 2008). The impact of HAART in modifying the incidence of the HIV associated lung cancer is minimal. Engel et al. has reported that the SIR for the lung cancer before and after HAART therapy remains 2.6 in their study cohort (Engels et al., 2006).

2.2.2.5 Prevention

The predominant intervention, which will reduce the incidence and prevalence of lung cancer in the HIV infected population, is the avoidance or reduction in tobacco exposition. It is highly recommended that non-smokers remain free of tobacco and that smokers reduce or cease tobacco use. This recommendation continues to be relevant even in the group in with a diagnosis of lung cancer has been established. In addition HIV infected persons need remain compliant with their HIV therapy in order to reduce the likelihood of recurrent pneumonia and other respiratory complications associated to HIV.

2.2.3 Hepatocelullar carcinoma

Hepatocellular carcinoma is the most common primary liver cancer, with an estimated incidence of 500,000 worldwide cases per year. It is more common in men and more frequently seen between the ages of 50 and 60 years old. Hepatocellular carcinoma is the third leading cause of cancer mortality worldwide. The incidence rates of this carcinoma in United States have historically been lower as compared to other tumors; nevertheless it has doubled in the past decades. In addition the trends of mortality associated to this tumor have increased at a faster rate than most other tumors of the body. Hepatocellular carcinoma often arises in the setting of a damaged liver, as seen in liver cirrhosis. As a consequence the risk factors for hepatic cirrhosis are also risk factors for this cancer. The most common external agents responsible for hepatic cirrhosis include prolonged abuse of alcohol, and chronic infection with the Hepatitis virus type B (HBV) and C (HCV) virus. The coexistence of HIV and HCV infection has been associated to a synergistic damage to the liver leading to a higher incidence of this liver cancer. The incidence of Hepatocellular carcinoma in HIV infected persons has increased with the introduction of HAART. With the growing armamentarium of anti retroviral interventions available for these patients, the survival and quality of life have markedly improved. This survival improvement has permitted re-exposition or continued expositions to drugs, alcohol, tobacco and viral agents, which will compound the extent of liver tissue damage in this high-risk population.

2.2.3.1 Pathophysiology

Hepatocellular carcinoma is an epithelial tumor that arises from the malignant transformation of the hepatocyte. In the majority of patients the tumor originates in the background of a cirrhotic liver suggesting the need of a damaged liver for the malignant transformation to occur. As a consequence all conditions, which lead to hepatic cirrhosis, increase the risk of this carcinoma. The conditions, which are considered risky factors for hepatic cirrhosis, include chronic HBV or HCV infections, chronic alcohol abuse, hemochromatosis, sialohepatitis, certain congenital hepatic disorders, and exposure to hepatotoxic agents. There are exceptional cases in which Hepatocellular carcinoma develops in the absence of liver damage. The exact mechanism for the genesis of this malignancy is uncertain in many of the scenarios described. In patients with chronic HBV infection, the integration of the HBV DNA into the hepatocyte genome produces a significant disturbance in the host tumor suppressor genes and an activation of oncogenes. This leads to a disruption in the cell's cycle, inhibition of the DNA repair mechanisms, and inhibition of hepatocyte apoptosis. These mechanisms contribute to the malignant transformation and tumor proliferation. In chronic HCV infection, immune mediated inflammation is present which results in inhibition of hepatocyte apoptosis. It has been postulated that the co-existence of HBV, HCV and HIV infection produces a significant increment in the risk in developing Hepatocellular carcinoma. These co-infections have also been associated with a reduction in the therapeutic efficacy for HBV and HCV, resulting in continued active co-infection with an augmentation in the incidence and the progression of this neoplasm (Fallon et al., 2006; McDonald et al., 2008).

2.2.3.2 Clinical manifestation and diagnosis

Hepatocelullar carcinoma usually presents with pain in the right upper quadrant of the abdomen, jaundice and hepatomegaly. Constitutional symptoms may include, fever, early satiety, lost of weight and anorexia. Occasionally some patients may present with hepatic function decompensation causing ascites, lower extremity edema, esophageal varices bleeding, acute portal hypertension, and encephalopathy. Laboratory findings related to liver failure may be present including elevated levels of alkaline phosphatase, total bilirubin, ALT or AST. The presences of an elevated α-Fetoprotein or des-gamma carboxyprothrombin are markers for the presence of the liver carcimoma and may be used as measures of tumor growth. Ultra sound (US), three-phase tomography (CT) or magnetic resonance imaging (MRI) is the imaging techniques that suggest the presence of this neoplasm. Histological evaluation of the hepatic mass is often used to confirm the diagnosis. Current guidelines suggest that in the presence of an elevated level of α-Fetorprotein and the presence of a hepatic mass in the context of a cirrhotic liver, a confirmatory biopsy is not necessary. Tissue confirmation is recommended for cases without elevated level of α-Fetorprotein or if the diagnosis remains uncertain (Fallon et al., 2006; McDonald et al., 2008).

2.2.3.3 Therapy

The prognosis of the Hepatocelullar carcinoma is variable and it largely depends whether complete surgical resection of the tumor is possible. Effective surgical interventions are compromised when the primary tumor is large, if there is vascular involvement, if the tumor infiltrates both hepatic lobes, and if there is evidence of metastatic disease. In addition, poor residual hepatic function may prevent hepatic resection. It is estimated that less than 15% of the patients with this cancer are surgical candidates and of these 60% have a tumor recurrence. Additional therapeutic interventions, which may be appropriate, include liver transplantation, hepatic chemoembolization, intratumoral injection of ethanol, and radiofrequency ablation. Hepatic transplantation is performed in patients with Hepatocelullar carcinoma without metastasis, which fulfills the Milan criteria. Systemic therapy with one of the tyrosine kinase receptor inhibitors such as sorafenid or sunitinib may be used. These therapies are not considered curative in nature but will increase survival (Fallon et al., 2006; McDonald et al., 2008).

2.2.3.4 Epidemiology

Hepatocelullar carcinoma is the fourth more common malignant tumor in men and the sixth most common in females in the United States. It is the third leading cause of cancer mortality worldwide. The incidence of Hepatocelullar carcinoma in HIV infected patients is higher than in the general population in great measure related to the common transmission related practices shared between HIV with HBV and HCV. Co-infected patients have been reported to present with more advanced Hepatocelullar carcinoma, and have a higher mortality as compared with patients who are HIV negative. The introduction of HAART has improved the life expectancy among HIV positive individuals but has allowed a greater risk for exposure to additional agents with oncogenic potential. In the HIV/AIDS Cancer Match Study of Simard and collaborators an increment in incidence of Hepatocelullar carcinoma of 90% (RR, 1.9: 95% CI, 0.9%-3.92%) was seen when comparing the pre HAART with the post HAART era (Simard et al., 2010). Other studies have confirmed this evolving increasing trend in the incidence and prevalence of this malignancy across time in different populations (Engels et al., 2008; Mayor et al., 2008b). Furthermore, the standardized incidence ratio (SIR) of Hepatocelullar carcinoma is significantly higher in the HIV infected patient as compared to the general population (Simard et al., 2010).

2.2.3.5 Prevention

The pathogenesis of Hepatocelullar carcinoma is intimately associated to alcohol abuse and chronic infection with HBV and HCV. Primary, secondary and tertiary preventive measures that reduce the risk for exposure to these agents or viruses will directly and indirectly reduce the incidence of this cancer. This is particularly true in the higher risk groups such as those with HIV infection. It has been shown that patients with HIV infection have high-risk practices that predispose them to co-infection with hepatitis A (HAV), HBV, and HCV. In addition alcohol abuse continues to be common practice in these patients. HAV infection carries a predominant fecal-oral viral transmission route that involucrate more commonly men who have sex with men and injecting drug users; HBV infection is predominantly transmitted by percutaneous or mucous contact with infected blood or body fluids including semen and saliva. HIV associated risk groups such as men who have sex with men, high risk heterosexual contact, or injecting drug use are the predominant group with this risk factor. Lastly, HCV infection is transmitted principally by percutaneous contact with infected blood, and this is a relevant issue in HIV patients who are injecting drug use (Samet, 2007) or who received transfusions of unscreened blood. Most patients with acute HBV or HCV infection are asymptomatic and early diagnosis rarely occurs. Approximately 4 % of the HBV mono-infected persons and 20% co-infected with HIV will develop chronic liver disease. Over 80% of HCV infected individuals will eventually develop chronic hepatic disease. In the majority of patients with either infection, the process will remain asymptomatic and undetected many years prior to the onset of liver damage and the development of cancer. All patients infected with HIV should undergo screening testing for HAV, HBV and HCV. In patients who are positive for the HCV serology and in those with unexplained liver disease determination of HCV virus load is suggested. Repeated testing after 4 months of follow up may be required in some cases if the infection was recently adquired. If high risk behaviors persist after an initial negative screening test, repeat testing on an annual basis is recommended. There is no HCV vaccine available. In patients where HBV infection is suspected, determination for the presence of the multiple viral components and antibodies in the serum is recommended. If the surface antigen (HBsAg) and the surface antibody (HBsAb) are negative, then vaccination against the HBV is suggested. This is particularly relevant for the HIV infected individual since the risk for HBV is high in this group. In individuals with detectable HBsAg, detectable HBsAb, or with elevated serum liver enzymes levels, the determination of the HBV viral load needs to be done. Chronic inactive viral infection is determined when the antibodies are positive and the viral load is negative. Both HCV and HBV require opportune therapy in order to minimize the extent of liver damage. HCV chronic infection is treated principally by the combination of peg interferon alpha and Ribavirin. Chronic HBV infection is treated with antiviral agents such as Lamivudine (3TC), Ettricitabine (FTC), Adefovir or Tenofovir. HIV co-infected persons on ART need to be monitored with liver function tests, since concomitant ART could cause liver damage and be responsible for metabolic disorders when used in combination with other medications.

Counseling and educational interventions directed to reduce the risk behavior associated to HBV, HCV and HIV transmission play an important role in Hepatocelullar carcinoma prevention (Center for Disease Control, 2001). One example of an intervention used in our cohort was a multimedia educational intervention, which was validated in Hispanic HIV injecting drug users in Puerto Rico (Mayor el al., 2010). This intervention motivated the participant to abolish their risky behaviors practices when injecting drugs. The Health Belief Model and Social Cognitive Theory were used as theoretical framework to modify the decision making process that led to the avoidance, or reduction of the risk factors relevant for acquiring new HCV infection (Mayor et al., 2008a). We are planning to extend this intervention to patients who are at an early stage of drug addiction in order to capture a larger cohort of patients who have not been infected with HBV or HCV. Counseling and educational interventions regarding alcohol use and abuse is an important approach particularly in the HIV infected person who has a high prevalence of both drug and alcohol use and abuse.

2.2.4 Squamous cell cancer of the anus

Squamous cell carcinoma of the anus is a tumor that originates from the epidermal cells of the hair bearing perianal skin. This tumor may develop outside and beyond the anal verge. The tumor is responsible for 3% of the malignancies of the lower gastrointestinal tract. It is intimately associated to infections with one of the carcinogenic types of HPV. The majority of patients with this tumor had anal intercourse as HIV risk factors, especially in the MSM group (Davis, 2008; Doweiko, 2007a; National Institute of Health, 2011).

2.2.4.1 Pathophysiology

Quite similar in pathogenesis to uterine cervix neoplasias, HPV infection has an important role in the genesis of the anal dysplasia or anal intraepithelial neoplasia (AIN) and its progression to squamous cell cancer. HPV is the most common sexually transmitted infection in the United Sates. The incidence of HPV infection is high and there is evidence of an increasing prevalence of infection in the HIV infected group of patients. HIV associated risk factor of MSM is associated to a high prevalence of anal HPV infection and at higher risk of developing anal cancer. The degree of anal dysplasia is inversely correlated with $CD4^{+}$ T lymphocyte count, suggesting an important role of the immune system in controlling the impact of HPV infection. With improvement in survival associated to HAART, the latency period for HPV infection has also increased, incrementing the risk of malignant transformation of the dysplastic tissue. Anal squamous cell cancer has a more aggressive presentation and clinical course in HIV infected persons when compared to HIV negative individuals. Other risk factors for the development of anal dysplasia include, heavy cigarette smoking, anal intercourse, and a greater number of lifetime sexual partners. These factors have all been associated to the increasing incidence of the anal cancer in men and in women across the world (Daling et al., 2004).

2.2.4.2 Clinical manifestations and diagnosis

Dysplasia of the squamous epithelium of the anus is a silent condition that becomes symptomatic as it evolves to the malignant stage. Anal carcinoma can induce changes in the intestinal habits, rectal bleeding, rectal itching, rectal irritation or the presence of lumps in the anal area. Low back pain and vaginal symptoms could be also part of the symptoms associated to these processes. In advanced stages the malignant process could ulcerate and infiltrate the anal sphincter muscle, incrementing the magnitude of the symptoms. A disruption of the integrity of the anal mucosa seen in these tumors may predispose to the development of infections in this area. The presence of anal dysplasia and invasive carcinoma require pathologic confirmation. The anal Pap smear is a screening test to evaluate cytologic changes in the anal epithelium in high-risk persons. High-resolution anoscopy (HRA) should be considered if the anal Pap smear shows atypical cytology and should be performed in patients who have low or high grade squamous intraepithelial lesions. Visible lesions should be biopsied to determine the magnitude of the histological changes and to rule out invasive cancer.

2.2.4.3 Therapy

Localized dysplasia requires clinical follow-up with anoscopy and colposcopic biopsy every 4 to 6 months. Lesions can be removed with photocoagulation. Frank carcinoma should be managed with surgical excision or a combination of chemotherapy with concomitant radiotherapy. Chemotherapy with 5-fluorouracil, mitomycin-C, platinum and other analogues has been used with success, particularly for early stage tumors. This modality will preserve anal sphincter function in the majority of patients. More advanced tumors will require an abdomino/perineal tumor resection with the placement of a permanent colostomy.

2.2.4.4 Epidemiology

Prior to the HIV epidemic, the presence of carcinoma of the anus was seen in the older patient, particularly women. With the onset of HIV infection in the community, anal carcinoma is detected in younger patients, and very often associated to HPV infection. Anogenital dysplasia and anal carcinoma are more frequently associated with HPV types 16, 18, 31, 33 and 35. Similar to other tumors influenced by external agents such as viruses, the incidence of anal carcinoma has increased significantly in the HAART era (Simard et al.,

2010; Engels et al., 2008; Long et al., 2008). Simard and coauthors in their United States HIV/AIDS Cancer Matched Study reported a 190% increment in the incidence of anal carcinoma (RR, 2.9: 95% CI, 2.1%-4.0%) in the HAART era when compared to pre HAART era. HAART associated increments in the survival of HIV infected patients will also prolong the HPV carcinogenic effects over the anal epithelium leading to an increased incidence of malignant transformation.

2.2.4.5 Prevention

Although formal guidelines recommending anal Pap smear screening have not been adopted, it is clear that anal cytologic screening for HIV-infected men and women at risk of HPV infection or with anogenital warts is warranted. Follow up exams are mandatory for patients with anal dysplasia, or history of anal cancer. Risk reduction education and intervention in sexual and smoking behaviors could have an indirect effect in the prevention of the anal cancer.

2.2.5 Oral cavity/pharynx cancer

The malignant processes of the cavities of the head and neck have different histological types. In this discussion we are reviewing the data associated to squamous cell carcinoma of the oropharyngeal tract. Other important histologies cancers of the oral cavity and pharynx, such as lymphomas, sarcomas, thyroid tumors and benign tumors are not addressed in this section. The squamous cell carcinomas, which originate in the oral cavity, oropharynx, hypopharynx, and larynx are strongly associated to the use of tobacco. The tobacco may be inhaled in several forms such as cigarettes or cigars, or it may be smokeless such as chewing tobacco or snuff. Tumors localized in the oropharynx may also be vinculated to infection with HPV (Posner, 2004). As anticipated the incidence of oropharyngeal cancer is higher in the HIV infected patient as compared to the general population and the incidence of this tumor is higher in the post HAART era.

2.2.5.1 Pathophysiology

Tobacco use in any form, alcohol consumption, HPV infection, a weakened immune system, micronutrient deficiencies, and poor oral hygiene have all been implicated in the pathogenesis of head and neck neoplasms (Kreimer et al.,2004; Marur et al., 2010; Posner, 2004, National Institute of Health, 2005). Smoking produces a direct exposure of the oral and pharynx mucosa to nicotine and other carcinogenic components of the tobacco, which increase the risk of squamous cell proliferation. Frequent and heavy consumption of alcohol produces local and systemic carcinogenic effect over the mucosa. It is well established the synergism associated between the use of alcohol and tobacco abuse and the risk of head and neck tumors. Infection with HPV types 16 has also been implicated in oropharyngeal tumors. The exact mechanism of HPV associated tumor transformation is unclear. It is postulated that HPV induces the inactivation of tumor suppressor proteins or genes, which promote cell immortality and dedifferentiation. HPV infection is very common and widespread in HIV infected patients. Damage of the HIV individuals' immune integrity may enhance the tissue susceptibility induced by HPV.

2.2.5.2 Clinical manifestations and diagnosis

The clinical manifestation are varied and related to the location and stage of the tumor. Lumps, masses, ulcers may be present in the oral cavity. Problems with swallowing, bleeding or pain may be some of the symptoms. There may be restrictions in the movement of the tongue, or difficulty swallowing certain products. Other manifestations my include, loose tooth, pain in the different bone structures of the face, difficulties with visual acuity, hoarseness, and lymph node enlargement. A diagnosis should be suspected on the basis of the clinical manifestations, physical examination of the head and neck region, endoscopy, computer tomography (CT) scan, magnetic resonance imaging (MRI), positron-emission tomography (PET). Histological confirmation with a needle aspiration and biopsy or excisional biopsy needs to be done. Complete staging of the tumor should follow a histological diagnosis (Posner, 2004).

2.2.5.3 Therapy

The management of these cancers is varied and may include surgery, radiotherapy, chemotherapy, neoadjuvant-chemotherapy, chemo-radiotherapy, and combination-modality interventions. Nutritional support to prevent significant weight loss is important. Associated morbidities such as lung, heart or liver dysfunction need to be identified in order to modify the cancer therapy to be instituted. Speech rehabilitation is occasionally required. Lifelong follow-up is suggested.

2.2.5.4 Epidemiology

Head and neck cancers account for 3 to 5% of all the tumors diagnosed in the United States. It is the sixth most common cancer worldwide. About 40,000 new cases are detected annually. The majority (95%) are squamous cell carcinomas with the oropharynx representing the most common anatomic site (Posner, 2004). These cancers are three times more common in men with a peak incidence over the age of 50 years of age. Approximately 13,000 deaths are attributable each year to these cancers. The patient with HIV infection is at a higher risk for oropharyngeal cancer with a SIR between 2.1 and 5.6 (Grulich et al., 2007; Patel et al., 2008). As with the other HPV related cancers, the impact of HAART in the natural history of these tumors remains unclear. Engels and co-authors have reported a decline in the rates of HIV associated oropharyngeal cancer with the introduction of HAART showing a reduction of the standardized incidence ratio (SIR) from 2.5 to 1.5. Nevertheless the risk of HIV associated head and neck cancer is higher as compared to the general population (Simard et al., 2010; Engels et al., 2008).

2.2.5.5 Prevention

There is no approved test for the early detection of oral cavity/pharynx cancers. Consequently the prevention of these tumors rests on improving the risky behavior patterns of patients. Smoking and alcohol abuse avoidance and cessation are the most important prevention measure for this type of cancer. Up today there is not an effective prevention protocol for HPV in relation to oropharynx cancer. Having a faithful relation with one person, limiting the number of sex partners, having a partner who did not have o had few sex partners, could limit the probability of HPV infection, but not eliminate it.

3. Conclusion

The use of HAART for patients with HIV infection has led to a partial restoration of the immune system prolonging the survival of these patients. The success of this therapy has dramatically altered the natural history and clinical course of infection. HIV/AIDS has become a chronic disease with the co-existence of co-morbid conditions, which have an important effect on the health of these patients. An increased likelihood of exposure to cancer promoters such as oncogenic viruses, increments in the exposure to tobacco and alcohol and continued risky practices have had a major role in the increased risk of developing malignant conditions in these patients. The incidence of most of the AIDS defining malignancies have decreased in large part due to immune restoration present in many patients. However, the incidence of other tumors such as uterine cervical cancers, Hodgkin's lymphoma, certain non-Hodgkins lymphomas, HPV related cancers, lung cancer, and liver cancer have all seen an increase in the HAART era. The synergistic effects of tobacco use, alcohol use, dietary elements and viral co-infections are having an effect in the malignant transformation of tissues in the HIV infected patient. Consequently, an appropriate and opportune management of the HIV infection needs to be supplemented with cancer preventive strategies in this high-risk group of patients. Implementation of recommended cancer screening techniques, educational intervention, and relevant vaccination in the HIV infected populations should decreased the morbidity and mortality rate of HIV associated malignancies. Furthermore, adequate and opportune cancer prevention efforts would be cost effective in the management of this high risk population. Researches into the barriers present, which are obstacles to the implementation of these important prevention techniques, are very relevant and require further evaluation.

4. Acknowledgement

This publication was made possible by the RCMI-NIH Grant number G12RR03035 from the National Center for Research Resources and the NIH Grant number U45RR026139. We would like to thank Christine Miranda for her help in the chapter preparation.

5. References

Bedimo, R., Chen, R. Y., Accortt, N. A., Raper, J. L., Linn, C., Allison, J. J., Dubay, J., Saag, M. S., & Hoesley, C. J. (2004). Trends in AIDS-defining and non-AIDS-defining malignancies among HIV-infected patients: 1982-2002. *Clinical Infectious Diseases,* Vol. 39, No. 1, (November 2004), pp. (1380-1384), ISSN 1058-4838

Bellan, C., De Falco, G., Lazzi, S., & Leoncini L. (2003) Pathologic aspects of AIDS malignancies. Oncogene, Vol.22, No 42, (September 2003), pp. (6639-6645), ISSN 0950-9232

Berretta, M., Cinelli, R., Martellotta, F., Spina, M., Vaccher, E., & Tirelli, U. (2003). Therapies approaches to AIDS-Related malignancies. *Oncogene,* Vol. 22, No 42, (September 2003), pp. (6646-6659), ISSN 0950-9232

Bierman, P. J., Lee Harris, N., & Armitage, J. O. (2004). Non-Hodgkin's lymphomas, In: *Cecil Textbook of Medicine,* Lee Goldman & Dennis Ausiello, pp. (1174-1183), Saunders, ISBN 978-0721696522, United States

Bonnet, F., & Chêne, G. (2008). Evolving epidemiology of malignancies in HIV. *Current Opinion in Oncology,* Vol. 20, No. 1, (September 2008), pp. (534-540), ISSN 1040-8746

Bower, M., Palmieri, C., & Dhillon, T. (2006). AIDS-related malignancies: changing epidemiology and the impact of highly active antiretroviral therapy. *Current Opinion in Infectious Diseases,* Vol. 19, No. 1, (February 2006), pp. (14-19), ISSN 0951-7375

Cáceres, W., Cruz-Amy, M., & Díaz-Meléndez, V. (2010). AIDS-related malignancies: revisited. *Puerto Rico Health Sciences Journal*, Vol. 29, No. 1, (March 2010), pp. (70-75), ISSN 0738-0658

Centers for Disease Control and Prevention (2001). A comprehensive strategy for the prevention and control of Hepatitis C virus infection and its consequences, In: *Centers for Disease Control and Prevention*, June 22, 2011, Available from: http://www.cdc.gov/hepatitis/HCV/Strategy/NatHepCPrevStrategy.htm

Crum-Clanflone, N., Huppler Hullsiek, K., Marconi, V., Weintrob, A., Ganesan, A., Vincent Barthel, R., Fraser, S., Agan, B. K., & Wegner, S. (2009). Trends in the incidence of cancers among HIV-infected persons and the impact of antiretroviral therapy: a 20-year cohort study. *AIDS*, Vol. 23, No. 1, (January 2009), pp. (41-50), ISSN 0269-9370

Daling, J.R., Madeleine, M.M., Johnson, L.G., Schwartz, S.M., Shera, K.A., Wurscher,M.A., Carter, J.J., Porter, P.J., Gallowway, D.A., & McDougall, J.K. (2004). Human papillomavirus, smoking, and sexual practices in the etiology of anal cancer. *Cancer*, Vol. 101, No. 2, (June 2004), pp. (270-280), ISSN 1097-0142

Davis, B. (2007). Men who have sex with men, In: *HIV*, Howard Libman & Harvey J. Makadon, pp. (304-308), American College of Physicians, ISBN 978-1930513730, United States

Dezube, B. J. (2007). Kaposi's sarcoma, In: *HIV*, Howard Libman & Harvey J. Makadon, pp. (271-281), American College of Physicians, ISBN 978-1930513730, United States

Doweiko, J. P. (2007). Anogenital squamous cell cancer, In: *HIV*, Howard Libman & Harvey J. Makadon, pp. (292-294), American College of Physicians, ISBN 978-1930513730, United States

Doweiko, J. P. (2007). HIV-related lymphomas, In: *HIV*, Howard Libman & Harvey J. Makadon, pp. (282-291), American College of Physicians, ISBN 978-1930513730, United States

Engels, E. A., Biggar, R. J., Irene Hall, H., Cross, H., Crutchfield, A., Finch, J. L., Grigg, R., Hylton, T., Pawlish, K. S., McNeel, T. S., & Goedert, J. J. (2008). Cancer risk in people infected with human immunodeficiency virus in the United States. *International Journal of Cancer*, Vol. 123, No. 1, (April 2008), pp. (187-194), ISSN 1097-0215

Engels, E. A., Brock, M. V., Chen, J., Hooker, C. M., Gillison, M., & Moore, R. D. (2006). Elevated incidence of lung cancer among HIV-infected individuals. *Journal of Clinical Oncology*, Vol. 24, No. 9, (March 2006), pp. (1383-1388), ISSN 0732-183X

Fallon, M. (2004). Hepatic tumors, In: *Cecil Textbook of Medicine*, Lee Goldman & Dennis Ausiello, pp. (1222-1225), Saunders, ISBN 978-0721696522, United States

Grulich, A. E., Li, Y., McDonald, A., Correll, P. K. L., Law, M. G., & Kaldor, J. M. (2002). Rates of non-AIDS-defining cancers in people with HIV infection before and after AIDS diagnosis. *AIDS*, Vol. 16, No. 1, (January 2002), pp. (1155-1161), ISSN 0269-9370

Grulich, A. E., van Leeuwen, M. T., Falster, M. O., & Vajdic, C. M. (2007). Incidence of cancers in people with HIV/AIDS compared with immunosuppressed transplant recipients: a meta-analysis. *The Lancet*, Vol. 370, No. 1, (July 2007), pp. (59-67), ISSN 0140-6736

James J. S. (2006). Lung cancer: very high death rate with HIV, huge reduction possible with CT screening for early diagnosis, In: *AIDS Treatment News*, June 22, 2011, Available from: http://www.aidsnews.org/2006/12/lung-cancer.html

Kreimer, A. R., Alberg, A. J., Daniel, R., Gravitt, P. E., Viscidi, R., Garrett, E. S., Shah, K. V., & Gillison, M. L. (2004). Oral human papillomavirus infection in adults is associated with sexual behavior and HIV serostatus. *The Journal of Infectious Diseases*, Vol. 189, No. 4, (February 2004), pp. (686-698), ISSN 0022-1899

Long, J.L., Engels, E.A., Moore, R.D, & Gebo, K.A. (2008). Incidence and outcome of malignancy in the HAART era in an urban cohort of HIV-infected individuals. *AIDS*, Vol. 22, No. 4, (February 2008), pp. (489-496), ISSN 0269-9670

Marur, S., D'Souza, G. D., Westra, W. H., & Forastiere, A. A. (2010). HPV-associated head and neck cancer: a virus-related cancer epidemic. *The Lancet Oncology*, Vol. 11, No. 8, (May 2010), pp. (781-789), ISSN 1470-2045

Mayor, A. M., Fernández, D.M., Colón, H. M., Thomas, J.C., & Hunter-Mellado, R. F. (2010). The effectiveness evaluation of a multimedia Hepatitis C prevention program for HIV infected individuals. *Ethnicity and Disease*, Vol. 20, No. 1, (December 2010), pp. (158-162), ISSN 1049-510X

Mayor, A. M., Fernández, D.M., Colón, H. M., Thomas, J.C., & Hunter-Mellado, R. F. (2008). Feasibility and acceptability of a multimedia Hepatitis C prevention program for Hispanic HIV infected persons. *Ethnicity and Disease*, Vol. 18, No. 2, (April 2008), pp. (195-199), ISSN 1049-510X

Mayor, A. M., Gómez, M. A. Rios-Olivares, E., & Hunter-Mellado, R. F. (2008). AIDS-defining neoplasm prevalence in a cohort of HIV-infected patients before and after highly active antiretroviral therapy. *Ethnicity and Disease*, Vol. 18, No. 2, (April 2008), pp. (189-194), ISSN 1049-510X

McDonald, D. C., Nelson, M., Bower, M., & Powles, T. (2008). Hepatocellular carcinoma, human immunodeficiency virus and viral hepatitis in the HAART era. *World Journal Gastroenterology*, Vol. 14, No. 11, (March 2008), pp. (1657–1663), ISSN 1007-9327

Miller, Y. E. (2004). Lung cancer and other pulmonary neoplasms, In: *Cecil Textbook of Medicine*, Lee Goldman & Dennis Ausiello, pp. (1201-1207), Saunders, ISBN 978-0721696522, United States

Mitsuyasy, R. T., Reddy, & D., Copper. J. S. (2011). AIDS-Related malignancies, In: *Cancernetwork*, March 25, 2011, Available from: http://www.cancernetwork.com/display/article/10165/1802726

Molpus, K. L., & Jones, H. W. (2004). Gynecologic cancer, In: *Cecil Textbook of Medicine*, Lee Goldman & Dennis Ausiello, pp. (1238-1241), Saunders, ISBN 978-0721696522, United States

National Institutes of Health. (2005). Head and neck cancer: questions and answers, In: *National Cancer Institute*, June 26, 2011, Available from: http://www.cancer.gov/cancertopics/factsheet/Sites-Types/head-and-neck

National Institutes of Health. (n.d.). Anal cancer, In: *National Cancer Institute*, June 22, 2011, Available from: http://www.cancer.gov/cancertopics/types/anal

Newcomb-Fernandez, J. (2003). Cancer in the HIV-infected population, In: *The Body*, June 22, 2011, Available from: http://www.thebody.com/content/art16834.html

Nguyen, M. L., Farrell, K. J., & Gunthel C. J. (2010). Non-AIDS-Defining malignancies in patients with HIV in the HAART era. Current Infectious Disease Reports, Vol.12 (January 2010), pp. (46-55) ISSN 1523-3847

Patel, P., Hanson, D. L., Sullivan, P. S., Novak, R. M., Moorman, A. C., Tong, T. C., Holmberg, S. D., & Brooks, J. T. (2008). Incidence of types of cancers among HIV-infected persons compared with the general population in the United States, 1992-2003. *Annals of Internal Medicine,* Vol. 148, No. 10, (May 2008), pp. (728-736), ISSN 1539-3704

Portlock, C. S., & Yahalom, J. (2004). Hodgkin's disease, In: *Cecil Textbook of Medicine,* Lee Goldman & Dennis Ausiello, pp. (1166-1173), Saunders, ISBN 978-0721696522, United States

Posner, M. (2004). Head and neck cancer, In: *Cecil Textbook of Medicine,* Lee Goldman & Dennis Ausiello, pp. (1195-1200), Saunders, ISBN 978-0721696522, United States

Powrie, R. O., & Cu-Uvin, S. (2007). Women, In: *HIV,* Howard Libman & Harvey J. Makadon, pp. (295-303), American College of Physicians, ISBN 978-1930513730, United States

Samet, J. H. (2007). Injection-drug users, In: *HIV,* Howard Libman & Harvey J. Makadon, pp. (317-324), American College of Physicians, ISBN 978-1930513730, United States

Simard, E. P., Pfeiffer, R. M., & Engels, E. A. (2010). Spectrum of cancer risk late after AIDS onset in the United States. *Archives of Internal Medicine,* Vol. 170, No. 15, (August 2010), pp. (1337-1345), ISSN 0003-9926

22

E-Health 2.0 Developments in Treatment and Research in Multiple Sclerosis

Peter Joseph Jongen
The MS4 Research Institute (MS4RI)
The Netherlands

1. Introduction

The treatment of multiple sclerosis (MS) is entering a new era, characterized by the availability of a broad range of disease modifying drugs (DMDs) for patients in the relapsing-remitting (RR) phase of the disease. Through interference with immune-mediated inflammatory processes the DMDs reduce the number and severity of relapses and the increase in relapse-related disability. Each DMD is characterized by a unique combination of mode of action, route of administration, degree of efficacy and potential side effects. In the past two decades the injectable drugs interferon beta-1a (INFb-1a), INFb-1b and glatiramer acetate (GA) have been proven to be safe first-line treatments. In more recent years, the intravenously administered monoclonal antibody natalizumab and the oral drugs fingolimod and cladribine have been demonstrated to be efficacious in RRMS. These DMDs are more potent, but also potentially more hazardous, which by and large restricts their use to patients who have very active disease or are refractory to first-line treatment. Lately, phase II/III studies showed beneficial effects of the oral drugs teriflunomide, laquinimod and BG-12, and the monoclonal antibodies rituximab and alemtuzumab in RRMS.

The advent of the new treatments coincides with the Web 2.0 evolution of the internet technology. Web 2.0 offers patients, doctors, and nurses unforeseen possibilities to fundamentally change, and hopefully improve, the ways in which care is delivered and clinical, patient-centered research is performed. The term Web 2.0 is associated with web applications that facilitate participatory information sharing, inter-operability, user-centered design and collaboration on the World Wide Web [1]. A Web 2.0 site allows users to interact and collaborate with each other, e.g. as creators of user-generated content in a virtual community, in contrast to websites where users are limited to the passive viewing of content that was created for them [2].

Basically, e-health 2.0 can be defined as the merging of the Web 2.0 phenomenon within health care [3]. However, e-health 2.0 goes beyond the social networking technology to include a reformative or even revolutionary change in the fields of health care and clinical research [3]. According to O'Grady the main point of e-health 2.0 is the use of social software and its ability to promote collaboration between patients, their caregivers, and medical professionals [3]. Thus, using the web to exchange information with others substantially relates to learning and education about an illness, what treatment options are available, how to make decisions, and for support [3]. In a broad sense, it can be conceived that Web 2.0 technologies enable and facilitate social networking, participation, openness, and collaboration, within and between health care consumers, caregivers, patients, health professionals, and biomedical researchers [4].

This chapter highlights actual developments at the crossroads of MS treatment and research and interactive applications of the internet, thereby focusing on online self-assessment, interactive web-based care and interactive phase IV research, and their potential for patient empowerment.

2. Multiple sclerosis

2.1 Disease characteristics

MS is a chronic disease of the central nervous system (CNS) that is pathologically characterized by multiple areas of inflammation, demyelination, axonal loss and gliosis, predominantly but not exclusively in the white matter. Compared to other chronic CNS disorders MS is distinguished by a wide range of symptoms and a highly variable course. Typical clinical features are optic neuritis, paresis, diplopia, paresthesias, incoordination, bladder and bowel disturbances, cognitive dysfunction, anxiety, depression and fatigue [5].

In most patients the onset of disease is between 20 and 40 years of age. In 80% to 85% of the patients the initial phase is characterized by relapses and remissions: RRMS. Relapse / remission episodes are alternated by relatively stable periods of months to years. During a relapse symptoms typically evolve over days to weeks, and after a plateau phase often spontaneously improve, completely or incompletely. The total duration of a relapse / remission episode, from initial symptom to final recovery, varies from less than a week to more than half a year.

To explain the etiology of MS it is thought that myelin-specific auto-reactive lymphocytes are primed in the periphery by unknown factors, after which they migrate to the CNS, leading to inflammatory demyelination and axonal loss [6]. Recent studies have suggested that the innate immune system also plays a role both in the initiation and progression of MS [6]. Inflammation composed of mononuclear cells, breakdown of the blood brain barrier, focal plaques of demyelination and axonal damage characterize the acute MS lesions and underlie relapses [7]. Importantly, the frequency and severity of the immune-mediated changes can be reduced by DMDs.

As the disease duration increases the tendency of relapses to recover diminishes, which results in a higher risk of relapse-related deficits and a step-wise accrual of disability. Eventually, after a period of 10 to 20 years, most RRMS patients transgress to the secondary progressive phase (SPMS), characterized by a relentless continuous progression of disability. In about 15% of the MS patients symptoms start insidiously and continue to slowly progress without relapses, the primary progressive course (PPMS). In both SPMS and PPMS clinical deficits mainly result from axonal degeneration, whereas inflammation plays only a minor role. Accordingly, DMDs are not efficacious in SPMS and PPMS.

2.2 Diagnosis

In the last two decades the sensitivity and specificity of the MS diagnosis has considerably improved due to two developments. Firstly, the wide-spread use of the magnetic resonance imaging (MRI) technique for detection of lesions in brain and spinal cord, and secondly, new diagnostic criteria proposed by McDonald et al.. The improved diagnosis in combination with the availability of DMDs has increased doctors' awareness of MS as a possible cause of an episode of CNS disturbances in young adults. In such patients ancillary MRI and cerebrospinal fluid (CSF) analyses may yield abnormal findings that, in combination with the clinical features, justify the diagnosis possible or definite RRMS according to the revised McDonald criteria [8]. Patients who do not fulfill these criteria and in whom other disorders have been adequately excluded are diagnosed as having a so-called clinically isolated syndrome (CIS) suggestive of MS, briefly CIS [8]. A CIS may be monofocal - when clinical abnormalities relate to a single CNS lesion - or multifocal, and often involve the optic nerve, brainstem, cerebellum, spinal cord, or cerebral hemispheres [8].

On T2-weighed brain MRI the great majority of MS patients show multiple hyper-intense lesions. These are typically ovoid shaped with the longitudinal axis perpendicular to the ventricles, of varying hyper-intensity, and located peri-ventricular, juxta-cortical or infra-tentorial in an asymmetric bilateral pattern [8]. In most MS patients MRI of the spinal cord also shows T2 hyper-intense abnormalities, and the absence of spinal lesions on a technically adequate MRI scan is considered a red flag.

2.3 Assessment and treatment of major symptoms

Fatigue

Fatigue is reported by over 80% of MS patients [9] and often interferes with family life, work or social activities [10]. It is a major determinant of impaired health-related quality of life (HRQoL) in MS [11]. Psychometrically validated questionnaires for measuring MS-related fatigue are the Fatigue Impact Scale (FIS), the Modified Fatigue Impact Scale (MFIS), and the Fatigue Severity Scale (FSS). Treatment options include a management program for a more efficient use of energy, progressive resistance training, cognitive behavioral therapy, and pharmacotherapy. Drugs that are believed to potentially improve MS-related fatigue are amantadine, 4-aminopyridine, 3,4-diaminopyridine, and modafinil. When 6 to 8 weeks after start of a drug treatment the patient has not experienced a relevant decrease in fatigue, the treatment is discontinued and a different drug is considered.

Bladder dysfunction

Symptoms of bladder dysfunction are uncommon at presentation but frequently develop in the course of the disease, and are often associated with spastic paraparesis and sexual problems [5]. The increased urge and voiding frequency result from detrusor muscle over-activity and detrusor-sphincter dyssynergia. Urinary tract infections, resulting from incomplete bladder emptying, are a frequent complication and may lead to worsening of MS symptoms. A 3-day Voiding Diary, the Urinary Distress Inventory (UDI-6) and the Incontinence Impact Questionnaire (IIQ-7) are validated tools to comprehensively assess bladder dysfunction in MS. Pharmacotherapeutic options include anticholinergics, cannabinoids and botulinum toxin.

Anxiety and depression

Anxiety and depression are increasingly being recognized as frequent symptoms in MS and as a major determinant of worsened HRQoL [11]. The Hospital Anxiety and Depression Scale (HADS) questionnaire is a validated assessment tool. In daily practice anxiety disorders, and to a lesser degree depression, are often under-diagnosed in MS patients. As a consequence, patients are deprived of psychological and pharmacological treatments that might be effective in reducing symptoms and disease burden.

Cognitive impairment

Cognitive disturbances are a prominent feature of MS, occurring in about half of all patients [12] and in one third of patients with early RRMS [13]. The most frequently impaired domains are complex attention, information processing speed, and memory and executive functions. MS patients with problems in cognitive performance have increased odds of becoming unemployed [12]. Importantly, cognitive symptoms in early RRMS are predictive of disability several years later [14], and in benign RRMS failure on neuropsychological tests predicts clinical worsening over a 3-year period [15].

The detection of cognitive impairment in a RRMS patient is a reason to evaluate the current policy. Routine evaluation of cognition is useful for helping patients to address ensuing problems and to detect cognitive decline as a sign of disease progression or treatment failure [16]. Two neuropsychological test batteries have been developed for use in MS patients, the Brief Repeatable Neuropsychological Battery (BRNB) and the Minimal Assessment of Cognitive Functioning in Multiple Sclerosis (MACFIMS) [for brief descriptions see reference 17]. The high rater and patient burden (the MACFIMS taking around 90 minutes to administer) and the high degree of expertise needed to administer, seriously limit the utility of BRNB and MACFIMS in patient care and clinical trials [17]. A recent study reported the preliminary validation of a brief computerized cognitive battery in RRMS [17]. Previous data supported the reliability of the Symbol Digit Modalities Test (SDMT) and the Multiple Sclerosis Neuropsychological Questionnaire (MSNQ) as potential tools for screening and monitoring of cognition in MS [18]. Studies investigating the utility of the SDMT as an online test are ongoing. Neuropsychological (memory) training, aiming to improve or stabilize cognitive performance, and adjustment of coping strategies are management options. Drugs for treatment of cognitive symptoms are under study, although presently no pharmacotherapy is available [17].

2.4 Disease modifying drugs

The DMDs exert their effect by modifying immune mechanisms related to the inflammatory disease process, and thus prevent demyelination and axonal damage. The first-line DMDs INFb and GA combine a moderate efficacy with proven safety, in both the short and the long term. In contrast, the highly efficacious DMDs natalizumab, fingolimod and cladribine are more likely to have potentially serious side effects on the short term, whereas their long term safety still has to be established. The ongoing debate on the optimal use of the DMDs in RRMS patients directly relates to their perceived benefits and risks.

In the escalating treatment approach naïve patients are first prescribed a moderately efficacious DMD, and in case of an insufficient response the drug is discontinued and a more potent DMD is started. This step-wise regimen is deemed appropriate in patients with low disability and a favorable prognosis. The alternative induction regimen is considered in treatment-naïve patients who, in spite of a short disease duration, already have acquired permanent neurological deficits due to frequent or severe relapses, and with a poor prognosis. The aim is to induce a substantial and long-lasting reduction in disease activity, in order that future relapses can be prevented by a moderately efficacious DMD. The inductive effects of the immunosuppressive agents mitoxantrone and cyclophosphamide

have been studied in clinical trials. Natalizumab is, strictly speaking, not an inductive agent, as it's discontinuation is followed by a reappearance of disease activity.
In either scenario, escalation or induction, there is a need to closely monitor disease activity, in order to prevent further increase in disability (escalation regimen) or unnecessary risk of serious side effects (induction regimen).

2.5 Concept of (very) early treatment

Pathological findings indicate that inflammation occurring early in the disease leads to axonal damage and permanent tissue loss. These histological changes are in due course mirrored by the appearance of permanent T1-weighed hypo-intense lesions, and brain and spinal cord atrophy on MRI. Recent epidemiological data indicate that as soon as a disability level of Expanded Disability Status Score (EDSS) 3 or 4 has been reached, the increase in disability during the further course of the disease no longer relates to relapses or treatment with DMDs. Interestingly, observational data indicate that start of DMD treatment within 24 months of disease onset, and even more so in the first 12 months, is associated with less long-term disability, later transgression to SPMS and a slower progression during SPMS. The concept of (very) early DMD treatment is based on these and related studies and proposes to start treatment after the first episode, including CIS, or at least in the first 12 to 24 months. However, the disease course and accrual of disability is highly variable between patients. So, in order not to unnecessarily treat patients who would have a benign course without treatment, the (very) early use of DMDs is restricted to those patients in whom prognostic features are unfavorable.

2.6 Prognostic features

There is a body of evidence suggesting that to a certain degree the short-term disease course can be predicted from the presence or absence of specific clinical, MRI and CSF findings. However, the methodological limitations of the investigations on the predictive value of parameters with respect to the long-term disability make that in individual patients a formal prognosis cannot be established. Yet, a comprehensive appraisal of the available patient data might justify an 'educated guess' on a patient's prospects, especially for the short term.
The following clinical characteristics of a first RRMS episode or of CIS are considered prognostically unfavorable: multifocal symptoms, pyramidal, cerebellar, or sphincter symptoms, need of steroid treatment, and incomplete recovery. In patients with two or more relapses a short interval between the first and the second attack is unfavorable, as is the occurrence of three or more relapses in the first three years. Some abnormalities suggestive of MS on diagnostic MRI also have a prognostic relevance: the occurrence of three or more T2-weighed hyper-intense lesions, two or more infra-tentorial lesions, corpus callosum lesions, cortical lesions, diffuse lesions in the cervical spinal cord, cerebral or cervical spinal cord atrophy, T1-weighed hypo-intense lesions, and one or more gadolinium-enhancing lesions. Finally, the presence of immunoglobuline G oligoclonal bands (IgG-OCB), intrathecal immunoglobulin M (IgM) synthesis, and a high concentration of light chain neurofilament on CSF analyses have also been associated with a less favorable course.

2.7 Therapeutic goals

Conventional clinical measures of the effectiveness of DMD treatment include the number and severity of relapses, need of steroid-treatment for relapses, and EDSS or Multiple

Sclerosis Functional Composite (MSFC) score (disability). In clinically stable patients new or enlarged T2-weighed hyper-intense lesions, new or enlarged T1-weighed hypo-intense lesions or gadolinium-enhanced T1- weighed MRI lesions, and (increase of) cerebral or spinal cord atrophy all reflect subclinical disease activity. Clinical and MRI parameters may be combined into a composite measure of disease activity or disease free status. Thus, in a recent study sustained freedom of disease activity was defined as the patient having no relapse, no 3-month sustained increase in EDSS, and no new MRI lesions (no T1 gadolinium-enhancing or new/enlarged T2 lesions) over a specified period [19].

The ultimate goal of DMD treatment is not only to prevent clinical and MRI disease activity, but also the transgression to SPMS. For DMDs to have a maximum chance to obtain this long-term goal, treatment should not only be started timely but also managed in such a way that EDSS 3 to 4 is not reached. To this end the following short-term clinical and MRI measures of disease activity may be monitored: occurrence of a relapse, change in disability (EDSS), new or enlarging T2-weighed hyper-intense or T1-weighed hypo-intense lesions, gadolinium-enhancing lesions, and (increase of) brain and spinal cord atrophy. It was recently found that early EDSS change and medication possession ratio are moderate predictors of long-term disability [20] [21]. A higher medication possession ratio predicted better long-term clinical outcomes, while greater early increase in EDSS score predicted worse outcomes. In contrast, change in MRI parameters were only weakly associated with long-term outcome [20]. So, it seems that short-term clinical changes and adherence to DMD treatment have a higher prognostic value than MRI measures. The added value of composite measures remains to be established.

3. E-health 2.0 in multiple sclerosis treatment

The availability of a broad range of DMDs for the treatment of RRMS, the prognostic relevance of early disease activity in CIS and RRMS, the prognostic relevance of early disease activity after start of treatment, the importance of the timing of treatment initiation, the potentially serious side effects of the newer drugs and our ignorance of their long-term risks, implicate that in the coming years MS treatment is increasingly being characterized by both complexity and personalization. In this context, the use of Web 2.0 techniques for interactive online monitoring and care might make a crucial contribution to the management of MS patients. Interactive online monitoring and care are believed to enhance the chances that the potential benefits of the DMDs are realized and that treatment goals are achieved.

3.1 Monitoring

Aspects of monitoring

Monitoring may be defined as repeated testing aimed at guiding and adjusting the management of a chronic or recurrent condition [22]. Minimum criteria for monitoring are that clinically significant changes in the condition or effect of treatment occur over time, that there is an available monitoring test that reliably detects clinically significant changes when they occur, and that cost-effective action can be taken on the basis of the test result [22]. As monitoring involves a series of tests over time a monitoring strategy needs to consider frequency and timing of tests in the context of a series of sequential results [22]. It should address the following questions: Who should be monitored? What outcome should be monitored? What test should be used? When, and at what interval? Who should do the monitoring? What action to take on the monitoring result? [23]. Only since the occurrence in 2005 of progressive multifocal leukencelopathy, a potentially lethal CNS disorder, as a rare side effect of natalizumab has monitoring become a topic in MS neurology. As monitoring of disease activity and adverse events in DMD-treated patients is a rather recent development, most of the fundamental questions regarding the optimal monitoring strategies still have to be answered.

Monitoring in multiple sclerosis

In view of the nature of the parameters for current or future disease activity mentioned above, the conventional monitoring of CIS and RRMS patients focuses on doctor-centered clinical and MRI outcomes. In fact, in daily clinical practice the natural course of the disease as well as the course after start of DMD treatment is monitored by means of assessments during the patients' regular visits to the out-patient department, with intervals that usually vary from 3 to 12 months. Doctors and nurses ask about relevant changes in symptoms, notably those suggestive of a relapse or progression, and ideally disability is measured using a validated clinical scale, e.g. the EDSS or MSFC. However, in general neurological practices the regular and standardized quantification of disability is probably an exception, rather than the rule. Moreover, it is doubtful whether CIS and RRMS patients have a T2-weighed and gadolinium-enhanced T1-weighed brain and spinal MRI scan performed on a sufficiently regular basis, given the costs of scanning time and of gadolinium. Importantly, practical circumstances, like travel distances and expenses, scarcity of qualified medical personnel, and restricted availability of MRI machines, often prevent the conventional monitoring process from being optimal, both in terms of the selection of patients, the tests used, and the frequency of assessments.

Monitoring by online self-assessment

Compared to doctor-centered or technical measures patient-reported outcomes have various advantages. Firstly, they have an intrinsic clinical relevance; secondly, data are less expensive to acquire; and thirdly, the assessment schedule is more flexible and can easily be adjusted to changing circumstances or unexpected outcomes. For example, the frequency of assessments can be increased if there is a narrow time window regarding the start of DMD treatment, or if a dose increase is associated with a risk of serious side effects. Traditionally, patient-reported outcomes are obtained via questionnaires on site, per postal questionnaire or per telephone. Prospective well-designed studies in MS patients using patient-reported outcomes via the internet are scarce. Yet, especially the web-based applications of accepted and validated measures have obvious advantages compared to doctor-centered outcomes obtained on site. Online questionnaires and diaries can be completed at home at time points convenient to patients; errors and missing data are minimized by instantaneous checks of completeness and consistency; and electronic data capture into a database prevents transmission errors. Moreover, as online questionnaires are ready available, assessment intervals can be short and flexible, and monitoring schedules can easily be tailored to individual needs, e.g. for detection of early changes. Finally, patient-centered data may provide information that complements or partially substitutes doctor-reported data, rendering monitoring less time-consuming for neurologists and MS nurses.

We investigated in an exploratory manner whether monitoring by online self-assessments with monthly intervals is feasible and informative in RRMS patients starting a DMD [24].

We included 167 RRMS patients in a 12-month observational study during which patients were asked to complete two short questionnaires, on HRQoL and fatigue, at monthly intervals. 73.7% completed both questionnaires at all 13 time points, whereas 85.1% of the patients completed both questionnaires in at least 7 of the 13 time points. For both questionnaires the mean changes between baseline and month 12 were similar to those found in studies using paper questionnaires completed on site or at home with 6-month intervals. These data indicate the feasibility and potential usefulness of monitoring by monthly online self-assessment. Intensive online monitoring appears to be an informative and patient-friendly tool for assessing short-term effectiveness. It can be argued that the full advantages of monitoring by online self-assessment are only realized in the context of an interactive care setting.

3.2 Treatment and care

In the past two decades the expanding knowledge on the inflammatory mechanisms leading to tissue damage in MS and the pathophysiological changes underlying the major symptoms have initiated a plethora of therapeutic studies, varying from placebo-controlled randomized trials to observational studies and anecdotal reports. Study data have given neurologists and MS-nurses ample opportunities to substantially lessen the disease burden in their patients. However, it is recognized that as yet most patients insufficiently benefit from the insights and therapeutic potential generated by research data [25]. The unmet needs in MS patients relate to the fact that the implementation of treatment options is hampered by limited resources and organizational insufficiencies and inefficiencies. One of the measures to improve both effectiveness and efficiency of MS care may be the introduction of Web 2.0 applications in the care process.

Interactive online care

To outline the potential advantages of interactive online care in MS patients a typical example, the MSmonitor project, is described here. This project aims to improve MS care in the Netherlands by interactive use of the internet on the basis of patient-reported outcomes, obtained via online self-assessment. MSmonitor started in 2010 and at present 12 MS centers and neurological practices participate. Basically, every six months patients complete the Multiple Sclerosis Impact Profile (MSIP) and the Multiple Sclerosis Quality of Life-54 (MSQoL-54) or the Leeds Multiple Sclerosis Quality of Life (LMSQoL) scale online 1 to 2 weeks before their regular out-patient visit.

The MSIP is a psychometrically validated outcome measure for disability and disability perception in MS patients [26]. The scale is based on the International Classification of Functioning, Disability and Health (ICF) of the World Health Organization (WHO). The MSIP disability data are complementary to the doctor-centered EDSS. In those neurological practices where the EDSS cannot be assessed (time constraints, lack of qualified personnel) the MSIP disability data may provide a validated patient-reported alternative. In addition, the disability perception part of the MSIP informs on the subjective dimension of symptoms and signs and provides a systematic, complete, detailed, and quantitative overview of experienced burden of disease. In the online application of the MSIP answers that represent a worsening compared to the previous assessment are automatically highlighted. Thus, the online MSIP gives a quick screen of both the current condition and of recent changes. The individual data are made available on the secured project website to treating MS-nurse and neurologist, and helps them to prepare the on site consultation. In fact, the MSIP overview may guide the conversation between patient and MS-nurse or neurologist, by focusing on changes with high disability perception. The inventory of symptoms according to relevance and the preview opportunity for caregivers are thought to enhance effectiveness and efficiency of outpatient visits.

The MSQoL-54 and the LMSQoL measure HRQoL. HRQoL is a multidimensional concept related to a person's perception of well-being and the level of role fulfillment across a range of dimensions, including physical, psychosocial, social and symptom-related dimensions [27]. It is a term that refers to an individual's assessment of how a health problem as well as its treatment affect his/her ability to perform activities and roles that he/she values [28]. A critical element of HRQoL is that it reflects the patient's assessment of the impact of his/her illness, not the physician's perspective, as most physiologically oriented measures and traditional clinical scales do [29]. As HRQoL comprises not only perceptions of physical functioning and general health, but also perceived psychological functioning and social/role functioning [30], its assessment is thought to provide a comprehensive evaluation of an individual's health [31]. Using the MSIP it was demonstrated that HRQoL impairment in MS patients was most related to emotional problems, cognitive dysfunction, and sleep disturbances [26]. In DMD-treated patients the HRQoL data help to assess the treatment's overall effectiveness from the patient's perspective [32] [33].

In addition to the 6-monthly assessments, MS-nurse and neurologist may in selected patients activate these scales at additional time points or activate symptom-related questionnaires for in-depth assessment of specific symptoms, e.g. when a subjective worsening has been reported by e-mail or by phone; or to obtain valid pre-treatment values by repeated measurements; or to closely follow initial changes after start of treatment; or to evaluate specific treatment effects. An example: the beneficial effect of symptomatic drug treatment of MS-related fatigue usually manifests itself within 6 to 8 weeks. The low chance of a relevant change in fatigue and the possibility of side effects urge a timely evaluation. The repeated online use of the MFIS informs on the baseline condition and the degree of short-term change in MS-related fatigue. Other symptoms can also be quantified online by symptom-specific validated questionnaires, such as depression and anxiety by the HADS, bladder symptoms by a Voiding Diary, and comorbidity by the Self-Report Comorbidity Questionnaire for Multiple Sclerosis (SRCQ-MS). The SDMT may be included for assessment of cognition, as soon as preliminary data on an the validity of the online version have been confirmed.

The combination of the instantaneous availability of patient-reported outcomes on disability, disability perception and symptoms prior to and during out-patient visits, the possibility of repeated assessments and of symptom-related in–depth measurements, the online evaluation by caregivers via the secured website, and the flexible feedback by short-message service (SMS) or e-email has the potential to improve effectiveness and efficiency of MS treatment and care. Moreover, an outcome value that represents a clinically minimally important change may be set as an alert level. As soon as the outcome variable reaches the predefined limit an alert pops up on the screen, a message is sent by e-mail to the neurologist or MS-nurse, or appears on their screen after log in, whatever is decided. E.g. patients with a tendency to depressive symptoms who start INFb treatment may use the online HADS for monitoring mood with a predefined alert set-point. Preliminary data from the MSmonitor project indicate that the use of Web 2.0 technology in MS care benefits both patient and caregiver in terms of flexibility and efficiency, as self-assessment, evaluation, and feedback do not depend on consulting hours or simultaneous availability of patient and caregiver. A next step will be the development of an interactive education program for patients and caregivers.

4. E-health 2.0 in multiple sclerosis research

4.1 Web-based phase IV research

Randomized placebo-controlled phase II/III trials provide data on a DMD's efficacy to reduce in the short term the frequency and severity of the clinical manifestations of inflammation (relapses) and of surrogate parameters (MRI lesions). Such trials do not inform on the long-term efficacy, in terms of preventing disability increase or conversion to SPMS, or slowing progression during SPMS; nor on long-term side effects. It is also of note that in fact the phase II/III results do not pertain to patients treated in real life, as data are typically obtained from selected patients, treated in dedicated MS centers in large, often academic hospitals.

Data on the long-term effectiveness and safety in patients treated in daily practice can be acquired in observational phase IV studies, and the internet enables virtually every MS patient to participate in such studies. Within the framework of a prospective observational study every patient who starts a treatment can be asked to regularly complete online a set of standard questions concerning aspects of effectiveness and side effects. In a web-based study a patient's participation does not depend on his/her geographic location or distance to out-patient clinic, and therefore an online study may include large cohorts in whole regions or even countries. Methodologically, the representative character of the online acquired data enables the external validation of the phase III data. As to drug safety, an online observational study covering a whole population or region with virtually no restrictive selection criteria yields an almost complete picture of adverse events in real life.

4.2 Interactive observational research

An important aspect of web-based phase IV research is that study data on effectiveness and safety from individual patients can be made available to treating MS-nurse or neurologist for monitoring purposes. We started in the Netherlands the Dutch MS Study, a prospective, online, patient-centred study of long-term disability, disability perception and HRQoL in patients with MS or CIS. Every 6 months patients complete the MSIP (disability and disability perception) and the MSQoL-54 (HRQoL). Disease characteristics and demographic, diagnostic and medication data are recorded online at the start of a patient's participation, and thereafter relapses and medication use can be updated every month. A patient may consent to give his/her MS-nurse or neurologist access to the study data for evaluation of treatment or the natural course of the disease. Actually, as the information provided by the study data may lead to an adjustment of the disease management, e.g. discontinuation or change of medication, we have created a setting in which there is an interaction between observation and daily practice. As a result, the study data may give insight not only into factors that relate to changes in the disease course, but also in those that drive the decisions regarding treatment and care processes.

The study's inclusion criteria are: having the diagnosis MS or CIS, and being willing and able to participate in the investigations. The latter criterion implies the availability of a computer for online access. In fact, as almost every patient with MS or CIS is eligible the Dutch MS study is developing into an interactive Dutch MS registry.

4.3 Adherence and adherence research

The effectiveness of DMD treatment depends on adequate adherence and implies year-long continued drug administration with a minimum of missed doses. The two aspects of inadequate adherence are: 1) missing doses, and 2) early discontinuation for other reason than insufficient response, serious side effects or persistent moderate side effects. Patients treated with the injectable first-line DMDs miss 30% of the doses [34], and the 6-month discontinuation rate may be as high as 27% [35]. It has been known that DMD discontinuation for more than three months is associated with a increased risk of relapses. Recent data show that in RRMS patients the degree of disability eight years after start of INFb-1a treatment is related to the medication possession ratio [21] Adherence is influenced by the socio-economic situation, health care and caregivers, disease, treatment and patient characteristics. In MS patients self-efficacy expectations are thought to be related to adherence, as are patient education and optimal support. A detailed knowledge of those aspects of care that significantly relate to adherence may lead to adherence-improving measures. Moreover, the identification of patients at high risk of inadequate adherence could lead to more efficient care.

The CAIR (Correlative analyses of Adherence In Relapsing remitting multiple sclerosis) study investigates in GA-treated RRMS patients the relationship between drug adherence and multidisciplinary care, as well as factors associated with adherence [36]. The study is a prospective, web-based, patient-centered, nation-wide, observational cohort study in the Netherlands. The primary objective is to investigate whether adherence is associated with specific disciplines of care or quantities of specific care. The secondary objective is to investigate whether adherence is associated with specific aspects of the socio-economic situation, health care and caregivers, disease, treatment or patient characteristics.

All data are acquired online via a study website (www.cairstudie.nl) and all RRMS patients in the Netherlands starting GA treatment were eligible. At pre-defined and random time-points patients are requested to complete a short questionnaire on missed doses and eventual discontinuation. Every two weeks patients record the care they received (discipline, frequency, duration). The Dutch Adherence Questionnaire-90 (DAQ-90), a 90-item questionnaire based on the World Health Organization (WHO) 2003 report on adherence, comprehensively assesses the five domains of evidence-based determinants of adherence: socio-economic, health care and caregivers, disease, treatment, and patient-related factors. Self-efficacy is assessed by the Multiple Sclerosis Self-Efficacy Scale (MSSES), and mood and HRQoL by the MSQoL-54.

Importantly, adherence data from online self-assessment can be used in an interactive web-based care setting, like the MSmonitor project. Access to individual data enables neurologist and MS-nurse to monitor adherence, whereas the regular completion of a short questionnaire may per se be an adherence promoting activity. Based on the online data caregivers will be able to give feedback to patients with inadequate adherence, whereas the choice of adherence improving measures can be guided by the pre-treatment online inventory of risk factors (DAQ-90). It is expected that in the near future online monitoring of adherence and interactive web-based care, tailored to the individual risk factors, may help to improve adherence and thus the effectiveness of DMD treatments.

4.4 Patient empowerment

The interactive use of the internet for monitoring and care purposes enables patients to better understand and evaluate their own conditions. As a result, patients become educated partners in the relation with caregivers and may take initiatives as to how their MS should be managed. Interactive programs that inform and educate on treatment options, e.g. using evidence-based algorithms, will help patients to position themselves as independent actors in the process of benefit-to-risk evaluation and shared decision making. As the Web 2.0 technology is likely to increase knowledge and awareness in many individual patients, it may thus collectively transform web-based patient communities into grassroots movements that initiate and drive research projects on topics that are relevant to patients but do not appeal to pharmaceutical companies and academia.

5. Conclusion

Current developments suggest that in the coming years Web 2.0 technologies will be integrated in the treatment and care of MS patients and in MS research. Monitoring of effectiveness, safety and adherence by online self-assessment is the basis of interactive online care and (interactive) observational phase IV research. E-health 2.0 developments are likely to increase patients' empowerment and will favor patient-driven decision making and research. In the context of ever diminishing health care resources and an increasing likelihood of drastic changes in the health care system, for MS patients e-health 2.0 could make the difference between, on the one hand, an ongoing suboptimal use of ever more efficacious drugs with persistence of unmet needs, and, on the other hand, personalized, more effective and safe treatments that may prevent long-term disability.

6. References

[1] http://www.techpluto.com/web-20-services.
[2] http://en.wikipedia.org/wiki/Web_2.0.
[3] http://health20.org/wiki/Health_2.0_Definition.
[4] Eysenbach G. Medicine 2.0: Social Networking, Collaboration, Participation, Apomediation, and Openness. J Med Internet Res 2008;10(3):e22; doi:10.2196/jmir.1030.
[5] Multiple Sclerosis. Clinical and pathogenetic basis. CS Raine, HF McFairland, WW Tourtelotte (eds). London, Chapman & Hall Medical, London, 1997.
[6] Gandhi R, Laroni A, Weiner HL. Role of the innate immune system in the pathogenesis of multiple sclerosis. Review. J Neuroimmunol 2010;221(1-2):7-14.
[7] Nessler S, Brück W. Advances in multiple sclerosis research in 2009. J Neurol 2010; 257(9):1590-1593.
[8] Polman CH, Reingold SC, Banwell B,Clanet M, Cohen JA, Filippi M, et al. Diagnostic criteria for multiple sclerosis: 2010 revisions to the McDonald criteria. Ann Neurol 2011;69(2):292-302. doi: 10.1002/ana.22366.
[9] Krupp LB. Mechanisms, measurement, and management of fatigue in multiple sclerosis. In Multiple sclerosis: clinical challenges and controversies. AJ Thompson, C Polman, R Hohlfeld (eds). London, Martin Dunitz, 1997: pp 283-294.
[10] Fisk JD, Pontefract A, Ritvo PG, Archibald CJ, Murray TJ: The impact of fatigue on patients with multiple sclerosis. Can J Neurol Sci 1994; 21:9-14.

[11] Ziemssen T. Multiple sclerosis beyond EDSS: depression and fatigue. J Neurol Sci 2009;277(Suppl 1):S37-41.
[12] Strober L, Englert J, Munschauer F, Weinstock-Guttman B, Rao S, Benedict RH. Sensitivity of conventional memory tests in multiple sclerosis: comparing the Rao Brief Repeatable Neuropsychological Battery and the Minimal Assessment of Cognitive Function in MS. Mult Scler 2009;15:1077-1084.
[13] Amato MP, Zipoli V, Portaccio E: Cognitive changes in multiple sclerosis. Expert Rev Neurother 2008;8:1585-1596.
[14] Deloire M, Ruet A, Hamel D, Bonnet M, Brochet B. Early cognitive impairment in multiple sclerosis predicts disability outcome several years later. Mult Scler;16:581-587.
[15] Portaccio E, Stromillo ML, Goretti B, Zipoli V, Siracusa G, Battaglini M, et al. Neuropsychological and MRI measures predict short-term evolution in benign multiple sclerosis. Neurology 2009;73:498-503.
[16] Benedict RH, Zivadinov R. Risk factors for and management of cognitive dysfunction in multiple sclerosis. Nat Rev Neurol 2011; 7(6):332-342. doi: 10.1038/nrneurol.2011.61.
[17] Edgar C, Jongen PJ, Sanders E, Sindic C, Goffette S, Dupuis M, et al. Cognitive performance in relapsing remitting multiple sclerosis: A longitudinal study in daily practice using a brief computerized cognitive battery. BMC Neurol 2011;11:68.
[18] Morrow SA, O'Connor PW, Polman CH, Goodman AD, Kappos L, Lublin FD, et al. Evaluation of the symbol digit modalities test (SDMT) and MS neuropsychological screening questionnaire (MSNQ) in natalizumab-treated MS patients over 48 weeks. Mult Scler 2010;16(11):1385-1392.
[19] Giovannoni G, Cook S, Rammohan K, Rieckmann P, Sorensen PS, Vermersch P, et al. Sustained disease-activity-free status in patients with relapsing-remitting multiple sclerosis treated with cladribine tablets in the CLARITY study: a post-hoc and subgroup analysis. The Lancet Neurology 2011;10(4); 329–337.
[20] Traboulsee A, Uitdehaag BMJ, Kappos L, Sandberg-Wollheim M, Li D, Jongen PJ, et al. Clinical and Magnetic Resonance Imaging Predictors of Long-Term Outcomes in Patients with Relapsing–Remitting Multiple Sclerosis: Additional Analyses. 63rd Annual Meeting of the American Academy of Neurology, Honolulu, Hawaii; 9–16 April 2011.
[21] Uitdehaag B, Constantinescu C, Cornelisse P, Jeffery D, Kappos L, Li D. Impact of exposure to interferon beta-1a on outcomes in patients with relapsing-remitting multiple sclerosis: exploratory analyses from the PRISMS long-term follow-up study. Ther Adv Neurol Disord 2011;4(1):3-14.
[22] Glasziou PP, Aronson JK. An introduction to monitoring therapeutic interventions in clinical practice. In Glasziou PP, Irwig L, Aronson JK (eds). Evidence-based medical monitoring. From principles to practice. Oxford, Blackwell Publishing 2008, pp. 3-14.
[23] Mant D. An introduction to monitoring therapeutic interventions in clinical practice. In Glasziou PP, Irwig L, Aronson JK (eds). Evidence-based medical monitoring. From principles to practice. Oxford, Blackwell Publishing 2008, pp. 15-30.
[24] Jongen PJ, Sanders E, Visser L, Zwanikken C, van Noort E, Koopmans P, et al. Automated on-line monitoring of health-related quality of life and fatigue in

relapsing remitting MS patients treated with glatiramer acetate. 1st International Congress on Clinical Neurology & Epidemiology, Munich, August 27-30, 2009.

[25] Bates D. Unmet Needs for People with Multiple Sclerosis. European Neurological Review. Touch Briefings 2008. http://www.touchbriefings.com/pdf/3248/bates.pdf European Neurology - Volume 3 Issue 2.

[26] Wynia K, Middel B, van Dijk JP, De Keyser JH, Reijneveld SA. The impact of disabilities on quality of life in people with multiple sclerosis. Mult Scler 2008;14:972–980.

[27] Zwibel H. Health and quality of life in patients with relapsing multiple sclerosis. J Neurol Sci 2009;287 S1:S11-S16

[28] Schipper H, Clinch JJ, Olweny CLM. Quality of life studies: de®nitions and conceptual issues. In Spilker B. (ed). Quality of life and pharmacoeconomics in clinical trials. 2nd ed. Philadelphia, Lippincott-Raven 1996, pp. 11-23.

[29] Hobart JC. Measuring health outcomes in multiple sclerosis: why, which, and how? In Thompson AJ, Polman C, Hohlfeld R, (eds). Multiple sclerosis: clinical challenges and controversies. London, Martin Dunitz 1997, pp. 211-225.

[30] Fischer JS, LaRocca NG, Miller DM, Ritvo PG, Andrews H, Paty D. Recent developments in the assessment of quality of life in multiple sclerosis (MS). Mult Scler 1999;5(4):251-259.

[31] Hopman WM, Coo H, Edgar CM, McBride EV, Day AG, Brunet DG. Factors associated with health-related quality of life in multiple sclerosis. Can J Neurol Sci 2007; 34(2):160-166.

[32] Jongen PJ, Sindic C, Carton H, Zwanikken C, Lemmens W, Borm G. Functional composite and quality of Life in Avonex-treated Relapsing multiple sclerosis patients study group. Improvement of health-related quality of life in relapsing remitting multiple sclerosis patients after 2 years of treatment with intramuscular interferon-beta-1a. J Neurol 2010;257(4):584-589.

[33] Jongen PJ, Lehnick D, Sanders E, Seeldrayers P, Fredrikson S, Andersson M, et al. Health-related quality of life in relapsing remitting multiple sclerosis patients during treatment with glatiramer acetate: a prospective, observational, international, multi-centre study. Health Qual Life Outcomes 2010;8:133.

[34] Lafata JE, Cerghet M, Dobie E, Schulz L, Tunceli K, Reuther J, Elias S. Measuring adherence and persistence to disease modifying agents among patients with relapsing remitting multiple sclerosis. J Am Pharm Assoc 2008;48:752-757.

[35] Tremlett HL, Oger J: Interrupted therapy: stopping and switching of the beta-interferons prescribed for MS. Neurology 2003;61:551-554.

[36] Jongen PJ, Hengstman G, Hupperts R, Schrijver H, Gilhuis J, Vliegen JH, et al. Drug adherence and multidisciplinary care in patients with multiple sclerosis: protocol of a prospective, web-based, patient-centred, nation-wide, Dutch cohort study in glatiramer acetate treated patients (CAIR study). BMC Neurol 2011;11:40.